VARIATION IN
Morphology of Teeth

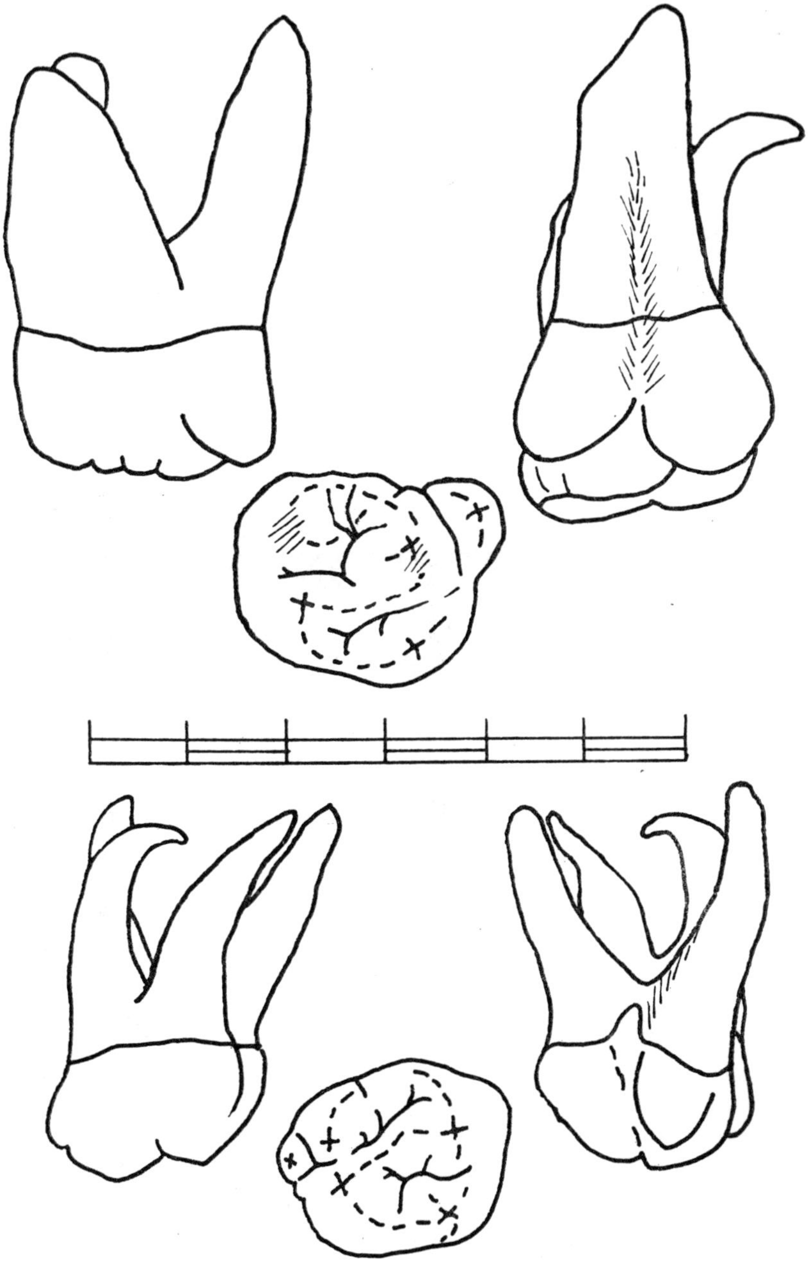

Above. Carabelli cusp and enlarged palatal root. See Figure 7-13 *a*, and p. 335.

Below. Three-cusped molar, having an additional element with two cusps and a separate root. See Figure 7-25 *c*, and pp. 271, 279, 283, 287.

VARIATION IN
Morphology of Teeth

ANTHROPOLOGIC AND FORENSIC ASPECTS

By

R. M. S. TAYLOR, D.D.S. (N.Z.), B.D.S.

Hon. Research Associate
Department of Zoology
University of Auckland
New Zealand

With a Foreword by

John E. Morton, D.Sc. (London)

Professor of Zoology
University of Auckland
New Zealand

CHARLES C THOMAS • PUBLISHER

Springfield • Illinois • U.S.A.

Published and Distributed Throughout the World by
CHARLES C THOMAS • PUBLISHER
Bannerstone House
301-327 East Lawrence Avenue, Springfield, Illinois, U.S.A.

ISBN 0-398-03697-7
Library of Congress Catalog Card Number: 77-12022

With THOMAS BOOKS careful attention is given to all details of manufacturing and design. It is the Publisher's desire to present books that are satisfactory as to their physical qualities and artistic possibilities and appropriate for their particular use. THOMAS BOOKS will be true to those laws of quality that assure a good name and good will.

Library of Congress Cataloging in Publication Data

Taylor, Richard Morris Stovin
Variation in morphology of teeth.

Bibliography: p. 371
Includes index.
1. Teeth. 2. Dental anthropology. 3. Dental jurisprudence. I. Title. [DNLM: 1. Tooth—Anatomy and histology. 2. Anthropology, Physical. WU101 T245v]
QM311.T39 611'.314 77-12022
ISBN 0-398-03697-7

Printed in the United States of America
C-1

Dedication

I would like to dedicate this book to my wife, Irene, for her patient endurance of my interest in "old bones," to my friend, Harry Dixon Erlam, to whom the reports of that interest owe so much through his encouragement and editorial skill and to Neil M. Officer, M.B.E., whose fine surgery saved my life when the manuscript was nearing completion.

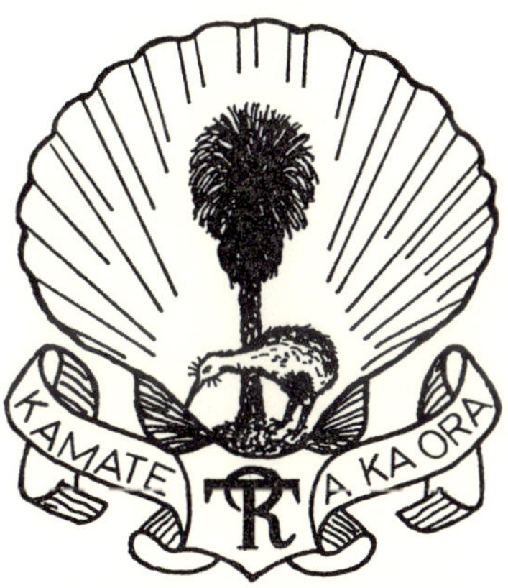

The author's missionary great-grandfather devised this seal from drawings of a scallop shell (which is part of a Taylor family crest), the New Zealand "cabbage-tree" (*Cordyline australis*) and the kiwi bird, which is now a New Zealand national emblem. The motto in the Maori language may be freely translated as "From death to life," or "From sickness to health," and it also comprises the opening line of a traditional "haka," or Maori chant. (See foreword to Mead, 1966.)

Foreword

OVER A LONG working life Doctor Taylor has been devoted to what we may appreciatively call the "natural history of teeth." When he retired from active dental practice in 1964, he came to join this department as a research associate; it has been one of his achievements to win a marine ecologist to enough of his own enthusiasm to be writing a foreword to this book. To begin to understand this large discipline's relevance to palaeontology, anthropology, sociology, and ecology is part of the liberal education of the fifteen years I have known Doctor Taylor.

It is against the memories of good companionship and laboratory coffee that I now read his finished book. From its title and subject matter one would take it to be a specialist work that few, perhaps—at a continuous reading—would follow right through. Yet it is not only a scholarly but also a readable book, and its author has a feeling for good writing and sensitive description. Seemingly technical chapters, going through dental variation from maxillary incisors to third molars, show how another man's expertise can interpret skeletal material not only genetically, but as a document of the ecology and life-style, even the stress psychology, of the individual it was once part of.

This book will not be primarily a text for dentists, although it has much that could be relevant to them in practice. Rather it shows the vast amount of information that can be obtained from teeth without sophisticated equipment. It sets out clearly what to see when looking at a tooth and how to describe it lucidly. A very considerable number of examples is accurately presented, and one cannot but be impressed by the careful attention to detail and the meticulous study that lies behind this report, in which a limitless variety in characters and their combinations is demonstrated. This is not just an important record of reality, but the amount of evidence brought forward invites a review of earlier hypotheses regarding dental morphology and variation. Many researchers would perhaps have begun by trying to select a small number of parameters for statistical analysis. Doctor Taylor has thought—I believe rightly—that such selection at the first stage would have obscured the initial richness and variety of the material to be assessed. Tooth description is still at a pioneering stage, even though the tooth—with the fingerprints—is bidding fair to become the most minutely recorded part of the human frame.

Doctor Taylor's own background and experience have been, for any professional man, extremely wide: from anthropological field work to the teaching of dentistry, including the early days of New Zealand's school dental service training. He also spent a considerable time in private practice, before returning—on retirement—to his earlier love of anthropological teaching and research, including university lecturing on physical anthropology.

I recommend this book, not as a dental scientist but as a biologist who has been able to appreciate the work it sets out. I want, too, to record as a zoologist my real pleasure that such a study should have been written in my own department.

John Morton, D.Sc.

Introduction

SOME TEETH ARE WELL described in textbook and atlas and superbly illustrated with the cunning arts of the photographer and printer. But it is always easy to find many teeth that by no means fit the description or illustration, and this lack of conformity to a pattern is distinctly unhelpful for the student, whether his interest is elementary or highly advanced. It should be made clear that this criticism does not refer to the abnormal tooth or even to that which lies on the subjective borderline of normality. The basic reason for this lack of adequate description must be the potential and actual infinity of variation in morphological characters of teeth. A more practical reason for the lack is the impossibility (in time, space and cost by present methods) of reporting all these variations. It is still common to present a "typical" tooth as a fair representative of its kind. More recently the fact of variation has been acknowledged in text and figure, but usually its presentation is relatively insignificant in relation to the extent of variation, and it would seem that such reports are based on examination of insufficient numbers of teeth.

Sometimes there has been an endeavour to report some details of variation statistically, with or without measurements. In nonmetrical characters it is important that categories be clearly defined. For metrical characters it is essential to define landmarks and describe procedure to cover variation. It is equally essential that measurements have some meaning. Faults in respect of any of these criteria cannot be offset merely by increasing the number of teeth examined. Elaboration of this aspect of the problem must show convincingly not only that variation cannot be described statistically but also that teeth themselves cannot be usefully described merely through measurement. This comment applies to crowns or roots or to whole teeth, and obtains for each one of the twenty-six kinds of teeth in the human dentition, deciduous and permanent. This does not discredit a great deal of work, mostly on crowns of teeth, that has been done from a qualitative or nonmetrical approach to variation. The conviction that such an approach is the most promising for analysis of morphological variation, and that individual teeth of the human dentition had not been adequately described in this way, was one reason for undertaking this work.

It should be made clear that the objection to measurement does not apply to examination of individual specimens, whether they are teeth, jaws, skulls or other bones. Such measurements not only record information about the specimen, but they also increase the investigator's awareness of morphological anatomy. The objection is to the use of particular measurements, and especially of their statistical treatment, as a basis for comparison and ethnic deduction.

The objective was set beyond the obtaining of more information concerning variation, with proposals to examine the possible application of such knowledge. The first and obvious practical application is in dentistry, and this field is wider than may at first appear. As in dental anthropology, in palaeontology and comparative anatomy the details of variation of characters when recognized may contribute important data. But it is in the forensic field that dental studies have acquired greatly increased importance, because such data may be crucial in problems of identification. This has been the case particularly where remains have been greatly affected by fire, and in these days the loss of a large aircraft, for example, may involve many such victims. Teeth may provide almost the only identifiable human remains in these cases.

An apparently sound tooth, however, may be deceptive unless it can be shown to have been part of a dentition. Evidence of function, such as a very small facet, may be important since some human teeth have never been in a jaw. Teeth formed in an ovarian teratoma could cause confusion after a mass disaster with fragmentation of bodies (Harvey, 1976, p.16). Therefore not only identification of the tooth is necessary but also recognition of its experience *in situ,* and this can be checked against dental records. Thus, although teeth may be the only identifiable human remains, they may be eloquent.

The availability and thoroughness of dental records made in an individual's lifetime are important in this respect, and improvement both in making records and also in examination of material could add greatly to the amount of data that can contribute to the solution of such problems (Taylor, 1971b, 1971c). The variety in kind of data that can be obtained from teeth is considerable, and perhaps one of the most productive sources of such data is found in morphological studies. Amongst these the recognition of particular characters of resemblance and of difference, and their interpretation, is of prime importance. The necessary abilities for this arise partly from familiarity with variation, and the need for this special knowledge is urgent. It may come from a long experience, coupled with a degree of continued interest that is sometimes called dedication. The mere fact of being a dentist or an anatomist, or either, with interests in the other's field or in dental anthropology, is insufficient in itself. It is necessary also to be able to illustrate and describe specimens in an acceptable manner. This requires that they can be related to an analysis of the characters of tooth crowns and roots but, except for some important studies by Dahlberg, no such analysis has been available. The present report arises from a rather different approach to the analysis of variation.

In spite of fine textbooks and atlases with diagrams and superb photography, including stereoscopy, with measurements and statistics aided by computers, the nature and extent of morphological variation remain largely unknown. Even the incomplete presentations just indicated often leave it to the reader or observer to interpret what is shown, and statistics create no useful image in one's mind. Explanation of this failure in presentation would appear to lie largely in the method. Apart from failure to interpret, a basic fault lies in the paucity of material presented. This may result from one or both of the following: (a) the limited amount of data on which the study is based; (b) the work, time or cost that could be required for a larger presentation in the same manner, making it impossible of completion. Allied to this is the probability that such a presentation would be too unwieldy to handle. This amounts to a dilemma for the worker and must account in some measure for the lack of information which has been shown as urgently required. The author has wrestled with this problem and presents this survey in the belief that it goes partway towards filling the gap.

As measurements, statistics and photographs have failed to analyze morphological variation in teeth, a new approach to the subject was necessary; essentially this new approach is qualitative, not quantitative. Variation has been analyzed and accepted for what it is, namely the interplay, within certain broad limits, of a multitude of characters which are themselves in large degree subject to variation. The characters may be grouped, but not among categories that may be clearly defined. For example let us consider curvature in roots. In a bent or curved root, where exactly does the bend start or finish? How much of the root is bent? How much does it bend? Is the bent part straight, or itself subject to other bends? Is the root really bent, or was the crown subjected to displacement? And so on. This kind of analysis does not appear to have been attempted before. Obviously it cannot be exactly measured or measurable, but it does convey an idea. It makes one examine a tooth in different terms, and it results in an appreciation of tooth form.

But how may these gradations within the characters of variation be indicated? It requires the illustration of a considerable number of teeth in a compact and inexpensive manner. Photography is unsuitable, not only through labour and expense involved, but also because it presents features unnecessary for the idea being conveyed.

When the author began teaching students in 1930, he found that they became more adept at drawing, and later at carving, a presentable likeness of a tooth if its form was described basically in a geometrical manner.

Thus cylinders, cones and wedges were related to roots and crowns of incisors, and their outlines to triangles, rectangles and circles, etc. A straight line was understood to represent a curve of larger radius in the natural object, and angles to represent arcs of various lengths, from circles of much smaller radii.

For the present report, diagrams and outline drawings would in theory admirably meet requirements, for the first are versatile and the latter are easily assembled and interchangeable for the making up of groups. In practice it was soon clear that accuracy and the time involved were the main problems with outlines, for freehand drawing and frequent checking with calipers could result in only a degree of accuracy and were extremely tedious. With the whole project once more in jeopardy (because of the number of outlines required), tests were made using a camera lucida. With much modification of equipment, and using specially made lenses, it became possible to present a scale with the outline drawings, and this set the seal on accuracy.

As for the time involved in planning and producing many hundreds of outlines, there was no prospect of quick results and the forbidding task was undertaken. Altogether this one-man project has involved a considerable number of years of work.

The sufficiency of numbers of teeth to validate the study is easily established. Apart from the vast numbers of teeth examined *in situ* over many years, the study is illustrated specifically from a collection of many thousands of extracted teeth. For each kind of tooth, a selection of some hundreds was mounted in groups on cards to illustrate the various features; characters were identified for reporting, the outlines required being traced from these through the camera lucida. Further details concerning the writer's dental collections and the relation of extracted teeth to the present report are given in Appendix 4.

If by chance a few persons of other races are represented in our material it could enhance the value of the study. It was intended to survey the variations that may be found in a community and there has been no thought of selecting or excluding any particular tooth. This community is predominantly European and has a growing minority of Polynesians and those of mixed blood. The important feature is that it is a community of *Homo sapiens.* As the science and practice of operative and forensic dentistry must continue, we hope that the present study will contribute to making the Homo just a little more sapiens.

The fact that this study is largely based on extracted teeth from a contemporary "western" society, and that so many teeth have contributed to the supporting collection, is reflected in the variety of observations reported. Thus, in addition to variations directly related to anatomical morphology, the study embraced also some conditions and effects that are seen by a dentist during many years in general practice. Familiarity with these *in vivo* features has greatly extended the data obtainable from extracted teeth, and so information has become available which is relevant in the forensic field.

Much of the information just referred to arises from the effects of dental pathology and of its treatment. Apart from this, dietary habits now lack the uniformity that characterized more primitive societies; since the concept of home care of teeth is carried out in such variety, much further data may be obtained when the effects of these habits are recognized.

It is well known that some pathological conditions and injuries produce permanent effects in developing teeth. Many examples of these and also of the effects of pathology and trauma experienced by the mature dentition are in the author's collection, but mostly they have been excluded from the present report. There are, however, some that are relevant in a study of morphological variation and of its bearing on identification of teeth or persons. For example, enamel hypoplasia may alter the apparent form of a cusp tip; dilaceration in a root may be mistaken for normal curvature; wear or abrasion, while altering tooth form, may also provide information concerning malocclusion or personal habits of the individual, especially if stain also is present.

As qualification for this study, the author has spent many years in teaching, in research and in administration. He has been involved in institutional practice, in public health dentistry, as well as in private practice. There has been extensive field work in New Zealand and in central Australia, and also in the museums and anatomical institutions in both countries, with participation in various science congresses. He has taught dentistry and anthropology, expanding and relating the fields of both to the interpretation of man's history and to the promotion of health.

As the writer was continually occupied with the dentition of man and of animals, and often intimately involved with it, familiarity with teeth was inevitable. The teaching of dental anatomy, both human and comparative, and of its relation through physical anthropology to archaeology, led him to a major interest in morphology of teeth and in the interpretation of their modifications as seen in life and in skeletal material, whether determined by function, injury or associated pathology.

A wide variety of topics in these related fields has been presented in previously published papers (see References). While these mostly refer to contemporary or to pre-European skeletal material from New Zealand, Australia and the Pacific area, there was also in 1937 a paper on the dentition of the Piltdown Man as represented in the then largely-accepted restoration of the fossil. Thus, many years before the hoax was revealed, the writer established that the Piltdown canine was an upper tooth, and that the dentition as represented in the restoration could not have existed in life. These claims were based on his appreciation of morphological characters and of the effects of function (Appendix 6).

Because such characters and effects provide valuable and useful data, the writer continued to collect teeth extracted by his colleagues as well as studying the dentition *in situ.* From the training of New Zealand school dental nurses his activities changed to administration and supervision of many clinics in the field and to dental inspections of great numbers of children, European and Maori in New Zealand, and European and Aborigine in Australia. Changed circumstances, some associated later with the war years, and then the responsibilities of private dental practice and part-time lecturing in anthropology, greatly restricted progress in this particular project; the way was cleared by the publication of other long-delayed material and by support from a research grant. Teaching and practice had focussed attention on detail, and on the great variation within the acceptable range of normality. With long experience in observing detail in teeth, and with a collection of many thousands of extracted teeth, the stage was set for an account of variation in morphology in human teeth. The results and conclusions arising out of an extensive study of this material are now presented.

By design the report is qualitative, the unsuitability of measurements for the purpose in hand having been established. It is not a textbook for dentists, although much of the study is relevant to their profession; nor does the work claim to present examples of variation that are "new" or unique. To be even more specific, it does not give prominence to teeth that might be considered abnormal, preserving an awareness nevertheless that the division between these and normal teeth is indefinite and subjective. Rather it aims to include everything possible, and to show that what appear as rather extreme characters are usually part of a demonstrable series which establishes their relation to the more common and easily recognized examples.

To sum up, this analysis of variation is based on examination of a very great number of teeth over many years during the teaching of dental anatomy and operative dentistry, coupled with both a considerable experience of dental examinations in the field and with the active practice in dentistry, associated with studies in a wide area of physical anthropology. It is illustrated extensively with accurate outlines of many hundreds of teeth taken from a very comprehensive collection. In short an intensive analysis of macroscopic morphological variation in normal human teeth is presented, carried out in a community of people predominantly European. The findings call for review of some long-held concepts, and they also have important practical applications.

Specific acknowledgments have been made in the usual manner. In addition, the writer acknowledges indebtedness to his teachers, to various authors and to the many other persons who, during a lifetime of experience and service through his profession, inspired him to "observe, compare, reflect and record" what is now reported. The profession of dentistry gives to its members knowledge and opportunities for unique services. One of these is the recording of dental information, potentially of critical importance in identification. In that respect this work shows how dentists could easily make better records, and indeed presents them with an obligation to do so.

Acknowledgments

THE WRITER GRATEFULLY acknowledges help of various kinds. He is indebted to Professor J. E. Morton and to the late Sir Douglas Robb for encouragement and advice over a number of years, and especially to the former for provision of working space and privileges in the Department of Zoology, University of Auckland.

He is indebted to Mr. H. D. Erlam, Librarian, School of Medicine, University of Auckland, for editorial supervision and advice with the manuscript, and to Mr. C. A. Schollum of the University's Anthropology Department for photography of the Figures.

Permission to incorporate into chapter 1 some material previously published in the *Journal of Dental Research* is hereby acknowledged to the editor of that journal.

A preliminary report on this project was presented in 1974 to the VI Congresso Paulista de Odontologia and the V Seminário Latino-Americano in São Paulo, Brazil, at the invitation of the Congress Committee. Acceptance of the invitation was made possible by grants from the Auckland Medical Research Foundation, Butland Medical Foundation, Medical Research Council of New Zealand and N.Z. Dental Association Research Foundation, all of whose assistance is gratefully acknowledged.

Working expenses in recent years have been assisted by support from the Golden Kiwi Distribution Committee for the Promotion of Medical Research, and from the University Grants Committee, Wellington, New Zealand, and lastly from the Dental Research Foundation mentioned above.

Contents

VARIATION IN
Morphology of Teeth

TO THE READER

Diagram showing the designation of cusps, surfaces, regions, dimensions and roots, according to their orientation in the jaws, as seen when facing a person or skull, with the jaws "open 180°."

See also Appendices 1 and 2.

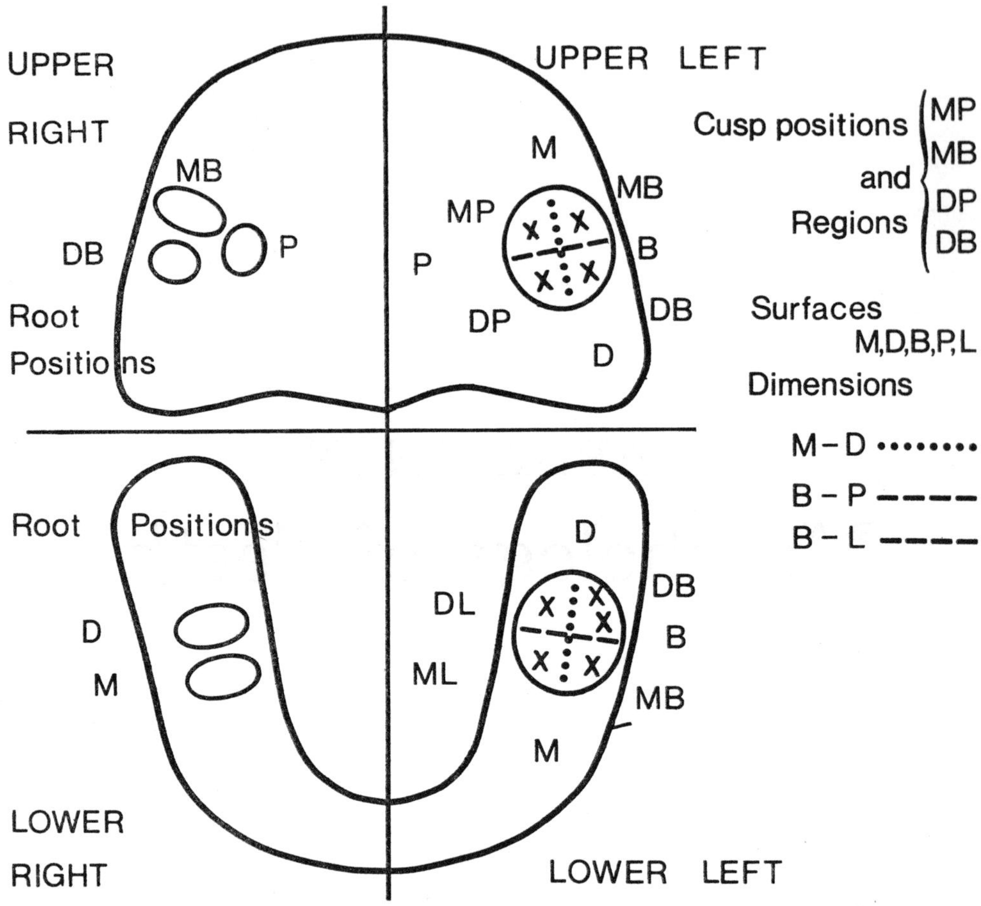

Since teeth are numbered from the midline in front, for each quarter of the mouth, tooth No. 6 is the first permanent molar. Upper, lower, left and right are indicated by the appropriate quadrant lines. Diagrams in upper jaw are as for 6⌋ (root positions), and ⌊6 (cusps, surfaces etc.). Diagrams in lower jaw are as for 6⌉ (root positions), and ⌈6 (cusps, surfaces etc.).

M=mesial, D=distal, B=buccal, P=palatal and L=lingual. In the upper jaw P and L are interchangeable, but in the lower jaw L only (never P) is used.

Although the relative orientations of front and back teeth change around the curve of the tooth row, M is always towards the midline of the front teeth. A good simile is to recall that the front of a railway carriage is always the end towards the engine, regardless of curvature of the track. "Proximal" is a collective term for M and D surfaces, like the contacting ends of the carriages in our railway train simile.

Chapter 1

Maxillary Incisors and Canines*

INCISORS

THE GENERAL and comparative characteristics of central and lateral incisors have been covered adequately in textbooks and are summarized here.

The central incisor is larger than the lateral and more robust while the crown of the lateral incisor is more rounded especially on the distal side. The root of the lateral incisor is more slender, relatively longer, and actually may be longer than that of the central incisor. Its root tends to bend distally, especially in the apical portion (Fig. 1-1 *a-d*†).

* Sections of this chapter were previously published in *Journal of Dental Research,* 48, 5-16, 173-182, 1969.

† Unless indicated otherwise, the outlines in Chapter 1 are drawn from the labial (La) aspect and are therefore frontal or facial views. In mesial and distal outlines (M, D) the labial or lingual side (La, Li) is indicated where this may not be clear. Linked outlines are views of one tooth. Pairs are not linked, but may be recognized by their symmetry or by the joined symbols as in *i* to *l* of Figure 1-3. Loss of substance may be shown by broken lines as for incisal wear, and worn facets by oblique shading (Fig. 1-6 *k*). Loss from tooth decay, trauma or fracture is shown by irregular outlines, but restorations (fillings) are shown by more regular outlines (Fig. 1-11 *a, b*). Shallow grooves in crown or root are easily recognized by their position. Where these retain stain through lack of friction, especially on lingual surfaces, light shading outlines these areas. Light shading may also indicate stain which reaches to the gingival margin (gum line) as distinct from the cervical line (Fig. 1-10 *c,f*) or it may indicate the extent of recession to the line of attachment (Fig. 1-22 *a,b*). Some other features are noted in the appropriate legends or text.

CENTRAL INCISOR

The basic form of this tooth is that of a wedge (crown) standing on edge with a cone (root) arising from its base. These component forms merge smoothly at the cervix, and the dimensions of either may be decreased or increased. Although the modification tends to correspond in both crown and root, this is not always so. There may be crowns of medium length with long roots, or, more often, large crowns with small roots (Figs. 1-1 and 1-3). In some, the roots may have become shortened by resorption (Fig. 1-4 *a,b*).

Seen from the labial side, the basic form for the whole tooth is a triangle (Figs. 1-2 *a,b,c* and 1-3 *i-l*). The triangle is almost isosceles, and the height may be more than three times the width of the base or just over twice the base measurement. The height of the crown is almost always greater than its width, although sometimes these measurements are almost equal. The root may be shorter than the crown if the crown is large or if the roots have been partly resorbed. The ability of an incisor to support a restoration or appliance depends on various factors, including the firmness of the tooth, which is largely dependent on the length of the root (determined radiographically) and its shape in cross section.

The crown has been described as basically wedge-shaped, or triangular when seen from mesial or distal sides. When an isosceles triangle is drawn with the cervical line as base, the incisal edge seldom coincides with the apex of the triangle but usually lies to the labial side (Fig. 1-5 *a*). When a perpendicular is drawn from apex to base, the base is divided unequally, the

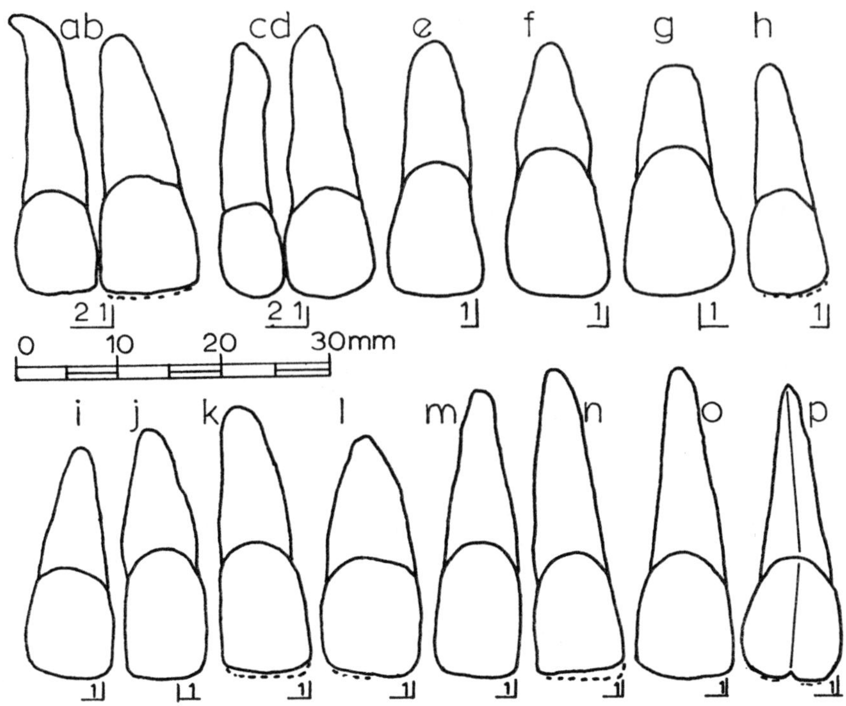

Figure 1-1. *ab* and *cd,* two central incisors with their laterals showing relative dimensions commonly found. *e* to *p,* central incisors showing some variations found in crown and root form, and in actual and relative dimensions of each part.

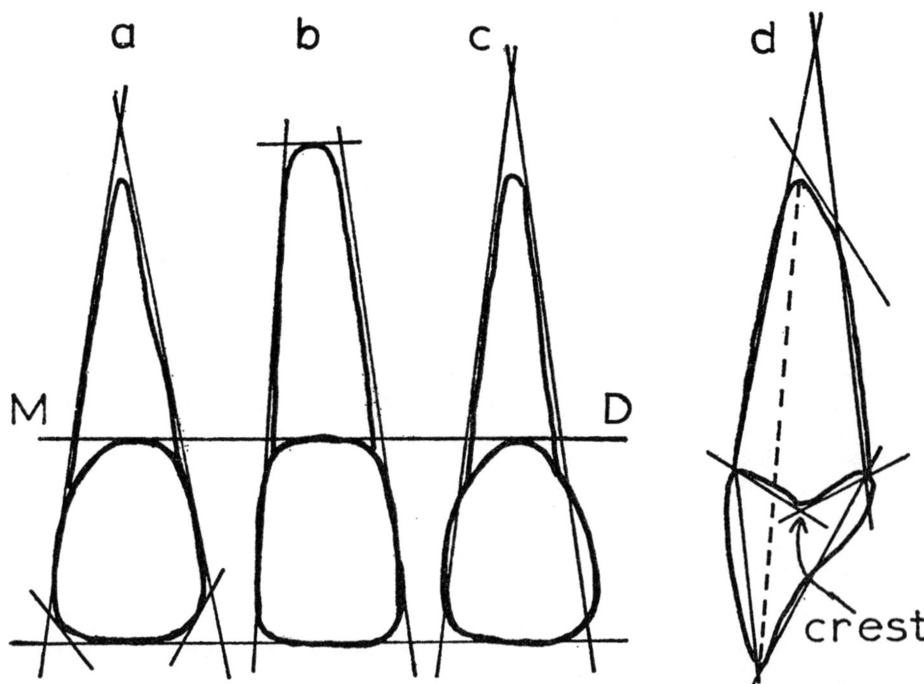

Figure 1-2. *a,b,c,* diagrams of the maxillary central incisor, labial view, to illustrate basic proportions, and the outline in relation to a triangle. *d,* maxillary incisor fitted to the straight lines of its basic form to show relation of the tooth axis to these when the root is not greatly curved. The tooth axis runs from the root apex to the incisal edge, which are both nearer to the labial than to the lingual outline. The cervical crest is approximately midway between labial and lingual.

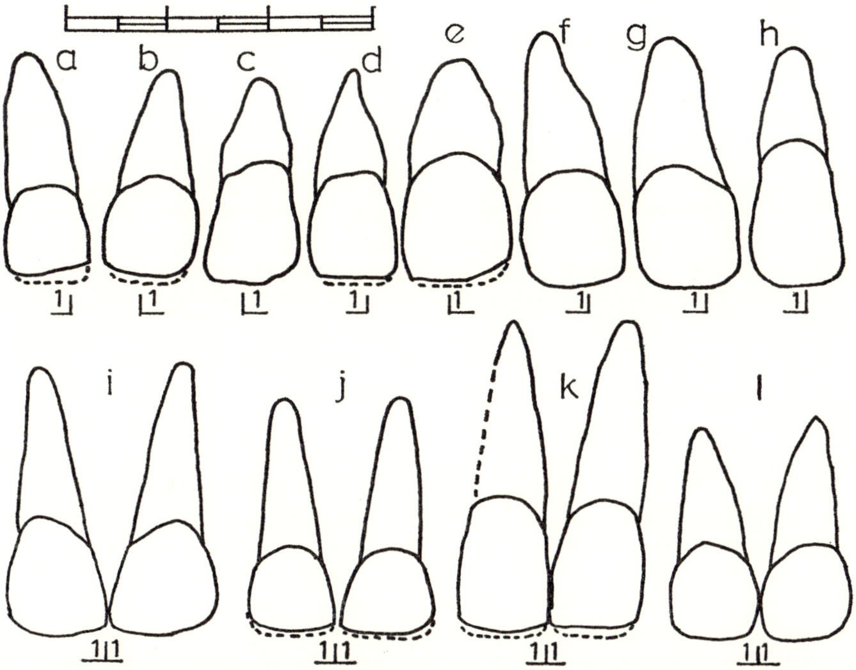

Figure 1-3. *a-h,* further variations as in Figure 1-1. *i-l,* pairs of centrals illustrating types of crown form: —*i,j,* tapering type; *k,* long square; *l,* ovoid type.

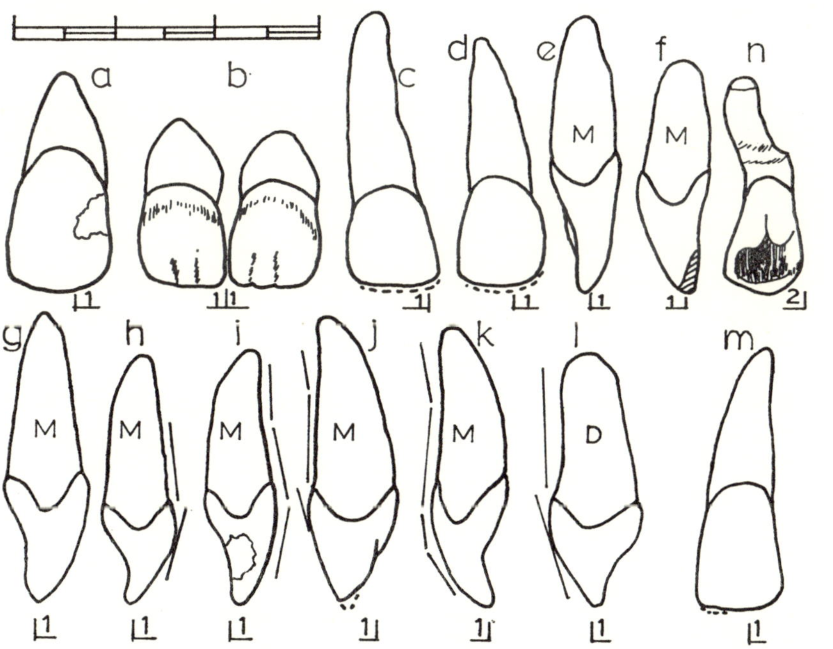

Figure 1-4. *a,b,* not small teeth, but teeth with very short roots. In *a* there is no wear of the crown, nor any sign of root shortening by resorption. In the *b* pair of centrals, the roots were not obviously resorbed, and the gingival level as indicated by stain suggested that these came from a not particularly old person. *c,d,* central incisors with roots tending to curve to mesial. The more usual curve to distal is seen in *m. e,f,* proximal views of centrals with contrasts in position of labial contour relative to tooth axis; that in *f* is common in lower teeth. (See also *g,h*). *g,h,* differences in thickness of blade of tooth crown. (See also *j,k,l*). *i,j,k,* roots tending to curve to labial. Contrasts in thickness of crown, and in crown form as regards blade and cingulum, and convexity of labial profile. *n,* an example of dilaceration or greenstick fracture of tooth root.

shorter portion being the labial segment (Fig. 1-5 *b*).

Although the crown of the incisor is basically wedge-shaped, conformity to the wedge-shape is modified by various curves in the outline. Thus the wedge outline is thickened in the lingual cingulum region and the crown may therefore be regarded as having two portions, the "body" and the "blade" (Fig. 1-5 *c*). In proximal profile, variations in degree of curvature appear to arise from differences in the relation of the blade to the body. This is viewed as a bending of the blade to the labial side (decreased curvature, Fig. 1-4 *i*) or to the lingual side (increased curvature, Fig. 1-4 *k*). Although this may seem contrary to the idea expressed in relation to Figures 1-2 *d*, 1-5 *a,b*, the differences are acceptable as variations on the basic form. Excessive lingual "bending" of crown may result from movement of a developing crown in its crypt after an impact on the deciduous tooth, but evidence of trauma easily identifies a case (Taylor, 1970a).

It is unsatisfactory to describe a crown as straight or flat but to give no further information. The crown of tooth *e* in Figure 1-4 is straight in that its axis closely aligns with that of the root, and it is flat as regards most of the labial profile. But a corresponding flatness is seen in teeth *j* and *l* of the same figure. Tooth *l* is a large tooth with a very convex labial surface when traced from M to D. Thus, the terms straight or flat should be coupled with reference to the axis or profile, or area to which they apply.

However, considerable variation is readily seen in proximal profiles. Body and blade of crowns and the range of direction of the blade have been noted. This is associated with convexity of labial profile, and with the S-curves of lingual profile, but it is by no means the only factor concerned. The lingual cingulum region and its counterpart at labial cervix often seem to vary independently. For linguals, compare teeth *f,j,k,l* of Figure 1-4 with *g,h,i,l* for labials. It is easy to find apparent contrasts if judged by ends of the cervical curve, as in Figures 1-4 *e,f,k* and 1-6 *a,c,d,f*, but this is not a valid procedure. In this view, the terminal portions of the cervical curve or wave are influenced by the convexity of root surfaces, as would be seen in a transverse section. Also, they are very sensitive to rotation of the tooth on its long axis. This last factor cannot be standardized, even for work with the camera lucida, because of the irregular and variable morphology of teeth—the subject of this study.

The height or depth of the cervical line or wave does, however, assist in drawing attention to another widely variable character in proximal view. This is the proportional thickness to length relation of the whole crown and of its body and blade components. This bears also on the direction of crown blade which has already been discussed in relation to axes of the crown and of the whole root.

Variation in thickness to length relation is well shown in many of the outlines. For the whole crown, attention is drawn especially to Figure 1-4 *e,f,i,l*, and for the blade to Figure 1-4 *e,g,h,j,k,l*.

The Cervical Line

The cervical line is established on completion of crown formation, and the alveolar border normally assumes a very similar contour when eruption of the tooth to occlusion is complete. The alveolar border may remain irregular if the tooth erupts into malocclusion, or it may become irregular by resorption in the presence of periodontal pathology, but the cervical line never changes its original form.

Insofar as its contour forecasts the contour of the alveolar border or interdental septum, it is of interest to note whether there is a difference between mesial and distal cervical contours that bears any consistent relation to the different widths of adjacent teeth. Such a difference was observed with a considerable degree of consistency in upper canines, as will be described in due course. In the case of incisors there is less contrast in B-L dimension of adjacent teeth, and any such association was not established, although differences between M and D contours were often found. It is clear that other factors are involved in establishing the cervical line, and while it may be believed that some can be recognized, the present concern is to describe some of the variations that result.

Although some characters of the cervical line have already been referred to, this feature merits analysis in greater detail. Unfortunately (and this applies throughout the present study), morphological details are three-dimensional, and one is practically limited to two-dimensional projections onto various planes to present them. Although some stereoscopic photographs have been published, their artistic and realistic attraction is far outweighed by their disadvantages. Apart from the labour and expense of production, they achieve little that cannot be better appreciated by projection of outlines. The superiority of outlines scientifically lies in the exclusion of unnecessary and distracting details and the inclusion (or feasibility of inclusion) of far more illustrations and much more relevant information.

Illustration of the cervical line therefore amounts to projections of portions of a closed irregular loop which is placed in three-dimensional space. The projections are made of the nearer portions as viewed from buccal, lingual, mesial or distal. In proximal view, small differences in the apparently terminal portions of the line arise from several facts. First, because the root outline at the cervix is more convex on the distal side, one may see further around a more sweeping curve so that the terminal portions may extend further into the central portion. Again, teeth differ in convexity, in size and in type so that these differences inevitably involve the cervical contours. A third reason already mentioned is the impossibility of placing each tooth in exactly the same position for tracing the outline through the camera lucida.

The last mentioned factor, slight rotation of a tooth on its long axis, could be expected to produce a result such as the "lopsided" cervical line of tooth *f* compared with *e* in Figure 1-6. It so happens, however, that this is not the explanation here. Tooth *f* has a small-radius ridge arising from the labial aspect of the root at both sides M and D, so that it has a wide, unusually flattened labial surface of the root, as well as a wide square crown (Fig. 1-1 *o*). Tooth *e* of Figure 1-6, also a square type (Fig. 1-1 *n*), has a much more rounded root. A transverse section at the cervices of these teeth would resemble a broad oval in one and a wide triangular outline in the other. It is clear that the form of cervical curves may result from several factors; these should be recognized, but their evident complexity should discourage confidence in explanation of form. Analysis, in consequence, is largely descriptive.

Therefore, being able to see a little "further around the corner" to the labial and lingual sides in a view from the distal side is one factor that increases the upper portion of the S-curve. Similarly the amount of this part of the S-curve that shows is less in a view from the mesial side and may be further reduced in views of both sides as the tooth becomes more nearly "square."

The proximal cervical outline may be analyzed as two S-shaped lines (one of which is reversed) that meet. Alternatively it is wave-shaped. When *in situ*, the tip of the interdental septum is by the wave trough in an upper tooth (and in a lower tooth the corresponding point is the crest of the wave). This is the point where the tails of each S meet, and their relationship in meeting (at the wave trough in upper teeth) may be likened to a small segment of a large circle (Figs. 1-5 *e* and 1-4 *j*) or a large segment of a small circle (Figs. 1-5 *f* and 1-4 *k*). Other acceptable descriptions of this feature are obtuse, flattened or U-shaped in the first case and acute, angular or V-shaped in the latter.

With this mixture of descriptive styles, the great variety of this feature in proximal view can be appreciated, as presented for incisors and canines in the various figures. One wave length is the labio-lingual dimension of the tooth at the cervix, and the measure of wave height is obvious. It is evident that neither of these bear any direct relationship to length of crown or of root. Neither does the other variable feature, namely the shape and steepness of the wave, but in this author's examination some of the characters that affect it have been shown.

In Figure 1-4, tooth *c* has wide and shallow cervices while in *d* they are deep and V-shaped, especially on mesial. In Figure 1-3, in the pairs *i,j,k,l,* all cervices are wide, and none are shallow. It seems, therefore, that neither tooth type nor crown length have a close relation to the style of the cervical curve.

Figure 1-7 presents in diagrammatic form the analysis of variations in cervical line which have been described. Figure 1-7 *d* depicts the S-curve for a tooth of wider labio-lingual dimension *(upper line)* and for one of narrower dimension *(lower line).* On one side of the diagram, the S-curves are reduced to straight line ele-

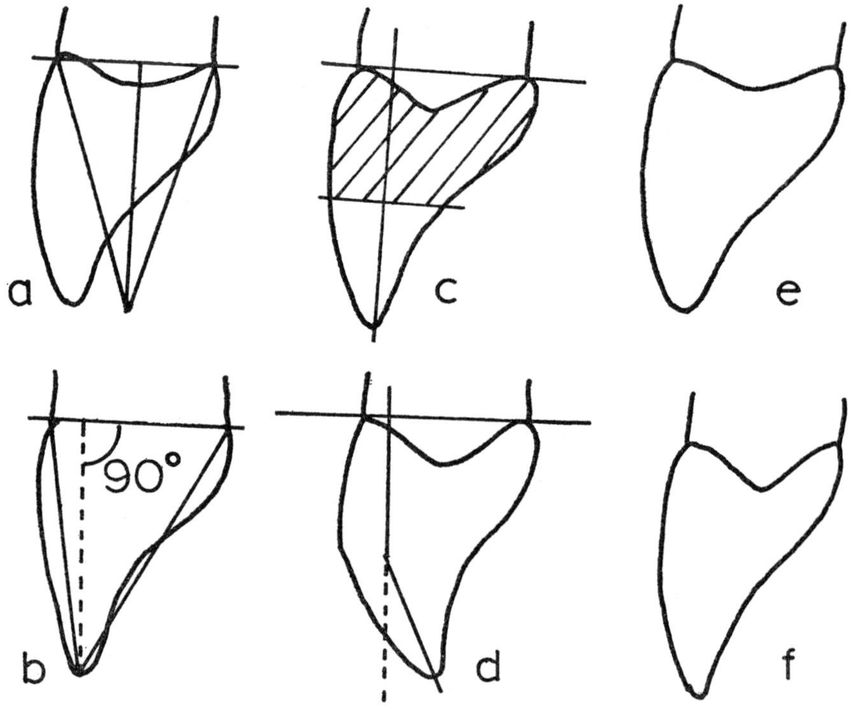

Figure 1-5. *a,* an isosceles triangle on the cervical base. The tooth crown appears to be "pushed" to the labial of the apex of the triangle. *b,* a scalene triangle on the cervical base and the apex of the triangle at the incisal edge. The perpendicular to the base, through this apex, is nearer to the labial. *c,* crown of an incisor. The shaded portion is the body of the crown and the unshaded portion is the blade. *d,* crown of an upper incisor. The blade of the crown has been bent to the lingual. (See Fig. 1-6, *a-d*). *e,f,* the cervical line; angular type and the somewhat flattened-curve variety.

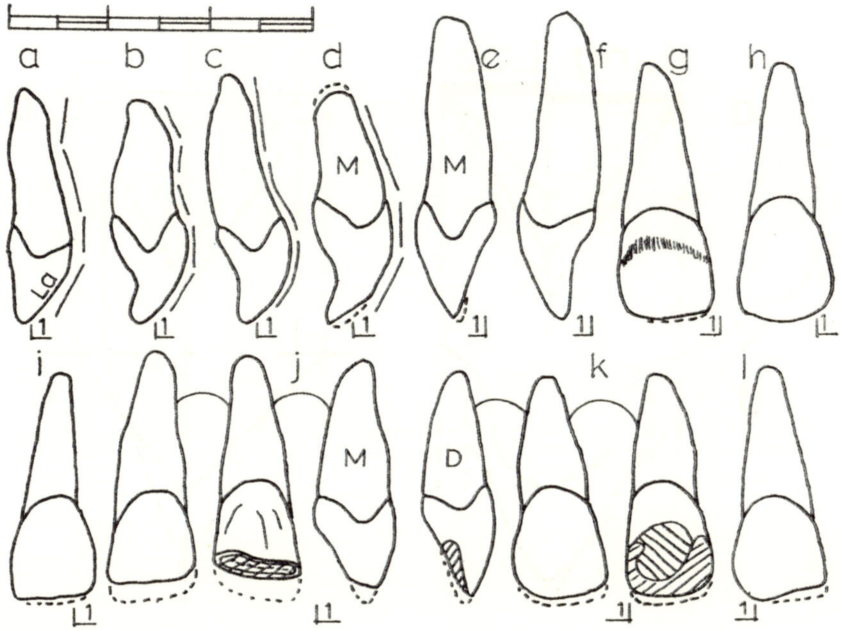

Figure 1-6. Curvature or bends in axes of crown and root as seen from proximal. *a-f,* mesial views. Note also variety in cervical arches. In tooth *a* the crown profile has so much reduction in labial convexity and lingual concavity that identification of these latter must be confirmed by other features. In *d* there is a labial facet of wear showing that the tooth was in lingual occlusion. Teeth *e,f* have many similarities in size and form of characters of root and crown, of convexities and axes, but cervical lines are very different. Tooth *g* illustrates features that could be of forensic interest: enamel is white for some distance below the cervix, there is then a markedly green band which changes to yellow for the remainder of the labial surface which terminates in an incisal facet. Reasonable deductions are that there was little incisal overlap, that the tooth belonged to a rather young person who completely neglected artificial prophylaxis. Teeth *i* and *j* show respectively light and moderate incisal wear from edge-to-edge occlusion. Tooth *k* presents wear from a deep overbite with free lateral movements which have combined to accentuate curvature of the M and D incisal angles. In tooth *l* the M angle only has been worn away.

ments of head, body and tail. The tail meets the almost "mirror image" tail on the same proximal surface beside the crest of the interdental septum.

Whether the cervical curve is shallow or deep, the labial portion tends to be shorter than the lingual (Fig. 1-7 *a,b,c*). In particular, Figure 1-7 *b* shows that the difference in labio-lingual dimensions does not necessarily alter the depth or angle of the cervical line but may follow from differences in actual size of the crown. Differences in proportion may accompany obvious differences in depth of curve (Fig. 1-7 *c*). These may be described by imagining the crown as plastic so that without change in bulk the crown may be stretched in length while compressed in cervical dimension.

Labial or Facial View

In the labial view, the upper central incisor presents wide variation both in root and crown. This is the easiest tooth for the recognition of variations of crown form, and most differences are readily seen *in situ*. These teeth, together with the lateral incisors and their arrangement,

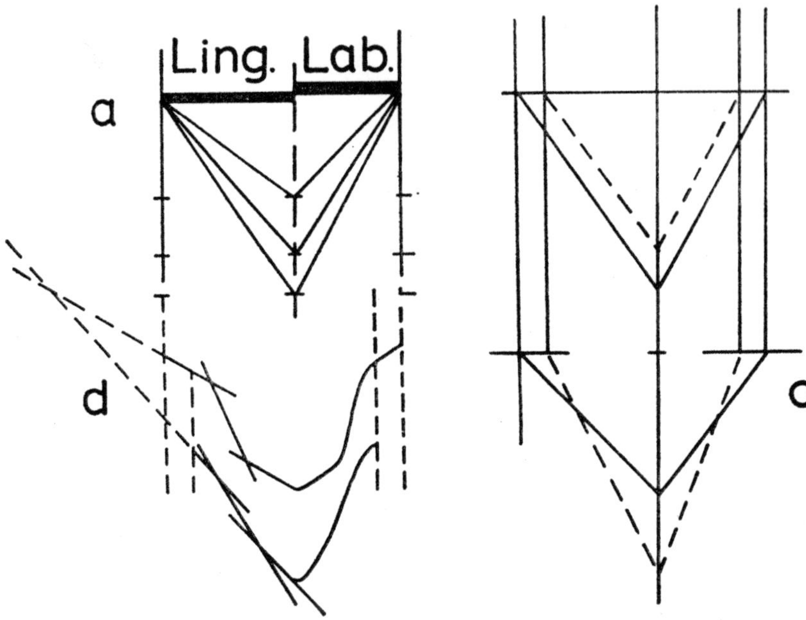

Figure 1-7. Analysis of the cervical line.

make the greatest contribution to the individuality of a dentition.

The labial view of the crown is contained within four lines: mesial, distal, incisal and cervical. Mesial and distal are collectively referred to as proximal, whereas the cervical outline may be covered by the gingival margin (Fig. 1-4 *b*), and the incisal may be altered by wear (Fig. 1-4 *c*, *d*). Both proximal margins are usually convex; the distal more so. Each joins the incisal margin at an angle. Both angles unless modified by wear are curves, where the distal angle has the larger radius (Fig. 1-1 *e-k*) and may be associated with a concavity in the distal outline (Fig. 1-1 *g*). Concavities in proximal outlines are sometimes associated with a narrow cervix (Fig. 1-8 *b*), which usually is a relatively short cervical and relatively wide incisal line although it is difficult to describe this feature in precise terms. Such a cervical line is sometimes more convex rootward (Fig. 1-8 *g*,*i*), and it may merge so smoothly with proximal outlines that termini cannot fairly be assigned.

The incisal edge may present notches which divide it into tubercles. There are usually three tubercles, but there is much variation (Fig. 1-8). Most often they are approximately equal in size, or the two outer tubercles may be progressively widened whereas the middle one is reduced (Fig. 1-8 *i*) or eliminated (Fig. 1-8 *g*). If there are only two tubercles, they may be unequal in size as though the middle one were incorporated in one or the other (Fig. 1-8 *e*,*k*). The distal tubercle may be wider than either of the other two, where all three remain distinct (Fig. 1-8 *f*).

There is sometimes a tendency for the identity of a tubercle to persist, if we may so interpret the prominent grooves seen on some labial or lingual surfaces (Figs. 1-8 *h*, 1-10 *h-m* and 1-21 *n*,*p*,*q*,*r*). As man is not alone in developing incisors from three genetic elements placed side by side, no doubt comparative dental anatomy would

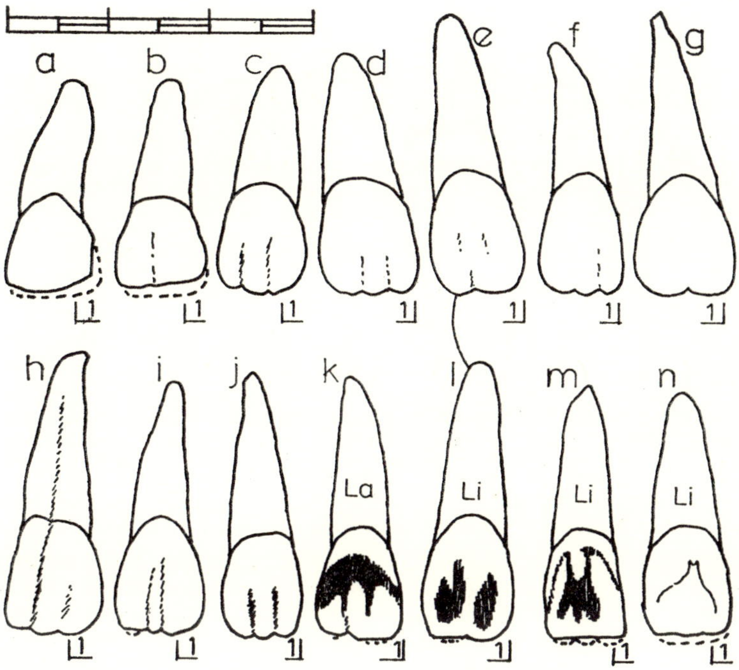

Figure 1-8. Mostly examples of variation in incisal mamelons or tubercles, and lingual features. *a,b,* modification of tapering and ovoid crowns by wear. *c-j,* labial views showing variation in number and relative width of incisal tubercles. The associated shallow grooves are often made more distinct by virtue of stain retained therein. Tooth *b* presents a crack rather than a groove in labial enamel. Tooth *h* presents a marked labial groove which continues (up on) to the root almost to the apex. (See similar grooves, but on lingual surface, in Figures 1-10 *h,i,j,m* and 1-21 *p,q,r*). *l,m,n,* lingual surfaces with low ridges and shallow concavities distinguished by stain areas. Much data may be obtained from the position and nature of stained or polished areas, relating to age, function, food, habits and oral hygiene of the person during life, or up to the time of extraction of the tooth.

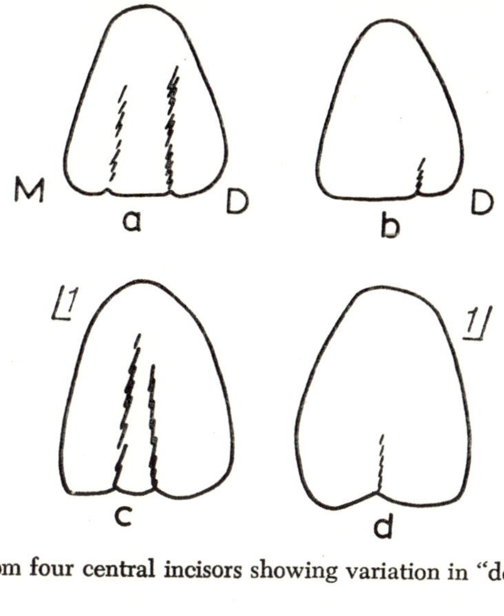

Figure 1-9. Outlines from four central incisors showing variation in "developmental" tubercles.

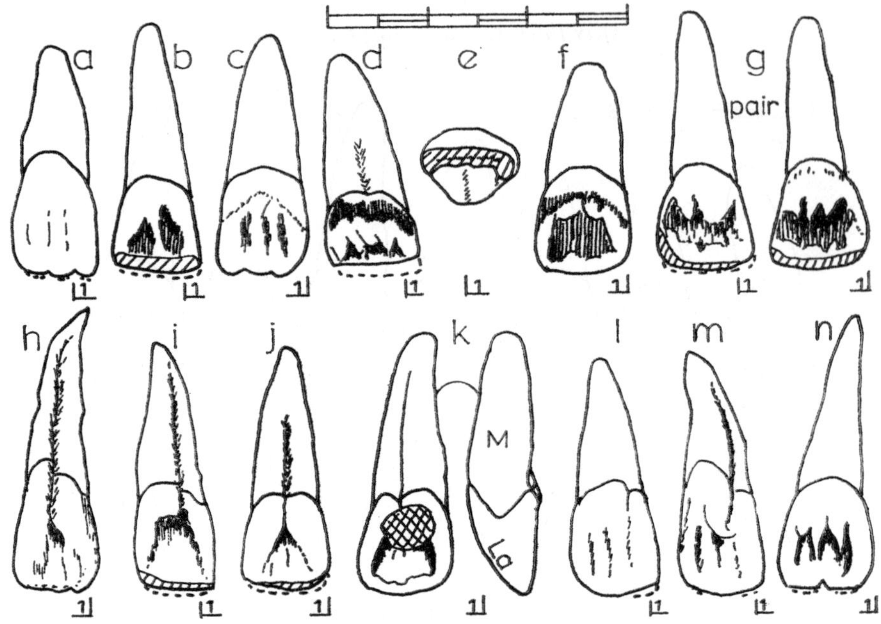

Figure 1-10. Lingual views of upper centrals where residual stain assists delineation of a great variety of lingual features of crown. *a,* almost featureless. *b,c,* slight ridges. *e,* incisal view where wear has given transverse section of lateral ridges in shovel-type tooth. *d,f,g,* some variations in the "tuberculum dentale" feature. It is seen that variation may occur between corresponding teeth in one person as in the pair of centrals in *g*. *h-m,* variations in groove dividing cingulum. This may be central *(j)* or lateral, usually on M side *(h,i,k,l,m)*. Tooth *k* is shovel-type, lingual and M views. There is an amalgam filling. *n,* lingual view of the tooth shown in Figure 1-8 *g*.

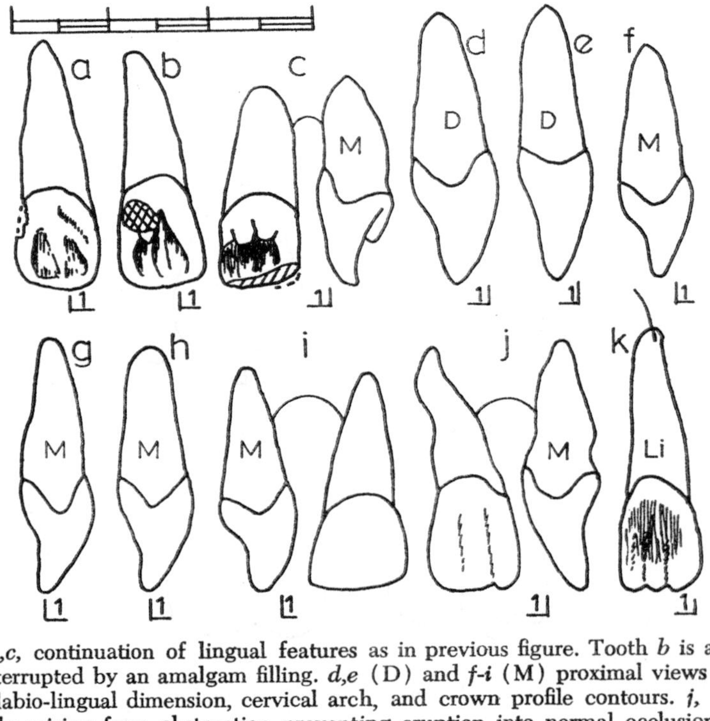

Figure 1-11. *a,b,c,* continuation of lingual features as in previous figure. Tooth *b* is a shovel-type with this character interrupted by an amalgam filling. *d,e* (D) and *f-i* (M) proximal views of centrals showing variation in labio-lingual dimension, cervical arch, and crown profile contours. *j,* variations in root direction probably arising from obstruction preventing eruption into normal occlusion. *k,* a bristle has been inserted to show that the apical foramen is not at the anatomical apex of the root in this tooth.

furnish useful data in a study of this character.

Corresponding to the position of the notches, shallow "developmental" grooves may divide the crown longitudinally (shadings in Figs. 1-8 and 1-9). The position of these grooves may be made more obvious by the tendency of stain to remain in them (Fig. 1-8). The grooves are not always easily discernible, but when present they are mostly confined to the incisal and middle third of the crown and do not reach the cervical third, although they may continue for varying distances up beyond the cervix to the root as already shown (Fig. 1-8 *h*).

Lingual or Palatal View

Lingual surfaces vary greatly. The junction of the two parts, body and blade, is most evident when there is a large cingulum, or when the blade of the crown bends lingually (Figs. 1-4 *k,l,* 1-10 and 1-11). The lingual surface may be smooth or marked by various longitudinal ridges and grooves. Sometimes there are two noticeable ridges, mesial and distal, with a depression between them, and this may continue as a groove or fissure more or less completely dividing the cingulum. When the condition is extreme with caries in a deep pit or fissure, treatment may present considerable difficulty as regards cavity preparation (Fig. 1-12 *d,e,f*). These grooves crossing the cingulum vary in position and may occur also in the upper lateral incisor (Fig. 1-21).

The groove may be more or less distinct but may not pass through the cingulum to the cervix. One or more grooves may divide this portion of the cingulum equally or unequally into small areas which may be raised into a tubercle known as tuberculum dentale (Figs. 1-10, 1-11 and 1-21). The tubercles are present in varying degrees of development and have been classified (Mühlreiter and de Jonge Cohen, 1928). Moorrees (1957) also refers to the condition called "shovel" teeth, in which teeth have fairly well-defined mesial and distal ridges on the lingual surfaces of upper incisors with a depression between them. Shovel teeth may or may not have lingual tubercles (Figs. 1-10 *k* and 1-21 *o*).

Incisal View of Crown

It has already been stated that the crown is wedge-shaped and is joined to a cone-shaped root. The quadrilateral base of the former and the circular base of the latter are modified to join at the cervix. The outline at the cervix, if a transverse section is made, will sometimes resemble more closely one figure or the other, but it is never bilaterally symmetrical (Fig. 1-13). In this figure attention is drawn to asymmetry: *(a)* by a broken line bisecting the lingual side at right angles; and *(b)* by producing the mesial and distal sides until they intersect, and drawing a perpendicular from this point to the labial line. The mesial and distal lines produced form a scalene triangle with the labial line as base. The greater slope of the mesial line in relation to the labial usually can be recognized without difficulty in the roots of extracted teeth. This asymmetry enables a left tooth to be distinguished from a right, even though other distinguishing features have been lost by wear or fracture. Similarly, if the whole crown has been lost by fracture, a root can be identified as left or right.

As no tooth conforms precisely to a basic geometric outline, some specimens may suggest a different geometric form. At the same time, certain characteristics tend to persist within the range of variation in the basic geometric form. The transverse section of this tooth in the cervical region is a case in point.

Associated with variations in crown form are variations in the cervical region which give rise to a variety of proportions and curvatures in the outline shape of a transverse section. In Figure 1-13 *a* distal and mesial sides are never parallel. It follows that a labial side is always longer than a lingual, sometimes so much so that the basic figure is changed from a quadrilateral to a triangle (Fig. 1-14).

In Figure 1-14, the upper diagrams relate to the basic quadrilateral form and the lower to the basic triangular form. In *a* and *c* the guidelines of the basic geometric form only are shown. In *b* and *d* the tooth outline is shown in relation to the guidelines; from the intersection of mesial and distal lines, a perpendicular is drawn to the labial line. As the perpendicular cuts the labial line nearer to the distal, the mesial line makes a more acute angle than does the distal line with the labial. Thus, even though the basic geometric form may differ, the same character is present to distinguish mesial from distal and left tooth from right tooth.

In Figure 1-15, two central incisors are viewed from the incisal aspect.

Variety *(a)* is found in teeth where labial "developmental grooves" are present and the labial outline is approximately parallel to incisal outline. In some instances the labial outline is arched *(b)*. The arch is then usually asymmetrical, the highest part being nearer the mesial; this may further assist in distinguishing a left tooth from a right one. A similar feature is more constant in canine teeth, where it represents the labial ridge usually passing from cusp tip to cervix.

Labio-lingual Thickness

In general this is the distance between labial and lingual surfaces at any point, when the tooth is viewed from M or D. In particular it is that distance where specified, and the most commonly selected position is between labial and lingual cervices. This was the distance named as cervical wave length when describing the cervical line. Another "thickness" dimension is that between the most prominent part of the lingual cingulum and the approximately opposite point. This distance may be appreciably greater than that at the cervix in such a tooth as *l* of Figure 1-4 as contrasted with tooth *e* of that figure. This distance at the cingulum is of no scientific value but serves to draw attention to variation of convexities at this region. Another thickness that is even less capable of precise or significant measurement, since there are no anatomical landmarks, is nevertheless worthy of attention. This is thickness of tooth blade, as in teeth *f,g,h,j,k,l* of Figure 1-4. Whether it is considered as a direct comparison between teeth, or as a "percentage" of the cervical thickness, its value lies in drawing attention to the considerable variation found in blades of incisor crowns.

But this is not all, for it must be pointed out that blade thickness, as judged in proximal view, is not necessarily what it appears to be; in fact it is sometimes an illusion. The impression one gets of blade thickness in proximal view is very much influenced by the absence, or degree of development, of ridges on the lingual surface. These have already been discussed along with some of their variations, shown in Figure 1-10 for centrals and Figure 1-21 for lateral incisors. In Figure 1-4 tooth *g* has moderate ridges but teeth *h,k* have no such feature. Tooth *e* has a strong distal ridge but none at mesial. Tooth *j* had ridges from the cingulum extending well down the lingual surface, and these were flanked by ridges arising midway and continuing to the tooth angles from which they were later worn away.

In sum, then, considerable variation in blade thickness does occur. It is not easy to illustrate graphically from any aspect, since it is affected by a number of other morphological characters. It is certainly not measurable in any meaningful way in relation to any other character.

LABIAL OUTLINE TYPES

It is the labial view of the crown which attracts most attention. Such features as tubercles, grooves and ridges, angles and convexity have been considered. It is now appropriate to examine variation in the

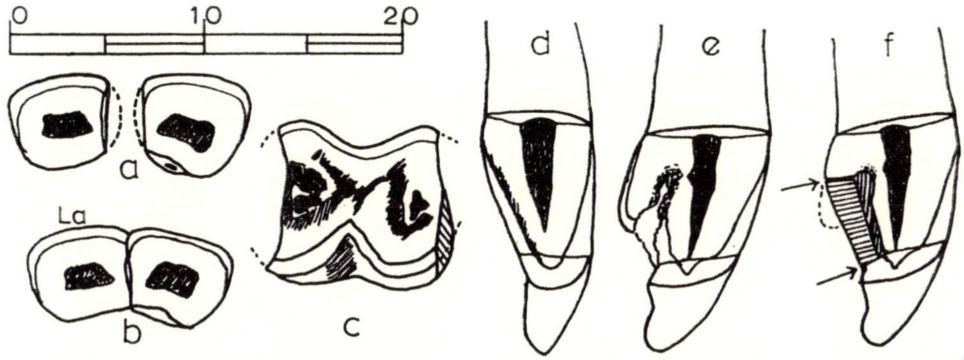

Figure 1-12. Occlusal view of teeth of sheep, showing advanced wear, and human incisors showing relation of lingual pit to operative procedures. *a,* the teeth have been parted and the lost proximal outline indicated by broken lines. *b,* the relation of the teeth to one another when the sheep died, showing that in spite of proximal wear, contact is maintained. *c,* premolar tooth of sheep showing similar severe wear of both proximal and occlusal surfaces. *d,* human incisor having no lingual pit, sectioned to show relation of lingual surface to pulp cavity. *e,* similar section of tooth with lingual pit, which has become carious. *f,* diagram to show style of cavity preparation and completed restoration, to avoid pulp exposure, or later thermal irritation from inlay or amalgam filling. Arrows show direction of drill for cavity preparation. Cement lining (vertical shading). Amalgam filling (horizontal shading). The outlines *a-e,* drawn with camera lucida, are approximately to the scale shown.

shapes enclosed by the four boundaries designated mesial (M), distal (D), incisal and cervical.

Williams (1914) demonstrated three basic types of outlines: square, tapering and ovoid. Variations and combinations within each basic type become increasingly complicated and therefore difficult to recognize. He showed that the majority of instances contained features of two, or all three, types, each of which might be modified into subtypes according to size and

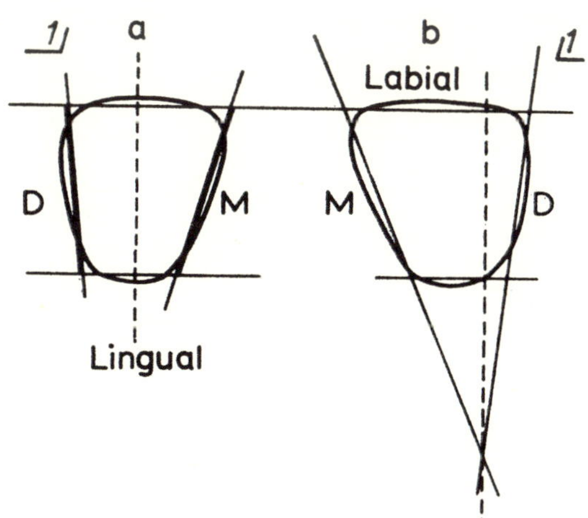

Figure 1-13. Maxillary central incisors, transverse sections at cervix. The straight lines indicate the general directions of the various surfaces, the lingual being drawn parallel to the labial. The resulting three- or four-sided figures are bilaterally symmetrical to one another (in left and right teeth), but they are individually asymmetrical. Asymmetry assists determination of mesial and distal from examination of the root; it also enables differentiation of a right root (or tooth) *(a)* from left *(b).*

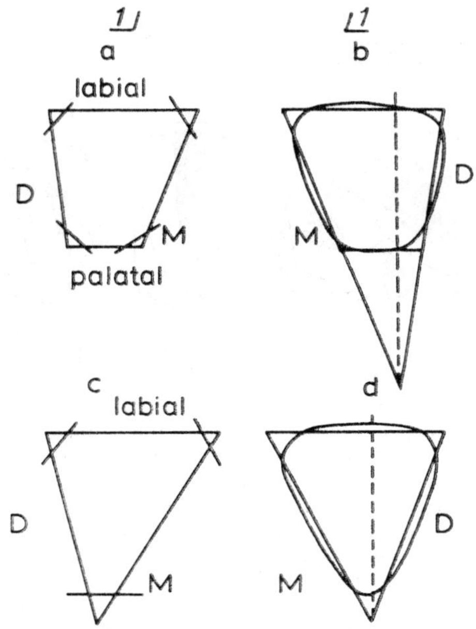

Figure 1-14. Transverse sections of central incisors at the cervix, showing variation in the basic form. *a,c* = right; *b,d* = left.

proportions of length and breadth. Thus there are large square, short square, long square and narrow square subtypes with a character of nearly parallel sides. Somewhat similar subtypes can be recognized for tapering and ovoid. The prospect of dealing with combinations of these however is far too daunting for this writer

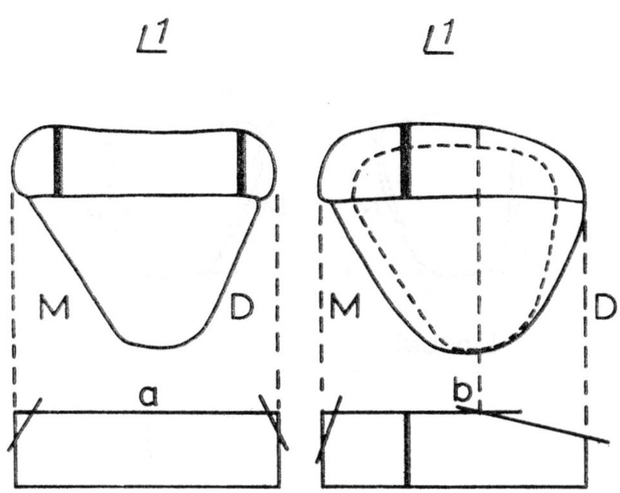

Figure 1-15. Upper central incisors from incisal aspect to indicate variations in labial contours. In some the tooth blade is of nearly even thickness *(a)*, as when incisal tubercles are present. In others the blade tends to be thicker towards the mesial side, as in *(b)*. In both diagrams lingual features such as ridges, grooves, tubercles and pits have been omitted. In *b*, the asymmetry of the root section at cervix has been added (broken line of shorter dashes).

and even more so in view of the many other morphological characters involved. Nevertheless, the writer is willing to agree that in theory the types must exist, but feels that the mixture must be even more complex than the ethnic groups of the genus homo.

Geometric symbols representing the three types named by Williams would be a square or rectangle, a triangle (either equilateral or isosceles), or a circle or oval (Fig. 1-16 *a,b,c*). The characteristics of these figures respectively are the almost parallel mesial and distal outlines, or the distinctly divergent outlines, and those that are more obviously curved. As the mesial and distal outlines are not strictly parallel, the widest dimension tends to be nearer the incisal. There is always a cervical margin so that the triangle is truncated; it would be preferable perhaps to visualize a trapezoid. The mesial-distal dimension (width) in an unworn tooth is less than the height. Again, the distal angle is more rounded, as is the whole distal outline, when compared with the mesial; the long axis of the crown, and of the whole tooth, is inclined toward the distal. This last feature may be illustrated by visualizing the basic figures (Fig. 1-16 *a,b,c*) made up with an elastic material, loosely jointed at the angles. If the top of each figure is pulled to one side, each assumes the bilateral asymmetry that is characteristic of the tooth crown (Fig 1-17 *a,b,c*). By taking off the angles (Fig. 1-17 *a,b*) in the manner shown in *d* and *e*, it is found that the basic straight line figures for a square-

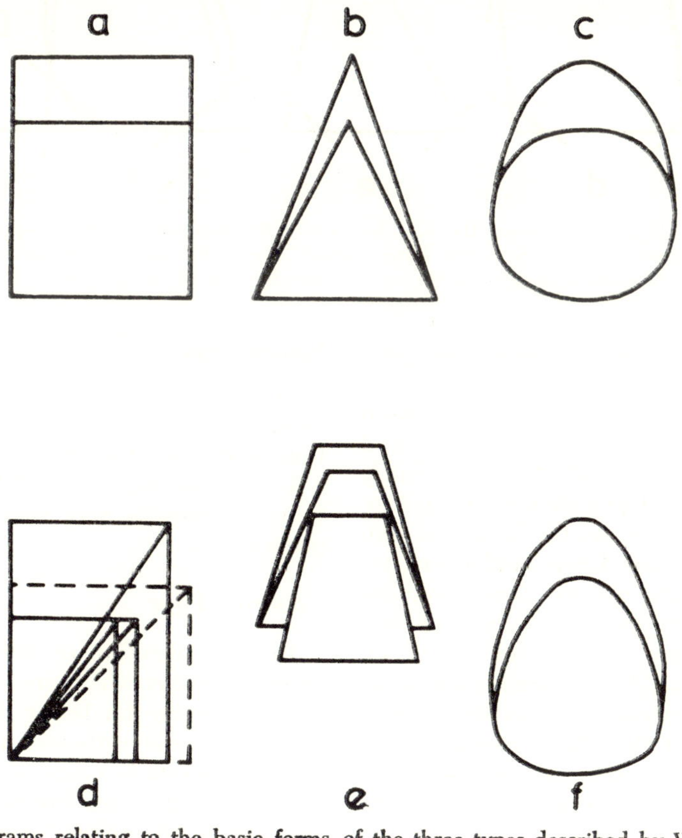

Figure 1-16. Diagrams relating to the basic forms of the three types described by Williams (1914) as found in the labial views of incisor teeth.

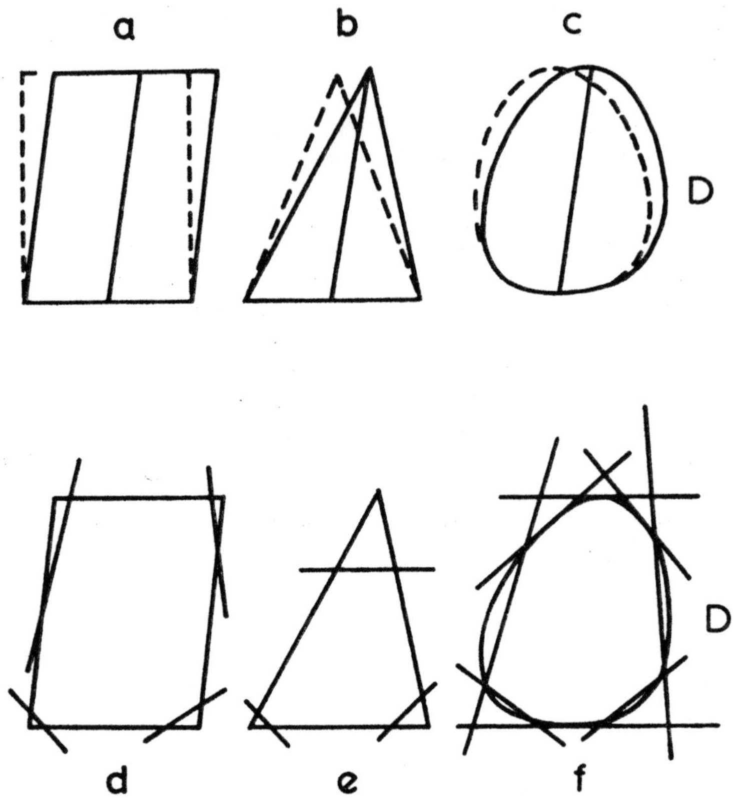

Figure 1-17. *a,b,c,* diagrams showing the modification of the basic forms to correspond with the asymmetry of a left-side incisor, seen from the labial aspect. *d,e,f,* the same, showing modification of the three typical figures to emphasize asymmetry in the rounding off of the angles.

type and a tapering-type tooth are produced.

As the height of the triangle is increased toward infinity (on the same base) and small angles are cut off to leave fairly straight sides, the form changes from tapering to square type. As the height is similarly increased and large angles are removed to indicate greater curvature, the changes in form provide much of the range of variation in morphology of incisor teeth. It has been shown that some teeth may be described as having features of two types, but that the recognition and naming of mixed types cannot be undertaken with sufficient exactitude to have scientific value.

Square Type

Many examples of the varieties of square-type teeth are in the author's collection and comprise parts of Figures 1-1, 1-3, 1-10 and 1-21 *a,b,c.* Figure 1-16 shows how the crowns may vary in size and in proportions.

Tapering Type

In the material of this study, upper central incisors which are easily recognized as tapering are far fewer than those which are square. Nevertheless, they are present in a considerable range of size, of proportion of length and breadth of crown, of proportion of crown length, and of root

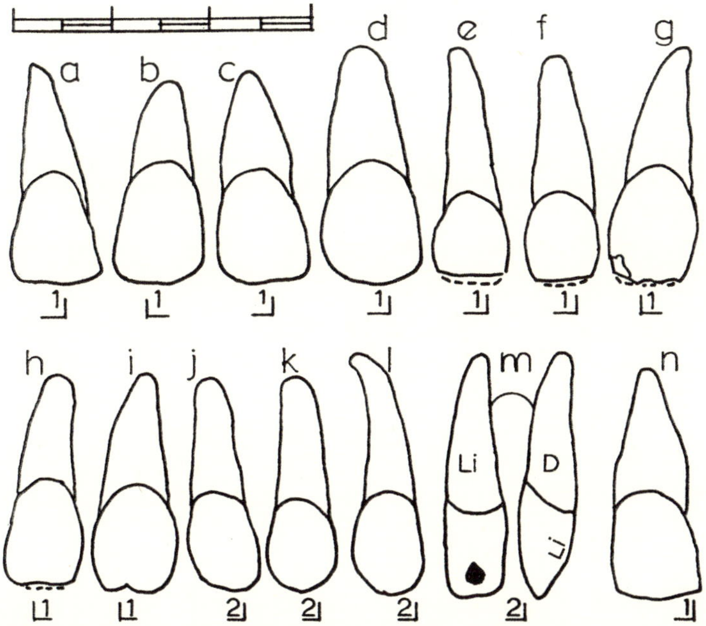

Figure 1-18. Variations in crown and root sizes and proportions, basic types, etc. *a,b,* tapering type crowns. *c-l,* ovoid-type crowns. *a-i* and *n,* central incisors. *j-m,* lateral incisors. Tooth *g* presents a chipped incisal edge and fracture lines in enamel indicating rough usage or trauma. Tooth *m* is the so-called "barrel" shape. Tooth *n* is large square type with a short root which tapers abruptly in its apical half.

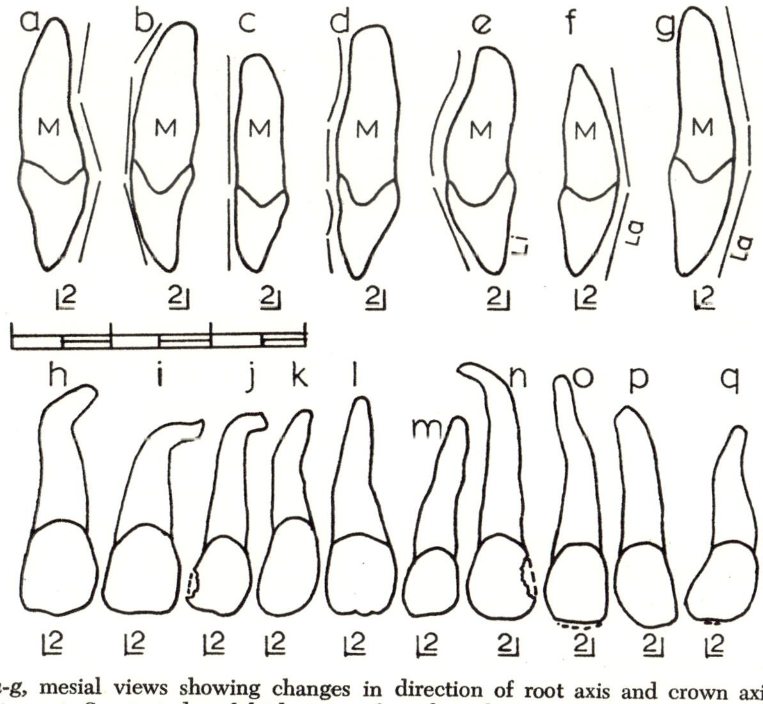

Figure 1-19. *a-g,* mesial views showing changes in direction of root axis and crown axis, and in relation of crown to root. See text. *h-q,* labial views of teeth with non-straight roots. Changes in direction may be abrupt or gentle, and may occur in any part of the root. The axis of a root may change direction more than once. The abrupt changes probably indicate close relationship to the floor of nasal fossa, perhaps associated with a short alveolar ridge. All these turn to D.

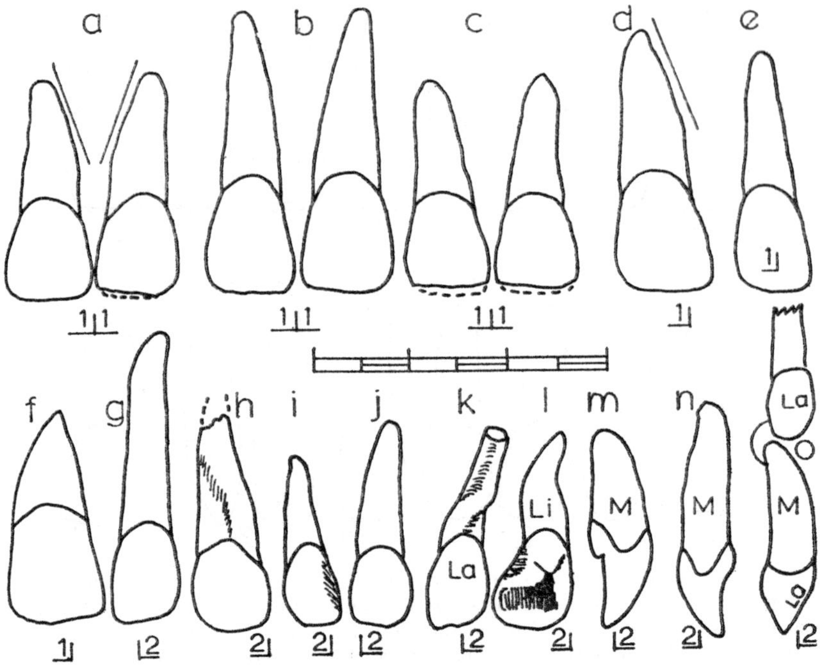

Figure 1-20. Features of crowns and roots. *a-d,* a root axis may appear to lean or curve, usually to D. This may result from asymmetrical taper in part of the root, *a,d,* or in the whole root, *b,c.* See also Figure 1-32. (*a,b,c* are pairs of central incisors). Tooth *c* in Figure 1-22 is apparently an exception in this character. *f,g,* a central incisor with disproportionately short root, and a lateral with disproportionately long root. Tooth *g* has a large ML facet worn by an unstable partial denture. *h,* a wide ovoid type lateral with groove on labial surface, and broken apex. *j,* type characters of crown well marked, but root unusually robust for a lateral. *k,l,* lateral incisors with distortions which appear to have been imposed by lack of space during development of crown *(l),* and of roots in both. These teeth must have erupted to malocclusion. *m,n,* lateral incisors with contrasting proportions of crown length to root length. *o,* a lateral incisor with reduced incisal edge and characters of a "barrel" type tooth.

size both in length and in thickness. Width of crown may occasionally equal its height (Fig. 1-11 *i*).

Two pairs, large and small, are shown in Figure 1-3 *i,j,* and others in Figures 1-18 *a* and 1-20 *a,b,d,e.*

Ovoid Type

Central incisors with contours of pure or predominantly ovoid type are very much in a minority in the present collection (Fig. 1-18 *e-l*). In labial view, these teeth present greater convexity of mesial and distal outline than do other types. The incisal outline also, when not changed by wear, is noticeably convex. These teeth also vary in crown size, in thickness of root, in acumination of apex, and in proportion of crown length to root length.

Whereas in tapering-type teeth the greater M-D dimension is close to the incisal edge, in ovoid type it is farther away, so that their M and D outlines may have a converging tendency below this point.

Examples of type combination may be recognized in Figure 1-8 *g,i* (ovoid with tapering types) and in Figure 1-8 *e,j* (ovoid with square types).

WEAR

Wear of incisors will be considered together with wear of canines later in this chapter.

ROOT APEX

Just as the morphology of tooth roots reflects personal dental characters such as length and breadth, sturdiness or slenderness, so also is the form of the apex related to these. It has been seen that roots of maxillary incisors and canines are often close to nasal fossae and maxillary sinuses, which are themselves subject to variation in form and extent. Moreover, the amount of alveolar and basal bone varies as between persons, so that the apex in these teeth is surrounded by anatomical variables. As the bulk and the morphology of these parts are largely established before completion of the tooth roots, it would seem that the position and form of the tooth apices must be influenced by those anatomical relationships. Thus, while each tooth root has its type characters, its final form reflects modification, not only by intrinsic personal characters but also by the morphology of its environment. The form of the apex therefore may present imposed characters in varying degree.

Studies of skeletal material with teeth *in situ,* and especially of fragments or sections of such material, facilitate one's appreciation of the possible effects on tooth form that might result from the interplay of these variable factors. Admittedly the author has assumed that such factors do indeed operate, and that their operation provides a somewhat *a priori* explanation of the morphological variation that is found. Be that as it may, the results of variation, in this case as regards apical form, are easily shown.

The root apex is defined as the terminal end of a tooth root, but the definition is far from precise, although sometimes it is used to imply a particular point. Often, however, it is used to refer to a region or portion of tooth root furthest from the crown, even though one cannot define the limits of that region. This is the sense in which the term has been used here in describing the form of the apex. When referring to an apex as a point, one has in mind either a geometrical position or an anatomical feature. The first is the point most distant from the crown. This may be difficult to locate on a blunt apex, or it may require modification of definition in a curved root, such as requiring that the distance be measured along the root axis rather than in a straight line.

The second is the anatomical feature known as the apical foramen, and although it is most often the "most distant point," this is not invariably the case (Fig. 1-11 *k*). A further complication is that there are often accessory foramina, although in such cases these are usually minor. (Their existence, however, presents a frustrating complication in efforts to place a satisfactory root filling. This "complication" is dealt with by the endodontist by partial pulp removal, by chemical treatment of pulp canal contents, or by resection of the root apex.)

This discussion will now return to examination of the form of the apex, or rather more precisely, the morphology of the apical region. In the figures of Chapter 1 there are outlines that record the form of the apex in 252 maxillary incisors and canines. In forty-four of these teeth there are presented additional outlines so that the apex is shown in proximal as well as in labial or lingual view. At first glance, perhaps the most obvious characters are sharpness or bluntness, and whether the region involves a curve or change in direction of root axis. At second glance it is observed that such differences may be found in proximal and in labial or lingual views. In general the acumination and curvature may seem to be personal and imposed characters respectively, but this is oversimplification and could not be sustained as a valid distinction. Neither acumination nor curvature is limited to long or short teeth, nor is either character necessarily found in different views of one tooth (Figs. 1-11 *c,* 1-21 *d,* 1-22 *e,* 1-23 *e,f,* 1-24 *f,* 1-26 *o,* 1-30 *l,* 1-31 *a,d,f,h*). Further study in these respects could be usefully pursued if some information were available concerning the physical characters of the persons concerned, but such is lacking for most of the teeth in the present collection. Alternatively, relevant data could be obtained from skeletal material with teeth *in situ*. Where such material was available to the writer, however, he was unwilling to mutilate it in order to obtain additional data. In the present case, therefore, it was necessary to be content with merely reporting what was found in the available extracted teeth.

Some of the factors which determine acumination are clearly the width of the tooth root at the cervix, the style of taper, and the root length. The style of taper presents many variations in detail, from which a few may be selected for description and illustration. In any tooth a proximal or a facial view will essentially comprise two principal profiles which usually present their maximum separation at the cervix, and this decreases more or less evenly as they approach the apex. It is the "more or less even" approach that comprises much of the variety of detail and necessitates the selection of suitable descriptive terms.

The taper may be equal and almost straight as regards both profiles and both views (Figs. 1-1*i*, 1-4 *g*, 1-8 *e,l*, 1-11 *i*, 1-31 *g*). It may be unequal but straight for both profiles of one view (Figs. 1-3 *i,l*, 1-8 *g*, 1-18 *a*, 1-22 *a*, 1-31 *b*). The taper may be between a straight and a curved outline (Figs. 1-18 *b,g*, 1-20 *f*, 1-26 *b* with curved lingual, 1-31 *f* with curved labial). The taper may be uneven with an abrupt bend in one (Figs. 1-22 *c* labial, 1-20 *a,d*, 1-24 *a,d*, 1-26 *n* lingual, 1-30 *l*, 1-31 *f* labial) or in both (Figs. 1-3 *e*, 1-18 *n*).

In roots with an abrupt terminal bend there is a variety of acumination of apex (Figs. 1-19, incisors, and 1-30, canines). Mostly in these the apex tends to be blunt, but length of tooth does not appear to be a decisive factor (Figs. 1-19 *n*, 1-21 *h*, 1-30 *n*, long teeth; and 1-19 *h,i*, 1-26 *e*, 1-30 *e*, shorter teeth). In labial view, long roots are often acuminate at the apex (Figs. 1-10 *h,n*, 1-21 *c,q*, 1-22 *g*, incisors; and 1-27 *g,n*, 1-28 *g,h*, 1-30 *b*, 1-31 *d,e*, canines). But again it is easy to find long teeth with a blunt apex (Figs. 1-8 *e*, 1-21 *h,s*, 1-24 *h*).

Since lateral incisors and canines usually have a somewhat flattened root, it would be expected that in proximal view the apex would appear less acuminate than in labial view, and this is common (Figs. 1-19, 1-23, 1-26, 1-31). But there are cases in these figures where the proximal view shows an acuminate apex (Figs. 1-19 *f*, 1-26 *b,n*, 1-31 *e*). As for the central incisor which usually has a less flattened root, there is much variety of apical acumination in proximal view (Figs. 1-4, 1-6, 1-11, 1-22). In this position also, even a pair of teeth from the same person may show appreciable difference in apical form (Fig. 1-27 *p*).

From this brief survey the apices of teeth with roots of complex curvature (Figs. 1-11 *j*, 1-19, 1-30 *f,k,l*) have so far been omitted, but they evidently share in the variety presented by other teeth of their kind. This variety has been shown to be considerable in these single-rooted teeth. In teeth with branched roots, some lower canines, premolars and molars, the branches tend to have their own type and personal characters. When to this is added the presence of imposed characters and of additional root elements, often with a separate apex, it is seen that description of apical variation would be a complicated and formidable undertaking. It is not proposed to attempt this beyond reference to such features as seem noteworthy.

ROOT CURVATURE

At first glance it would appear to be easy to judge whether a root is straight or curved, but to set down clearly what one does find after examination of a considerable number of teeth is by no means simple. Even the term "straight" applied to a root is not at all precise, because a root is tapered. The taper may proceed evenly but at different rates on different surfaces, so that the root appears to lean. A similar adjective applies when the axes of crown and root are not parallel, as in tooth *p* of Figure 1-1 (see also Fig. 1-32).

The degree of taper may increase at a particular point, on one side (Fig. 1-3 *f*), on each side (Fig. 1-3 *c*) or by an even curve on each side (Fig. 1-3 *d,e*). Are these straight roots? The outline may be straight on one side and curved on the other (Fig. 1-18 *f,g*). Are these curved roots?

Roots vary considerably in actual and in relative thickness. They may be wide in one view and narrow in another. Tooth *i* of Figure 1-11 is an unusual example because it is the B-L dimension that is more often disproportionately wide. This may give strongly curved outlines in one view but not in the other, especially towards the apex. Apart from such detail, which may be specified, these are not regarded as curved roots.

In the present study the writer has endeavoured to use the term "curve" for a recognizable continuing change of direction of the root axis. The direction is indicated by the usual terms M, D, lingual and labial or buccal, and it is applied as from the cervix towards the apex. It will be appreciated that curves are not limited to any one of these directions any more than is the wind to the cardinal points of the compass. A single tooth root may curve into more than one direction.

A distinction may well be drawn between the continuing curve defined above and that which changes direction more or less abruptly and finally, as it were, rather than continuing to change direction. This will be called a bend, but it must be understood that the distinction is merely one of convenience for description and that many tooth roots conform precisely to neither style.

It is usual for a central incisor to have a relatively short root. Reference to a skull and examination of the relation of incisors to nasal fossae will show why, in the orthognathic face, there is little space, or rather bone, to accommodate a long central incisor root curving to M or D. But there is more room for the root to curve to labial or lingual, and these are the predominant directions of curves in central incisors (Figs. 1-4, 1-6 and 1-19). In the prognathic maxilla there is more bone to accommodate root length. It would be of interest to check this feature in ancient skulls. The writer, working with plaster casts, found that the Rhodesian skull, although orthognathous, had unusual length in this part of the maxilla (Taylor, 1962a).

The roots of the lateral incisor and canine are often in close relation to the bony pillar between the nasal fossa and maxillary sinus and this gives more scope for variation in root length and curvature. It seems reasonable to regard variations in those relationships and in the lateral, anterior and vertical extent of these cavities as largely responsible for the curves and bends which can easily be visualized in relation to the various anatomical structures mentioned.

It could be noted that the root of the lateral incisor almost invariably turns distally in these cases. Bends such as those in Figure 1-19 *h,i,j* might well indicate that the root was directly below the nasal floor. Less abrupt bends and curves in the other cases could arise where the root was directed more laterally or where the nasal cavity was relatively narrower.

In the case of the canine, while root curve is often to D, curves or bends to M are by no means rare. In Figure 1-30 roots of teeth *d,e,i,k,l,n* are directed to M, and *b,c,g,j,o* to D. But there are complications. Teeth *h* and *o* tend first to lean to D, and then curve back to M. Teeth *k* and *l*, while both showing a distinct curve to M as seen in the partial views from labial, also curve in the same regions to labial and palatal respectively.

Curvature of canine roots in these varying directions is understandable when one observes variation in the form of nasal cavity and maxillary sinus, and in their resulting relationships to one another. The nasal cavity varies in lateral extent. The maxillary sinus (in its anterior portion, which is of particular concern at the moment) varies in its form and extent anteriorly, laterally and inferiorly. In the last respect its "floor" may be above, level with, or below that of the nasal cavity. The height of the alveolar ridge and depth of palate (by no means necessarily the same) and the amount of basal bone are some of the other variables that collectively affect the developing tooth root and greatly increase the scope for morphological variation.

If the maxillary sinus extends below the nasal cavity and forward, the canine root may adapt by curving to M and labially. If the sinus does not extend so far forward and laterally, and there is less basal bone, a curve to D and perhaps also to P may well take place. But this is not all, for the personal dental character that may tend in a particular person to produce large or small teeth, long and slender, or robust roots, and so on, has not been considered.

Root curvature has been discussed so far in relation to normal developmental anatomy, but there is another aspect of change in root direction that is relevant to this study. Whether it is regarded as abnormal development, or related to trauma or pathology (as was the presence of hypoplastic enamel), this further aspect is certainly of forensic interest. And it is made more so because recognition and interpretation of additional data provided by stains, deposits or loss of tooth substance by wear, trauma and pathology may proceed beyond deduction and lead to the establishment of facts which can often be checked.

Tooth *n* of Figure 1-4 is a case of dilaceration as shown by the abrupt change in root direction, and this could be confirmed by microscopic examination of a section through the damaged region. The age at which the injury took place can be estimated by reference to an appropriate table of dental development, in this case 5 years ± 9 months. The estimate can often be confirmed by a relative. A great variety of effects is produced by such injuries in childhood according to the stage of development (Taylor, 1970a).

Teeth *k,l* of Figure 1-20 are deformed, probably by having insufficient space during development of the crown *(l)*, and during root formation and eruption in both cases. As a result, the emerging crowns have been deflected in varying degrees while they erupted into malocclusion. The rotation of crown *k* during this process has caused a twisting of the root.

A somewhat similar case of deflection in a canine tooth is shown in Figure 1-30 *f*. In this tooth the root has developed into a spiral curve rather than a twist. That this tooth functioned for a considerable time is indicated by the presence of facets (not shown), but the unusual position of polished enamel, stain, and a carious cavity establish that the tooth was in malocclusion and rotated about 45 degrees from normal. The wear facet, partly seen in the figure, is not from occlusion but was caused by the clasp of an unstable partial denture. Its position on the anatomical distal but functional lingual surface confirms the rotation of the tooth and the crowded relation with adjacent teeth.

Tooth *g* of Figure 1-30 bears testimony to the difficulty experienced by the dental surgeon in its removal, and to the reason why this was so. There are areas of abraded enamel and dentine from movement of tightly held but ill-fitting dental forceps, ill-fitting because they had to be applied to the anatomical M and D of a crown which had been rotated and forced into buccal occlusion. As a result there was insufficient width for the lingual blade of the forceps which must repeatedly have slipped off the tooth during the operation.

The unusual position of the facet of tooth wear confirms the functional position of the tooth.

Tooth *m* of Figure 1-30 has a piece of thin labial alveolar plate adherent to the anatomical D surface of the root. Like tooth *g*, this tooth also was rotated, but tooth *m*, by contrast, was in lingual occlusion. The anatomical D surface of the crown which faced labially was largely protected from functional friction and was covered with stain where exposed. The stain pattern, and the unusual position of the small facet of wear, give further support to this interpretation of the tooth's position when *in situ*.

These five examples of root curvature serve to show that there are circumstantial or mechanical factors, additional to the more strictly anatomical factors, that increase the complexity of morphological variety found in tooth roots. Apart from their obvious susceptibility to early trauma, central incisors seem less affected by these additional factors than are laterals and canines. If this is in fact the case, part of the explanation may lie in the earlier formation and eruption of central incisors. Laterals and canines may be obstructed or "handicapped" by the earlier establishment of adjacent permanent teeth, or by jaw growth that has been checked by loss of functional stimuli, through caries or early removal of deciduous teeth.

LATERAL INCISOR

The upper lateral incisor is basically similar to the central in that it has a flattened crown (modified wedge) with an incisal edge. In labial or lingual view the wedge flares from its butt at the cervix to its thin edge at the incisal. As with the central incisor, the butt is wider at the labial than at lingual aspect so that the transverse section at the cervix tends to be oval. The long axis of the oval runs from labial to lingual, and the difference in axes is relatively greater than in the central. In the labial view, as with the central incisor, the distal angle is more rounded than the mesial, and the rounding is relatively greater in the lateral incisor. To describe the tooth as smaller than the central incisor is true for the crown but misleading for the root, whose relation to its crown is relatively longer and often is actually longer than that of the adjacent central incisor (Fig. 1-1 *ab,cd*).

The lateral incisor is sometimes reduced in size. All degrees of reduction, through diminutive and so-called "peg" teeth to complete absence of the tooth, are found, and one tooth or both may be involved. This trait, which some have regarded as a tendency towards suppression, is sometimes found in relatives, which shows that it is heritable. Its manifestations add considerably to variations found in this tooth.

Although this wide variation is found in maxillary lateral incisors, there are characteristics which enable a tooth to be described as presenting the usual features of a lateral incisor. Small specimens are easily identified, but large specimens may cause difficulty, since they are within the size range of central incisors (Figs. 1-19, 1-20 *g-o*, and 1-21). Large lateral incisors are larger than small central incisors from another person. If the root is not visible, the crown in labial view is relatively narrower for its length, and the outlines are more convex than in the central incisor. In proximal view the cingulum convexity is less prominent, and the root, when visible, provides additional identification; it is relatively slender, longer and (as already noted) appears as a more flattened oval in transverse section.

It is easy to distinguish whether a tooth is from the right or the left side if both crown and root are present and intact.

Distinguishing features in the crown are similar to those in the central incisor and are directly concerned with the more rounded distal incisal angle. The root tends to curve distally, either in the whole tooth or in the apical region. The long axis of the crown may be tilted from the

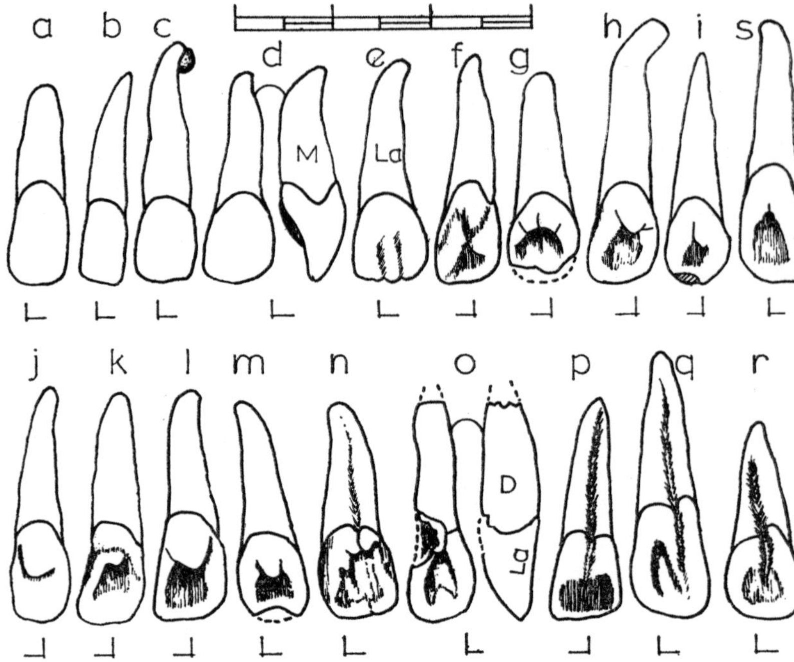

Figure 1-21. Lateral incisors. *a,b,c,* square-type crowns, with blunt and sharp apices. *c,* long root with small cementoma at apex. *d,* contrasting incisal angles in crown, and apex of root bends to M and labial. *e,* well-developed mamelons or incisal tubercles. *f-s,* lingual surfaces with great variety of ridges, tubercles and grooves as in central incisors of Figures 1-8, 1-10 and 1-11. *m,* the concavity in the incisal edge, now smooth, may originally have been chipped, or worn by a pipe stem.

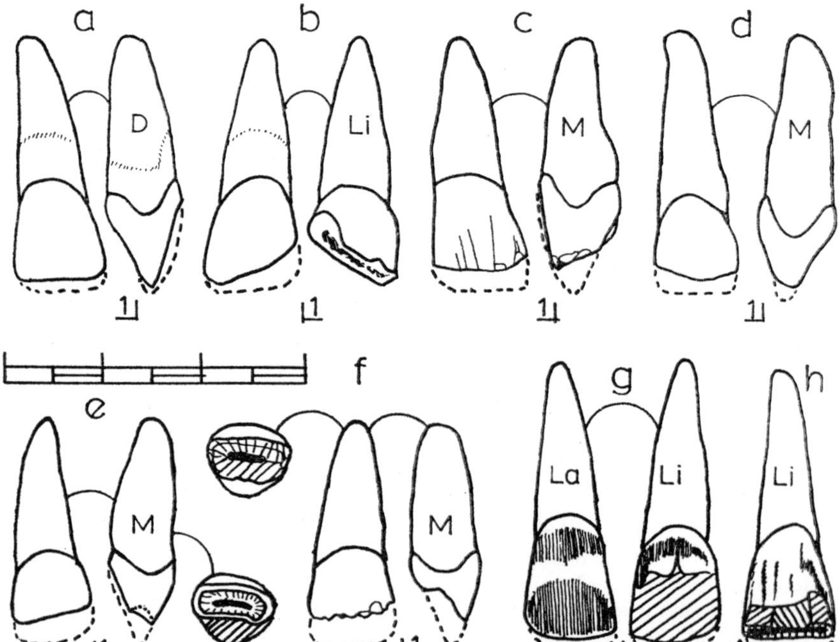

Figure 1-22. Upper incisors. Loss of tissue by wear, etc.

cervix toward the central, so that in labial or lingual view, the long axis of the tooth may suggest a flattened S-curve (Fig. 1-19 *k,p,q*). This effect is sometimes exaggerated by apparent deformity of the tooth during development (Fig. 1-20 *l*).

Similarly, the axis of the crown may appear to be bent lingually (Figs. 1-19*e*, 1-20 *m*), partly from greater convexity of the labial outline. The crown may range from a distinctly wedge-like shape to those with much greater curvature (Figs. 1-19 *a-g*, 1-20 *m-o*).

The crown outline in labial or lingual view in the majority of laterals suggests the basic forms (square, tapering and ovoid) or combinations of these. It is not always possible to determine type form from lateral incisors alone, since they may be examples of the reduction trait mentioned above. Thus some lateral incisors look like extremes of long, narrow square types, but if seen *in situ* alongside their central incisors they could be recognized as diminutives (Figs. 1-20 *i,o*, 1-21 *a,b* and 8-23 *b,c*). The pairing tooth may be reduced to a different degree, to a "peg" type (a diminutive tooth with one more or less sharp point or cusp), or it may be congenitally absent. It may suggest an incisal edge which is shorter than the mesial to distal diameter at the cervix. These teeth usually are found in the incisor region and may be supernumeraries or diminutive lateral incisors. They always have a flattened root, as distinct from those found in the midline and called fissural odontoids by Herbst and Apffelstaedt (1930).

As with central incisors, the labial surface of lateral incisors may present longitudinal grooves. Where these meet the incisal edge as notches, they may divide it into tubercles (Fig. 1-21 *e*).

The lingual surface of the crown presents features similar to the central, i.e. mesial and distal ridges meeting at the cingulum and enclosing a more or less concave area depending on the development of the ridges (Fig. 1-21). The ridges may be sufficiently prominent to form the shovel-type tooth (Fig. 1-21 *o*). Where the ridges meet at the cingulum, there may be a pit or fissure which may pass upward for varying distances through the cingulum on to the root (Fig. 1-21 *p,q,r*). Clinical complications associated with similar grooves are illustrated in Figure 1-12 *e,f* and have been described by Lee, Lee and Poon (1968).

In tooth *m* in Figure 1-18 the cingulum region is over-developed, extending approximately two-thirds of the distance to the incisal edge, where there is a deep pit and almost an occlusal surface. This is an example of the "barrel"-shaped incisor mentioned by Dahlberg (1963).

Some reference has already been made to the root of the upper lateral incisor, which is slender, relatively longer than the root of the central incisor, and has a tendency to bend distally. The root may vary from extremely slender to fairly thick, as the length of the root bears no constant relation to the length of the crown. The apex varies from a fine sharp point to blunt and rounded (Fig. 1-21). The root is almost invariably greater in its labio-lingual axis than in the mesio-distal axis at any part where a transverse section may be made.

Although the crown varies in convexity, the tooth axis from crown through the root (excluding any small curve in the apical region) runs nearer to the labial as described for the central incisor (Figs. 1-2 *d* and 1-5) than to the lingual. However, considerable variations arise, partly as the crown is apparently bent to the labial or lingual aspect and partly through curvature of the root (Figs. 1-19 *a-g* and 1-20 *m,n,o*). Sharp bends in this region probably are related to proximity of the floor of the nasal fossae (Fig. 1-19 *h,i,j,n,o*).

Lateral incisors were included in the earlier discussion of root curvature.

Wear in lateral incisors will be discussed later together with that in centrals and canines.

MAXILLARY CANINE TOOTH

Both crown and root of this tooth are larger than those of the lateral incisor, and the root is also relatively larger in the canine. Labially and lingually the crown outline is basically pentagonal instead of quadrilateral because the incisal edge consists of mesial and distal portions which meet to form the single cusp (Figs. 1-24 *h,i*, 1-25, 1-26, 1-27).

The canine ranges considerably in length, at least from 18-35mm and occasionally much longer (Fig. 1-26 *a-d*). Large or small teeth may have either long roots tapering to a slender apical region and point, or sturdy roots with the apical region thick and blunt. The proportionate size of crown to root also varies considerably. When a root is very thick and short it may appear to have been shortened by resorption, but this is not necessarily so. Two such teeth, with tracings of pulp cavities superposed on the outlines, are shown in Figure 1-26 *i-l*, and these do not suggest that resorption has taken place.

The pentagonal crown is seen best when almost straight sides meet at rounded easily recognized angles. When greater convexity results in merging of sides and angles the form becomes oval (Fig. 1-27). The base of the pentagon is the cervical outline. This may be very convex, i.e. a relatively large arc of a small circle, or less convex or even straight (Fig. 1-27). Variation in the convexity and length of the cervical outline is associated in some degree with the relative thickness of the root, with the length/width proportions of the crown, with the curvature or straightness of outlines in general, and with the divergence of mesial and distal outlines in particular.

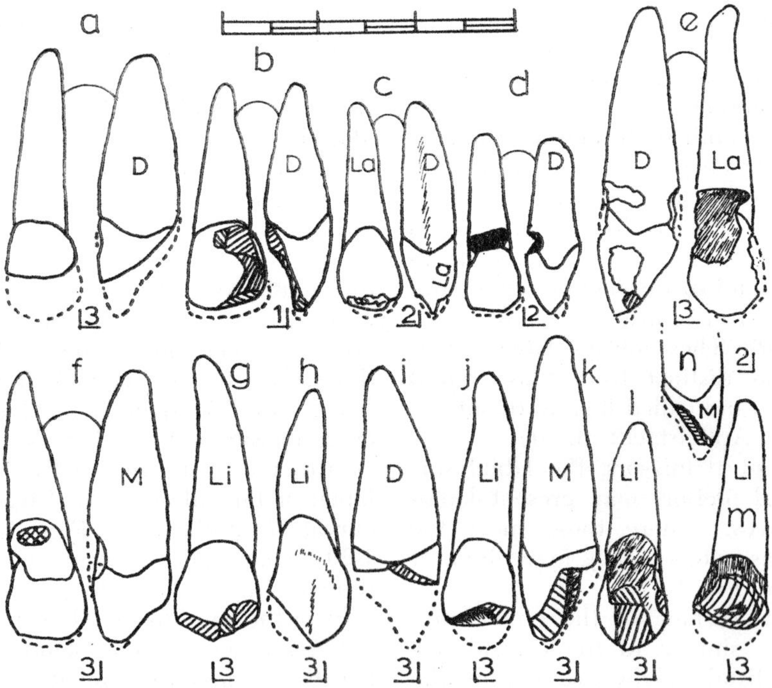

Figure 1-23. Patterns of wear etc., in incisors and canines. *c*, hypoplasia of enamel. See also Figure 1-27 *o*. *l*, fine shading is abrasion from denture. *m*, fine shading is an area of heavy stain deposit. *n*, horizontal shading is dentine, exposed but not worn.

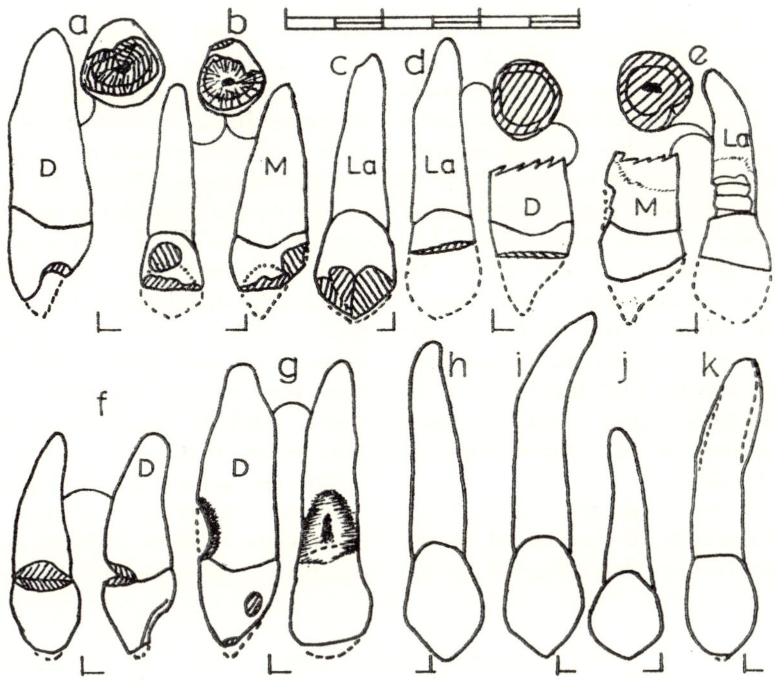

Figure 1-24. *a-g,* wear and abrasion in canines. *h,i,* similar pentagonal crowns, but not a pair. *j,* small tooth. *k,* apical half of root thickened by cementosis. See also Figure 1-30 *c.*

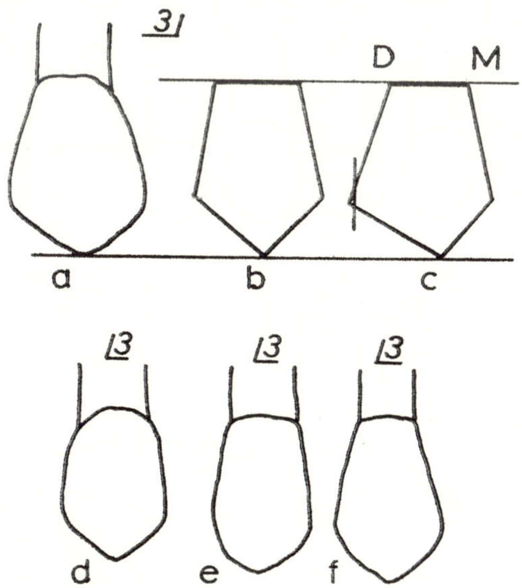

Figure 1-25. *a,b,c,* basic pentagonal labial view of an upper canine. *d,e,f,* crown outlines, rather straight-sided but varying in divergence and in relative widths at cervix and at cusp shoulders.

These proximal outlines when almost straight may be nearly parallel or more divergent (Figs. 1-26 *o* and 1-24 *h*). The character of curvature appears to be modified by, but is not dependent upon, variations in dimensions. In the case of incisors, relative dimensions could be visualized at the incisal or cervical region reasonably well. With canines, this is more difficult because of the presence of the cusp. Although it is sometimes easy to note maximum breadth, the variation in the length of the cusp or its acumination or pointedness, or both, means that the position of maximum breadth varies over a much greater proportion of the crown between cervix and cusp tip.

Acumination, seen labially, varies from a true point through all degrees of bluntness to almost the cuspless edge of an incisor (Figs. 1-27, 1-30, 1-31). The slopes of the cusp meet the mesial and distal outlines at the shoulders. This meeting place is seldom a definable point and may be indistinguishable on one or both sides, usually because the curves of each portion form a continuous arc (Figs. 1-27, 1-30, 1-31).

The mesial shoulder is usually more definite than the distal, and it is often farther from the cervix. The mesial slope is shorter than the distal and is less rounded (Figs. 1-25, 1-24 *h-k* and 1-30 *i*). The long axis of crown and root passes through the cusp tip; the mesial shoulder and "contact point" tend to be closer to this axis line than are the distal.

The mesial and distal slopes of the cusp may be very convex, slightly so, straight, or concave. Either or both slopes may be complex, consisting of two convex por-

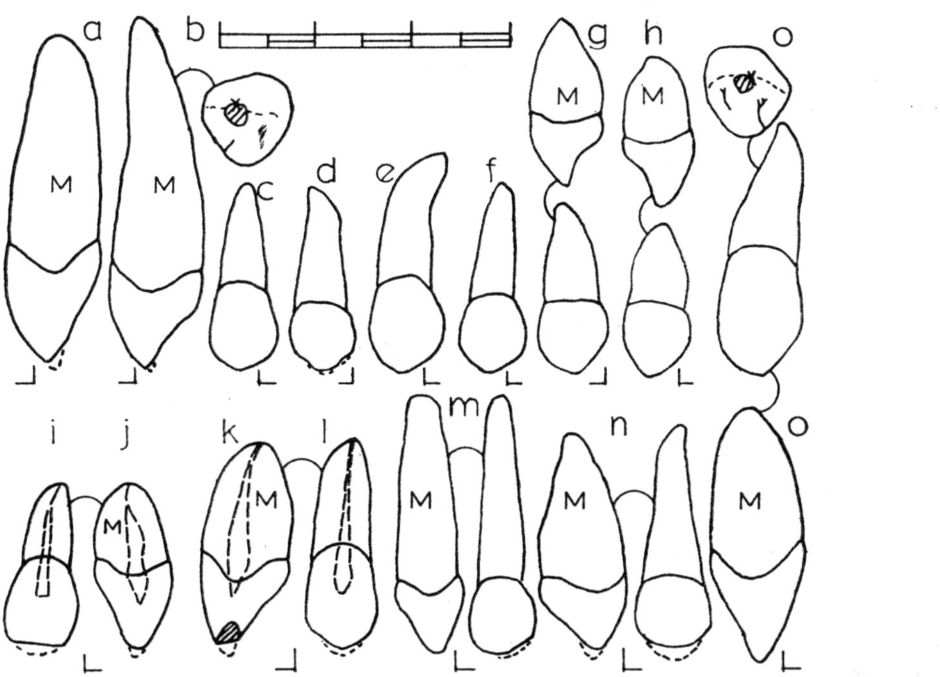

Figure 1-26. Upper canines. Variation in form of crown and root, and in crown/root proportions. *i-l,* labial and proximal outlines of two canines with superposed outlines of pulp cavities traced from radiographs. *b,o,* outlines include occlusal views to show character of bilateral asymmetry which assists differentiation of M and D, and of left and right teeth. See Figure 1-33. *m,* small crown with long, straight, flattened root. *n,* small crown with relatively very wide labio-lingual dimension. *o,* short robust tooth with relatively long crown.

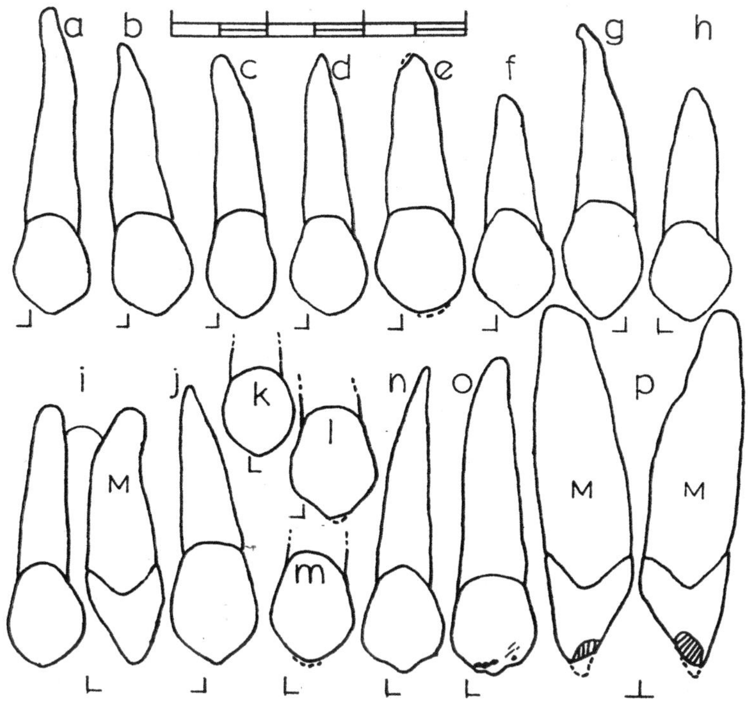

Figure 1-27. Upper canines. Crown form, cusp acu mination and labial cervix. Root form, length taper and apex. *o*, cusp tip malformation with hypoplastic enamel. See also Figure 1-23 *c*. *p*, pair of large canines with low convexity of crown profiles and dissimilar apices. Crown outlines; compare *e,g,h,k,n*. Cervical lines (labial); compare *e,f,i,k,n,o*.

tions (Fig. 1-28 *b*, distal slope), or of a convex and a concave portion (Fig. 1-28 *a,c*).

The concave slope may be unilaterally exaggerated, which may cause marked asymmetry of the cusp (Fig. 1-28 *m*). Such variations might have a similar origin to the variations in developmental tubercles (p. 10); investigation of both features could be combined.

Acumination and length of cusp relative to crown length are independent of the size of the crown or of the root. Although relatively long and narrow crowns tend to have long or sharp cusps, these latter are also found with relatively short crowns (Figs. 1-27 *f,h*, and 1-31 *d*).

The labial surface of the canine differs from the incisor in that the canine has a broad vertical ridge from the cusp to the cervix, which is convex both longitudinally and transversely. It is often made more distinct by a longitudinal groove on each side. In most cases the grooves do not divide the crown equally, but the medial portion is much wider than the lateral portions. Usually, the grooves are more prominent in the cusp region than in the cervical portion of the labial surface, and the distal groove is more distinct. The grooves meet the slopes of the cusp where concavities have been noted in the outline of the slope, although they may also be present when the slope is straight or convex.

Sometimes the grooves tend to be closer together near the cusp tip, and then diverge. When they are parallel the greater width of the central ridge is more obvious. Corresponding ridges and grooves are found on the lingual surface, which like

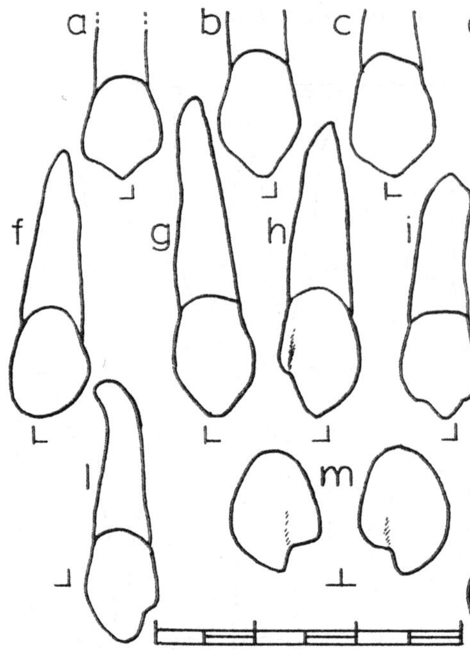

Figure 1-28. Upper canines. Further variations in cusp acumination and asymmetry. In most of these there is no evidence of wear. There is slight wear in the pair *n*, and wear in *k* on each side has changed a blunt convex cusp into an acuminate cusp with concave shoulders. Tooth *l* is one of a similar pair to *m*. Pair *m*, for which the scale is approximate, was drawn from radiographs, made by the writer, of teeth found in a girl aged eleven years. The "notch" is mesial in these, and in *l*, but distal in *e,h*.

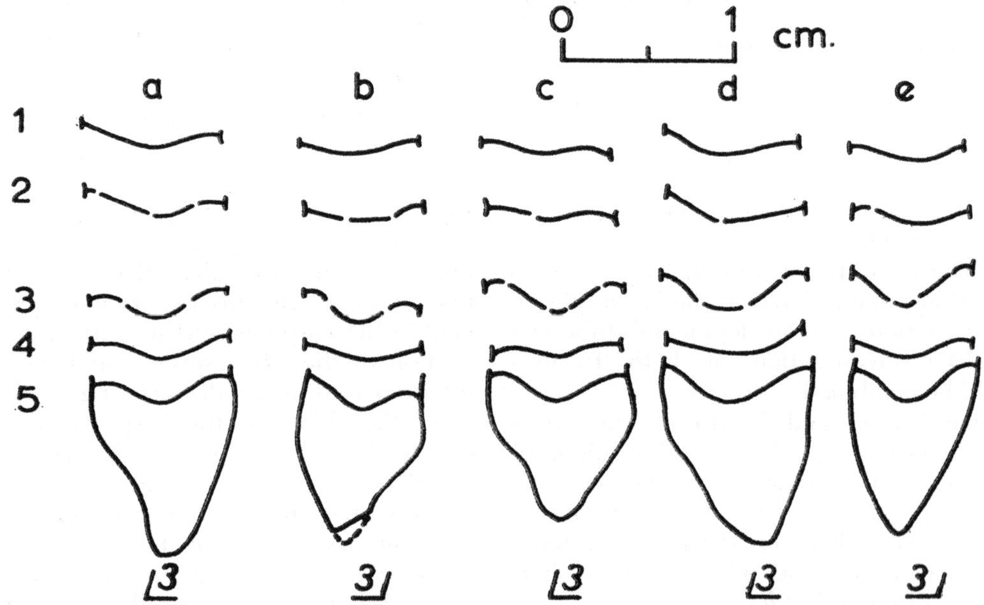

Figure 1-29. Comparison of cervical outlines in proximal views of five upper canines. *1, 5,* distal and mesial outlines respectively, traced with a camera lucida; *2, 3,* the same outlines in semidiagrammatic form of straight lines and arcs; *4,* the same outlines as in *1,* but reversed for comparison with *5,* and as if seen through transparent teeth.

the incisors presents much variation in these and in the "tuberculum dentale" (Fig. 1-31). The labial grooves, and sometimes lingual also, may present pits. The fact that they are found at the same "level" suggests pathology as the cause; they probably indicate enamel hypoplasia caused by an exanthematous illness. If similar pits are found on the other canines of that person, such diagnosis receives strong support. It is not suggested that such evidence would be limited to the canines but rather that in them, the checking of similarity of developmental stage may be easier, especially if the illness occurred after the completion of enamel in incisors.

The lingual surface of the crown, like the labial, tends to be pentagonal in outline, but the base of the pentagon at the cervix is narrower than it is on the labial. Thus the lingual view of the crown often includes parts of the mesial and distal surfaces within the outline (Fig. 1-31).

The Canine Cingulum

The cingulum region is usually prominent and convex, and it often presents a small lingual cusp, as has just been mentioned. But this cusp varies considerably and may range from a true cusp, separated by a groove or fissure from the main cusp, to a diminutive trace of a cusp; it may also be absent (Fig. 1-31). Somewhat prominent ridges may extend to each shoulder of the main cusp regardless of the presence of the small cusp. They may enclose a pit at the cingulum or be separated there by a small groove or fissure. Prom inent small cusps or ridges may embrace an irregularly concave area. In addition, the labial outline may present a prominence at the cervix, although in other cases there is a smooth continuous curve from crown to root (Figs. 1-26, 1-27, 1-30 and 1-31).

The Canine Cervical Line

The cervical outline in proximal view varies from a much flattened curve to one which presents a rounded, near right angle as it dips crownward. This dip tends to be greater on the mesial than on the distal side. Thus the radius of the curve of the cervical outline is like a small arc of a larger circle on the distal but includes a greater arc of a small circle on the mesial side (Figs. 1-23, 1-24, 1-26, 1-27, 1-30 and 1-31). In Figure 1-29 the mesial and distal outlines have been traced with a camera lucida from five upper canines. To facilitate comparison the outlines have also been broken into straight lines and arcs, presented diagrammatically.

In the great majority of upper canines it was not difficult to recognize this difference between the M and D cervical lines, namely that the wave trough line of the cervix is relatively deep and narrow on M but less deep, and wider, on D. This finding is significant, since it provides a fairly consistent character that can be used to assist identification of an upper canine as left or right. It may be specially useful where decay, wear or fracture have removed the features that are more commonly used for this purpose.

This character was mentioned above when discussing the cervical line in central incisors, and some suggestions were made to account for the difference noted in M and D of canines.

Root Curvature and Tooth Identification

The curves and bends seen in canine roots were discussed above with curvature in incisors. Other studies have given attention to root curvature in general, as well as in particular teeth, and this will be done also in the present survey. Carter (1914) wrote that root curvature may be described according to origin, location and direction. He went on to say that it may be "simple" (with only one bend in the length), "compound" (with more than one bend), or "complex" (if associated with root or teeth fusion, hypercementosis, perforation of maxillary sinus, nasal fossa, mandibular canal, etc.). His classification is not precise enough to be satisfactorily illustrated. It conveys no idea of degree of curvature, or when a curve is better described as a bend, or in what part of a root it occurs. The necessity to include some indication of direction is a further complication. It was felt that Carter's classification was in the nature of oversimplification and not really applicable to what actually exists.

Earlier in this study it was shown that curvature is but one aspect of variation in morphology which, in tooth roots as in crowns, is extremely complex. Asymmetry in root characters is often a feature in root curvature. Some aspects of the asymmetry are part of the study of morphological variation. The same applies to tooth crowns. By a study of the whole tooth, characters are found that can be used in identification of a tooth, first as a canine (or whatever tooth), then as an upper canine, and then as left or right.

In many canines there is a shallow longitudinal groove passing up the mesial and distal surfaces of the root. The groove is centrally placed and tends to be more noticeable on the mesial surface.

In some teeth, the root is truncated at some point in the apical region. This may result from fracture during extraction, or it may indicate that the root is not yet completed. The age of the patient should indicate the more likely explanation because a malposed canine removed in late childhood should be incomplete. In such case the end of the root is wide open, with a thin edge enclosing a conical area, and the margins are transverse to the long axis of the root. With a fractured apex in an older person the root end presents no conical opening but a solid surface perforated by the root canal. In these cases the line of fracture may be transverse, oblique or uneven.

If the subsidiary curves or bends in the root are ignored and the axis of root and crown is observed, the features described for the incisor (Fig. 1-2 *d*) apply also for the canine. Thus the position of the cusp and the long axis of the tooth, as viewed from the proximal, are nearer to the labial than to the lingual side (Fig. 9-3 *b*).

Distinction between left and right canines is usually easy. Viewed labially, although each tooth tends to be a mirror image of the other, each in itself is bilaterally asymmetrical. As just mentioned, the long axis through root and cusp, or of the crown alone, is nearer to the mesial than to the distal side. The distal shoulder is less distinct, or more rounded and further from the axis, than is the mesial shoulder. The longitudinal ridge on the labial surface of the crown is nearer to the mesial.

From an end view, the crown outline is approximately oval. The long axis of the oval is nearer to the mesial than to the distal side (Fig. 1-33). This form is an asymmetrical pentagon, the labial surface representing two sides of the pentagon and the angle between these sides representing the longitudinal ridge of the labial surface, with the mesial portion shorter than the distal. If nonadjacent sides of the pentagon are compared, it is clear that the mesial side is longer than the distal. Such asymmetry applies also to the outline of a transverse section at the cervix. The cervical outline is of course much narrower from mesial to distal, and the narrow end of the oval is always the lingual part (Fig. 1-33). Although these characters are less obvious they have been noted in crowns, and they are easily recognizable in cervical outlines also. Thus it is not always necessary to have the crown of a tooth to distinguish left from right, and, if most of the root is present, the tendency to bend distally may provide an additional aid in identification. But since it has been shown that a minority bend mesially, more reliance should be placed on the character of asymmetry, especially if it is well marked in that particular tooth.

When a perpendicular is taken to the cervical base, the long axis of the whole tooth or of the crown is nearer to the labial in proximal view. In a few cases this character is exaggerated so that the labial outline of the crown lies in an almost straight line, continuous with the labial outline of the root (Fig. 1-27 *p*).

Differential Identification of Upper Incisors and Canines

This section largely summarizes findings in the foregoing part of this chapter while showing their practical application.

In this study of a great number of each kind of tooth in the permanent dentition, variation is analyzed not only in main features but also in minor ones. In this first chapter, relating particularly to maxillary incisors and canines, twelve of the thirty-three figures present forty-six diagrams. The remaining twenty-one figures contain approximately 345 outlines accurately drawn to scale with a specially adapted camera lucida. These relate to some 279 mounted teeth from the much larger collection of incisors and canines which comprise 968 teeth mounted on 146 cards.

Some lower incisors and some upper lateral incisors may show a resemblance, although proximal profiles of lower incisors tend to be more arc-like on the labial side and so bring the tooth axis nearer to lingual. Upper lateral incisors are more likely to have a prominent lingual cingulum or lateral lingual ridges (in the same

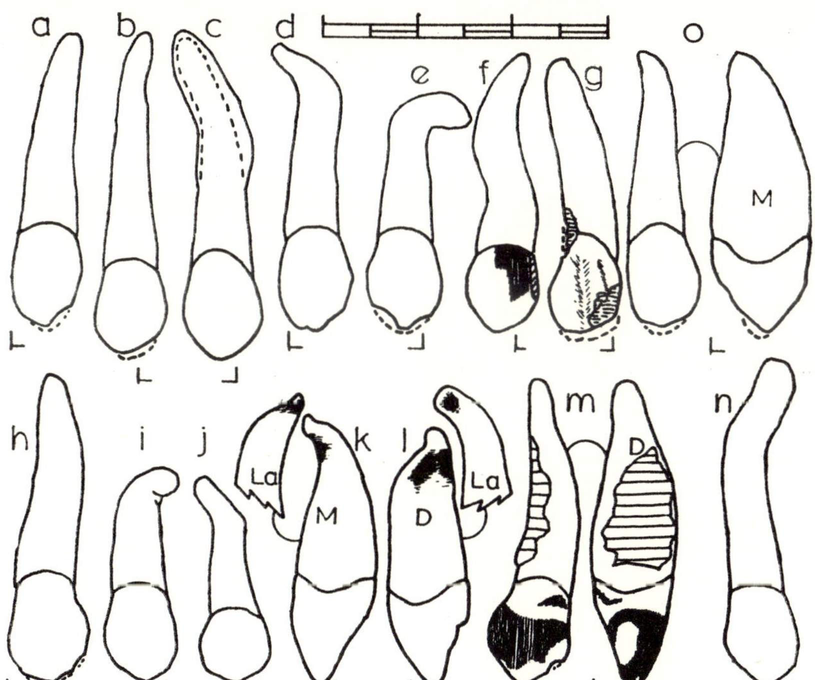

Figure 1-30. Upper canines. In roots, compare lengths and curves. In crowns, note size, shape, stains etc., and interpretation of these in the text. *c,* root thickness increased by cementosis (See also Fig. 1-24 *k*). In *d,e,i,n,* the root bends abruptly to M, and in *j* to D. *f,* spiral root, with clasp facet and significant stain area. *g,* forceps trauma. *m,* attached alveolar bone, root curve, stain and calculus are source of data. *n,* small crown with long thick root. *o,* tooth with some characters of upper, and some of lower, canine.

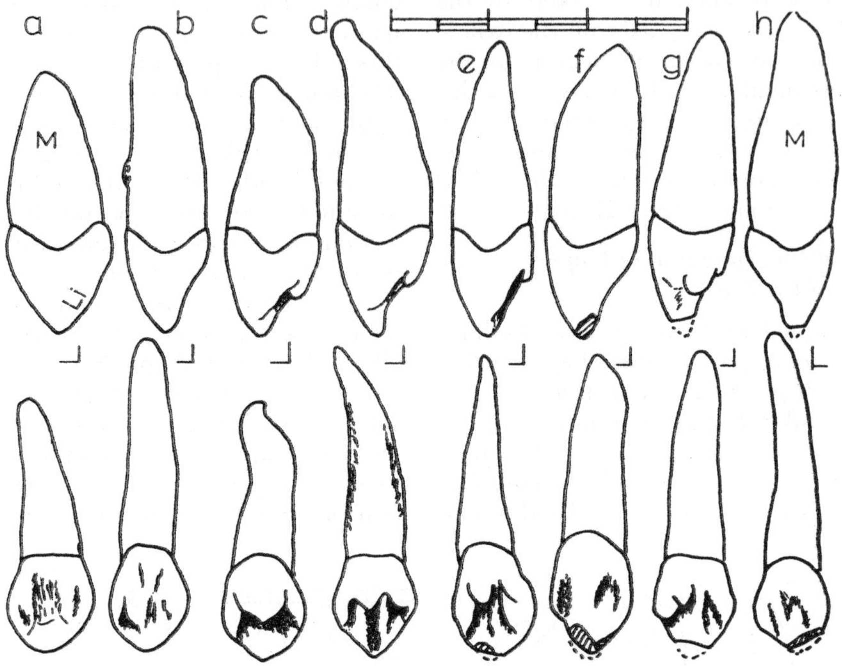

Figure 1-31. Mesial and lingual views of eight upper canines. *a-g* are right side, *h* is left. Compare labio-lingual dimension and tooth length, as in *a,b;* direction of taper, to labial in *c,d,* and to lingual in *f;* lingual profiles of crowns mostly concave *(b,f,h),* sometimes convex *(a),* and often complicated in varied style and degree by ridges, grooves and tubercles, the latter sometimes in the form designated "tuberculum dentale." There is a small cementoma on *b*.

position as shovel-type ridges), often with a pit or fissure between them. Attritional facets in normal occlusion are more labial in lower and more lingual in upper incisors.

Upper central incisors and lateral incisors, when complete and free from decay or severe wear, should be easily distinguished from one another by (a) overall size, the central being heavier, especially when from the same person; (b) length of root, relatively longer in the lateral incisor; (c) at the cervix, a cross-section of root is more nearly an equilateral triangle in the central incisor and a compressed oval in the lateral (this last difference is very useful when part of the root or crown is missing); and (d) the central incisor is more likely than the lateral to present developmental grooves on the labial surface.

Identity of the central incisor may be checked as follows: (1) in the crown, the distal angle of the incisal edge is more rounded than the mesial, except where incisal wear may have altered the outline; (2) at the cervix, a transverse section appears more "drawn out" toward an acute angle on the mesiolabial than elsewhere. Compare this with the basic quadrilateral (Figs. 1-13 and 1-14). This feature is more reliable than root bend; (3) in the great majority of central incisors, the root tends to lean or curve (or even to taper in an otherwise straight root) to the distal (Fig. 1-32 *a,b*). Occasionally it may bend to the mesial (Fig. 1-4 *c,d*).

In the case of a small central and a large

lateral incisor, the lateral incisor's root would probably be much longer than that of the central. A further check that should facilitate differentiation may be made at the cervix. The central incisor should present the asymmetry referred to earlier, whereas the cervical outline of the lateral incisor would probably be a flattened oval with less asymmetry.

Whether a lateral incisor is a left or right tooth should be readily determined if crown or root are intact. From the crown in labial view it should be easy to identify the more rounded distal angle. From the root, the almost invariable bend or curve to distal, usually more obvious than in the central, is perhaps the most reliable guide.

If a very shallow longitudinal groove is more readily distinguishable on one proximal surface of the root or if it is present only on one surface, then that surface is likely to be the mesial. This groove is not present in a number of lateral incisors, but when present in a straight root with damaged or missing crown, it may enable the root to be properly identified.

The upper canine may vary a great deal in crown and root and may sometimes be confused with a lower canine, especially if the crown has a low degree of convexity

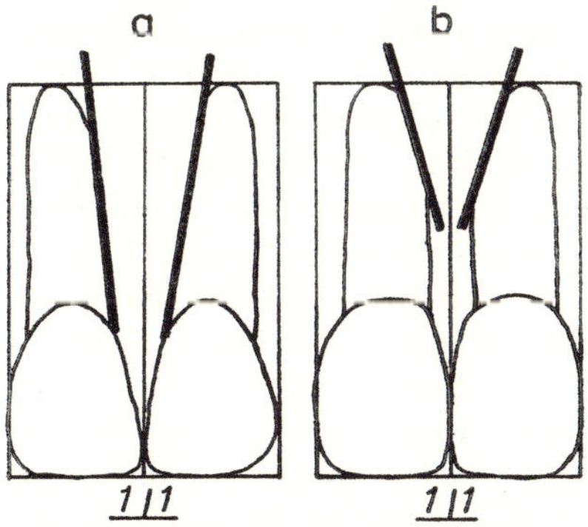

Figure 1-32. Diagram illustrating the apparent tilt of the root of incisors and canines to D, caused by tendency to taper more from M aspect. See examples in Figures 1-20 *a,b,d,* 1-26 *o,* and apparent exceptions in Figures 1-22 *c* and 1-28 *f*.

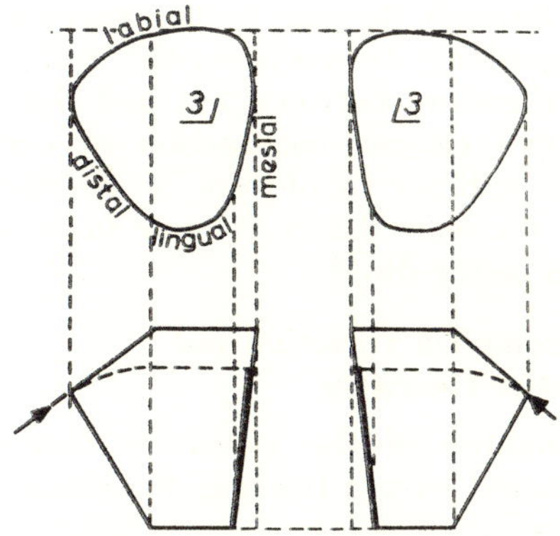

Figure 1-33. Diagrams to illustrate the basic form in transverse section of canine roots at the cervix. This diagram is taken from the writer's 1937 paper, in which the identity of the "Piltdown canine" was established (Taylor, 1937b).

of proximal outlines and a relatively long crown or reduced acumination of the cusp (Fig. 1-30 *o*). However, the crown is usually quite different from central or lateral incisor crowns, and the root is heavier and larger than either if from the same person. Where the root only is intact, a small canine and a larger central incisor may resemble one another in some features, but transverse sections at cervix should indicate basic differences which also should enable identification as left or right. These basic differences are essentially *(a)* in the central incisor, the labial outline is flattened by contrast with the angle in the labial outline of the canine; *(b)* in the central incisor, there is little appreciable difference in the lengths of mesial and distal portions, whereas in the canine the mesial portion is obviously longer (Figs. 1-13, 1-14 and 1-33). The frequency of a distinct distal curve or bend in the root of the canine is a useful diagnostic feature. However , it may (as in the case of the central incisor) present a mesial bend, particularly in the apical portion; thus more reliance should be given to crown shape and to outline of cervical transverse section if these clearly are not in accord with determinations by root curve alone. If there is difficulty through damage to the specimen in distinguishing between mesial and distal (and therefore between left and right) in an upper canine, comparison of cervical enamel outlines should not be overlooked, where the more flattened curve in proximal view is on the distal.

Morphological Variation and Operative Dentistry

A number of the variations that have been noted have a bearing on clinical procedures.

The loosening of a tooth in forceps extraction is not by pulling but by rotation and rocking movements, according to the expected shape of the root. Root fracture during the procedure results not only from excessive force on a slender root but also from attempting to rotate a flattened or curved root. Thus a knowledge of possible variation in morphology and of actual form in a particular case is very relevant. The greatest aid in the latter respect comes from radiography, but it is equally important to know its limitations as well as how to obtain maximum information from this medium. Thus root curvature in line with the X-rays is easily overlooked.

Direct lingual access to a pulp cavity is complicated if labial convexity of the crown is increased, as when the blade of the tooth curves lingually (Fig. 1-6).

Lingual pits and fissures may need modified techniques as well as extreme care in cavity preparation (Figs. 1-10, 1-12 *e,f*, 1-21). Instead of a fissure passing through the cingulum there may be a well-defined pit, even in teeth which do not present a shovel form. These cavities should be prepared with the bur approximately at right angles to the lingual surface to facilitate obtaining strong walls and even depth, and deep caries should be removed afterward. If the bur is inclined toward the long axis of the tooth, poor visibility may easily lead to pulp exposure.

It has already been shown that variation in proximal cervical lines may occur in teeth of similar size and proportion, but a clue as to the likely form may be gained by inspection of tooth type. Where the crown is long and narrow and where the labio-lingual dimension of the alveolus is similarly reduced, it is more likely that the curve will be deep, or acute-angled. In these cases preparation of a proximal cavity may easily approach closely to the interdental crest so that greater care is necessary to avoid injury to soft tissues and bleeding into the cavity. Further, it is also likely to be more difficult to apply a rubber dam and to place ligatures effectively.

Similarly, the contouring of the gingival margins of preparations for partial or full crowns is made more difficult. Here again the difference in the M and D cervical curves has a practical application, for since the cervical enamel curve has a greater radius on the distal side, a band to fit an upper canine should be cut away more deeply on the mesial side.

When discussing this particular observation regarding cervical lines, it was suggested that it is associated with the thickness of the alveolar ridge. On the mesial side a canine is adjacent to a narrow tooth labio-lingually, but on the distal side there is the much wider first premolar. The shape of curve of the interdental alveolar crests reflects these differences in tooth widths but is not determined by them entirely, because canine variation in cervical curves is not according to size alone. The cervical outline is completed long before the root is formed, and probably bears some forecast of the ultimate bone shape. In other words, the cervical line as well as the labio-lingual dimension may carry some indication of the genetic potential for bone formation. Such information would be useful to the orthodontist, but it is hardly obtainable by radiography, and it is not accessible by visual examination at the time it is needed.

The apical foramen may open at an angle to the long axis of the root, and this is one of the factors responsible for failure of some root fillings. Mechanical clearing of the apical part of the canal, impossible in these cases and also in those with accessory foramina, has been replaced by apical resection, or by sterilization of canal contents *in situ*.

In addition to such detailed considerations the ability to recognize characteristics of type of tooth (square, tapering or ovoid) has a bearing on conservative dentistry. Curvature of proximal surfaces is often a factor influencing ease of cavity preparation and the useful life of a restoration.

Characteristics of tooth morphology and arrangement are important to the individual's oral hygiene. When these physical factors are not recognized they may also introduce significant variables in the interpretation of research findings.

There is much evidence that the cause or causes of dental troubles are not nearly as obscure as many would have us believe. Certainly it is known that in pre-European times the Maori of New Zealand were almost entirely free of tooth decay and periodontal troubles (Taylor, 1962c), although there is now a very high incidence of dental caries in the New Zealand population, both Maori and European. The role of physical factors has not received sufficient attention. Among these neglected physical factors are not only those concerning the condition of food and the manner of its mastication (Taylor, 1962c, 1963a, 1975, 1976) but also variations in morphologic characters and arrangement of teeth (Taylor, 1971a). The association of known cariogenic conditions with some of these variations and the inability to recognize the association appear to account for dental troubles in some of the cases that so far have been difficult to explain. This study draws attention to the nature and extent of variations in form and arrangement of teeth and shows how they may sometimes be critical factors in the prevention and treatment of dental conditions.

It was found that roots varied in such characters as actual overall size; size in certain dimensions such as length, breadth, and thickness; and size relative to the crown of the tooth. All these variations may produce different appearances according to whether the root was short or otherwise; a totally different effect may result from viewing the tooth in profile from proximal or labial. In the character of root curves, there is great variety presented by a single-rooted tooth, for aspects of curvature may be combined with aspects of taper, of thickness, or of length and so on.

Similarly, with the crown, it was found that quite apart from overall size there is much variation in relative proportions among any of the three principal dimensions. A counterpart to taper in roots is seen in crowns, and its study was facilitated by using the idea of types, of square, tapering and ovoid, with their characters of straightness or curvature, divergence or near parallelism of outlines, and of the nature of angles formed by adjacent outlines.

Thus it has already been shown how one might distinguish among the three kinds of teeth and how any of them might be identified alone. It has also been shown that certain characters (which may be called type characters) are so often combined in a particular tooth that they may greatly assist in its identification, and that this may sometimes be possible when only the crown or root of the tooth is intact, while additional information may be deduced from facets of wear or the presence of stain on teeth.

Although discussion of wear in anterior teeth is appropriate to this chapter, wear is in the nature of an acquired variation as distinct from formative variation. Since the subject of wear recurs as each type of tooth is studied, it is preferable to deal with it in a general way at this introductory stage. It may therefore be excusable first to present a brief summary of the analysis of formative variation found in maxillary anterior teeth. The aspects of acquired variation, collectively called wear, will then be outlined and their significance in this study explained.

SUMMARY OF FORMATIVE VARIATION IN MAXILLARY ANTERIOR TEETH

It is concluded that the range of normal variation in any kind of tooth is much greater than has hitherto been suggested or illustrated in textbooks. Much of this information cannot be presented metrically or quantitatively. It cannot be fairly claimed that any particular tooth is "typical" of its kind, although some characteristics do tend to be found in a particular tooth, and others in many teeth of one individual. The former are referred to as type characters, and the latter as personal characters. In addition to identification of an isolated tooth, therefore, it is often possible to say that a particular tooth could, or could not, have belonged to the same person as other known teeth. Thus data of anthropologic or forensic importance may be obtained from naked-eye studies of morphology, as indicated in this chapter.

Schroeter's *Atlas* (1966) presents photographs of selected and polished teeth, together with stereo pairs. Some variations are seen in his group panels, but they are not coordinated with comments, and the emphasis is on generalization. The present study rather emphasizes variation, although the search for common or basic features is by no means reduced.

Examination of facets on teeth may have forensic significance (Taylor, 1971c) and may assist identification especially where isolated teeth are found in the debris where fire follows such fatalities as aircraft crashes. Practical applications of this study include identification of skeletons or other remains in archaeological and police work.

The roots of teeth are virtually unknown to those whose acquaintance with the dentition is limited to visible parts in the living mouth or in skeletal material, but they cannot be ignored. In many fields, not only in dentistry, anthropology and forensics, it is the biology and morphology of the whole tooth that is important. Essential information cannot be obtained from tooth crowns only, and data so limited may easily lead to faulty conclusions. This may well be the case, as will be shown later, concerning the cusp of Carabelli.

Similarly a full appreciation of data concerning tooth roots requires an awareness of their relation, not only to the crown, but also to other anatomical structures. This applies both during development and later while functional. In other words, tooth crowns are not significant in isolation, but the whole tooth as part of a whole individual bears witness to that relationship. In such a setting is placed this analysis of morphological variation.

ACQUIRED VARIATION IN FORM—WEAR

There is so much that could be included under this heading that tooth wear might well become a separate study, but it must be considered here because of its relevance. It is involved in tooth form, and in changes in form. Its effects are relevant in the three main fields to which this work applies. For the dental surgeon the causes of wear, and their effects, are intimately concerned with oral health, and with stresses that determine the success or failure of operative procedures.

In physical anthropology tooth wear provides a great amount of data, and its interpretation is also important in the allied fields of palaeontology, archaeology and ethnology. The subject interests anyone involved in such studies and some of the causes and effects are well known or obvious. Beyond this the subject is an irresistible source for speculation, so that apparently similar effects are interpreted as supporting or disproving some particular hypothesis. While training and experience in dental and biological science should enable some of the pitfalls to be avoided, it is felt that confusion has also arisen from unsound experimental procedures. Among these are failure to recognize variable factors and the tendency to generalize from the particular case, or at least from too few cases.

For example, a number of workers recently expressed strongly varying interpretations concerning aspects of incisor wear on a particular fossil skull (Wallace, 1975). In the first place we have no proof that the condition of that ancient man's dentition was typical of his unknown contemporaries. It is known that widely different effects are seen in any group in modern times. The conditions are not known under which that fossil man lived; he may well have been a loner, more of a hunter than his fellows. Certainly he was in some way nontypical for the "accident" that preserved his skull. Secondly it is relevant to mention that there was much argument as to how that man may have divided meat (no mention of bones) so that he might swallow it. In our own times some people like to "pick a bone"; in those ancient times the picking of bones might well have been vital to the survival of some individuals. The writer has in his collection the skull of a dog in which the much worn incisors occlude to an open V-shape, very similar to wear in the particular fossil skull mentioned. The dog skull is that of a working collie dog, fed mostly on sheep meat on a New Zealand farm, and those dogs certainly know how to pick meat from bones. Very similar V-shaped wear in a Kalahari Bushman is figured in van Reenen (1967).

The writer offers these comments, but would not enter into a controversy concerning prehistoric peoples of whose living conditions he knows little. However, he is familiar with skeletal material of the much more recent Australian Aborigine and of some pre-European Polynesians, also with the dentitions of their living descendants and of the contemporary population. A lifetime of study, including field work and teaching in physical anthropology and dental sciences, institutional and private clinical practice of dentistry, research and publications, has ensured that examinations of many thousands of dentitions comprise the setting for this report. Such a study is relevant in view of the increasing importance accorded to dental forensics.

The degree of wear varies between recognizable evidence of friction and gross loss of tooth substance. Familiarity with tooth morphology and its variation facilitates awareness that tooth substance is missing, but something more in the nature of clinical experience and ethnological knowledge may be needed for correct diagnosis. Tooth tissue may be "missing" for other reasons than wear or fracture, and these cases may be overlooked if the observer lacks clinical experience or training in dental biology and pathology. Thus tooth substance may be missing because it has actually been lost, or because it failed to form. For example, it is normal for deciduous teeth to lose root substance by resorption, but a similar process may occur abnormally in permanent teeth. Again, tooth substance may be deficient because it has been formed defectively. An example is the hypoplastic enamel whose formation in a permanent tooth was affected by the local sepsis of an abscessed deciduous tooth root, or by the systemic effects of severe illness.

The manifestations of hypoplastic enamel are many and varied according to the cause, its severity and duration, and the age of the child. The age determines the area of the tooth that will be affected. *In situ,* information can often be deduced by examination of other teeth, but in the case of an isolated (extracted?) tooth without known history, data may still be obtained. Thus tooth 2| in Figure 1-23 *c* presents a small area of defective enamel at the incisal edge. Naked eye examination shows that this has neither been worn away nor chipped away, but is apparently hypoplastic. This could be an effect of an exanthematous illness, or of trauma. Enamel would be forming in this region of the permanent tooth between approximately fifteen months and three years of age, at which time the apex of the deciduous incisor would be close to it and could readily cause damage from a blow on its crown—not a rare happening for a younger child.

Evidence of missing tooth substance as a result of wear occurs in great variety, especially where the amount lost is moderate or small. But wear of occlusal surfaces, even of moderate severity, is much less common in contemporary society where people have sophisticated habits. This has assisted the present study by making available more adult teeth in which anatomical details have not been obliterated by wear.

Among ethnic groups of less sophisticated or of primitive culture severe tooth wear is common. The nature, effects and significance of this have been discussed in previous papers (Taylor, 1934, 1937b, 1955, 1962b, 1963a, 1970c, 1971b, 1975, 1976).

The most common causes of wear in contemporary society are friction from abrasive substances or materials consciously applied to non-occluding tooth surfaces, or moved between occluding surfaces during masticatory movements, or friction between tooth surfaces themselves. The last mentioned leads to a wide variety of effects, but our report must be limited to effects visible on teeth. These include facets or worn surfaces which are found in wide variety as regards position, form, size or extent, facets which for the present are designated as simple or complex. Some facets may be small and difficult to find and yet have considerable significance in diagnosis, for they confirm habitual, though often unconscious, clenching of teeth in momentary malocclusion associated with extreme mandibular movements as reported by Every (1960). But other facets in unusual positions, and sometimes of considerable size, arise from malocclusion. The malocclusion may be of long duration and relatively stable, such as the upper incisor in lingual occlusion (Fig. 1-6 *d*), or it may develop as a result of "mutilation" or extraction of one or more teeth without prosthetic replacement. Again, malocclusion may follow tooth decay, but in either case the drifting or tipping of remaining teeth may be associated with such wear.

While the style of wear just mentioned is not rare in contemporary society, it did occur also under some primitive conditions. In the pre-European culture of the Maori and Chatham Islander, where tooth decay and extractions (in the modern sense) were unknown, exposure of the dental pulp by excessive wear was common. This often initiated a train of pathological changes, the nature and effects of which have been described (Taylor, 1962b, 1963a, 1970c, 1975, 1976).

Returning to consideration of causes and effects of tooth wear in contemporary society, a distinction was drawn between those involving occluding and non-occluding tooth surfaces. In the latter, the effects are mostly associated with frictional habits of "artificial prophylaxis," but a chemical factor is sometimes also present. This may be dealt with briefly by reference to the decalcifying action of "soft drinks" upon tooth enamel, easily demonstrated by placing a shed deciduous tooth in such liquid. Some citrus drinks or juices taken habitually have a similarly destructive effect, so that tooth enamel is then more easily worn away by brushing. The so-called "erosion" cavities have been ascribed to acid reaction, but their etiology does not appear fully understood. Tooth *n* of Figure 1-23 could be a case of accelerated loss of lingual enamel by decalcification by acid drinks. (See p. 46.)

Habitual routines or "patterns" in artificial prophylaxis vary considerably. In essentials there is usually a brush or thread, and in some cases the piece of cloth on a finger or other support is still favoured. With these some form of dentifrice is used by most people. Seldom used now, favourites have been such materials as soot, cigar ash, baking soda, chalk and salt (the latter still recommended if used in dilute solution). Much more common is some form of paste or powder combined with fillers and flavours, and including the currently favoured additions in accordance with the latest hypothesis of commercial or other research.

Although morphologically much alike, the two right central incisors of Figure 1-1 *n,o* bear witness to contrasting history, although there is no confirmation available. Tooth *n* is that of a middle-aged person. Gingival attachment had receded well above the cervix; there is calculus deposit and dark stain, especially on proximal surfaces, and appreciable wear from a normal overbite. The labial surface has stained longitudinal enamel cracks and is highly polished, while the lingual surface is less polished and has light stain in shallow grooves. The person was probably a cigarette smoker devoted to regular light tooth-brushing of visible or easily accessible tooth surfaces mainly as a gesture to appearance. A hand-held lens reveals fine scratches in all directions, and much finer scratches from horizontal polishing.

Tooth *o* is from a much younger person as shown by the low gingival line and virtual absence of any wear. The subgingival enamel is clean and white and there is no tartar deposit. The exposed parts of the crown are lightly covered with a grey-green stain, and there are deep proximal cavities. This person neglected regular brushing or other prophylaxis.

Tooth *a* of Figure 1-22 has a highly polished labial surface. The line of gingival attachment has receded well above the cervix and much higher on the labial aspect of the root. There is some calculus deposit but none on labial. There are stained fracture lines in enamel and appreciable incisal and lingual wear. The striking feature, however, as seen in the proximal outline, is the considerable loss of thickness of labial enamel. The area has a well-marked border below the cervix and is actually concave from here to the incisal region. The tooth is one of a pair, and the condition of each is identical. A hand-held lens shows parallel horizontal scratches throughout the abraded areas. It is apparent that this middle-aged person had conscientiously, but with more zeal than understanding, scrubbed the teeth in an habitual and invariable side-to-side manner. The abraded areas do not suggest either that stiff bristles or a coarse dentifrice was favoured, but nevertheless gingival recession was aggravated, if not largely initiated, by this habit.

A less uncommon result of habitual traumatic tooth-brushing is the notch worn at the lingual cervix of anterior teeth, and sometimes right to the molar region. A difference in depth of notch between left and right side, especially when the canines at the angles of the arch must bear the brunt of the attacks, has enabled the writer successfully to recognize left-handedness in a new patient. Examples are shown in Figures 1-23 *d,f* and 1-24 *e,f,g*.

In these cases it is assumed that the form of the notch-like abrasions is basically the result of the greater resistance offered by the harder enamel. But there are several variable additional factors (choice of bristle, of dentifrice, individual technique, etc.) that lead to differences in the result. Tooth *d* of Figure 1-23 suggests a much more consistent or precise manner of work than tooth *f* of that figure. The unusual stepped notch in Figure 1-24 *e* certainly suggests vigorous and consistent attacks, and the advanced occlusal wear bears witness to a vigorously used dentition with freedom of lateral masticatory movements.

The contrast in the form of notches produced in Figure 1-24 *f,g* invites speculation. It is suggested that the first, as with tooth *d* of Figure 1-23, is more likely to arise through using coarse or hard-bristled brushes, and the second through contact with softer bristles, perhaps combined with a less abrasive dentifrice. The notch in tooth g does not have sharply defined margins and angles, but all surfaces are smoothly rounded. Some authorities insist that it is the dentifrice and not the brush which causes abrasion. The writer has for many years used natural bristle of medium stiffness, and no dentifrice. Brushing has been in all directions with light pressure, but labial enamel has worn thin, and some cervices smoothly concave. On this evidence there is high abrasive potential in "scrubbing" with stiff or synthetic bristles alone, and the more so when loaded with dentifrice.

Wear of non-occluding surfaces is not caused only by prophylactic activities. Ritual and decorative filing described in ancient and more recent ethnic groups will not be considered here, but functional effects are relevant. Two distinct functional effects have been described for the pre-European New Zealand Maori and Chatham Islander (Taylor, 1963a, 1970c). What the writer called "Fern root planes" never involved occluding surfaces. The wear on dislocating surfaces often involved buccal surfaces in a functional occlusion as the tooth turned over, crown inwards, towards lingual (Taylor, 1970c).

In contemporary society, wear on non-occluding surfaces of teeth arises frequently from the use of prosthetic dental appliances. Needless to say, this results from ill-fitting or unstable devices, usually partial dentures. They may originally have been of faulty design, or, if satisfactory, had not later been checked or adjusted to meet changing conditions in the mouth. Such wear on natural teeth arises from movement of the denture base or of clasps intended to support it.

Other troubles in the nature of trauma and pathology of soft tissues, tooth decay, etc., and their causes, cannot be discussed here. It is sufficient to say that the wear produced is found in great variety of form, position and degree. It must be added, however, that wear often occurs in considerable degree where partial dentures are not worn, but where decay or mutilation from extractions has caused remaining teeth to drift into malocclusion. Some such circumstances have probably contributed to the complex or unusual facets of wear which may be found in extracted teeth of unknown origin, and also in skeletal material.

Wear of occluding surfaces in incisors and canines occurs with as much variety of form, position and degree as anywhere else in the mouth, and it seems unlikely that any satisfactory system could be devised to classify and describe the complex manifestations that are found, particularly in contemporary material. Physical anthropologists appear to approach classification of wear with a "tongue-in-cheek" attitude, as though it were sufficient to select from primitive or other skeletal material only those cases where wear is even, or limited to the "normal" occlusal plane. Nevertheless the present writer has not hesitated to use the classification of Broca (1879) as a convenient, albeit inadequate, indication of depth or degree of wear. Broca's scale, which really should be limited to wear in normal occlusion of edge-to-edge bite, is as follows:

I. Enamel worn, without cusp obliteration or exposure of dentine.
II. Cusps worn down and dentine exposed.
III. Stage in which quite an appreciable amount of the tooth has been worn away.
IV. Extreme stage in which most of the crown of the tooth has disappeared, and the wear has extended to the neck of the tooth.

Earlier work (Taylor, 1962b) proposed a modification of the foregoing classification, limiting third-degree wear to teeth in which the original outline of the pulp chamber has been reached. Either secondary dentine, or an opening into the pulp cavity, will be visible.

The writer sees no advantage in limitation of the word attrition to imply a special kind of wear between tooth surfaces, as distinct from wear caused by toughness or fibre in the food itself. The term "abrasion" however is useful to imply the involvement of an additional or foreign factor, whether it be a gritty contamination of food, a bristle brush or other implement with or without a dentifrice. Other causes of abrasion are artificial dentures, something frequently held between teeth such as a pipe stem, or an article associated with one's occupation or cultural activity. The greater damage of chipping of incisal enamel through holding pins, nails or "bobby pins" between the teeth is well known.

The incisors of sheep and cattle, having no upper antagonists, must be worn by the toughness of their food fibre contaminated in varying degree by soil abrasives. Other factors, such as substances which act on enamel or dentine, may be involved (Rouiller et al., 1952; Barnicoat, 1957, 1959; Barnicoat and Hall, 1960). In these animals interproximal wear also causes considerable loss of tooth substance, and yet contact with adjacent teeth may be maintained (Fig. 1-12 *a,b,c*). Similar interproximal wear in human teeth in varying degree is a source of data regarding function and may also be useful in distinguishing between certain teeth. On the other hand, interproximal wear is one of the factors that invalidates deductions from measurement of teeth (see Chapter 10).

A facet over which wear has taken place may be very small or it may be considerable, and it may involve more than one surface of a tooth. It may be flat but is usually curved. It may be concave or convex. Concavity may result from more rapid wear of dentin than of adjacent harder enamel.

A facet may be described as simple where it has only one light-reflecting surface (Fig. 1-31 *e,g,h*), or compound when there is more than one (Fig. 1-23 *b*). There seems little merit in this distinction, either on the grounds of size or of shape. In Figure 1-22, tooth *g* has one facet and tooth *h* has three lingually, yet each is the result of wear between overlapping enamel surfaces that have no lateral movement. Here the amount of overbite is different and the relationship of lower incisors must have been different. In Figure 1-23 *a* the large curved facet indicates only protrusive movement from an originally deep overbite, but Figures 1-23 *m* and 1-24 *d,e,* with their large and almost flat facets, testify to free lateral and protrusive masticatory movements.

The details of occlusion in a particular mouth may vary considerably from those in another, but both may be relatively stable and satisfactory. The facets of wear record details of occlusal relationship and movements at a particular time. These relationships and the functional habits will largely determine the changes that take place in the course of time. In some mouths there is an increasing freedom of movements, and in others the reverse.

A feature of wear associated with facets and not necessarily covered in the above remarks has been referred to as "cupping." Examples are in Figures 1-22 *e*, 1-24 *b*, and they are concavities in occlusal or incisal dentine which are surrounded by an enamel rim. They do not indicate appreciable lateral movement of mandibular teeth as do the slotted facets (Figs. 1-22 *f*, 1-23 *i,l* and 1-24 *a*). Explanation of the cupping might appear to be simple if some substance acting more on dentine than on enamel could be demonstrated. Alternatively, explanation in terms of crushing of fibrous food between facets of dentine bordered by more resistant enamel seems acceptable. This assumes the prior development of flat occlusal facets which later become concave or cupped. If this does in fact occur, explanation of unevenness between dentine and enamel in other cases of wear is facilitated.

In Figure 1-22 *b* and 1-23 *h* the oblique wear suggests rotation or other malposition of the tooth or of its antagonist. Tooth *c* of Figure 1-22 had been subjected to repeated severe strains resulting in cracks in labial enamel and chipping of enamel edge. In regard to cracks in enamel this may also arise from sudden changes in temperature. It is easy to see many fine cracks in the enamel of teeth which make contact with frozen foods.

In tooth *l* of Figure 1-23 the area of fine shading has been worn by the clasp of an unstable partial denture, but in tooth *m* the fine shading is an area of heavy stain deposit. In tooth *n* there is a facet of lingual wear from a deep overbite, but much of the remaining lingual enamel has disappeared as though by chemical solution, and dentine is fully exposed. It is suggested that this might happen from habitual sucking of a medicinal tablet "parked" in this region, or from the use of a straw for a favoured "soft" drink.

In the majority of upper anterior teeth the first facets of wear appear on the incisal and lingual aspects, because slight incisal overlap is the usual occlusal relationship, and such wear has been indicated in many of the figures. In adults of a contemporary western-style society, from which the teeth here described have mostly been taken, relatively few teeth reach the most advanced stages of wear. However, because many people have malocclusion and mutilated dentitions, the variety of facets of wear and abrasion is very much greater than is usually seen in skeletal material from less sophisticated people. In this discussion attempts have been made to illustrate a fair sample of that modern variety while avoiding extreme cases. Such, of course, do occur and carry their own evidence of exceptional conditions.

To sum up, in the forensic field, tooth wear and loss of tooth tissue by other means, the presence of stain in a "sheltered" area, or its absence through friction or abrasion are all sources of data. In combination with other morphological or anatomical characters it may be possible to identify positively an isolated tooth. Furthermore, information may be deduced concerning the rest of the dentition and also concerning the habits of the person concerned. This has relevance in identification of an individual, for it will be seen that it may be possible to say that the tooth could, or could not, have formed part of a dentition for which some previously recorded information is available. It is unfortunate that dental personnel seem largely unaware of the importance of their opportunities in this respect. The present report aims to draw attention to features and characters that can be recognized with the naked eye, without the need for time or facilities for making sections or microscopic examinations.

Chapter 2

Maxillary Premolars

IN MAXILLARY or upper premolars there are so many characters that are commonly found in first and second premolars that it is convenient to deal with both teeth together. When it is necessary to distinguish between them, reference is made particularly to one or the other.

VARIATION IN ROOTS

This may be discussed under a number of headings such as size, root curves or bends, root division, taper, shape of apex, etc., and these characters occur in varying combinations in a particular tooth. Discussion of variation in first and second upper premolars together is complicated by the tendency of the root not only to bifurcate in one and not in the other, but also to present almost any degree of division in both of them.

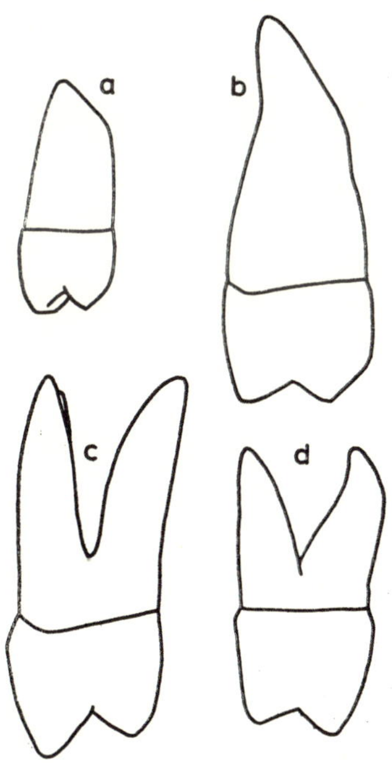

Figure 2-1. Variation in crown and root and in actual dimensions (length overall and width at cervix in mm approx.) *a*, 16 and 7; *b*, 28 and 9.5; *c*, 25 and 10.5; *d*, 18.5 and 8.5.

Root Size

Although premolars may be small overall (Fig. 2-1 *a,d*)* or large (Fig. 2-1 *b,c*) others have large crowns and small roots (Fig. 2-2 *a,b*) or small crowns and large roots, better described as small crowns and long roots (Fig. 2-2 *c,d*). Therefore crown and root vary in size independently of one another. In many cases, however, there is a general relation between crown and root. It is easy to find long or short, wide (B-P)† or narrow teeth, and combinations of these such as long wide or long narrow teeth, with no disharmony between crown and root. These comments apply not only to upper premolars, but also to all teeth in the dentition. Some variations are more easily demonstrated in upper incisors.

---

* The outlines in figures of this chapter were drawn through the camera lucida, as were outlines in all other chapters, and to approximately the same scale. Unfortunately at this stage it had not become the writer's practice to draw in the scale as each figure was drafted. Since there were likely to be small differences of magnification between figures when drafting, and more so in the photographic procedures for subsequent reproduction, it was not feasible to add the scales later.

The presence of scales in the figures for Chapter 1 is explained by the fact that the text and figures for that chapter were revised after completion of other chapters.

† See Appendix 2.

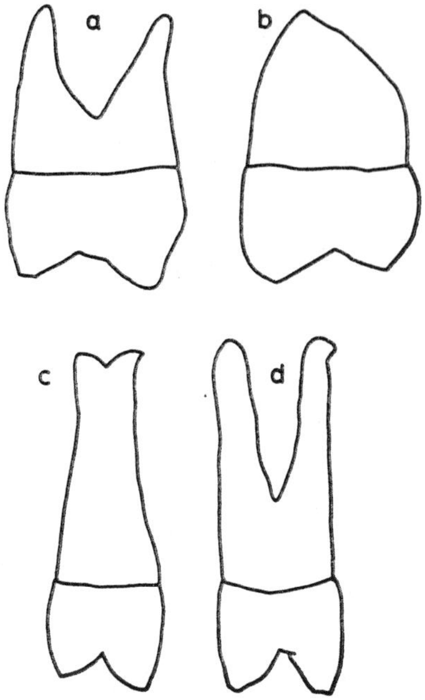

Figure 2-2. Further examples of variation in upper premolars. Drawn to same relative scale within each figure. Dimensions indicated in mm as for overall length and B-P at cervix. *a,* 17 and 10; *b,* 17 and 10.5; *c,* 25 and 7.5; *d,* 27 and 8.

Curves or Bends in Roots of Upper Premolars

These frustrate one's efforts at concise classification on account of the great variety of form and degree of presentation. As with upper incisors and canines, roots of upper premolars may be closely related to anatomical features. With the former it was chiefly the nasal fossae, but with premolars it is mainly the maxillary sinuses. As both features are subject to considerable variation in size, sometimes either or both could be associated with root bends. Thus the floor of the maxillary sinus may be superior to the nasal floor, or inferior, its anterior limits and form also varying considerably. Other factors are the width and height of the palate, also the length and width of the alveolar process. Height or depth of palate and length of alveolar process are not strictly just different names for the same feature (see also

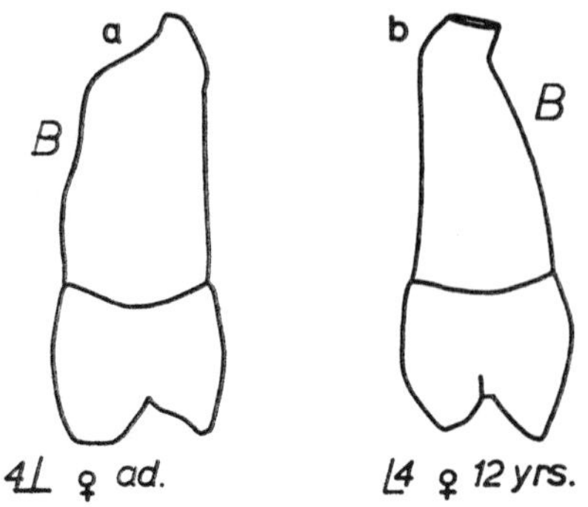

Figure 2-3. Curves or bends in roots.

p. 273). Some of these variations are illustrated by Cryer (1901).

A single-rooted tooth may occasionally curve to the palatal side. The left tooth shown in Figure 2-3 *b* curves initially to palatal, and then at the apex bends sharply to buccal. It was one of four first premolars removed to relieve crowding in the mouth of a girl aged twelve years. As the right tooth is not correspondingly curved to palatal it seems probable that the curve is related to deflection of the tooth while

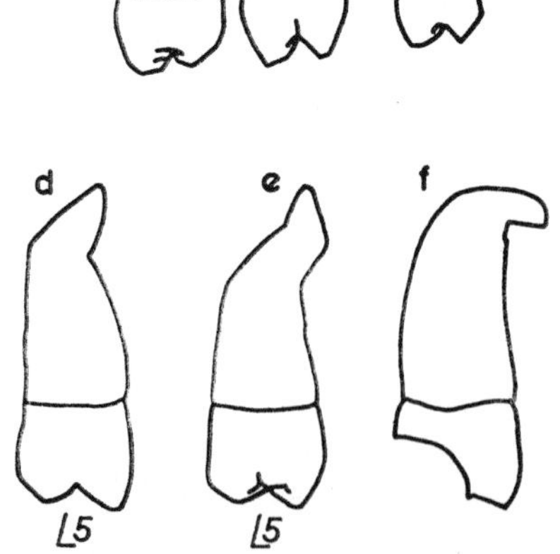

Figure 2-4. Curves or bends in roots.

erupting. A root may appear to curve towards palatal when it is broad at first but tapers rather abruptly towards that side when near the apex (Fig. 2-3 *a*). It is common for a single-rooted tooth to curve towards buccal (Fig. 2-4 *a,b,c*). When the curve is abrupt it is reasonable to assume that the change in direction could have arisen from close proximity to one of the sinuses, in the case of premolars the maxillary sinus (Fig. 2-4 *d,e,f*). But this is not the only explanation for an abrupt change in direction of the long axis of a root, as will be shown presently.

In buccal view an upper premolar often presents a curved root, and mostly the curve is to distal (as is common for every tooth in the human dentition), but it may curve to mesial (Fig. 2-5 *d*). The curve may be slight and involve nearly the whole root or it may be confined to the apical portion, in which case it is well demonstrated in a pair of first or second premolars from the same person (Fig. 2-5 *a,b*).

The curve to distal may be much more obvious (Fig. 2-5 *c*) and in some cases so abrupt that one suspects approach of the developing root to the maxillary sinus as a cause (Fig. 2-5 *d,e,f*). The latter tooth presents both stain and slight subgingival tartar so that it has certainly been fully erupted. The abrupt bend is similar to that sometimes found on an unerupted premolar, but that would not make it impossible for the bend to be related to the sinus.

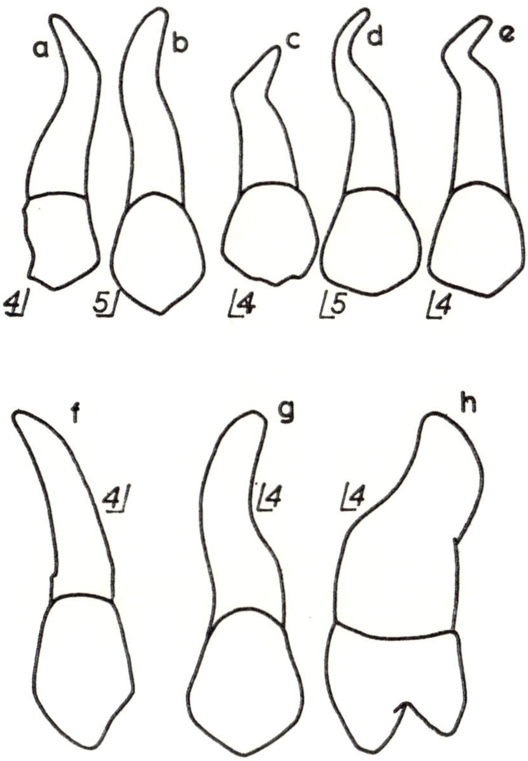

Figure 2-6. Curves or bends of S-type in roots.

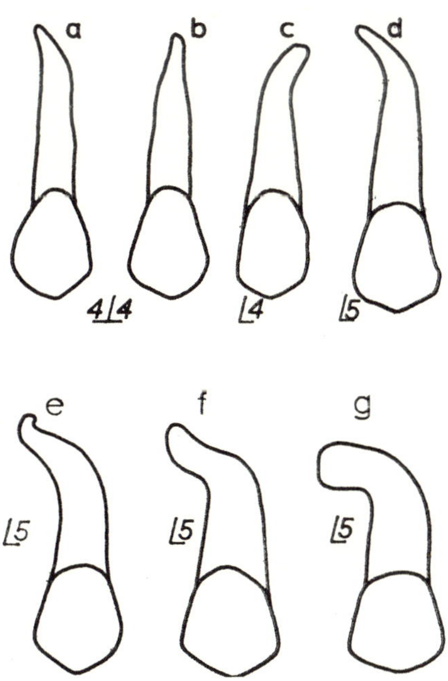

Figure 2-5. Curves or bends in roots.

Another variety of root bend in upper premolars is a double bend in the nature of a flattened "S" when seen from buccal, illustrated by five teeth, each from a different person: two right (one each first and second premolar), and three left side (of which two are first premolars). In four of these the root curves first to M, and the apical section curves to D. The exception is the 5| where the bend is reversed. In each of these teeth the bend differs in de-

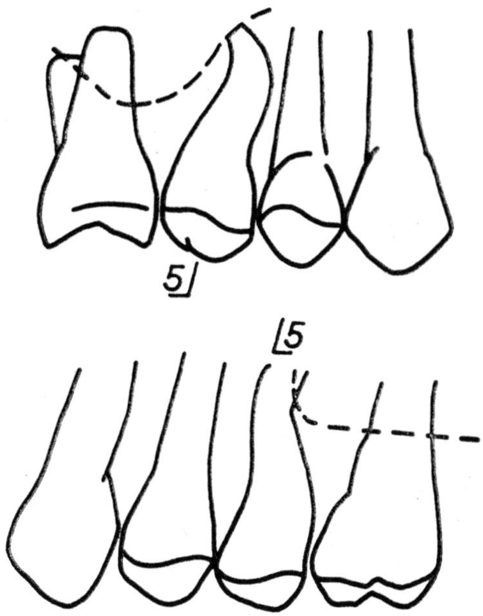

Figure 2-7. Instead of the more common curve to distal, the reverse may occur. Outlines drawn from radiographs of 5|5 in a girl aged 14 3/12 years, showing root curving to mesial in each case. The broken line is the floor of the maxillary sinus.

tail from all the others, their only common feature being the S bend. No explanation of the double bend is offered (Fig. 2-6 *a-e*).

One possible cause of root bend is dilaceration. In upper premolars it would occur during extraction of a deciduous molar, most likely before root absorption and especially where the deciduous molar's roots are closely related to, or "embracing," the developing premolar. At about the age of seven or eight years for the first and second deciduous molars respectively, extraction might easily disturb the almost completed crown of the premolar, and the period of risk extends to the time of partial formation of the root. With the normal range in age periods associated with calcification in permanent teeth and resorption of deciduous roots, the calendar ages of seven and eight could apply for the average child who may never be seen. For the child that is examined, his approximate relation to the hypothetical average may be found from a number of clues. Among these are the degree of development of the mixed dentition in relation to calendar age, records of past shedding and eruption of teeth, and information obtainable from X-rays. In such quests one has for many years been able to refer to useful charts. Those of Schour, Massler and others (1940, 1941, 1958) extended the information provided by earlier workers; further detail has more recently been presented by Fanning (1961).

In Figure 2-6 *f*, is an 4| that suggests this condition by presenting first a straight portion of root, then a slight ledge at the start of the root curve. Figure 2-6 *g,h* gives B and D views of an |4 which also looks like a case of dilaceration. The curvature seen in both views of this tooth draws at-

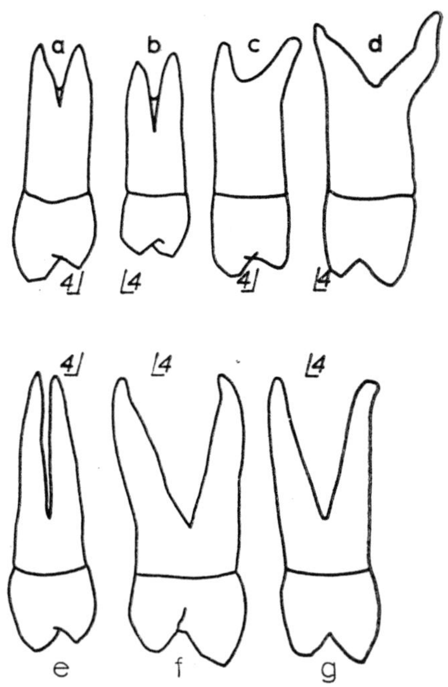

Figure 2-8. Characters of root division in upper premolars. Root trunk and the root branches; position of bifurcation, and depth and width of cleft; divergence of root branches; their taper, and sharpness of apices; relative sizes, thickness and length of root branches; direction and curves in root branches.

tention to another feature of root curvature, namely that the bend is by no means confined to M-D or B-L planes. The root axis may curve in almost any direction, also changing direction in the same root so that the curve may not be well represented by a projection onto any particular plane. Thus an X-ray picture may give a misleading idea of root curvature, as it so often does of root length. Additional radiographs at different angles may indicate the presence of curvature, but may give very little positive information concerning its details.

It has been noted above that in buccal view the root of an upper premolar curves to the distal much more often than to the mesial. A case of the unusual mesial curve is presented in Figure 2-7. This figure is drawn from radiographs of the left and right premolars and shows the root of each second premolar curving anteriorly in close relation to the outline of the maxillary sinus. A similar case is figured in antero-posterior section through the orbit and sinus by Cryer (1901, p.64, Fig. 41).

Discussion of root curvature has so far been confined to single-rooted teeth, but as both upper premolars may present a root that divides into two or three branches, the possibilities for variation in curvature are many. A study of bends or curves in other than single-rooted teeth must therefore attempt to analyze the varieties and degrees of root division at the same time.

Root Division in Upper Premolars

Before a developing root actually divides, the impending division has been forecast by thinning or grooving. The groove may be shallow or deep and present increasing depth until furcation takes place. A straight root may not vary in direction after division; or, one or more branches may curve or bend away from the line of the trunk (Figs. 2-8 *a,b* and 2-8 *c,d*). With division near the cervix there may be relatively long branches, straight in themselves, but one or both may deviate from the general long axis of the tooth (Fig. 2-8 *e,f,g*). Thus division of roots introduces the further factor of divergence, but it is not feasible to consider divergence separately from bends or curves.

External and internal factors must determine whether, or in what manner, division of a root may eventuate, but it is not clear which have the greater influence. It has already been seen that root shape may apparently be influenced by the form and nearness of anatomical structures, but it seems that determination of form and size of root should be predominantly effected through the pulp. Be that as it may, it is much more convenient to study variation in form, both in human and in comparative dental anatomy, by observation of the calcified or completed tooth, both crown and root, than by study of the enamel organ, dental papilla and epithelial sheath. A study of these specialized tissues and of adjacent structures during development and growth may well illuminate the reasons for variations and the manner of their development. The present study is concerned with the end results and their more obvious associations and implications.

In upper premolars the groove before division is often present, or prominent, in proximal surfaces where it is related to formation of B and P roots, but the root may be completed without bifurcation actually taking place. In many of these teeth it is obvious that the pulp cavity must have divided into two canals, B and P, and where this is not obvious it will sometimes be found on opening into the pulp cavity (especially in 4) that such division has occurred. As the root cannot divide unless the pulp has already done so, it is concluded that division is effected through the pulp, modified by factors external to the pulp, but of course initiated by hereditary and genetic factors. As the effect of pulp division is visible in the un-

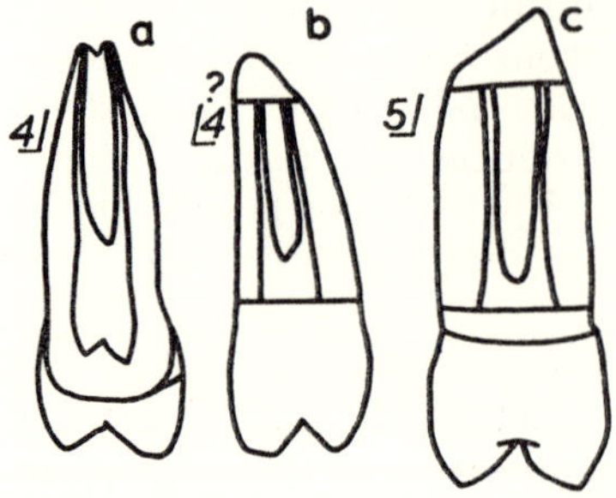

Figure 2-9. Relation of pulp canals to grooved single roots.

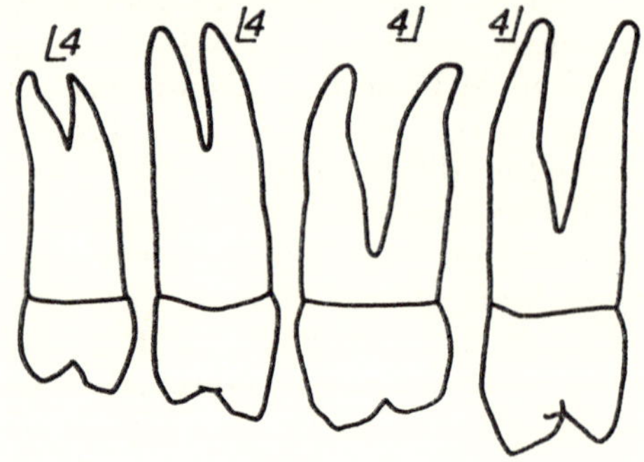

Figure 2-11. Direction of bend or curve in root branches; both to palatal.

divided root, the study of root division in upper premolars begins in single-rooted teeth. In these the grooves on proximal surfaces nearly always divide the root evenly so that B and P sides are approximately equal in size. This applies also when division actually takes place, and is in contrast to what is found in two-rooted lower canines. The groove is usually deeper on the mesial, especially in 4 compared with its 5; in fact a concavity at the mesial cervix of 4 is one of the most reliable characters for identification of a 4. The concavity and the groove merge so smoothly that the latter may be described as commencing in the concavity. In a branched root, the point of visible division may vary from somewhere in the cervical half of the root to so near the apex that the root is virtually single. In longitudinal section there will be an area of cementum varying in extent according to age and other factors; between the cementum and the pulp there is dentine which also varies in extent. A transverse section of the root trunk therefore may or may not present continuity of dentine between the root canals, according to the position of the section. Single-rooted teeth with a deep groove may present only cementum as a "bridge" between the root elements, according to the position of the section; in others the pulp may divide into two quite separate canals but dentine may join the root elements for their whole length (Fig. 2-9 *a,b,c*) where only dentine is visible between the canals in the sectioned areas.

Mummery (1924), discussing the first maxillary premolar, wrote "When the root is not bifurcated there is, according to

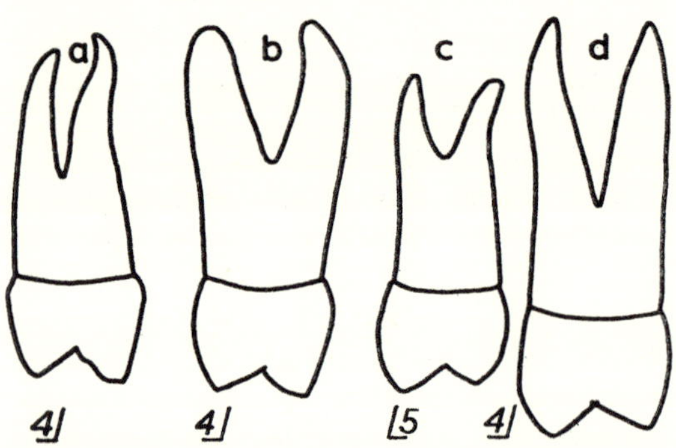

Figure 2-10. Relative size of crown and root where root division has taken place.

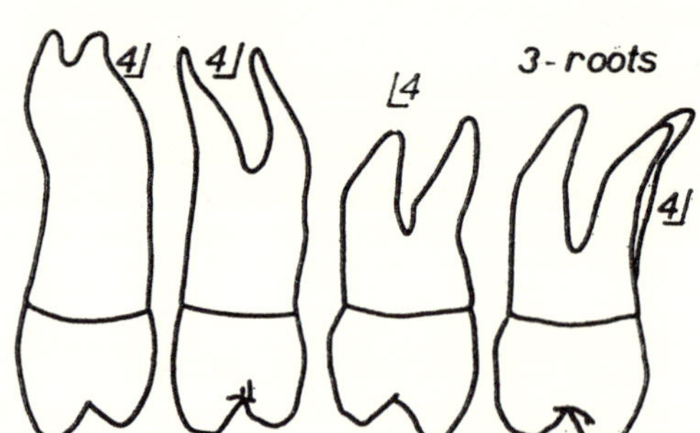

Figure 2-12. Direction of bend or curve in root branches; both to buccal.

Amodeo, no dentine between the two root canals but only cement." The present study does not support this particular statement attributed to Amodeo, for this study has shown that there is wide variation in form and that it is easy to find dentine and no cementum between the canals far from their commencement.

Although B and P roots are approximately equal in size in most cases of two-rooted teeth, the B root may be thicker than the P root in its M-D dimension, and somewhat flattened on its B surface. This may be regarded as a tendency towards the three-rooted tooth. The flatness referred to may in other cases be replaced by a groove, nearly always on the buccal aspect, and of varying degrees of depth right through to complete division of the B root. When there is a third root it is always the B root that is bifid. To return to the two-rooted tooth, the two branches vary from relatively thick to very fine, although in two such different teeth the crowns may be approximately equal in size (Fig. 2-10 *a,b*). The root may be short or long (Fig. 2-10 *c,d*). The bifurcation may occur anywhere in (approximately) the apical three fifths of the root length.

Both branches of the root may curve towards palatal (Fig. 2-11) or towards buccal (Fig. 2-12).

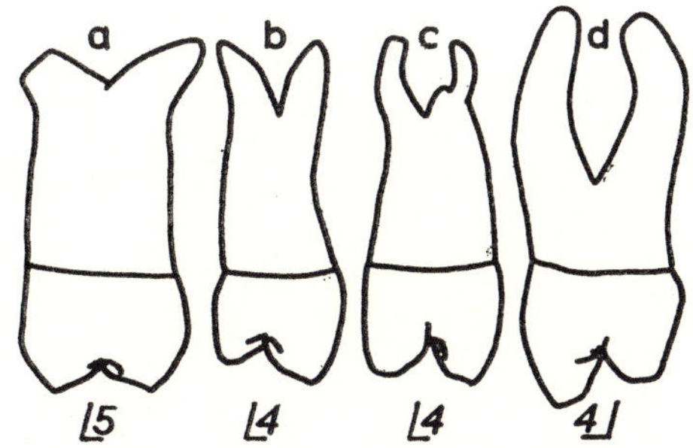

Figure 2-14. Direction of bend or curve in root branches; both may diverge or converge, or diverge and then converge towards one another *(d)*.

One root may appear straight and the other curved. Thus the P root may curve to P or to B (Fig. 2-13 *a,b*) or the B root may do likewise (Fig. 2-13 *c,d*).

Both branches may diverge from the bifurcation of the root (Figs. 2-8 *d* and 2-14 *a,b*) and may then converge (Fig. 2-14 *c,d*). As with single-rooted teeth, a two-rooted upper premolar viewed from B may present in its root a double curve or S bend (Fig. 2-15 *a*).

The variations in bends in two-rooted upper premolars so far described have been observed in teeth in which both of the roots and the bends lie mostly in one plane so that they can be seen almost entirely in buccal or proximal view. As with single-rooted teeth, a divided root may be

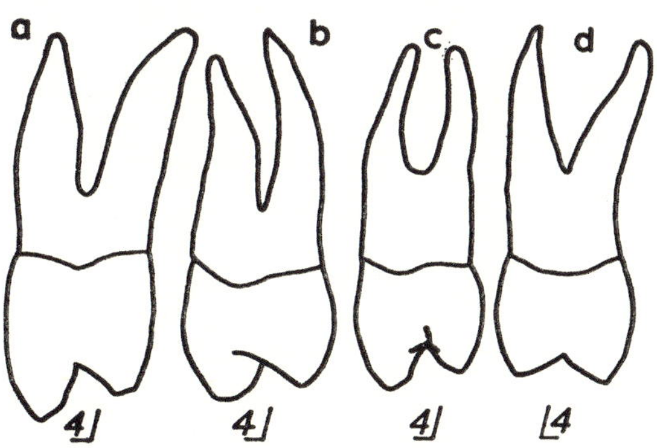

Figure 2-13. Direction of bend or curve in root branches; either branch may be fairly straight while the other may curve towards it or away from it.

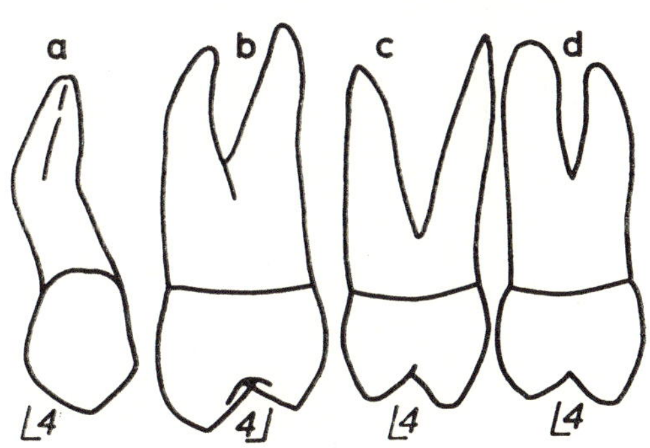

Figure 2-15. *a*, an S-bend in buccal view of a two-rooted upper premolar. *b,c,d*, differences in length or thickness between the root-branches in multi-rooted teeth.

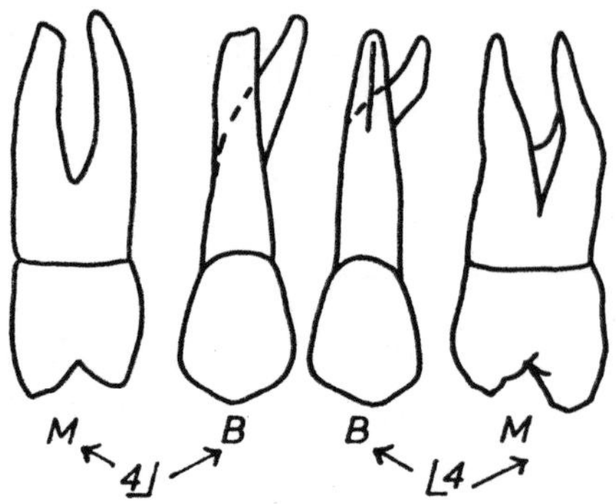

Figure 2-16. Root bends that cannot be represented in a single view, and bends in one branch that contrast with bends in the other. Mesial and buccal views of a left and a right first premolar.

curved in more than one plane and further, the two branches may be curved quite independently. Such different bends in varying degrees occur frequently in the collection on which the present work is based, and two examples are shown in Figure 2-16. In the first the P root curves to M and P. In the second the P root bends abruptly to D as though related closely to the sinus. Where the B root is divided into M and D branches, the varieties of root curve may be even more complex.

The two roots of an upper premolar have been described as approximately equal in thickness, with the buccal tending to be wider when it is grooved as for an early stage of division. Infrequently however the two roots are visibly unequal in length. Figure 2-15 *b,c,d* shows three such teeth. In one the B root is the longer; in the other two the B root is shorter; and in one of these it is almost divided into two. This last case draws attention to those upper premolars that are three-rooted or almost so. In these there is often a difference in root size, both in length and in thickness. The P root is usually the longest and the thickest (Figs. 2-13 *a*, 2-17 *a,b*) but not always (Fig. 2-17 *c*). Sometimes one of the B roots is fused to the P root giving the appearance of one very wide root and one very slender root, which was always the MB in the specimens of the present collection (Fig. 2-18 *a*). This is an unusual variation but it is similar to the most common pattern of fusion of upper molars, both deciduous and permanent, where if the palatal root is fused to a buccal root, it is nearly always the MB root that remains separate. In the great majority of upper premolars, however, there is no division of the B root unless there is already a separate P root. An apparent exception even to this was presented by a premolar from

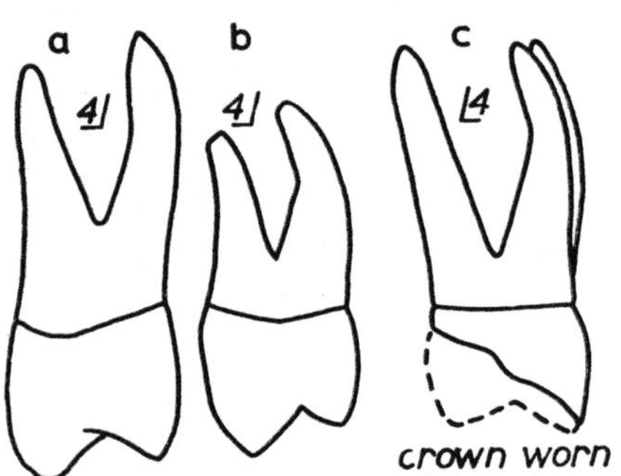

Figure 2-17. Division of buccal root into branches that tend to be smaller than palatal branch but are not always so.

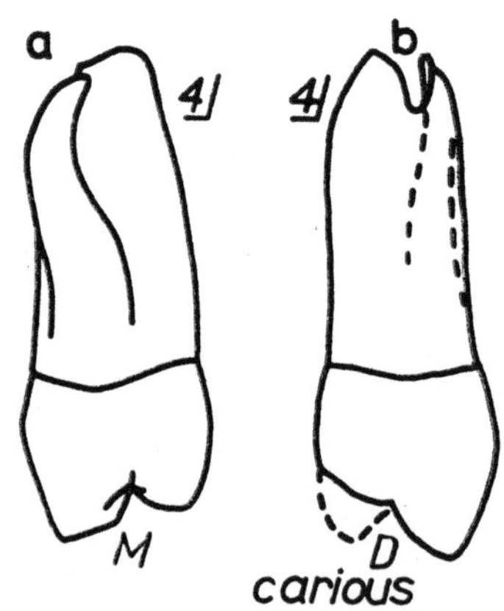

Figure 2-18. Two "three-rooted" upper premolars showing "fusion" of palatal and disto-buccal root branches as is often found in upper molars, both deciduous and permanent. There were four such cases, two like *a* with complete fusion and two like *b* presenting a small cleft separating P from DB element. All were 4|.

a young person. The root was not quite complete, and the single open apex was U-shaped. The single root of this 4 was lightly grooved on M and deeply grooved on B aspect as for two buccal roots. The completed tooth could easily have presented three root canals in a single U-shaped apex.

Having noted the great variety of root forms and root curves in upper premolars, what is the significance of the knowledge?

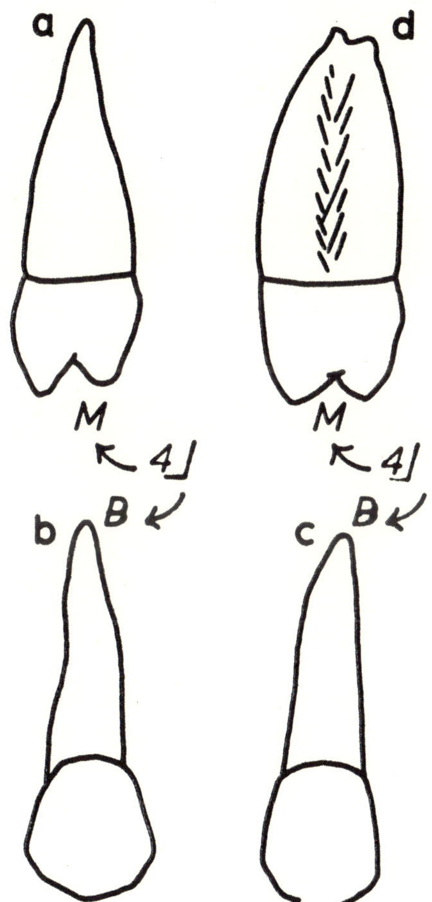

Figure 2-19. Contrasts in root taper. Two 4| with roots similar in buccal view, *b* and *c,* as regards length and thickness, but completely different when the single roots are viewed from proximal as in *a* and *d.* Tooth *cd* is deeply grooved on M and one mm wider at cervix B-P, but both teeth are the same length. See also Figure 2-20, tooth *ab.*

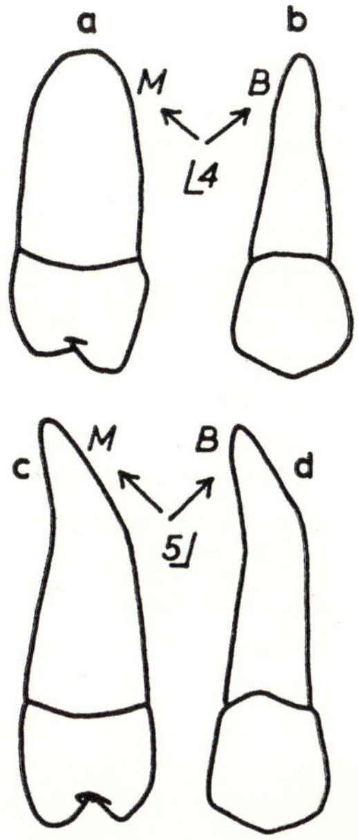

Figure 2-20. Another contrast in root form. In buccal view teeth *b* and *d* are comparable in thickness of root, but in proximal view, *a* and *c,* one is relatively short and very blunt while the other is long and tapers to a fine apex.

For the dental operator contemplating pulp surgery it is necessary to proceed cautiously. Obviously the older methods involving mechanical clearance of root canals are doomed to failure in many cases. Where extraction is necessary it is equally wise to be cautious, especially with first premolars. An aid to diagnosis of form of root or pulp canals is of course provided by X-rays, but there are many cases where the information obtainable from the radiograph is very limited, and in some cases a correct reading of the film is almost impossible. Thus if the root curves in the same plane as that in which the X-rays are projected, the image should appear straight; but a further distortion may result if the film itself is curved to fit the palate. The unrecognized curvature is a factor that may lead to failure in root canal work, or to fracture during extraction. Similarly the image of two root canals or of two root branches may be superposed so that only one is assumed to be present. In another case it may be overlooked that the image has not distinguished between a single root that has two canals and one that is actually bifid. The bifid root of course is more likely to fracture during extraction and leave an apex that is difficult to recover, especially if the radiograph indicates that it may be closely related to the maxillary sinus. Study of partial division of roots shows that a short separate apex may break off and remain *in situ,* leaving the operator unaware that the root was bifid. The tooth with a single root, especially if it is fine, may leave the operator unaware of a fractured apex, or faced with similar difficulty in recovery. Obviously the extracted tooth or major fragment should be carefully inspected immediately after it is removed. If there is any doubt it should be washed to facilitate examination. The writer removed an $\underline{|4}$ which appeared to have two roots, but closer examination after washing the tooth established that the buccal root was bifid and that one small apical fragment was missing. This was located *in situ* and recovered. The tooth is mounted on card E26 in the collection supporting this study.

As root division is into B and P branches, rather than mesial and distal, the widest dimension of the root is nearly always B-P. Variation is considerable in this direction, especially in the apical portion. It follows therefore that variation in shape of apex, particularly in a single-rooted tooth, will occur mainly in the B-P dimension, and of course this is the dimension in which we are given least information in the radiograph. When the image of the apex is relatively wide or rounded it is to be expected that the apex will be fairly solid in the B-P dimension also, but apart from a clear outline we may have to obtain such information as we can from variation in density of the root image from cervix to apex.

Root Taper and Shape of Apex

These characters might at first seem to be closely related in that the more the root tapers the sharper will be the apex. But this feature is not so easily dealt with. A root that is much flattened on M and D could present a wide or blunt apex from proximal view but be fine or sharp when seen from B or P. In Figure 2-19 *a,d* are shown two teeth, each being $\underline{4|}$. They are of equal length and both have single roots. From proximal aspect the roots are quite different, but when viewed from B, the root widths and taper are almost identical (Fig. 2-19 *b,c*). Another single-rooted $\underline{4}$ is shown in Figure 2-20 *a,b*. It has a very rounded blunt apex in proximal view, but is almost identical in B view with the two teeth of Figure 2-19. In the same Figure 2-20 *(c,d)* is shown a single-rooted premolar, this time $\underline{5|}$. This tooth is larger both in crown and in length of root. The root is rather thick in B view *(d),* but in proximal view *(c)* it tapers to a relatively fine apex. From these differences and the demonstration that the B view of a root is no guide to the B-P width there arises a practical point already indicated, namely that the density of the X-ray record of the root apex should be carefully compared with the record of the rest of the root. This may give a clue to root thickness or taper (B-P), useful information where surgery is involved. In general it can thus be expected that a single root which tapers to a thin or pointed apex in proximal view will present an image on the film that fades from cervix to apex. Some of the variable factors that may upset this generalization are (a) the direction of the X-rays in regard to tooth axis and film, (b) their direction in relation to frontal, sagittal and horizontal planes of the skull, (c) bends in tooth root and (d) twist in tooth root. Apart from such variables, a clear even image from cervix to apex is likely to indicate a more sturdy root. In Figure

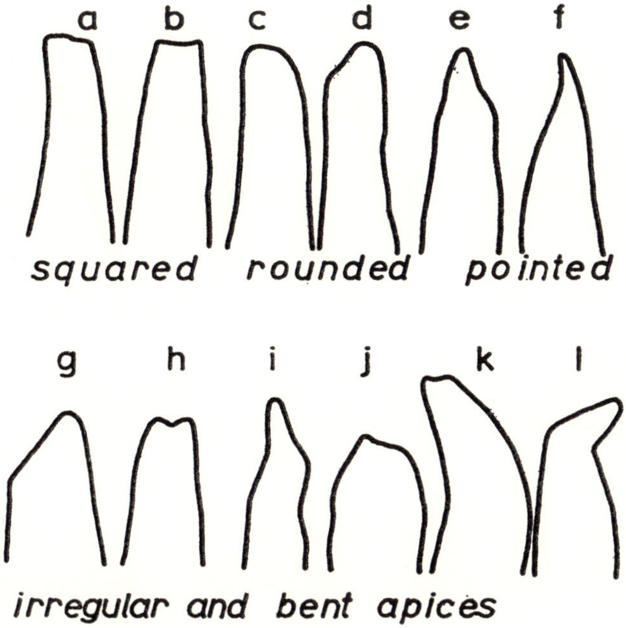

Figure 2-21. Proximal views of a variety of shapes of roots and apices of single-rooted upper premolars. In each case the outline terminates at the cervix.

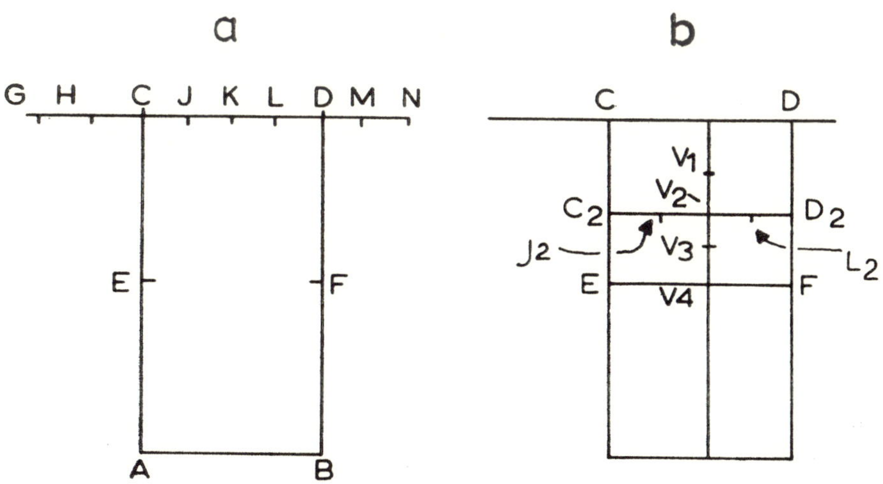

Figure 2-22. Scheme for analysis of root form whereby taper and curvature or bending is represented by a diagram of straight lines. See p. 60. *a,* a rectangle erected on the cervical base line AB, and showing the main points to and from which the lines are drawn. This may be used to represent a single root in buccal or proximal view; *b,* method of subdivision of the rectangle to establish additional landmark points. In this way shorter teeth and proximal views of two-rooted teeth may be shown in straight-line diagrams.

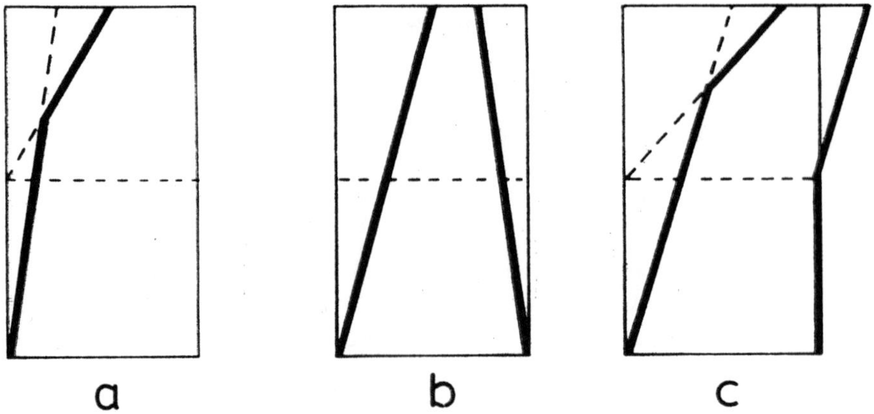

Figure 2-23. Method of using the rectangle and straight lines to represent root shape in straight-line diagrams. *a,* the representation of taper and root bend for one side of the root outline; *b,* representation of a straight, tapering root that appears to lean slightly to one side; *c,* a root that both leans and bends.

2-21 in proximal view is shown a variety of shapes of root and apex. In each case the outline is drawn to end at the cervix of the tooth.

These comments and diagrams have referred to single-rooted premolars. Variations in taper and apex just described were also found in two-rooted upper premolars. As with root curvature, so also with root taper and form of apex, the presence of an extra root branch adds to the variations that may be found. Unlike the two-rooted variations in lower canines and lower first premolars, the two roots of an upper premolar were seldom appreciably different in length or thickness. A few such cases in the present collection have already been referred to (Fig. 2-17).

The variety found in roots of upper premolars is so great that exact description or classification is not possible. There are some obvious major characters such as length, breadth (in two directions), thickness throughout the root and taper of sides to sharp or blunt apex. Single or divided root and root curves or bends are

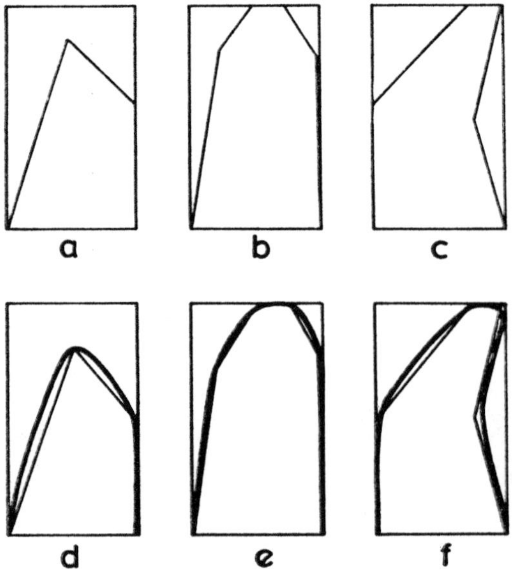

Figure 2-24. Relation of the straight-line diagram to the root outline. *a* and *d,* a short thick root with a sharp asymmetrical apex; *b* and *e,* a broad and slightly tapering root with a rounded apex; *c* and *f,* an unevenly tapering root with a reverse bend in the apical half.

other main characters. However, a study of specimens soon convinces us that there are many degrees in almost every character, and many possible combinations of different characters. For example, a root may be curved after a straight portion has been formed and may curve in more than one direction, or curve gently or bend abruptly; again, a single root may present a groove that is shallow or deep (or both, in different parts); root division may affect a considerable portion or a small apical portion of the root; root branches may lie close together straight or curved, or diverge straight or curved, and so on. The bewildering variety may account for the brief and inadequate descriptions in textbooks. The problem will be approached with due caution and an analysis and classification of these variations will be attempted here.

The author's method is to visualize the root outline as composed of straight lines and to select or present the principal lines. These are related to the sides of a rectangle. The same plan is used for buccal view as for proximal view, except that the buccal view is based on a more narrow rectangle, and does not include the palatal root in multi-rooted teeth. Certain points on or within the rectangle are assumed to be centres on which radii may pivot to form angles, and these permit the representation of taper, bend or curve. The short sides of the rectangle represent the root diameter of the cervix and the apical end of the root. The long sides of the rectangle rep-

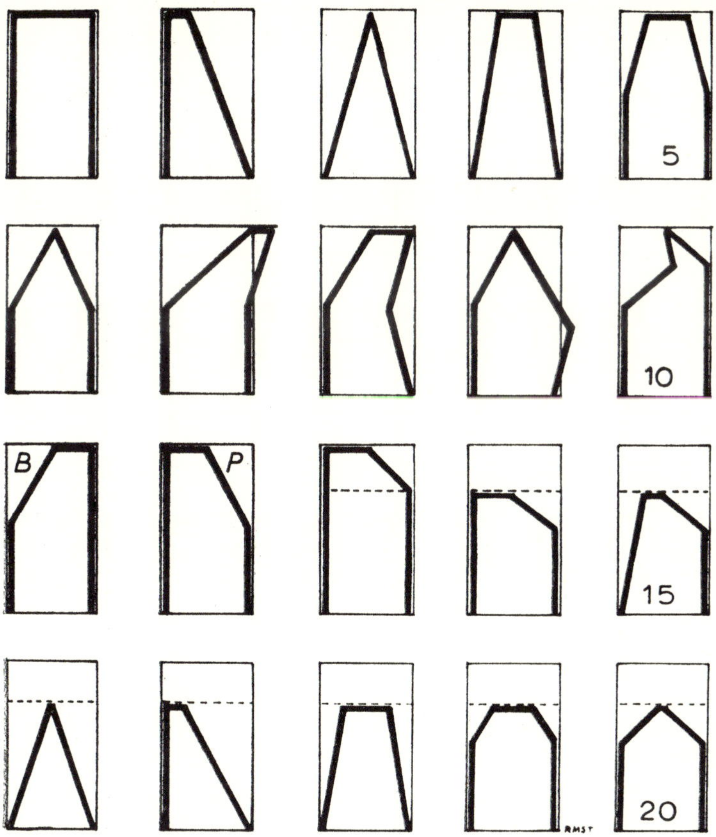

Figure 2-25. Variation in root form shown by diagrams. These are proximal views representing actual specimens of single-rooted upper premolars.

resent root length and may be shortened to represent short teeth.

Such a working rectangle is shown in Figure 2-22 *a* where AB is the cervical line and CD is the apical line. The line CD is divided into four equal parts and the extensions are marked at intervals equal to those fourths. Working from C, the divisions at J, K, L, D, M, N are ¼, ½, ¾, Unit, 1¼, 1½ respectively while H and G are −¼, and −½. Working from D, C is Unit and H or M are 1¼ or −¼. A "long external radius" always starts from the cervix and pivots on A or B, while a "short external radius" pivots on E or F which are approximately the mid-points of AC and BD. The radii are always drawn to one of the points on line GN and make angles such as CAJ or CEJ which are called "quarter angles" (although unequal to one another). A radius falling along the side of the rectangle makes a "nil" angle, and a radius that falls outside the rectangle makes a "minus" angle unless the radius has already passed across the rectangle when it could make a 1¼ angle, for example, in an abruptly bent root.

Figure 2-22 *b* shows how the basic rectangle and some pivot points for radii may be modified to facilitate representation of a much greater variety of root forms. The half rectangle EFDC is divided to give the points V_1 to V_4, which are the pivots for the internal radii which are used to represent the "cleft," so that V is the actual point of bifurcation of the root. Point V therefore may be used in representing a proximal view of a two-rooted premolar (Fig. 2-26), or the buccal view of a three-rooted premolar (Fig. 2-27, bottom row). The depth of the cleft may be varied by use of the quarters at V_1, V_2, V_3, V_4, and

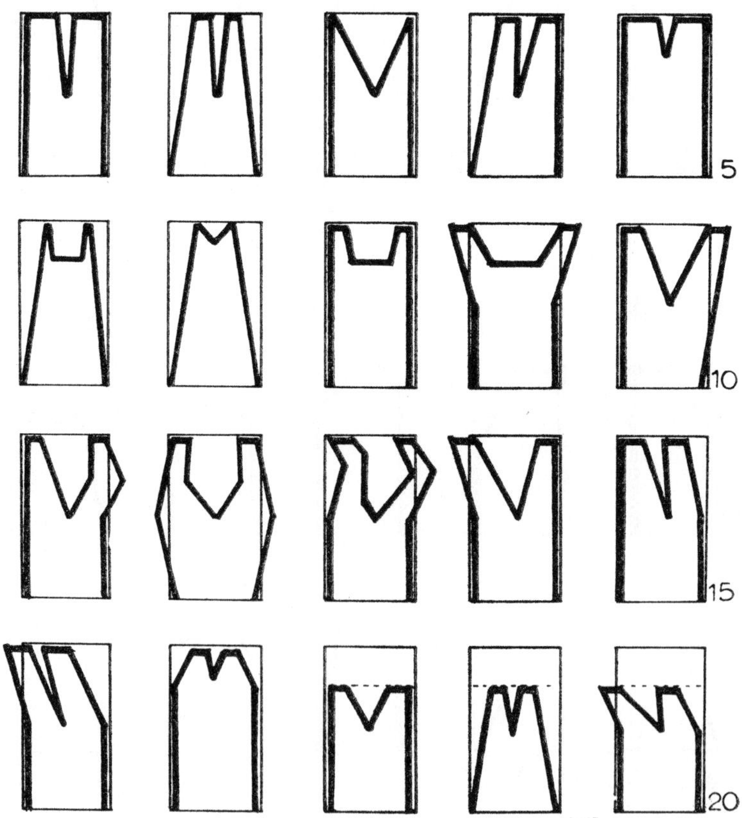

the width varied by use of such points as J_2. The length of the root may be similarly reduced by placing the apical line at C_2D_2 etc. Thus a long tooth with a shallow cleft could have its apical line at CD and its cleft point at V_1; a short tooth with a deep cleft may use the apical line C_2D_2 and cleft point V_4, and so on.

In Figure 2-23 are three rectangles with lines drawn to illustrate the method. In *a* the line is described as "long external radius with angle ¼ and short external radius, angle ½." In *b* it is "one long external radius, angle ½, plus one long external radius, angle ¼." In *c* we have "one long external radius, angle ½, short external radius, angle ¾; the other long radius, angle nil, short radius, angle minus ¼." Diagram *b* indicates a fairly strongly tapering straight root but leaning to one side, and apex medium sharpness. Diagram *c* indicates a root bending rather strongly. These diagrams could represent buccal view of a single- or two-rooted, or proximal view of a single-rooted premolar. Such identification and direction of bend are easily added. A few modifications easily applied to the basic rectangle are illustrated in Figure 2-24. In diagram *a* the rectangle is shortened at the expense of short radii and the form shown is "one long external radius, angle ½, no short radius; other long external radius, angle nil, and short external radius, angle ½." In diagram *b* the long radii are increased at the expense of short radii, and the form is "one long radius ¼ with short radius ½; other long radius, angle nil, short radius, angle ¼." Diagram *c* shows a reversed short radius—"one long radius, angle nil, short radius, angle ¾; other long radius, angle ½, short radius reversed pivot with angle ½." In describing *b* and *c* the adjective "external" applied to long and short radii has been omitted. It

---

←

Figure 2-26. Variation in root form as shown by diagrams. These diagrams represent proximal views of *two-rooted* upper premolars. Main characters of the twenty variations represented are as follows:

Variety No.	*Main Characters*
1.	Profile tapers little, cleft narrow, apices thick or blunt.
2.	Profile tapers evenly, cleft narrow, apices fine.
3.	Profile tapers little, cleft wide, apices fine.
4.	Profile tapers more on one side, cleft narrow, apices medium.
5.	Profile tapers little, cleft short and narrow, apices blunt.
6.	Profile tapers evenly, cleft short and wide U-shape, apices fine.
7.	Profile tapers evenly, cleft short and wide V-shape, apices fine.
8.	Profile tapers little, cleft short wide U-shape, apices fine.
9.	Profile tapers little on root trunk, cleft wide and short, root-branches widely divergent, apices medium.
10.	Profile hardly tapers, cleft wide V-shape, one root branch divergent, apices medium.
11.	Similar to No. 10, but divergent root branch recurves.
12.	Profile divergent in root trunk, cleft prominent, both branches divergent, then recurve.
13.	Trunk profile hardly tapers, cleft prominent, both branches bend to same side, then recurve to other side.
14.	Trunk profile hardly tapers, cleft prominent, one branch straight, other branch divergent, apices strong.
15.	As with No. 14 but instead of diverging, one branch recurves.
16.	Profile of trunk as for No. 15, both branches bend to same side so that cleft is narrow.
17.	Profile long straight trunk hardly tapers. Root branches short and strongly tapered, cleft short and narrow, apices medium.
18.	Resembles No. 5 but whole root short, cleft wide and short, apices blunt.
19.	Resembles No. 2 but whole root relatively short.
20.	Resembles No. 16 but shortening of root is mostly in branched portion leaving cleft prominent and aspices strong.

is useful for more precise description but is essential only where internal radii also are involved, namely where bifurcation of a root must be described.

Figure 2-25 presents a series of such diagrams illustrating some of the varieties of root form in the present material. These are proximal views of single-rooted premolars. In general, where a diagram could have a mirror image, examples in right and left teeth have been recorded together. So also for buccal and palatal, but to illustrate this point varieties 11 and 12 represent one pair of mirror images, "external long radii, both angles nil; one external short radius, angle ½." In Figure 2-26 a corresponding set of diagrams represents proximal views of two-rooted upper premolars.

It now remains to illustrate buccal views of upper premolars. Only the buccal root is recorded and it will be remembered that buccal roots may present all stages from grooving to division into two separate branches. Any of these together with the single buccal root of a two-rooted tooth and the buccal aspect of a single-rooted tooth, may be represented in one set of diagrams with slight extension of detail in the method. This has been done in Figure 2-27.

The convergence of corresponding radii indicates tapering of the root. If taper appears to be bilaterally uneven it may

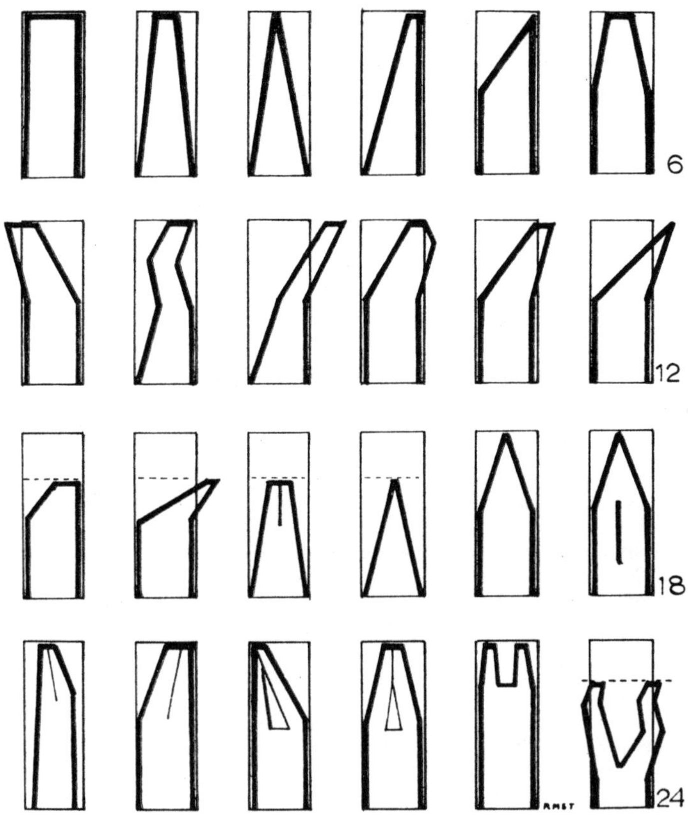

Figure 2-27. Variation in root form shown by diagrams. These are buccal views of buccal roots of actual specimens of upper premolars and include teeth with one, two or three root branches.

give the effect of leaning of the root to M or D as in Figure 2-27, No. 4, by contrast with No. 2. If we visualize the axis of the root in such cases it will of course lean or bend as indicated.

DISCUSSION WITH PARTICULAR REFERENCE TO ROOTS OF UPPER PREMOLARS

It is sometimes said that information on certain studies is unacceptable unless it has been expressed in mathematical terms. A study of teeth for example, particularly of variation in teeth, might be expected to be based on measurements and to be reported statistically giving coefficients of variability and indications of the significance of certain results. But when the nature of some such material is examined, one may well question whether statistics based on certain measurements do in fact have value or significance.

While engaged in a study of skulls and palates the writer became aware of difficulties involved in measurements of anatomical material where data were sought for comparative purposes (Taylor 1962a, b, c) and examination of teeth confirmed the very limited number of measurements that may be made.

It is believed that the present study does provide useful information, over a wide range, in spite of its essentially qualitative methods. The reason for the virtual rejection here of a metrical approach therefore is that important morphological features and characters in teeth vary in ways that preclude their analysis by measurement.

The fact that there is variation in roots of upper premolars is well known and comments most often refer to the size of the root, whether it is curved and whether it is single or divided. Our study shows that plain statements about these characters give very little information; all of them, and other characters also, may present so much variety that more detail is essential in description. Thus, with regard to size, a root may be large or small as compared with other premolars, or when compared with the size of its crown, so that it may be large without being actually long. Again, the root may be described as large because it is long. And yet again, a root may be quite long but not really large if it happens to be a slender root (Fig. 2-2 *c*).

We find also that such characters as slenderness or robustness are not necessarily a matter of measurement as between teeth, but may be terms that are applicable when we change our viewpoint. It was shown for example that two roots may be very similar in buccal view and quite different in proximal view (Fig. 2-19). Are these roots respectively slender and robust, or thin and thick, or narrow and wide? It requires several adjectives related to size therefore to give even an approximate description of a root in this respect, and how might these roots be measured in a way that would record their different forms?

The character of root division adds many difficulties to the analysis of variation because there are not only many varieties of division as regards direction of root branches, but also degrees of division as regards the position of the bifurcation or the width or depth of grooves. Grooves are often closely related to the characters of slenderness or robustness of roots, and some single but grooved roots cannot be excluded from a study of root division. There is no more easily definable borderline between single and divided roots than there is between slender and robust roots.

Analysis of root division is complicated by its obvious lack of relationship to characters of root size, and it inevitably involves description of divergence or otherwise of root branches. But root curvatures or bends are by no means confined to divided roots and may be found in the root trunk as well as root branches. The roots that are single but not straight present in themselves ample scope for study of variation, and root division extends that scope considerably. A study of nonstraight roots would be very complicated even if changes in direction were confined to one viewpoint. But they cannot be so confined even to facilitate description, for it must be accepted that they may in fact involve several directions; and so also may the branches of a divided root. An analysis of root bends and curves alone could therefore involve a really infinite number of variations. Metrical studies of material with such characters are not feasible.

One might well search for a definition of a straight root and then conclude that there is no such root. Impressions of straightness are closely concerned with root taper, and taper is an important factor in both root thickness or slenderness and in the bluntness or sharpness of the apex. In buccal or proximal view the amount of taper may not be the same on each profile and so it may give an impression of root bend. But along any root profile the amount of taper may vary in different regions, giving some degree of curvature to the outline. This use of the word "curvature" implies something different from that usually implied by the term "root-curvature"; but as a change in root profile is involved, it may be a factor influencing an assessment of root curvature.

Here again it is evident that measurement has no place, but descriptive analysis fairly adequately presents the wide range of variation. This is a picture of things as they are, and shows that no set of measurements, statistical symbol of variation, or illustrated specimen claimed as average, or as typical of these teeth, has any relation to reality. This conclusion is evident from a study of the root alone; the added complexity when the tooth crown is included in the study will merely add emphasis.

CROWNS OF UPPER PREMOLARS

If one were asked to identify a tooth root without a crown, the root of a single-rooted premolar might often be confused with that of some other tooth. Much less

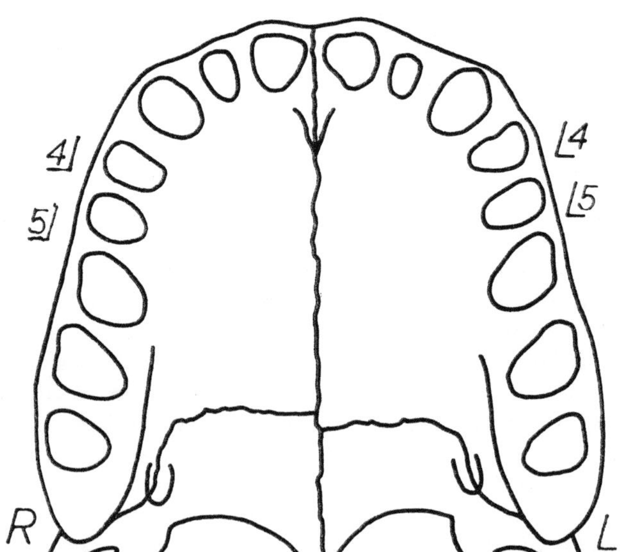

Figure 2-28. Diagram of human palate with socket outlines of permanent teeth. The appropriate symbol for each upper premolar is shown alongside its own position in the dental arch (Appendix 1). Ability to visualize this diagram (and its counterpart for the lower dental arch in the U position) is of great assistance in orientation or identification of an isolated tooth.

difficulty arises with crowns, for the crown of an upper premolar, even without its root, is seldom likely to be confused with the crown of any other tooth. Further, it should be possible to identify the crown as a first or second premolar and from left or right side. The author has found identification facilitated by visualizing a tooth's orientation in relation to a jaw, or diagram of a jaw such as in Figure 2-28. This will be referred to later, but it serves here to emphasize that each individual tooth in the dentition has characters that tend to differentiate it from any other. Each kind of tooth has what may be regarded as its group characters. For upper premolars these are the two cusps placed buccal and lingual, and so constantly present as to justify the alternative term bicuspid. Associated with these main group characters are the relative size of the cusps and the convexity of surfaces and outlines. Variations in these give some of the individual characters to first and second, and to left and right upper premolars (Figs. 2-29, 2-30, 2-31). These, and other characters such as ridges, grooves, cusp slopes, profiles, angles and cusp acumination, are the subject of this analysis of variation in crowns of upper premolars. Attention may be drawn to variation in actual size or shape or curvature, or some of these qualities may be compared in relation to other features in the same tooth, such as proportionate dimensions in the crown and its own root. It may then be shown that these features

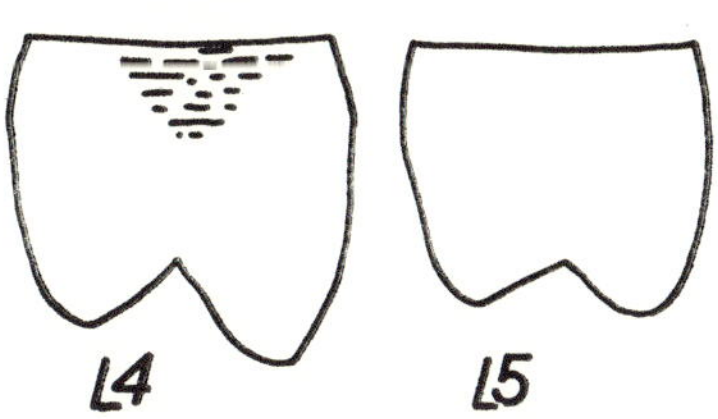

Figure 2-29. Differentiation between the crowns of upper first, |4 and second, |5 premolars. Mesial views of teeth from the left side. In |4 the buccal cusp is noticeably longer, and there is a concavity at the mesial cervix (shaded).

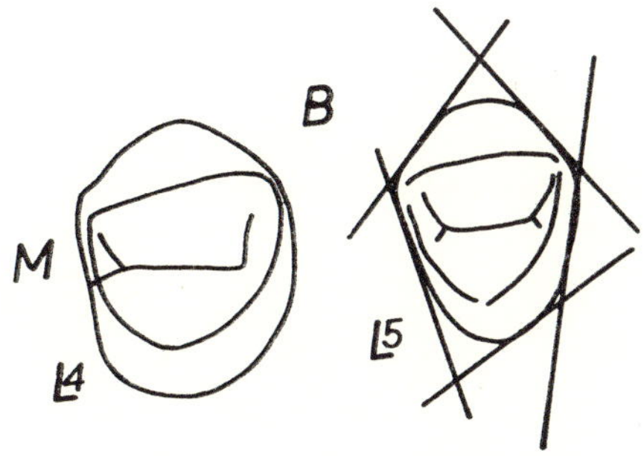

Figure 2-30. Differentiation between upper first and second premolars seen from occlusal aspect.

bear a different relation to one another in other teeth of the same kind.

Thus when commencing the study of roots it was observed that there were large and small roots not only in the sense that they varied in length from cervix to apex, or in thickness, but also in length or thickness compared with those dimensions in the crowns of the same teeth (Figs. 2-1 and 2-2). From the standpoint of the crown some of these variations will be looked at again, and others related to the crowns only will be viewed also.

Three contrasting teeth are shown in Figure 2-32. The tooth with the smallest crown has the longest root and the narrowest B-P in actual measurement. In this tooth the B-P measurement is the same in crown and root, and from the small size of the crown the relatively large root might not be expected by the operator who had to extract it. Such a possibility should be remembered. The first tooth would certainly be difficult to extract, for its sturdy root is even wider B-P than the crown, and this could easily be missed in the X-ray. The third tooth has a root that is narrower than the crown, relatively short and sturdy, and it should have been easy to extract. In this tooth the contours of the crown are more noticeably convex than usual, but in the tooth with the small crown those contours are unusually flattened.

Turning now to M-D diameters of crowns and roots it is easy to find teeth presenting much variation in this propor-

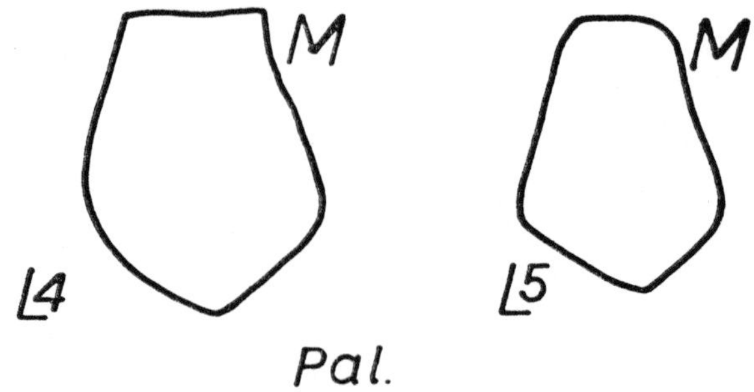

Figure 2-31. Differentiation between upper first and second premolars by outlines of crowns in palatal view.

tion also. In Figure 2-33 *a,b,* the crown of the first tooth is wide relative to the root, and in the other it is narrow.

Again, using M-D diameter of crown as a basis of comparison we find this varies not only in its relation to the M-D diameter of the root at the cervix but also to the length of the root. In Figure 2-33 *c,d* are two upper first premolars of approximately equal M-D diameter of crown. The much shorter root is bifid, and thicker M-D at the cervix. These four crowns in buccal view have little in common regarding details of outline form, or in length—breadth relations, or in these proportions compared with those of their roots.

An upper premolar which is narrow M-D at the cervix presents difficulties to the operator. If a class II cavity is prepared it is more difficult to do good work because of the smaller thickness of dentine to work in, and the filling itself as well as the restored tooth may be less resistant to stress on these teeth. As reduction in this cervical dimension implies a similarly narrow root, the risk of fracture during extraction is greater, and even more so in a bifid root, each branch of which will tend to be slender even if reasonably straight. Narrowness at the cervix, therefore, is a character that may well be looked for in a radiograph when operative work is to be undertaken.

Crown Profiles

One can usually visualize a point which may be called the cusp tip. In proximal views of upper premolars the cervical diameter is greater than the distance between the two cusp tips (in a direction parallel to the two cervical points) because of the curvature of the B and P outlines. Figure 2-34 is a diagrammatic representation of the mesial view of an upper right first premolar, with the outline drawn first in the normal manner and then as a series of straight lines meeting at various angles. It is easy to visualize curved outlines as made up of a number of adjacent arcs. The arcs may be of different length of radius as well as having different centres. In the

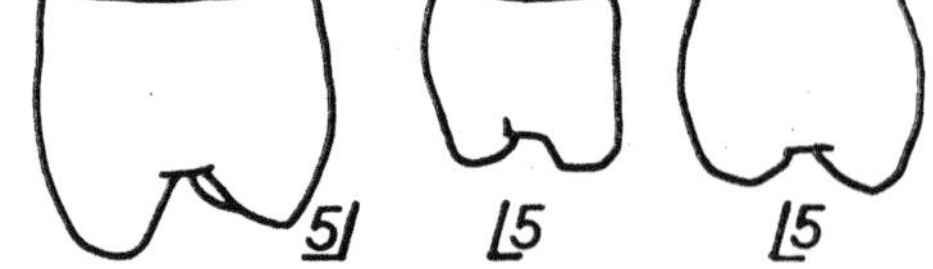

Figure 2-32. Variety in size and shape of crown and root, and in crown size relative to root size in upper second premolars.

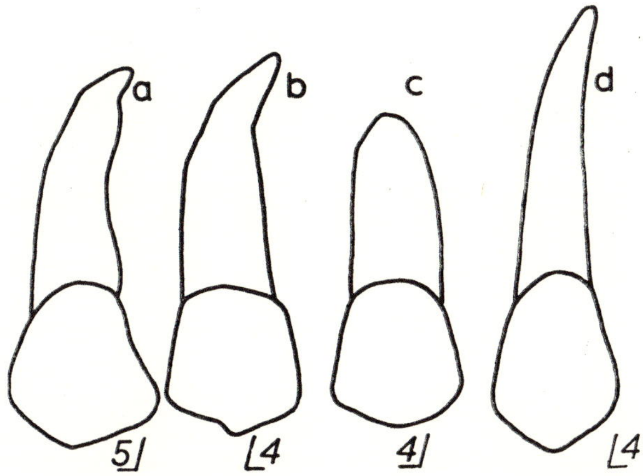

Figure 2-33. *a* and *b*, comparing M-D dimension; crown *a* is wide compared with thickness of root, and the reverse is the case in tooth *b*. Convexity of crown outlines also is a contrast. Using M-D dimension again as basis of comparison, root *c* is very short and sturdy, while root *d* is long and slender.

diagram the principal arcs are represented by their chords, and CL, the cervical line, is the baseline. Cusp tips become definite points, such as B for the buccal cusp. Through B is drawn a line AD parallel to CL, and perpendiculars are drawn through B and the shorter palatal cusp to cut CL at b and p. The distance pL is greater than bC, because the palatal cusp is nearer than the buccal cusp to the central axis of the tooth, and partly because of the greater convexity of the palatal surface. Perpendiculars through A and D are tangential to the buccal and palatal outlines, and

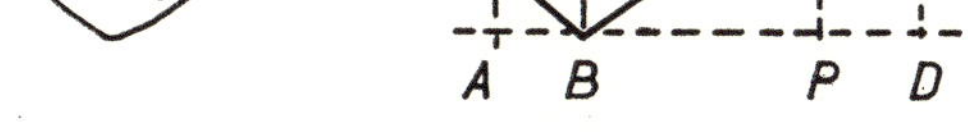

Figure 2-34. Diagrammatic representation of proximal view of upper premolar to facilitate study of convexities and of relation of cusp tips to B and P surfaces.

make contact with these outlines at different distances from the line CL produced.

Let us imagine a series of transverse (approximately horizontal) sections through the crown and root of a single-rooted upper premolar. These will be somewhat oval in outline and we can accept that the outlines will have a short and long axis, or a minor and a major axis, and these will correspond to the M-D and B-P "diameters" at the levels of the transverse sections referred to. The short axis in each case will be nearer to buccal than to palatal surfaces. Neither of the axes will be of similar length to those of an adjacent section, nor will the lengths of the two axes be likely to bear a constant ratio to one another, particularly in sections through the crown. The section with the longest major axis will be nearer to the cervix than the section with the longest minor axis. This last section will pass through one, if not both, of the contact points and will be fairly close to the shoulders of the buccal cusp on the cervical side of the mesial and distal marginal ridges of the occlusal surface.

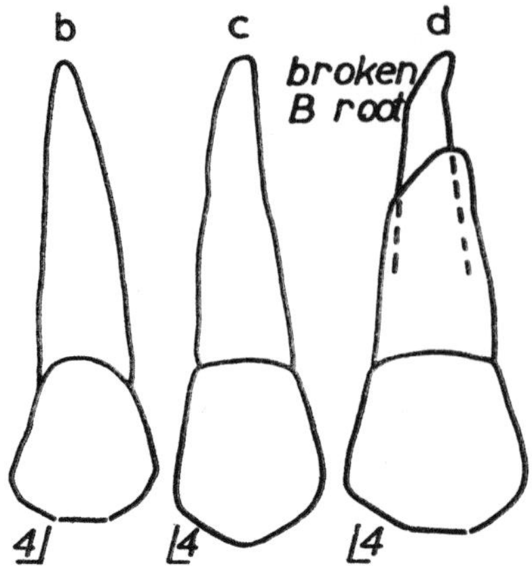

Figure 2-35. Relative size of crown and root. Three upper first premolars with roots of similar length but with considerable differences in length and breadth of crowns as seen from buccal.

Appreciation of form has been made easier by visualizing its relation to geometrical figures, either imaginary or in diagrammatic form. In this way attention is easily drawn to deviation from a regular figure and to asymmetry. Bilateral symmetry in nature, including tooth form, although it may be closely approached in some cases, is seldom if ever achieved in fact, if one is strictly accurate in comparison. This use of diagrams with straight lines and angles, or arcs of different radius to represent curvature, was developed by the present writer when teaching dental anatomy to New Zealand Student School Dental Nurses in Wellington, commencing in 1930. The author's original diagrams have been used in similar training courses in other countries and some are used in the present work.

Crown and Root Axes

In Figure 2-34 one may visualize a central axis of the crown as intersecting CL at right angles. In the case of a single-rooted premolar, whether the root be straight or curved, this axis may be visualized as extending through the centre of the root, following such curve as may be present but not necessarily passing through the apex or its foramen, which would often lie to the buccal side of the central axis. In a two- or three-rooted tooth it may be difficult or impossible to visualize such an axis beyond the furcation.

Another hypothetical axis, useful for descriptive purposes, might for convenience be called the geometrical axis. This would be visualized as passing through the intersections of the major and minor axes of the infinite number of transverse sections mentioned above. In the root portion of the tooth this conception would meet difficulties similar to the central axis in multi-rooted teeth. This axis would be to the buccal side of the central axis and in

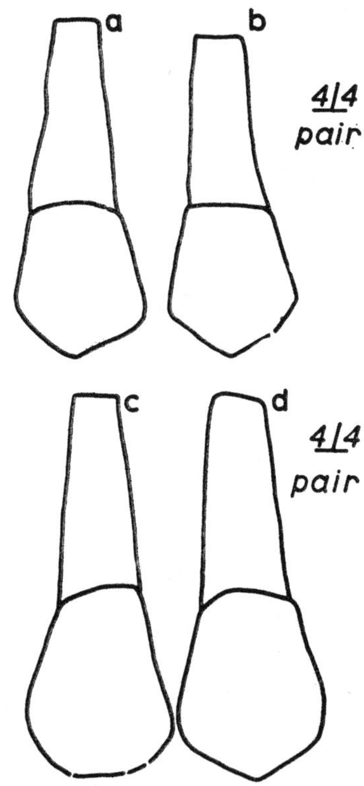

Figure 2-36. Two pairs of upper first premolars from young persons. One pair relatively straight-sided and the other pair larger and more rounded. These contrasts in curvature are not so readily discernible in proximal or occlusal views. (See Fig. 2-37.)

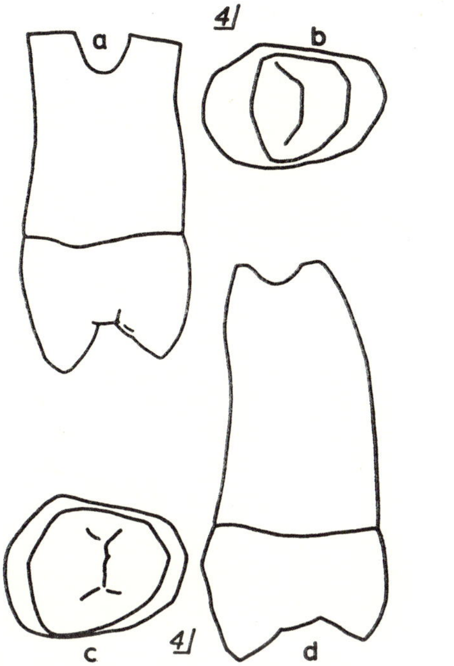

Figure 2-37. Comparison of curvature in crowns of teeth of Figure 2-36 *a* and *c*. Both teeth are the same in B-P dimension at cervix, but the distance between cusp tips differs considerably, being greater in *d*. As a result, the occlusal surface proper covers a relatively larger area of the occlusal view outline in *c* than in *b*.

the diagram would pass through or close to the contact point (Fig. 2-34, point x). It would not pass through point B; in fact it would terminate just beyond point x in a transverse section which was not cut by the occlusal groove.

As the mesial and distal contact points may be at different distances from the cervix, both the contact point and the geometrical axis are much more easily visualized for a proximal view, or diagram, of the tooth than for the actual tooth. Herein lies the usefulness of these visualized points, sections and axes: In trying to define their limitations and relationships one must have a clear concept of the very irregular three-dimensional body being described; then the ways in which details vary are more easily grasped. They are difficult to describe because there are no constants in any dimension or ratio to which they may be related. Similarly, the straight lines and angles, arcs of different radius, and geometrical figures to which shapes and outlines are likened, all assist in creating the image of the actual tooth form and the approximate nature and range of variation.

In Figure 2-33 were shown four teeth, all different in crown size and shape, and in root length and thickness. In Figure 2-35 are three first premolars with roots of similar length but crowns of different size, mostly in the M-D dimension.

In Figure 2-36 are two pairs of first premolars taken from children (roots not complete). In each case the crowns are large, especially *c* and *d*, but in buccal view the outlines differ; the first pair are relatively straight-sided and irregularly pentagonal while the second pair are much more rounded. Such contrast in curvature is not discernible in proximal or occlusal view (Fig. 2-37, where *a* and *b* are of tooth *a* in Fig. 2-36, and *c* and *d* are of tooth *c*). These views do, however, show a consider-

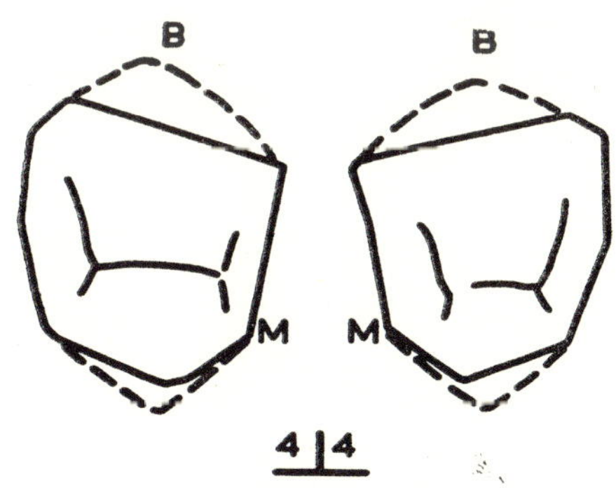

Figure 2-38. "Straight-line" drawings of the occlusal views of the lower pair of first premolars shown in Figure 2-36 *c,d*. The relation of occlusal surface (continuous outline) to occlusal view outline (broken lines) is asymmetrical as far as each tooth is concerned but approximately bilaterally symmetrical when one tooth is compared with the other. Recognition of this character facilitates identification of a tooth as left or right.

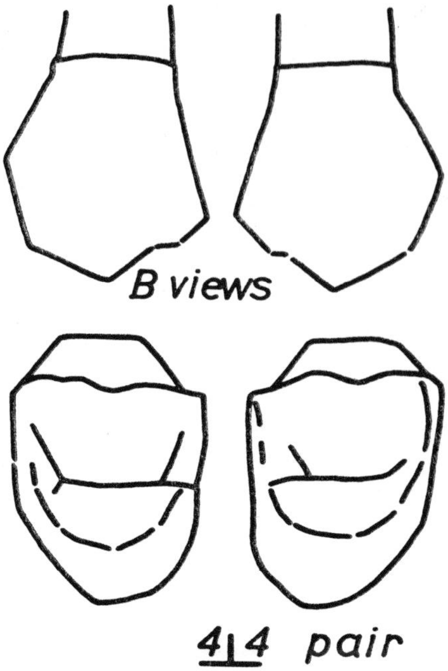

Figure 2-39. A pair of upper first premolars. B views (above) in straight-line drawing, and occlusal views (below) showing the individual asymmetry of each tooth as in Figure 2-38.

able difference between the two teeth. Although each is the same width at the cervix, the tooth of the second child has a greater distance between cusps and a larger occlusal surface. There are, of course, visible differences in these outlines to correspond, but it is emphasized that the differences are not of the degree of straightness or roundness as was seen in the buccal views.

The large occlusal surfaces of this second pair give an opportunity to see more clearly the differences between left and right. In Figure 2-38 such differences are shown by straight-line diagrams. The continuous lines represent marginal ridges and main cusp ridges enclosing occlusal surfaces (and also occlusal grooves). Broken lines represent the outline of the occlusal view of the crown. The occlusal surfaces are wider towards the distal. The distal portion occludes with the lower second premolar which is wider than the lower first premolar.

Another pair of large upper first premolars presented almost identical dimensions of major and minor diameters of crown and cervix, as the second pair in Figure 2-36. This third pair is slightly

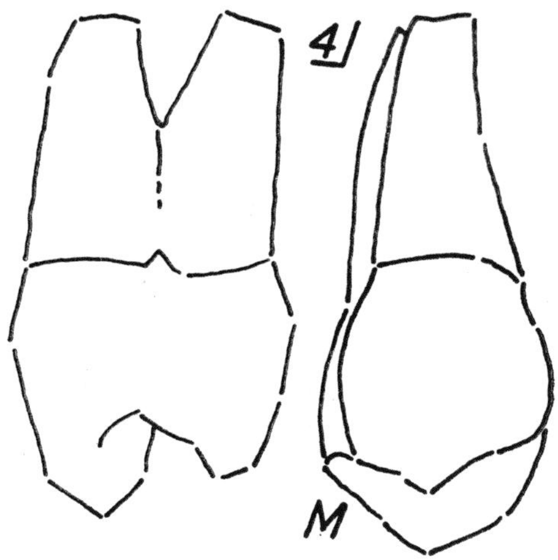

Figure 2-40. The upper right first premolar of Figure 2-39 in M and P views. In proximal view the "fosse" angle is that formed by the medial occlusal profiles of each cusp, from cusp tip to medial occlusal groove. The profiles are curved and their junction is often hidden by the marginal ridge (see Fig. 2-41). The root of this tooth is deeply grooved and the cervical enamel enters the groove. In palatal view the palatal cusp is seen to be smaller and the asymmetry which places its cusp tip nearer to M than to D assists in identifying the tooth as left or right.

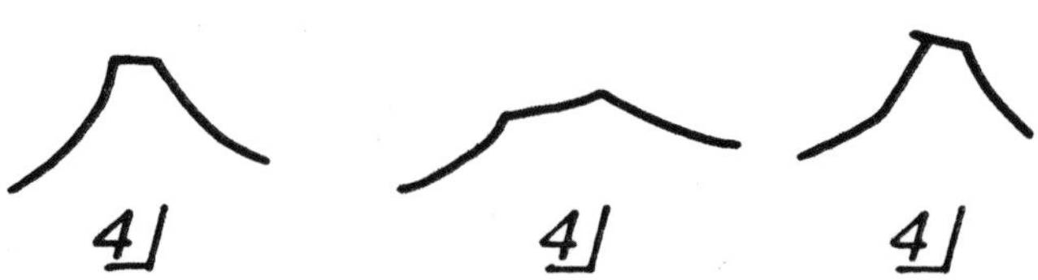

Figure 2-41. Variation in the "fosse" angle. (See Fig. 2-40.)

greater in minor diameter at cervix and has some very rounded outlines. Some features in which they differ strongly from the second pair are: (a) the root bifurcates early into robust branches, (b) the cusp tips are closer together and the occlusal surface is therefore smaller, and (c) the cusps, especially B, are thicker B-P so that the occlusal angle between cusps is less. These teeth are shown in Figures 2-39 and 2-40.

Fosse Angle

This occlusal angle, which I prefer to call the "fosse" angle (as seen in proximal views, Figs. 2-37 and 2-40) depends on several factors such as cusp length and distance between cusps, both of these in relation to crown size; another factor is cusp thickness which is increased in the presence of a ridge ascending from the buccal cusp tip to the central groove or fissure (this is the triangular ridge). Where the angle is much reduced the tooth is somewhat vaguely stated to have a deep fissure. The term "fosse angle" also is a term of convenience rather than of precision for it relates to the meeting of two irregular arcs, the profiles of the occlusal slopes of the two cusps as seen in proximal view. The actual meeting of the arcs to form the central groove is often obscured in proximal view by the marginal ridge.

In Figure 2-41 the fosse angles have been taken from the diagrams of Figures 2-37 and 2-40. It is easy to see what is meant by a narrow fosse angle or a wide one. Also, if the arcs are continued beyond the points where they are cut by the marginal ridge a "deep fissure" is easily visualized in the two outer tracings. It will be seen further that the angle is not satisfactorily represented by straight lines from cusp tips to central groove, for this would eliminate the angle-reducing effect of the cusp-thickening ridge of such teeth as that shown in Figure 2-40.

It has been shown that the fosse angle is not dependent directly on the size of the tooth (see also Figs. 2-8 to 2-20 inclusive).

In the operative treatment of dental caries, cavity design and filling of class I and class II cavities should take account of fosse angles. Where the angle is reduced the cavity margin should be taken further towards the cusp in order to obtain sufficient width for instrumentation and strength in the filling, but without weakening either cusp. The filling should not restore the anatomical fissure but be left as full as possible so that maximum margin strength may be retained. In general, it is more difficult to do good work where the fosse angle is reduced.

The fosse angle here discussed is a particular transverse contour or section of the irregular depression which Black calls a sulcus. In his nomenclature, the sulcus of an upper premolar appears to consist of two fossae, anterior and posterior, "which pass mesio-distally entirely through the occlusal surface" (Black, 1901).

Curvature and Convexity

Figure 2-34 demonstrated the diagrammatic use of straight lines to represent curvature and it was shown that one can easily visualize the curved outline of a tooth as being made up of many chords of arcs which have different centres and different radii. Although the diagrams make use of lines and angles to indicate curvature, the different lengths of line may also draw attention to asymmetry as well as to differences in convexity. A few crown outlines were presented to show certain features and then the method was also applied to root variety. With crowns also both methods of representation are used, straight lines as well as true copies of curvature, to illustrate the features and differences discussed.

The three teeth shown in Figure 2-32 presented clearly recognizable differences in crowns as well as in roots. In Figure 2-42 *a,b,* and *c* are shown the crowns of these teeth as in the previous figure and below in *aa, bb,* and *cc* the same outlines

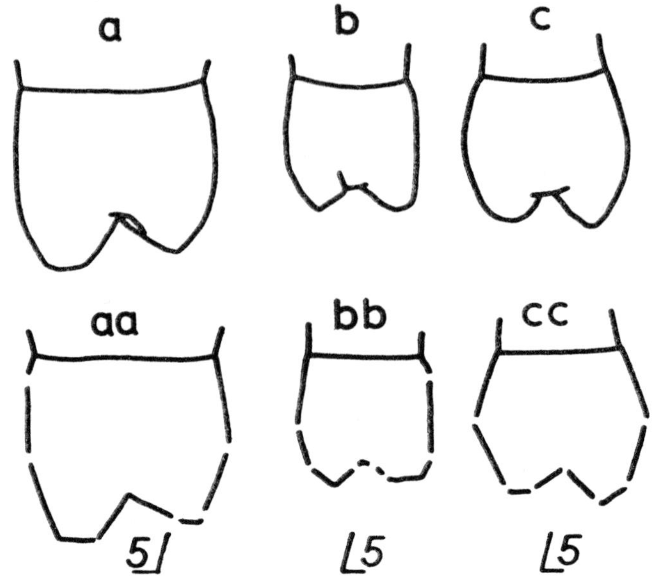

Figure 2-42. Variation in size and convexity of crowns of three second premolars seen from mesial. In *a,b,c* the drawings are conventional but they are re-drawn in *aa, bb* and *cc* in the author's method of straight-line representation. This facilitates appreciation of differences in curvature of outline, acumination of cusps, fosse angles (and other features such as tooth roots, when desired).

are represented in the straight-line style, but without relating the outline to any geometrical figure.

These three crowns present differences in absolute size and in curvature. Crown *a* is large, and *b* is small; this applies both in buccal and proximal views. For relative size of crown to root these three teeth must be described by using another order and set of terms.

Figure 2-43 shows an even greater range in crown size and curvature in nine single-rooted teeth selected from a certain group in the collection. Tooth *c* has a large crown but only moderate-sized root, and the smaller-crowned *d* has a small root which is very narrow in M-D dimension. Tooth *f* has a thick heavy root and the very convex crown is quite short, the cervix curving low on B side, so that the cervix is actually closer to the cusp tip on the B side. The teeth in the middle row present much less curvature. Tooth *g* has a small crown and the occlusal outline has been somewhat flattened by wear of enamel, but tooth *h* is not worn and has a relatively long B cusp. Tooth k_2 has a long crown in both cusps. The last three teeth have small crowns but relatively long roots, especially *n*. All three have unusually straight outlines, and while the greatest B-P diameter is close to the cervix in *l* and *m*, it is widest at the occlusal of *n* and gives this tooth a wide fosse angle in spite of a rather deep central groove.

In another group in the collection (but not figured) are twelve two-rooted upper premolars (two with almost three roots), including several which appear to be second premolars. This group presents a considerable range in many features, length of roots, length of cleft between root branches, size of crowns, crowns short or long relative to width B-P, very convex or straight-sided outlines with varying degrees of convergence to give wide or nar-

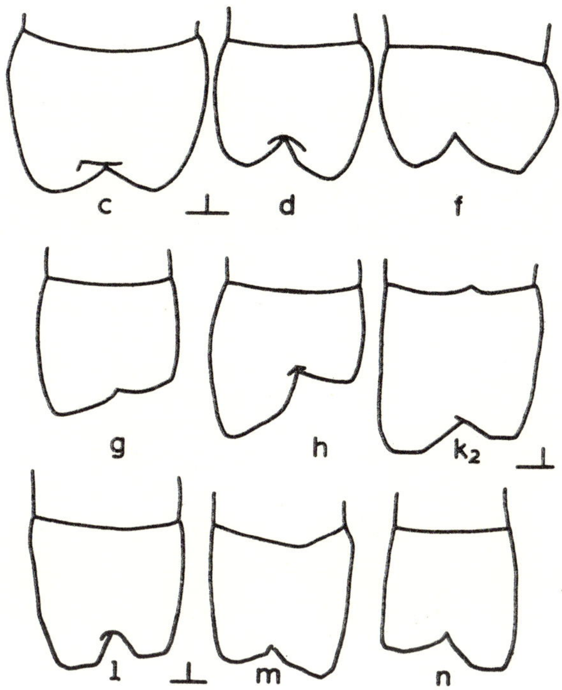

Figure 2-43. Variation in mesial outlines of crowns of nine single-rooted upper premolars.

row fosse angles, varying cusp length, depth of central groove, cusp ridges, relative size of occlusal surfaces and so on (Card E18a). Collectively their variations could present many different problems to the surgeon whether in filling or extraction, and much of interest to the scientist. The fact of wide variation is very apparent already but there are a few more features that will be shown to add further evidence to this theme of variation.

Occlusal Surfaces

If anterior teeth are omitted, one can define the word "occlusal" in general terms as meaning "towards corresponding parts of teeth in the opposite jaw." If occlusal "surface," is specified and defined as that surface facing the corresponding parts of the opposite teeth we have a different conception, and it is more precise because it excludes buccal and lingual surfaces from participation. Those surfaces face the named directions, but portions of them are certainly included in the areas normally involved in the trituration of food. These portions have no particular outline that can be defined, so if it is desired to visualize a particular area that may be defined anatomically, the "occlusal" must not be associated with masticatory function. The occlusal surface may then be defined as that area bounded by ridges passing from cusp tips through the shoulders of the cusps, and meeting those from the opposite cusps in marginal ridges. It is an area sometimes called the "occlusal surface proper" and it is the area which, in operative dentistry, is meant by the term occlusal surface. It is the area the author has in mind when, in dealing with unworn teeth, he refers to the occlusal surface. It is a convenient conception and a convenient term, but it is of limited use in dental anatomy because the defined boundaries lose precision as soon as a cusp tip becomes worn. From this stage onwards, and because the worn surface must be included, the boundary of the occlusal surface now extends on to a buccal or palatal surface, or both. It is suggested that there is justification for the conception of a "functional" occlusal surface which, although it cannot be precisely defined, will include those parts of buccal or lingual surfaces which participate in trituration of food whether tooth substance has been worn away or not.

This functional occlusal surface is unlikely to involve just the same areas in corresponding teeth of different individuals, even in unworn teeth, nor will it necessarily involve exactly similar areas in the corresponding teeth (left and right) of the same individual at the same time. Some of the factors that may account for such differences between individuals are size of teeth, curvature of tooth surfaces, arrangement of teeth (including minor malocclusions and direction of tooth axes) and masticatory habits. These last two factors, arrangement and habits, would apply also to differences in left and right in the same mouth. When wear of tooth surfaces has begun, the effect of some of these factors begins to change and it may become more difficult or even impossible to draw fair conclusions from observed differences. Thus, as more of the crown is worn away, curvature of tooth surfaces may have a decreasing effect, and even be eliminated, as a factor in determination of boundaries of a functional occlusal surface. This was often the case in Maori and Moriori skeletal material the author has examined (Taylor, 1962b,c; 1963a). In those skulls the nature of the food and the masticatory habits and age of the individual had been important factors in the wear of teeth. Extreme stages of wear found in individual teeth or groups of teeth (no doubt complicated sometimes by pathological changes in bone and soft tissues) resulted in changes in position of these and adjacent or opposing teeth and even of teeth on the other side of the mouth. In the studies just referred to, the conditions of dislocation of teeth and fern root planes were described (see also Taylor, 1970c). Some teeth presented one of these conditions, sometimes both were present in the same tooth. The worn areas were certainly part of the functional occlusal surface even though anatomically they might extend obliquely and irregularly beyond the cervix on to the root of the tooth. These are extremes but as they are provided for in the conception of a "functional" occlusal surface the usefulness of that term is emphasized.

So there is the "occlusal surface" of the dental surgeon, a term which can be made more explicit by changing it to the "occlusal surface proper." A larger area, which is not limited by anatomical landmarks, with boundaries that are determined by a number of factors, and which tends to alter as conditions change, is the "functional occlusal surface."

Occlusal Views

A third conception which assists the study of variation is the "occlusal view" and it could be described as those parts of the tooth crown that can normally be seen from a viewpoint lying on the produced long axis of the tooth. Its shape and area will be that of a projection of the crown on to a plane passing through the buccal or lingual cervix, and perpendicular to the long axis of the tooth. It will include within it the projection of the occlusal surface proper on to the same plane, and will usually include also the whole functional occlusal surface. Portions of the functional occlusal surface may not be included under the definition just given, where there is dislocation of teeth and extreme or oblique wear extending beyond the cervix. Examples of such cases, illustrated in Taylor (1963a) are as follows:

(a) Dislocated and worn obliquely—Plate 5, Figures 29 and 31, 6| in each case. Also Plate 10, Figures 55 and 56, lower first molars, and Figure 57, $\overline{6|6}$ in middle specimen.

(b) Excessive wear. Plate 8, Figures 45, 46, 47 and 48, all upper premolars present.

(c) Oblique wear beyond cervix but not dislocated. Plate 10, Figures 59 and 60, 5| and Plate 11, Figures 61 and 64, 4|.

For these special cases two definitions are suggested for occlusal view. The first is a modification of the previous definition and would be "all that is seen from a viewpoint on the long axis produced, the long axis to ignore an abrupt bend in the root." This definition would apply to a tooth removed from the alveolus, or *in situ*. The second definition, to apply only to a tooth *in situ*, and to be specified as such, would include such parts of the tooth as could be seen from a point on a line through the approximate centre of the dental arch and approximately perpendicular to the occlusal plane. This would give a view as in the photographs of palates referred to above, approximately the same as *norma basilaris* which is perpendicular to the Frankfurt Horizontal Plane. The definition could therefore be stated concisely as "the view of the tooth *in situ*, as seen in *norma basilaris*." The area thus seen, apart from what was covered by gingival tissue in life, would be very closely similar to the "functional occlusal surface" described above.

We now return to the study of variation in its relation to occlusal views and to views of occlusal features in upper premolars. From Figure 2-43 it is easy to see that the outlines of occlusal views will fall at relatively different parts between cervix and cusps in different teeth according to curvature. Teeth *c,f* and *h* are repeated in Figure 2-44, in order to illustrate this. The points on B and P outlines at which perpendiculars to the plane already described are tangential have been joined by broken lines. It is seen that these lines are not at the same relative distance from the cervix, nor are they necessarily parallel to the cervix.

Such differences are much more evident when similar treatment is applied, in Figure 2-45, to another group of outlines from Figure 2-43. The buccal sides of these outlines have been indicated. These four teeth are less convex in their outlines than usual, and they make it easier to appreciate that another factor in addition to curvature really determines the point between cervix and cusps where the tangent touches. This factor is taper. The proximal view of most upper premolars is bounded on B and P by curves which are approximately arcs of varying convexities, and the main chords of those arcs often tend to diverge as they leave the cervix and proceed towards occlusal, but this is not always so. One or both of these chords may tend to converge towards the central axis. In these four teeth the B outline diverges in k_2 and n, and converges in l and m. The P outline diverges in n and converges in k_2,l,m. Thus both converge in l and m and the broken line is almost parallel to the cervix and close to it; both diverge in n and the broken line is far from the cervix; in k_2 there is a divergent and a convergent outline and the broken line runs obliquely from near the cervix on one side to the base of the opposite cusp.

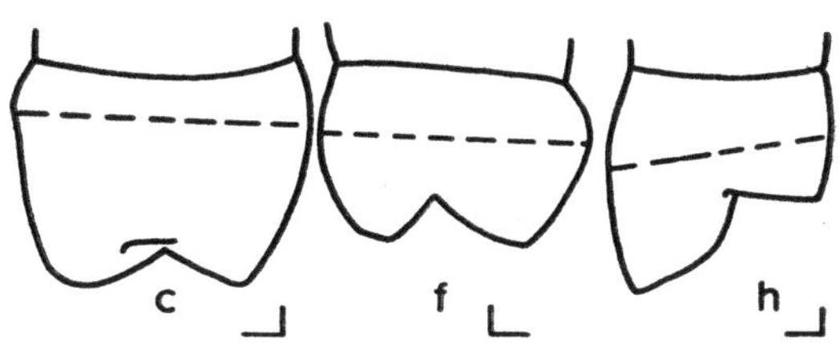

Figure 2-44. Relation of outline of occlusal view of tooth to view of occlusal surface.

It should be emphasized that the broken line in these diagrams does not indicate where the outline of the occlusal view would pass across the mesial surface in these proximal views. Only the points at each end of the line will surely be on that outline, but the rest of the outline of the occlusal view may be found with a dental surveyor. This device marks the contacts while a straight surface or a margin passes around the tooth crown parallel with its long axis. A stick of pencil lead (graphite) can serve well as a surveyor and was used on the seven teeth which have just been under consideration. The mesial outlines of their crowns are repeated in Figure 2-46, and between terminal points used in the two preceding figures the outlines so obtained are seen to be very irregular and often consist of discontinuous segments. In occlusal view the segments would appear continuous. Between the broken ends of segments the areas traversed by the broken connecting lines will represent concavities on the tooth surfaces. As the diagrams represent mesial surfaces it is to be expected that first premolars will present such concavities, especially where lack of convergence brings buccal and lingual terminals near to the cervix, as in teeth *l* and *m*. Places where two lines appear (h,k_2,n), or where broad areas are marked by the surveyor, represent areas which are almost flat to the surveyor.

In the present collection I have formed the impression that of those upper premolars which have less convex and more nearly straight outlines (as in k_2,l,m,n of Fig. 2-46) most have rather smaller than average-sized crowns. The same was my experience in dental practice, also that such cases tended to have spaces between teeth. Whether this arrangement would constitute a physical factor that would assist the initiation of carious cavities or otherwise one cannot say, for the degrees of curvature or flatness, the width of interdental spaces, the nature of the food and many

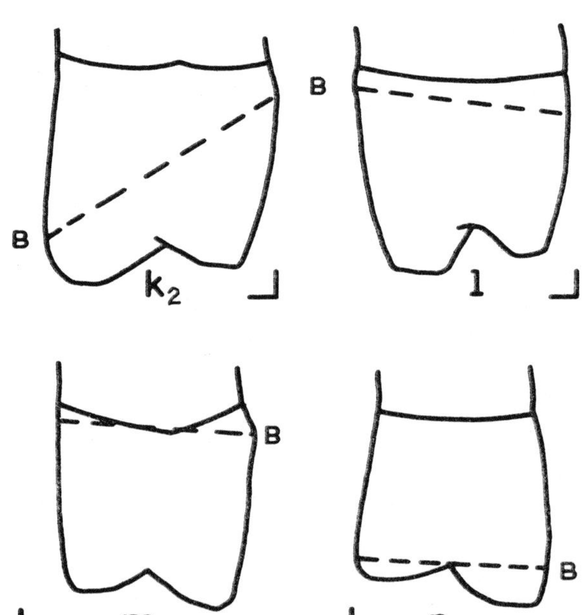

Figure 2-45. Further to Figure 2-44, these drawings from teeth show that outline of occlusal view may be near cervix or near occlusal or pass obliquely from one to the other.

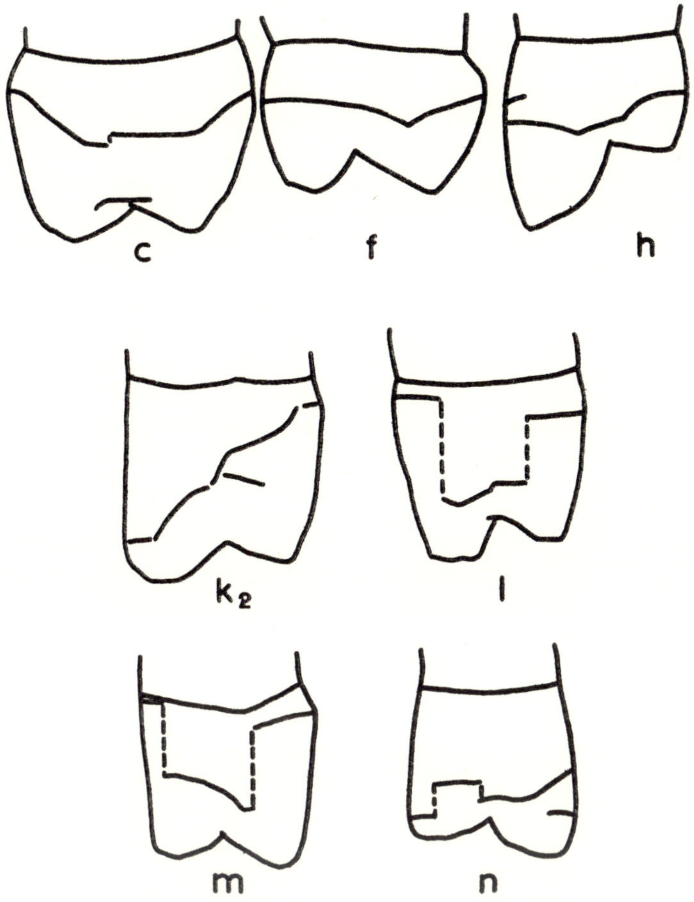

Figure 2-46. Variation in actual position of greatest convexity of proximal surfaces of upper premolars.

individual differences in mastication could all act as variables, which in sum total might conceivably influence conditions in either direction. The same might be said for their effect on the efficiency of oral prophylaxis by the individual person, but here it would be easy to suggest many additional variable factors. It is certain, however, that variations in curvature and in positions of approximal contacts have a bearing on operative, restorative and prosthetic procedures undertaken by the dentist; among other details they may influence the desirable or practicable location of cavity margins, the fitting of matrix bands and the design and location of supports for bridges or partial dentures. The existence of these variables or the need to consider them when advising on prophylactic or operative procedures is not, of course, confined to upper premolars. The whole of the denture is most likely to be involved, and usually the existence of this kind of variation is most easily recognized in the upper incisors. As for explaining the occurrence of such variations in morphological characters, there is reason to suspect that some may at least have been aggravated by pathological conditions during the time of tooth formation. In most cases, however, as with many other variations already noted, it seems most likely that they must have a genetic origin, and it is desirable that data be gathered to assist studies of this. In the meantime, it is convenient, even if unsatisfactory, to regard the majority of these variations as "within the normal range."

Occlusal Features

GENERAL CHARACTERS. It is inevitable that occlusal features have had to be considered in part while studying other details of form. Thus, in proximal views, the writer has studied the occlusal slopes of cusps, finding them usually convex when unworn, sometimes nearly straight, and meeting in the central fissure although the marginal ridge often obscures this part. In general, the two slopes were visualized as containing an angle between them called the fosse angle. This was shown to be important in operative dentistry, but it is also a physical factor with a bearing on the susceptibility to dental caries and on the success or otherwise of prophylaxis against caries, whether the prophylaxis is natural or artificial, or whether it is chemical or mechanical, or both. This association exists because the "fosse angle" is a character of the dental sulci (Black, 1901, p.11).

In dental anatomy and anthropology, and in dentistry, the terms groove and fissure are very frequently used, and fossa and sulcus less often, but seldom are any of them used with the conciseness of meaning desired by Black. Most admit that some vagueness persists around these terms, probably because the features concerned do not readily fit into precise definitions that may be mutually exclusive. The familiar occlusal groove or fissure would evidently be "sulcate groove," "sulcate fissure," or "sulcate fault" in Black's terminology. Presumably then, the corresponding feature of two teeth must bear one of these names but not necessarily the same one in each case. In actual fact, however, it is easy to find a tooth where more than one of these terms could be applied to different parts of the same feature. The difficulty in choosing the correct term thus appears to depend, in part, on ability to recognize histological as well as anatomical characters, an unnecessarily fine distinction in the great majority of instances. The claim that differences can be determined by use of a fine probe or explorer this writer rejects emphatically, as there would still be variable factors apart from the impossibility of maintaining an explorer point of standard fineness and taper. The author therefore accepts that the terms fissure and groove are reasonably interchangeable and convenient, and that almost all risk of confusion will be avoided if such terms as buccal, occlusal, developmental, etc., are added when it seems advisable.

It appears that Black gives the name sulci to the occlusal depressions in upper teeth which receive the buccal cusps of the lowers, and to the occlusal depressions in lower teeth which receive the palatal cusps of upper teeth. Sulci of two adjacent teeth form between them a very irregular, somewhat cone-shaped depression. An upper premolar may be visualized as having one half of each of two of these cone-shaped depressions extending from mesial and distal marginal ridges, and "intersecting." The line of intersection forms the crests of the triangular ridges of palatal and buccal cusps, and these crests together make up the profile of the fosse angle. A wider fosse angle indicates the likelihood that the sulci are more open and therefore more easily kept clear of food debris. Some of the factors concerned in natural prophylaxis are the physical condition of the food, the nature of the salivary response, the masticatory movements, length of time of mastication, sequence of different kinds of food, and the occlusion. Occlusal factors include those of dental anatomy such as length of cusps in opposing teeth, the manner and the depth of their inter-digitation. This, in turn, bears on fosse angles. A wide fosse angle, short cusps, normal occlusion, fibrous or "natural" foods and vigorous mastication individually and collectively favour wear of cusps and more effective prophylaxis, natural or artificial. On the other hand, teeth with reduced fosse angles, and usually also with deep fissures, are less efficiently self-cleansing, more difficult to cleanse by artificial prophylaxis and thus more retentive of food debris. In the presence of certain cariogenic factors such as carbohydrate debris, and in a caries-susceptible person, these features will facilitate dental caries.

The fosse angle has been shown to depend on cusp length, cusp thickness and distance between cusps.

Cusp length is a convenient term and it is fairly obvious what is meant when it is said that a tooth has long cusps. But it is quite a different matter to define the term in such a way that a cusp can be measured, or the cusps of different teeth fairly compared. In the case of the four teeth of Figure 2-47, one gets the impression that *a* certainly, and *c* probably, would be called long-cusped teeth. By contrast *b* and *d* are short-cusped, but the cusp length is partly hidden by marginal ridges, so that even a visual impression of cusp length may not give a fair basis for comparison between teeth. Moreover, marginal ridges themselves vary considerably in different teeth, and even in a particular tooth more of the occlusal surface is likely to be obscured (in proximal views) by the mesial than by the distal marginal ridge. Therefore fair comparisons would also demand that teeth be viewed from similar proximal aspects. None of these observations

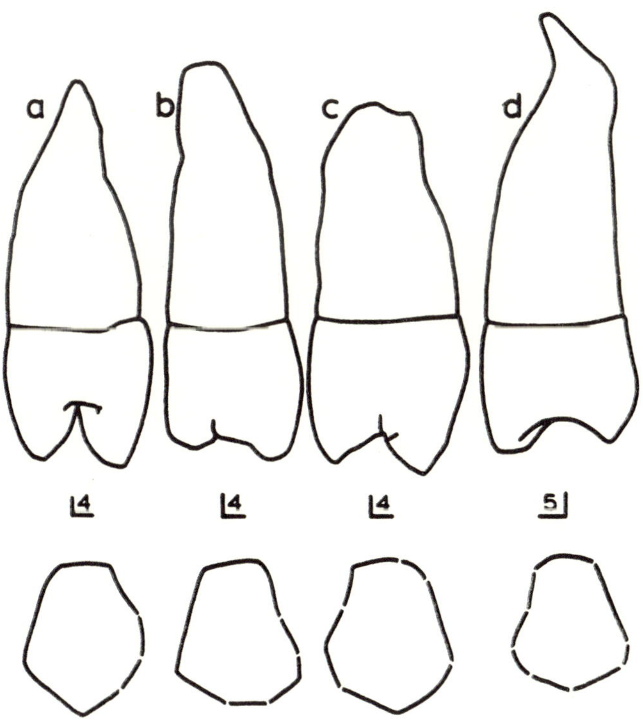

Figure 2-47. Cusp length, marginal ridges, fosse angles. The buccal outline of each crown is also shown and facilitates comparison of curvature and cusp acumination.

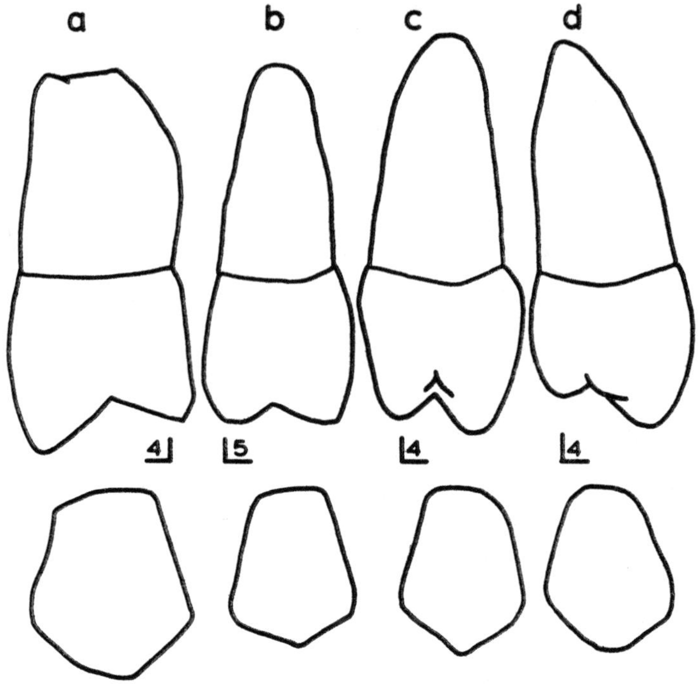

Figure 2-48. Buccal and palatal cusps; distance apart, relative lengths and fosse angles. As in Figure 2-47, buccal views of crowns are shown also.

encourage one to attempt actual measurement of cusp length.

In Figures 2-47 and 2-48 the buccal outline of each crown is shown beneath the proximal view of the tooth. In Figure 2-48 *a* the crown is large but the B cusp is not relatively long. The P cusp is proportionately short, but as it is set towards the P side with a wide fosse angle this P cusp is prominent. In tooth *d* there is also a wide fosse angle and a short P cusp. In this case, however, the P cusp is very small, so the shape contrasts with tooth *a*, quite apart from their difference in size. Tooth *d* in this proximal view has an outline not unlike a lower premolar. Tooth *b* is a small tooth but with a wide fosse angle and short cusps, while *c* is quite different. Both cusps are relatively long and set close together. This gives convergent B and P outlines, a narrow occlusal surface and reduced fosse angle. It is evident from these two figures and eight teeth that cusp length is not a character that can be clearly classified or compared because it depends on tooth size, closeness of cusps, and fosse angle which, when reduced, tends to give the appearance of a longer cusp or a deeper central groove. Any attempt to judge cusp length in B view fails because of difficulty in finding a base line. The cusp shoulders are too indefinite to serve as such, and a line joining the most M and most D points of the outline is too remotely associated with cusp length to be useful. Even in proximal view the estimation of cusp length is subjective rather than real, for it is largely an "impression" compounded of crown size, or height and width together with separation of cusps, size of fosse angle and position of marginal ridge. This notion leads to the belief that cusp length is a rather minor factor in fixing the amount of overlap when jaws are closed. Width of sulci would appear just as important, and in general these would tend to be narrower where the fosse angle is reduced. Other factors such as relation of long axes of teeth in one jaw to those in the other jaw and relative width of dental arches must also be important and would also have an influence on the manner in which wear of teeth could take place, sometimes facilitating and sometimes hindering this desirable change in the dentition.

Cusp thickness as a factor affecting the fosse angle is a less definite character than cusp length and therefore more difficult to deal with. It is another of those features that are easier to assess subjectively than to measure, and the assessment is made in relation to the size of the crown, if not to the whole tooth. Shorter cusps, prominent triangular ridges, and greater B-P diameter of the crown are factors favouring a thick cusp, and of course they favour a blunt cusp tip also.

In proximal view prominent triangular ridges reduce the fosse angle, so that it is possible to have thick cusps even though the cusps are relatively long and their cusp tips not widely separated.

In Figure 2-49 tooth *b* appears to have thick cusps because of prominent triangular ridges, especially on the B cusp, but the sulci are much wider than the fosse angle would suggest. Tooth *c* is a contrast with no triangular ridges, a wide open fosse angle and occlusal surface and thin cusps, but as nearly as can be judged the cusp tips are the same distance apart in each. Teeth *a* and *d* have very short and relatively thick cusps, but *d* is unusual in that the B cusp is distinctly smaller than P. Tooth *e* is amongst the larger upper premolars in this collection when judged by its crown, but it has convergent outlines, and the "tips" of its cusps are less than 1.0 mm wider apart than those of *b* and *c*. The B cusp is thick with a prominent triangular ridge, but the P cusp thickness measured from the central fissure is the same as that in tooth *d*. This fact is not obvious in the diagram because of the longer cusp in the larger crown.

In proximal views of crowns we have noted convergence or otherwise of B and P outlines and distance apart of the cusp tips; triangular ridges were easily seen to be related to fosse angles, and so also were length and thickness of cusps. That none of these characters could be studied without reference to most of the others clearly established their close relation to one another. Less frequently involved have been the marginal ridges, and they can be studied both in proximal and occlusal views.

Marginal Ridges. In upper first premolars in proximal views the M marginal

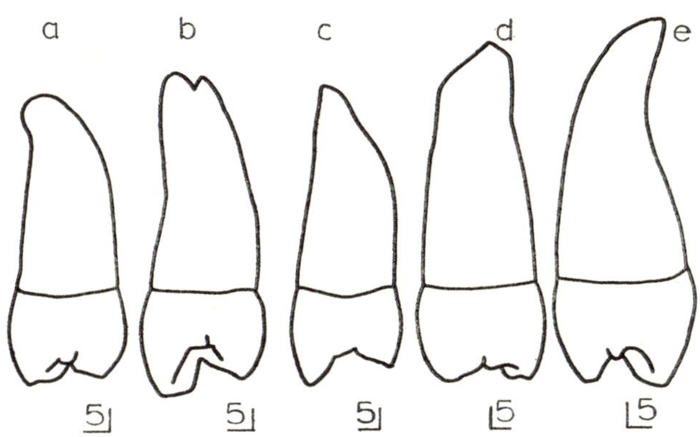

Figure 2-49. Buccal and palatal cusps; cusp thickness and triangular ridges, crown size, marginal ridges and fosse angles. Also, variety in bend and apex of root in single-rooted upper second premolars.

ridge is further from the cervix than is the D ridge. The M ridge also is usually crossed by a small groove which is in line with the central groove. This traversing groove is not as pronounced or as long as that seen on a lower first premolar, and it may be almost imperceptible but tends to take its character from the central occlusal groove. If that groove is deep and fissure-like and has well-marked accessory grooves the small traversing groove tends to be more noticeable. When very noticeable there may be a somewhat similar but less prominent groove on to the D marginal ridge.

In the second upper premolar also the M marginal ridge may be further from the cervix, but the difference between M and D ridges is less noticeable in this respect than in the first premolar. These small details may assist in the identification of a tooth where some of the more obvious features have been lost through wear, decay, filling or fracture.

In occlusal view the chief difference between the M and D marginal ridges is in the portions of the occlusal outline they occupy. Again, the difference is usually more noticeable in the first premolar. The M ridge is shorter, more nearly straight and forms the shoulder of the B cusp at a more definite angle. On the P side the marginal ridges join the cusp ridges in a more sweeping curve, especially on the DP side.

Marginal ridges permit greater efficiency during mastication and also assist in maintaining the health of the gingival tissues. By providing an angle which more or less abruptly terminates the proximal surface near the contact, and gives maximal extension to the occlusal surface, food may be broken up more effectively. Marginal ridges help to retain food on occlusal surfaces so that tough particles do not pass readily between the teeth. In this way soft tissue is protected from compression stresses, and so also when a dental restoration is contoured to present an angle between occlusal and proximal surfaces.

OCCLUSAL GROOVES. The feature referred to is that groove which passes M-D between the cusps and is terminated by the marginal ridges. It is most often called the central, or occlusal, groove or fissure. Less often it is apparently what is meant by the terms occlusal sulcus, or fossa, but these terms more correctly include the whole of the occlusal surface between the cusps. Whatever term is used for the occlusal groove, it is certain that it presents a great variety of form. This fact and the obvious difficulty of determining the exact boundaries of the groove (as with the banks of some streams or watercourses) no doubt accounts largely for the variety of terms used for the feature.

In Figure 2-50 are shown sixteen variations of this feature, but it is not claimed that these are individually distinct from one another, and they certainly do not exhaust the possible variations. These are outlines seen in occlusal views of the teeth, and the position of cusp tips have been shown by intersecting or joining lines, forming a modified "plus" symbol, or a T, which may be inverted. The cross-bar of the T indicates the direction of cusp ridges proceeding to join marginal ridges; the stem of the T (or the vertical stroke of the plus sign) indicates that ridges are present on B or P, i.e. triangular ridges, but a small mark or dot signifies that no such ridge is easily recognizable. If, however, there is a prominent triangular ridge, its direction is shown by a double line.

A groove that could fairly be called a fissure, or is definite enough to retain stain, is shown by a continuous line, and a broken line indicates a very shallow groove which is open so that its base is visible. Pits or deep fissures have been "blacked in" or shown in a heavier line, as in teeth *j,f,g* and *m*.

Comments are as follows:

(a) There is a fine fissure passing straight

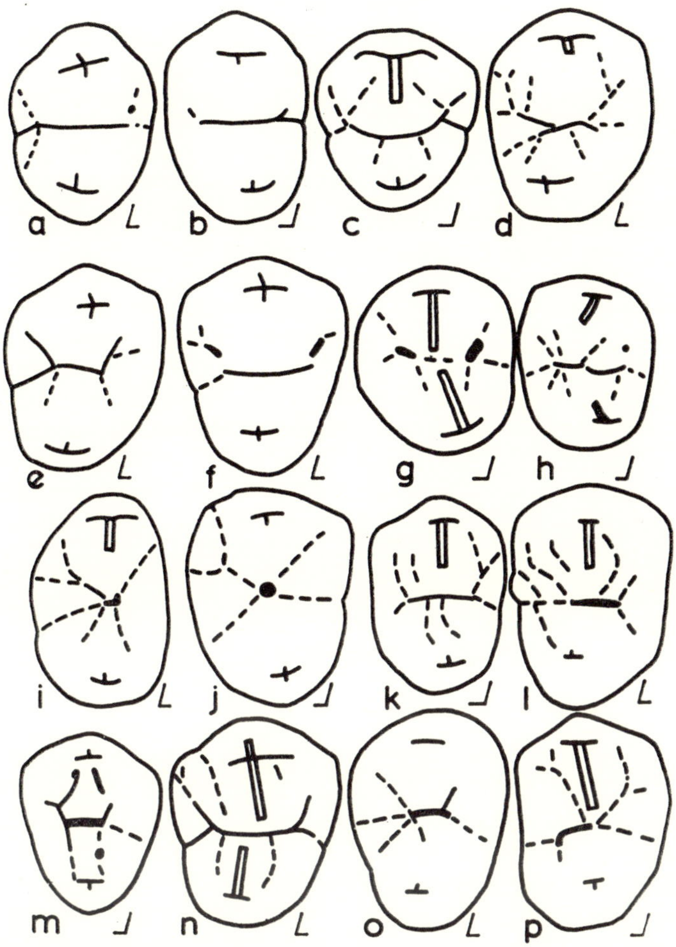

Figure 2-50. Variation in occlusal grooves, fissures and pits, in triangular ridges and in occlusal view outlines in upper premolars.

through between the cusps and over the M marginal ridge, and there is a very small pit offset at DB.

(b) Similar to (a) but the fissure is deeper and there is an offset fissure at MB.

(c) Long deep fissure, cuts M marginal ridge deeply, terminal occlusal pits, very prominent B triangular ridge.

(d) Short central fissure, two offset B fissures, one long; many subsidiary grooves.

(e) Short shallow fissure and offsets; M marginal ridge traversed; wide marginal ridges.

(f) Deep central groove with two offset B pits.

(g) Prominent triangular ridges from both cusps almost meet to interrupt fissure into two offset B pits.

(h) Short triangular ridges from each cusp; irregular shallow fissure with small offset pit; a number of short subsidiary grooves; small crown.

(i) Compressed crown (M-D) with small B cusp; small central pit with radiating grooves.

(j) Very uncommon form with one large central pit and four long radiating grooves.
(k) Small crown, prominent B triangular ridge; short central fissure, irregular subsidiary grooves, and wide M marginal ridge.
(l) Large crown with prominent B triangular ridge; very short fissure and a number of subsidiary grooves.
(m) Small crown with absence of both triangular ridges; small deep central fissure with subsidiary and offset fissures and pits on slopes of both cusps.
(n) Prominent triangular and marginal ridges; deep fissure with subsidiary terminal fissures on B; large crown.
(o) Large crown, very short fissure with one subsidiary fissure DB and radiating grooves.
(p) Wide crown compressed M-D, marked asymmetry, long triangular ridge on B, very wide M marginal ridge, very short fissure curves to DP.

The usual teaching is that Black (1901, p.46) adapted his cavity outline to conform to his statement that "the central groove . . . sinks into a triangular pit at either end." In our experience this is not acceptable for many upper premolars, although it is acknowledged that the differences between a fissure and a groove and a pit are sometimes a matter of degree and of subjective judgment. Among the specimens just illustrated, however, it is difficult to find more than one or two where the central fissure is terminated by pits. Short subsidiary fissures are more common, but by no means always present. Subsidiary fissures or grooves or offset pits are more common on the B side than on P side. The B cusp more often presents a triangular ridge than does the P cusp, and one or both ridges may be absent. Subsidiary grooves in nearly all cases may be found at each side of the B triangular ridge, and they are usually wide and shallow, but they may be fissured for a short distance from the central fissure. Both marginal ridges are often traversed, at least part-way by subsidiary grooves tending to veer towards P side. That on the M ridge more often tends to be a fissure than the groove on D ridge, especially in the first premolar.

CUSPS: ACUMINATION, RIDGES AND GROOVES. Both cusps vary in degree of acumination. The P cusp is shorter than the B cusp, particularly in the first premolar, and it is often more rounded or blunt. But the P cusp may have a fairly definite point, as in Figure 2-51 *a,b*. This particular tooth has unusually sharp cusps, and its B cusp is shown in outline *c*. It is proposed to study acumination by buccal views only, which means that P cusps will be omitted.

It is appropriate here to recall that certain physical characteristics such as length and breadth (and in some degree curvature also), which are noted in an individual as a general observation, are found in many details of parts of the body. Thus apart from some variations between those of different racial stock, one would expect a tall slim person to have long slim bones in some contrast to those of a person who (also in normal good health) tends to be short and plump. Somewhat corresponding differences would be found in the bodies of the vertebrae and in the teeth. Admittedly there are found instances of apparent disharmony where teeth seem to be too large, or too small for the bone type, as expressed in the jaws. The explanation of these cases where parents of dissimilar physical type have a child presenting orthodontic disharmony may be found through genetic studies, but it is easy to suggest other factors that should also be considered. What concerns us at the moment, however, is that characters of form such as length and breadth, actual and relative, degree of curvature, complexity of roots or of fissures and grooves, or acumination of cusps, tend to be consistent throughout a dentition. So also with the two cusps of an upper premolar. Therefore it seems a reasonable observation that the P cusp resembles the B cusp in the character of acumination, as it does in other characters. Thus a crown that is short and rounded with a blunt cusp in B view may be expected to show similar characters in P view. Similarly with outlines that are less convex, or relatively long compared with M-D diameters, a straight-sided or narrow B cusp is associated with a P cusp of similar character. This is the reason for concentrating on the B cusp in presenting variation in acumination.

A full study of acumination even for one cusp should reasonably include proximal views but it has already been shown that variation in marginal ridges is one factor that prevents reasonably accurate determination of the base of cusps in these views. Although it is therefore not feasible to consider the proximal view of cusp outlines as such, this has of necessity been covered while studying curvature in crown outlines. These present a very considerable variety of form as regards degree of convexity, length, position of greatest prominence on B and P, and position of cusp "tips" in relation to central axis of crown. In this last respect the P cusp often appears to be nearer the axis, and accordingly the P outline often appears to be more convex. These features are often factors concerned in the initiation of pathological changes in the hard tissues of the teeth and periodontal tissues, and are factors in the prognosis of treatment by the dentist and by the individual himself. Their significance in these respects arises from their relation to occlusion and to masticatory habits and stresses. It has already been shown that they act in part as physical factors in relation to retention or ready removal of food debris, to the manner in which food debris meets soft tissues (impinging on it or sliding over it), and similarly they have a bearing on the stresses and strains to which restorations and prosthetic structures are submitted. It is seen, therefore, that in addition to conscientious and skilful operative technique, good dentistry depends in part on the operator's ability to recognize and assess the significance of these features and factors in the case he is treating. It is also evident that in spite of the best intentions and ability there will be cases where anatomical features and functional factors combine to reduce the efficiency and the period of service of some dental restorations.

In the unworn or partly worn tooth, in which state are found the majority of adult teeth examined here, the shape of cusps and the manner of their occlusion are among the important and more easily recognized features just considered. In B view the "thickness" of the cusps cannot be seen for it is dependent not only on the cusp length but also on the triangular ridge passing from cusp tip to central groove. These ridges have been referred to frequently, and also shown in some of the diagrams, even though not separately mentioned. They are completely absent in a few cases, but are nearly always recognizable in some degree, especially on the B cusp. Recognition is often facilitated

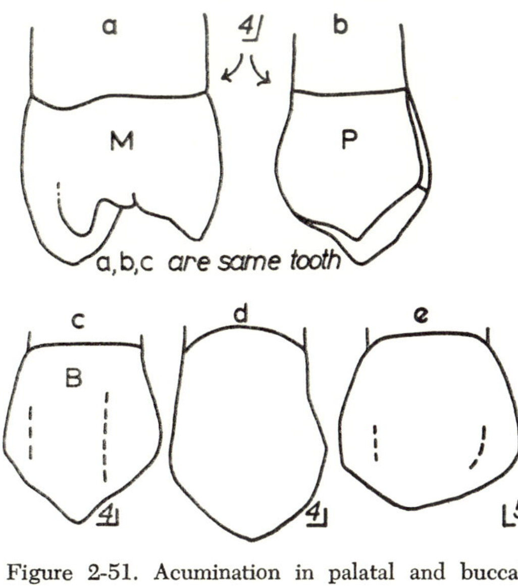

Figure 2-51. Acumination in palatal and buccal cusps.

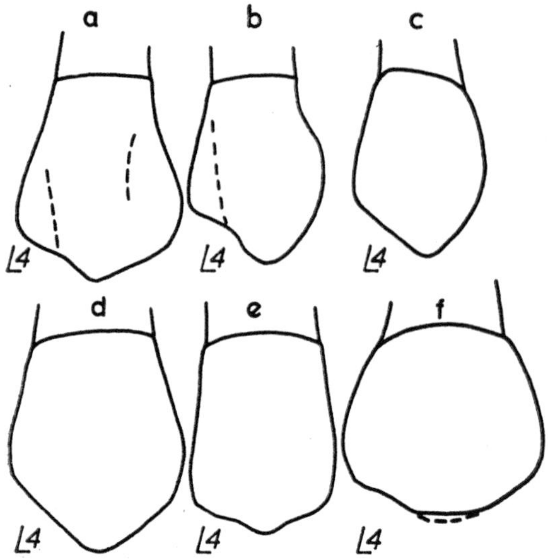

Figure 2-52. Buccal views of crowns of upper premolars. Variation in convexity and in cusp acumination and in presence of developmental grooves.

by the presence of a shallow groove on one or both sides of the ridge. The grooves tend to converge towards the cusp tip, so making the ridge somewhat triangular both in section and in extent. On the B cusp it may be possible to trace these grooves, especially the mesial one, up on to the B surface and in these cases the tip of the cusp is more obvious. According to Black (1901, pp. 13 and 46) these are developmental grooves corresponding to those in incisors and canines, and they mark the confluence of three lobes in which calcification of the buccal enamel commenced, the palatal cusp representing the fourth lobe in these teeth. The shoulders of the cusp extend from the developmental groove to that point of termination at the marginal ridges which Black called the triangular groove. As the purpose of this study is to observe variation, it is emphasized that some of these finer details may not be readily identified, even in an unworn tooth.

It is not easy to represent such features in diagrams but an attempt has been made to add developmental grooves to B outlines in Figures 2-51 and 2-52. Where these were more distinct the broken lines were longer. Where the broken line has only one or two segments the grooves were hardly discernible, or very short, and in other teeth shown the grooves were absent. As with other characters, there is much variation in these grooves, and in the more obvious cases they may be associated with prominence of cusp shoulders and cusp tip in buccal and occlusal views of a tooth.

DISCUSSION WITH PARTICULAR REFERENCE TO CROWNS OF UPPER PREMOLARS

Although this chapter deals separately with roots and with crowns of upper premolars, some characters had also to be considered for both together. Apart from their common outline at the cervix it was desired to ascertain whether there was a size or proportionate relationship between the two parts. Beyond the rather general observation that a large crown tends to have a large root, and a small crown a small root, it is found that there is not a consistently close relationship in some characters. Indeed, one must stress that the tendency just mentioned applies both to frequency and to degree; that is to say, a crown that is long and wide will usually have a long wide root, but the root may be thickened and sturdy rather than appearing fragile, and this applies even though the root is divided. Exceptions are found, but these may be more apparent than real, because it is not possible clearly to define or to distinguish between degree of root development and linear measurements in relation to sturdiness or fragility of a root. This follows from the infinite variety in which the single or grooved or divided root of an upper premolar may be presented. Variation in the crown has been shown to be almost as great, with perhaps one outstanding difference—namely, that in both premolars there were without exception two cusps in the material examined, and they were distinct and readily recognized as cusps. Although teeth that differ morphologically from this two-cusp crown type are found in the same region of the mouth, they present as an addition to, rather than in place of, a recognizable first and second premolar, and are regarded as supplemental or supernumerary teeth.

The consistency with which these cusps are placed buccally and palatally, and the relative sizes in length, as well as in both width dimensions, give rise to the most constant characters that enable differentiation between first and second, and between left and right premolars. To these might be added such characters as relative convexities of profile outlines. Here then are most of the data necessary to illustrate these characters in diagrammatic form, using straight lines and angles, to represent curvature by chords of arcs of varying length and radius. Outlines from actual teeth were presented to demonstrate variations in convexity and taper.

These characters were shown in relation to the conception of occlusal surface and occlusal view, and these latter in turn were distinguished from the functional occlusal surface which related tooth anatomy and tooth position to friction during mastication. It was found useful also to use the term "occlusal surface proper." This was shown to vary in extent according to whether the cusps were set more apart or closer together, and furthermore it was shown to extend into the functional occlusal surface as the cusps became worn.

The term "fosse angle" was suggested and explained, and the use of such terms as fossa, sulcus, fissure, groove, and pit were discussed in relation to morphology of occlusal features. It was shown how these may present very considerable variety and they were illustrated with drawings from actual teeth.

Variation in crown morphology was found to have a wide range, and while this analysis of variation is essentially anatomical as regards features and characters, some of the variations have special significance for the dental surgeon. It is unfortunate that some of these, or their importance to the operator, do not always receive attention in textbook descriptions of dental anatomy. For example, in the first premolar the concavity at the mesial cervix calls for special attention in adjustment of matrix bands and in condensation of amalgam, and it reduces working space within the cavity. In both premolars a thin cervix will make good work more difficult or will increase the risk of fracture during extraction. Again, a reduction in distance between cusps, or in the fosse angle, calls for careful placing of cavity margins for access, and for resistance to stress by both filling and tooth substance. The situation is further complicated by changing conditions in the presence of tooth wear.

Although variation in size is obvious, whether it be in particular dimensions or in bulk, it was shown that there is much variation also in the form of anatomical characters such as convexity of surfaces and of profiles, in pits and grooves and ridges. These also should be recognized and allowed for in the course of operative procedures. It was found that these morphological variations did not occur in any definite grouping of association or degree, and therefore could not easily be classified or measured. This fact and the wide range of variation in size and form shown to exist within an almost entirely European community are important because it is not uncommon for measurement of teeth to be presented in statistical form for various ethnic groups. As teeth are merely parts of the body, surely such statistics, even if satisfactory in themselves, would have to be associated with further information before comparisons between groups could be acceptable. It would be necessary to have statistics for the same groups of individuals as regards stature, for example, and weight or physical type, but these are not given. Even if they were given one would still have to deny the usefulness of the data because of the nature of the material. Thus, apart from dimensional changes in teeth resulting from occlusal and interproximal wear, this study of crowns gives further support to the writer's contention that tooth morphology and normal variation render teeth unsuitable for quantitative or dimensional measurement and comparison. It follows that statistics based on these are not acceptable. By the same token, the value of qualitative studies leading to that conclusion is enhanced.

Chapter 3

Aspects of Variation in Tooth Morphology

THE TEETH DESCRIBED and depicted in this study are assumed to represent much of the normal range of variation found within a community. Specimens which seem to be abnormal, or affected by pathological conditions, have been excluded, for many such teeth have been described in the literature or preserved in museum collections. The present writer has aimed to analyze or describe the nature of "normal" variations in tooth morphology rather than to explain them.

This has served as a general guide in presenting results of the study, but there are some aspects of variation to which attention should be drawn. While not presented as causes of variation they are pertinent thereto, and although their relevance is not confined to upper premolar teeth there are reasons for considering them here.

One of these aspects is the relation of sex to variation in tooth morphology. It is not a matter for intensive investigation in this study, but data of sex and age were available for premolar teeth extracted from young persons.

Another aspect of variation in tooth form relates to pulp cavities and root canals. It has been convenient to study these in young premolar teeth with incomplete roots, and as upper premolars frequently have root branches, they were chosen as presenting more variety than lower teeth.

It would be difficult to define a borderline between abnormality and normal variation and therefore some teeth with unusual morphological characters have been included. Wear is found in all kinds of teeth, but as it is sometimes related to tooth morphology it is relevant to the study. These are the aspects of variation considered in this chapter.

VARIATION WITHIN KNOWN SEX

It was impossible to sex the material on which this study is based because the dentists who saved the many thousands of extracted teeth provided no such records. The great bulk of the material was received in batches of perhaps a few hundred teeth at a time. Some teeth, with information concerning them, were saved by individual dentists especially for the writer, and further specimens were added from his own practice. This group of teeth with data concerning sex, age, race (where not European) and also the records of operative treatment, has widened the scope of the study and partly removed the disadvantage of working mostly with unsexed material.

For example, without such data one may

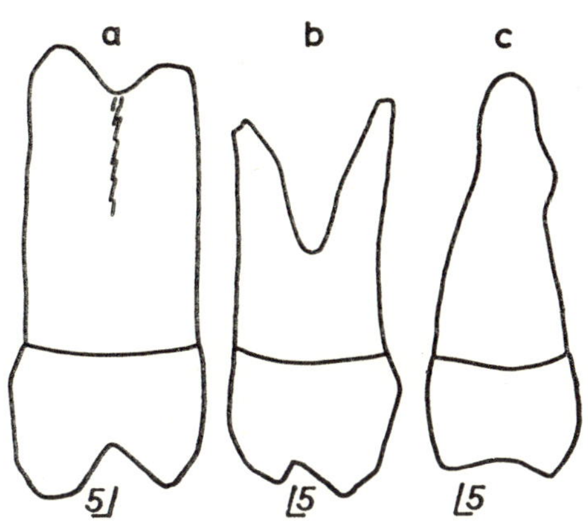

Figure 3-1. Variation in teeth within known sex (male).

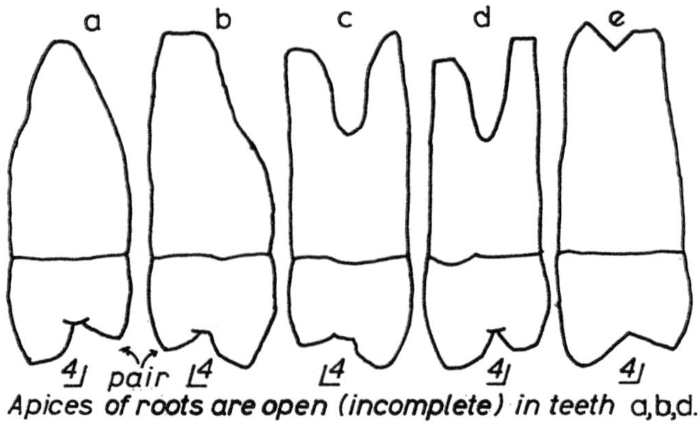

Figure 3-2. Upper first premolars from males.

be tempted to assume that robust teeth and large teeth have come from males, and slender or small teeth from females. With the accepted fact of variation within the sexes these assumptions would sometimes be correct, but experience gained in years of dental practice and in examination of teeth with recorded data shows that this is often not so.

In Figure 3-1 are shown three teeth, all upper second premolars, extracted from males.* Teeth *a* and *b* are from young adults and *c* from a man aged about forty years. The differences in these teeth are considerable and involve crowns as well as the obvious differences in the roots. Figure 3-2 shows upper first premolars from males. Teeth *a* and *b* are a pair from a boy aged $10\frac{10}{12}$ years. They, and tooth *d* (approximately 10 years), have open apices. Tooth *c* (14 years) has closed apices, and tooth *e* is from a man of about 48 years. As with the second premolars in the previous figure, these first premolars show single-rooted, bifurcated and intermediate forms, and in the crowns differences in fosse angles are

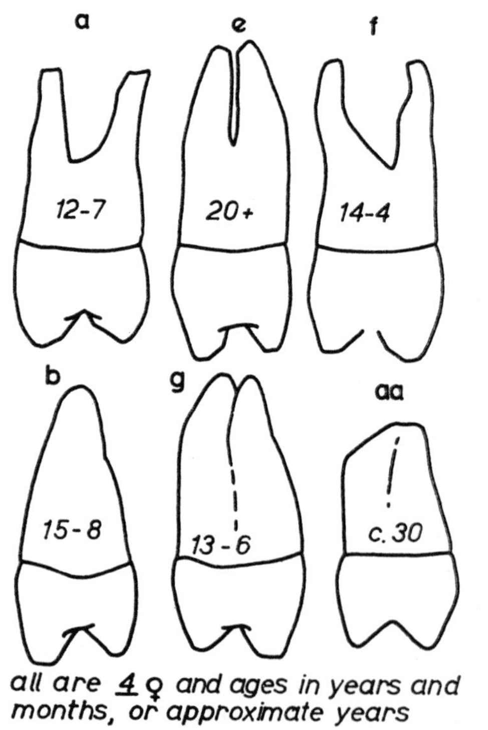

Figure 3-3. Upper first premolars from females. (An occlusal cavity preparation accounts for the break in the outline of tooth *f*).

* The outlines in figures of this chapter were drawn through the camera lucida, as were outlines in all other chapters, and to approximately the same scale. Unfortunately at this stage it had not become the writer's practice to draw in the scale as each figure was drafted. Since there were likely to be small differences of magnification between figures when drafting, and more so in the photographic procedures for subsequent reproduction, it was not feasible to add the scales later.

The presence of scales in the figures for Chapter 1 is explained by the fact that the text and figures for that chapter were revised after completion of other chapters.

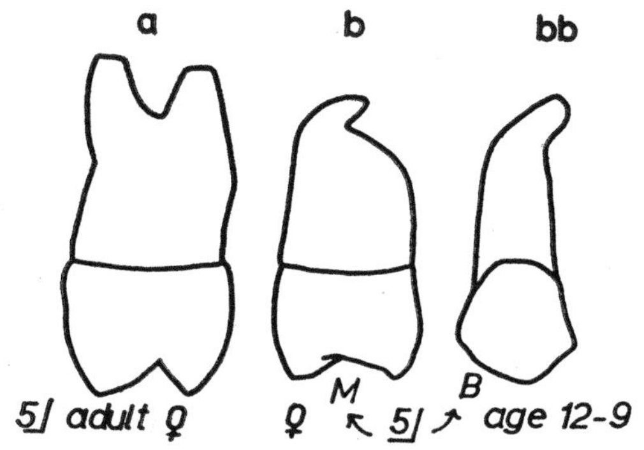

Figure 3-4. Two second premolars from females. Tooth *a*, adult. Tooth *b* and *bb* from girl in her thirteenth year.

again evident. An interesting detail is the difference in palatal outlines of the two teeth from the one boy.

Figure 3-3 shows first upper premolars from females, and again there is visible variation in a number of features. Specimens *a* and *g* are relatively large teeth, especially in regard to crown size, but both girls are of slight build; in fact girl "*a*" is from a family who are all of unusually slight build—both this girl and her brother were keen participants in ballet dancing as children. Tooth *aa* is from a woman of about 30 years of age, and although it has a small single root this root is lightly grooved as for three canals.

Figure 3-4 shows two upper second premolars from females. Both are short-rooted, and tooth *a* which has a quite large crown and is from an adult, has a bifid root. Tooth *b,* shown in buccal view in *bb,* is one of a pair, and was extracted at age 12⁹⁄₁₂. The left tooth which is not shown is very similar, and was extracted six months later. Both were erupting palatally through crowding and both have closed apices.

FORMATION OF ROOTS AND PULP CANALS

This study is not concerned with the process of formation of the whole root or canals. Recent work by Fanning (1961) has provided much information concerning the stage of root development at various ages, as obtained from serial X-rays. In the present study there were many premolars that had been extracted at various stages of root formation for orthodontic reasons. In those from the author's practice, records were kept of the name, age and sex of the child, but with the others there is no such record. These immature teeth are of special interest for examination from the apical aspect, for instead of presenting a transverse section of the root and canal outline with a thickness of dentine between these double outlines, they present thin single outlines of root form with indentations or folds representing grooves. Some of these grooves presumably anticipate root division, but no particular feature has been found that would provide reliable evidence as to whether division would or would not have taken place

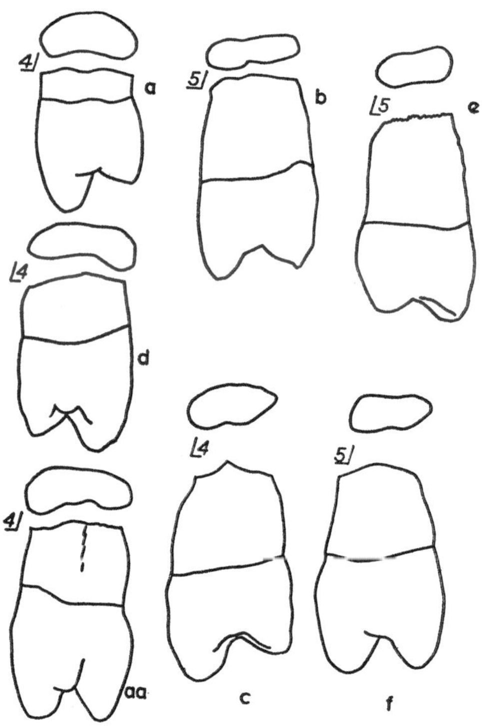

Figure 3-5. Proximal outlines of upper premolars extracted during period of root formation, together with outlines of their open root ends, drawn with a camera lucida. These teeth are in the C– group defined in the text, but with pulp cavities undivided or only lightly grooved.

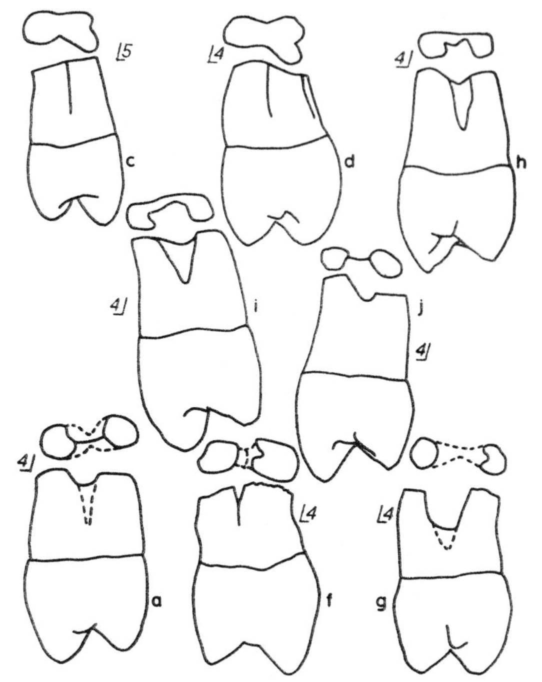

Figure 3-6. Further outlines in the C– group, with roots grooved or already bifurcated.

by the time the root was complete. In many cases (but certainly not all) a groove tends to become wider or deeper, or both, as formation progresses towards the apex, but this change may be more apparent than real. It is just as true to say that the root tends to become less bulky as formation progresses and obviously these characters are involved in the description of final root form. They may be thought of as related and somewhat reciprocal in their effect, if it may be said that the increasing depth of the groove could be cancelled out by the decrease in bulk of the root. Obviously there is no justification for such a statement for it is not known how the bulk decreases, or why it does so more in some teeth than in others. Such a notion is merely a convenience for purposes of description.

In talking of root taper and divergence of root branches, one conveys a notion of form, well aware that it cannot be explained. It has been observed that divergence bears no obvious relation to such characters as root bulk or position of furcation or even to depth of grooving of root trunk before division. The ultimate form could not therefore depend on the shape of the root in its early stage of formation. After examination of these incomplete roots and of fully formed teeth it can be concluded that, until completion has been reached, it cannot be said that a root will in fact divide, or whether the grooves will continue to the apex without division. If the corresponding tooth on the other side of the mouth is examined (as

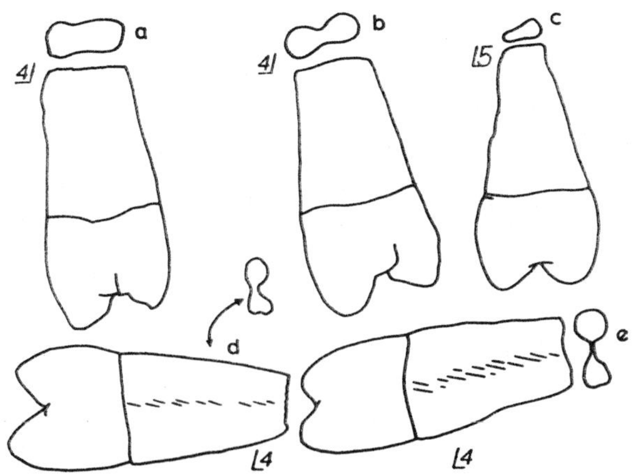

Figure 3-7. Outlines from the C+ group; varieties with undivided pulp cavity, and those with bifurcated pulp cavity but no furcation yet in root.

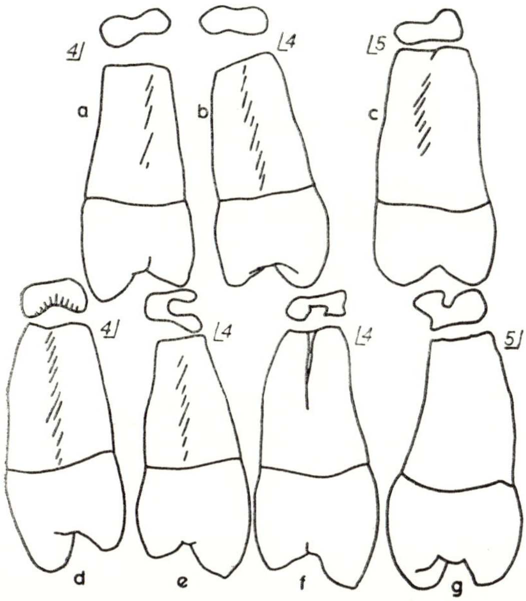

Figure 3-8. Outlines from the C+ group; varieties with deeply grooved pulp cavities but no furcation in pulp or root.

is possible when both are to be extracted) it is most likely that both will be very similar in this respect. But there are exceptions, or differences as to the point of bifurcation, as the author has found in a few cases in his own practice. Differences in root curvature are even more likely to be found (and might well be expected) if one of the teeth has erupted more lingually than the other and both remained for much of the root to be formed. Corresponding differences may be found in the roots of lower premolars.

To return to the "apical" view of incomplete roots, the thin single outlines mentioned above represent the form of the completed outside surface of the root at this position. For the present examination of anatomical form it will be assumed that appreciable addition of cementum to the surface in later life, especially if irregular, is to be regarded as abnormal or pathological. Such irregular thickenings do sometimes present difficulties to the operator when removing teeth. At that age they may partly fill or obscure the indentations which we now observe as indicative of grooving, and sometimes of impending division, in the forming root of young teeth.

Thirty-five of these immature teeth are used to illustrate variation in formation of roots and pulp canals, and eighteen mature teeth in section are added to illustrate the formation of two or three pulp canals in single-rooted upper premolars.

For convenience, the immature teeth are divided into two groups representing earlier and later stages of root formation. The earlier stage presents a length of root formation up to approximately the crown height from cervix to tip of buccal cusp, and is represented by the symbol C−. The later stage is from C− to completion of the root and is represented by C+. In apical view these present varied outlines, but they have been grouped into four main varieties with a symbol for each as follows:

Symbol	*Variety of outline represented by symbol*
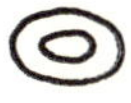	Single. Wide pulp canal, with no deep grooving.
	Grooved. One or more deep grooves.
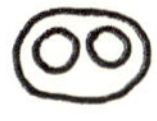	Double. Two (or three) separate canals but not actual furcation of root.
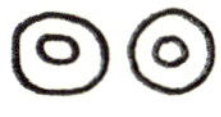	Separate. Actual furcation of root established.

For illustration, these immature teeth are analyzed in two ways as follows:

Group	Teeth selected	Variety of outline	Shown in Figure
a	All C- specimens	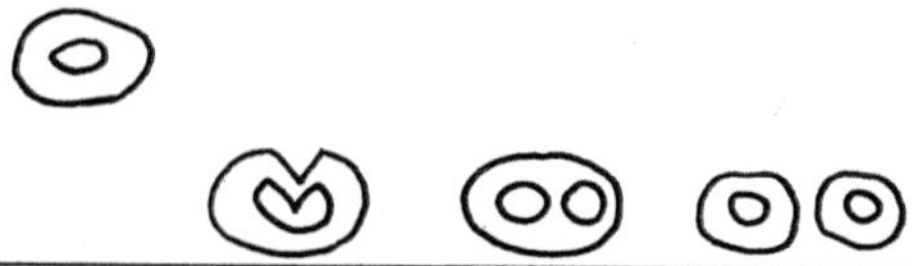	3–5 3–6
b	All C+ specimens	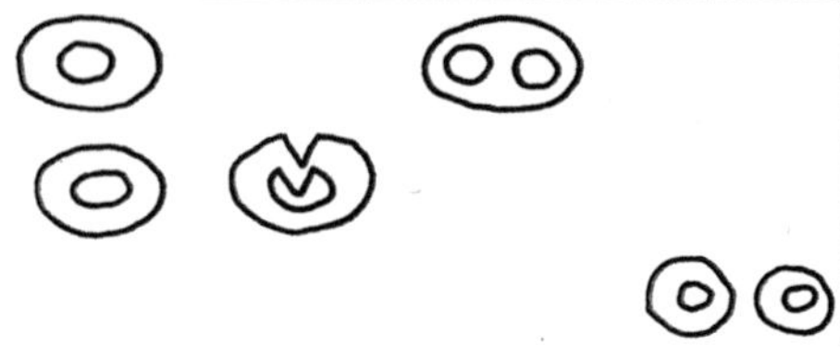	3–7 3–8 3–9

1. Giving apical and proximal views of each tooth.

Group	Nature of groove	Probable number of canals when root completed	Shown in Figure
I	Shallow, or nil	one	3–10
II	Deep	one	3–10
III	Deep	two, or three	3–10
IV*	Shallow, or nil	two	3–11

2. *Presenting relation of root grooving to division of pulp cavity. Single C+ roots. Apical views in Groups I, II and III.*

* These are illustrated by proximal views of sectioned, single-rooted, mature (C+) teeth.

Figures 3-5 to 3-12 inclusive have been drawn with a camera lucida. The outlines, particularly in regard to crowns, are a good illustration of the variability already described for proximal views. Features that may be compared are length and breadth proportions, length of cusps, curvatures of B and P, fosse angles, width between cusps, and cervical lines. In each figure all outlines are drawn to the same scale so that actual dimensions also are comparable within that figure.

The outlines of the incomplete roots are shown with the tooth outlines in Figures 3-5 to 3-9, and grooving of proximal surfaces is indicated with light shading. In

Figure 3-5 all have end outlines that are simple and not deeply grooved. In Figure 3-6 teeth *c,d,h* have deeply grooved end outlines, but the pulp cavities are not divided into separate canals. In teeth *i,j* division is virtually complete. In *j* a point of bifurcation of the root appears to have been reached, but not yet in *i*. Tooth *a* is almost identical with *j* in this respect and also in the very thin sharp ridge forming the actual bifurcation, but it contrasts with tooth *f* where the two parts of the pulp canal are closer together. In proximal views one is V-shaped and the other more rounded and U-shaped. Both varieties of form at the bifurcation are common. In one, the bifurcation may be described as a narrow ridge joining the roots whereas the V-shape is a narrow groove separating the roots. Between these extremes the V has widened to U-shape, and the narrow ridge has become thick and rounded.

It is not intended that these differences be regarded as distinctions, but rather as convenient ways of description, for both the V and U features may be found in one tooth, such as that in Figure 3-10V, where *a* is the feature concerned, as seen from apical aspect. The U-ridge joins the roots on mesial aspect and the V-groove separates them on distal. Between the roots at the bifurcation there is therefore a depression which is bounded on the mesial by the side of the U-shaped ridge, and it is made more cup-shaped by the groove on that palatal surface of the buccal root. This groove in the uncompleted root causes the end outline to be crescent-shaped, and the same may be seen in the corresponding outlines of several other teeth in this series. In Figure 3-6 *g* the formation of separate roots is clearly established and the outlines have become quite separate.

Figures 3-7, 3-8 and 3-9 present examples of C+ teeth and their open end outlines. In Figure 3-7 *a,b,c* are single, and *d,e* are double variety. Figure 3-8 shows grooved specimens. In the first four of these teeth the constriction is greater in the pulp cavity than appears in the outlines; an endeavour has been made to indicate this in outline *d*. None of these teeth appear likely to have established a furcation by the time the apex was formed, but the pulp cavities in *f* and *g* could possibly have divided into two by then. In Figure 3-9 root bifurcation has been accomplished at an earlier stage so that each branch presents a separate outline. Tooth *a* presents two very deep grooves so that the point of bifurcation is formed by a sharp ridge. Tooth *b* is the same as that in Figure 3-10V and attention is drawn to the groove on palatal aspect of the buccal root. A similar feature is seen in teeth *d-g*, of this figure, and also in Figure 3-6 *f,g*. Attention may well be drawn also to the variety in divergence or otherwise of the root trunks and branches in the teeth of Figure 3-9. In *c,d,f,h* the trunk outline converges rootwards but in three of these the buccal branch tends to diverge. In *e* the divergence of palatal root is marked, but buc-

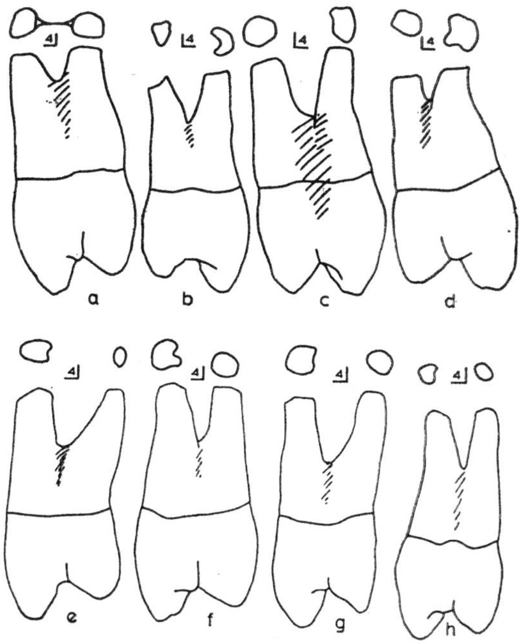

Figure 3-9. Outlines from the C+ group with bifurcated roots.

cal crown and root are almost straight in line, as are both outlines of tooth *g*.

In the second analysis an endeavour is made to relate grooves in single roots to probable division, not of the root, but of the pulp cavity into more than one canal by the time the root is complete. (This study is not concerned with the small accessory apical foramina that are sometimes present.) Of the twelve teeth that are illustrated in Parts I, II and III of Figure 3-10, nine are first premolars. In Figure 3-10 Part I are end outlines of teeth that have only a shallow groove, or none, and these might reasonably be expected to retain one undivided canal. In Part II teeth *b,e,* while having deep grooves (*b* on mesial and *e* on buccal), might easily retain their single canal. Whether this were the case or not, tooth *e* would present considerable difficulty to any operator attempting to remove mechanically the contents of its pulp cavity. Part III shows outlines for teeth deeply grooved and likely to present more than one pulp canal when complete in root formation. Tooth *m* has a deep groove on distal, and shallower grooves on mesial and on buccal aspect of the buccal root, but one could not say whether the buccal canal would eventually divide into two. It is a second premolar. (See also Figs. 3-11 *j* and 3-12 *g,h.*)

Part IV is presented differently and separately in Figure 3-11. It is concerned with single-rooted teeth with only a shallow groove, or no groove, in which two canals were present, and is illustrated in fully mature teeth instead of in teeth with uncompleted roots. Ten teeth are depicted and three of these are second premolars. Parts of the roots of these teeth have been ground away so that portions of the pulp cavity are shown in longitudinal B-P section (M-D section in one case), and the cervical line is shown (cervix indicated in tooth *i*). It should be noted that the level of division of pulp cavity into two canals varies considerably, but in all these teeth

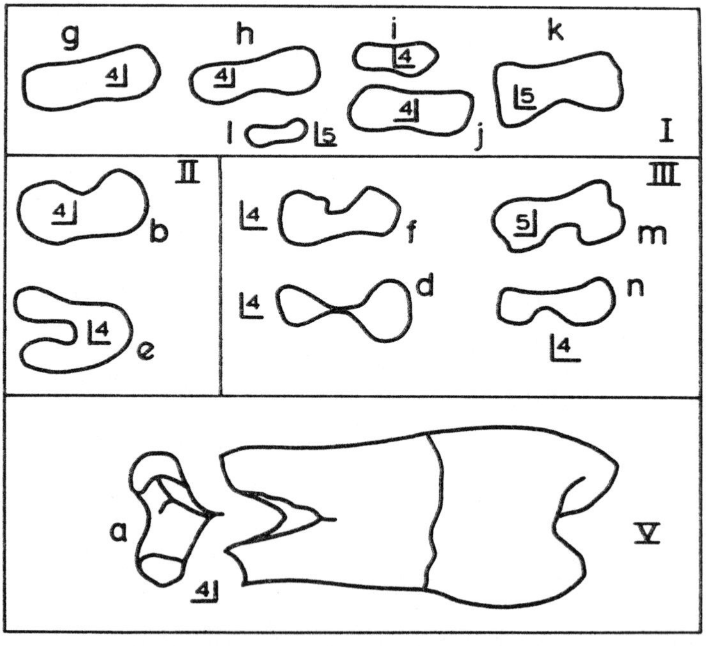

Figure 3-10. Relation of root grooving to division of pulp cavity. I-III, end outlines of single-rooted C+ teeth showing shallow and deep grooving and probable completion with one canal, or division into two or three canals. V, tooth from Figure 3-9 *b* presenting groove on palatal aspect of buccal root.

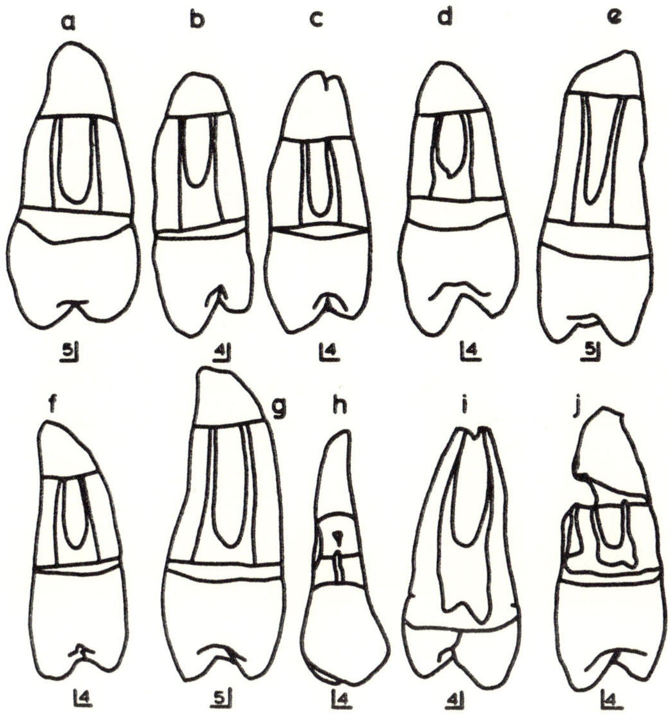

Figure 3-11. Single-rooted upper premolars, presenting a shallow groove or no groove at all, but with division of pulp cavity into two canals. These are drawn with camera lucida from mature sectioned teeth and represent Group IV of the second analysis.

it is in the cervical half of the root. It is of interest to note also that those with the relatively shortest pulp chambers (and longest canals) include the three second premolars. These are the teeth in which the pulp cavity has divided into canals at an early stage of root formation, even though the root did not bifurcate. In tooth *h* the two canals are seen, buccal in transverse and palatal in longitudinal section, but the place of division of pulp cavity has been removed in making the section. Tooth *j* presented a shallow groove on the buccal surface of the root, but the additional section showed only one buccal canal. (See also Fig. 3-12 *g,h.*)

In Figure 3-12 *a-d* are four teeth in which the root bifurcated at a late stage into short and rather divergent branches. The teeth were X-rayed and the outlines of pulp cavities added to the tooth outlines in which the level of the cervices are indicated. In *a,b,c,* which are first premolars, the pulp cavities have remained wide until a late stage and then divided into canals just before root bifurcation. This condition resembles the "taurodont" character found in Neanderthal Man. Tooth *d* does not show this character but it has a short pulp chamber and long canals, as also has tooth *e* where the root bifurcates at a late stage into two short but scarcely divergent branches. Both of these teeth with short pulp chambers and long canals are second premolars. Attention was drawn to a similar pattern in the pulp cavities of second premolars in the previous figure (Fig. 3-11 *a,e,g*). Teeth *f* in each Figure 3-11, 3-12 are left first premolars seen from distal; they also have

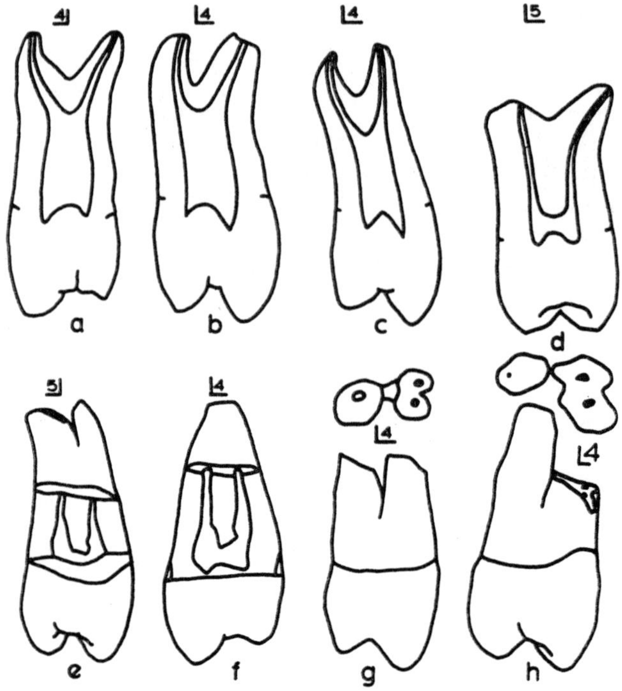

Figure 3-12. Division of pulp cavity at late or early stage of root formation is evidently not dependent on whether the root will divide at a later stage or even remain undivided. Teeth *a,b,c* resemble the taurodont condition, but teeth such as *d* and *f* emphasize that whether (or where) a pulp cavity divides into canals may not be determined visually from the form of the root. The fractured roots of teeth *g,h* present in each case a grooved buccal root branch with two separate pulp canals therein.

short pulp chambers and long canals. These teeth are of the same length but they differ in many other morphological characters such as B-P width, curvature of surfaces and of outlines and apex, marginal ridges and position of B cusp relative to tooth axis.

Teeth *g* and *h* of Figure 3-12 each presented a bifurcated root but the B branches of each root were grooved on the buccal aspect. The P root of tooth *h* is intact but the other roots have been fractured during extraction. In each tooth the B root presented two separate canals, whereas this was not the case with the buccal groove on the root of tooth *j* in Figure 3-11. It is evident that such a groove does not necessarily indicate the presence of two canals. It is also evident that X-rays of upper premolars should be examined carefully as regards root canals. It may be difficult to recognize two main canals placed B and P because of superposition of images. It may be even more difficult to recognize two canals in the buccal part of the root, partly because of superposition on the palatal canal image and partly because these two buccal canals are close together and very fine. The importance of finding multiple canals when present is obvious for certain endodontic techniques. The possibility that they may be associated with actual division of the root is of special interest also to the exodontist.

This study of end outlines of immature teeth, and of grooves in immature and mature teeth, has demonstrated that one cannot do more than guess whether a grooved root contains a single canal or whether it divides. Similarly the point of division into canals cannot be determined by external morphology. Further, it is evident that knowledge as to whether the tooth is a first or second premolar may increase the chances of a judicious guess proving correct, more so if first and second premolars from the same person can be compared. In any case one must recognize the possibility that the guess may easily prove wrong, and that the odds could hardly be determined in the presence of so many variable factors.

UNUSUAL FEATURES

It has already been mentioned that this study does not include gross anomalies in form, but there are a number of cases which justify the use of the adjective unusual. It has been seen that some features and characters vary in the degree to which they have developed or are noticeable. Although there may be no precise limitations in the range of that development, there are some teeth that are obviously different from the great majority. These are the cases that we call unusual.

Some have already been referred to when considering variations such as root thickness, root length and root division. In crowns there were very rounded outlines and almost straight outlines. In several cases the palatal cusps were so short compared with the buccal that one was reminded of lower premolars. In one of these, the palatal cusp tip presents a small irregular depression which could have resulted from hypoplasia of enamel formation associated with abscess of the deciduous molar at about three or four years of age.

In other cases there is no suggestion of a pathological factor being involved in the development of an unusual feature, and the occlusal surface provides good examples. In several teeth a small prominent ridge interrupts the central groove, but it is not the usual triangular ridge ascending from the cusps, for on the buccal cusps, where it is more prominent, it ascends rather from the shoulder of the buccal cusp. It passes somewhat obliquely towards the middle of the groove (Fig. 3-13 *a,b*).

In several teeth the triangular ridges from each cusp were so prominent that the central groove passed over a ridge and was almost divided into two pits as in some lower premolars (Fig. 3-13 *c,d*). In another, by contrast there were no triangular ridges and the two cusps were close together with a small fissure between them. As a result the occlusal surface proper was much reduced and in proximal view the B and P outlines approach the central axis much more than usual (Fig. 3-13 *e,f*).

In two other teeth there was a distinct third cusp placed centrally with a groove or fissure surrounding it. This cusp is larg-

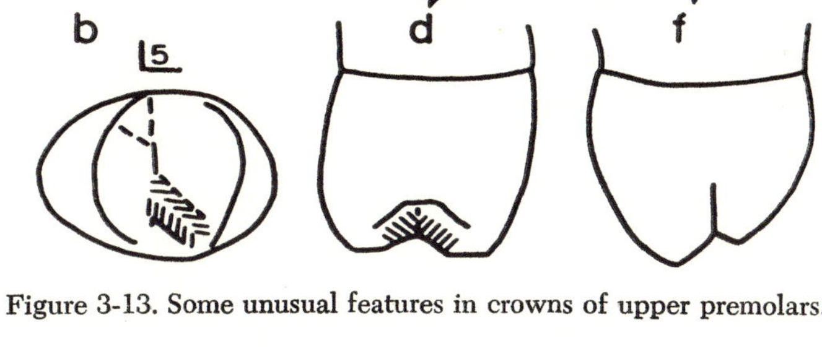

Figure 3-13. Some unusual features in crowns of upper premolars.

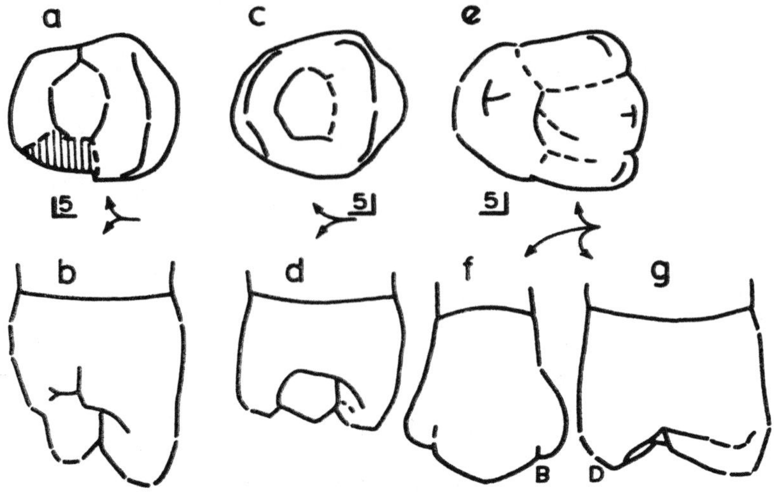

Figure 3-14. Further examples of unusual features in crowns of upper premolars. (The shaded area in tooth *a* is a carious cavity.)

er in one tooth than in the other. The larger one is associated with a much reduced P cusp (Fig. 3-14 *a,b*), but in the other the P cusp is reduced in thickness but not in height (Fig. 3-14 *c,d*). Tooth *a,b* is carious on D and has been drawn from M in *b*.

In another tooth the developmental grooves on the B cusp are very prominent, especially where they pass from buccal to occlusal surfaces, giving prominent shoulders in B view (Fig. 3-14 *e,f,g*). I have presented very few cases as unusual crowns considering the many hundreds that have been examined for this study and considering the very wide variation noted in so many features.

This may prompt enquiry as to what are the usual features of the crown of upper premolars. The answer could be that they present two fairly well defined cusps placed buccally and palatally, and separated by a groove or fissure lying more or less mesial to distal. Seen from buccal, the outline tends to be pentagonal in the unworn tooth; three sides being formed by proximal and cervical outlines, and the cusp forming the other two sides. In buccal view also, features on all other surfaces of the crown are obscured. Insofar as the palatal view can be concentrated on palatal features, the crown outline is again basically pentagonal but the cusp portion is less prominent and more rounded compared with the buccal. The cusp is also asymmetrical, the mesial slope being shorter.

As for the root of upper premolars, the writer has been reluctant to describe any particular feature as unusual. This is because the wide range includes almost every possible variation one could imagine, and in the many hundreds of premolar roots in this collection there were a number of specimens to represent almost every variation found.

WEAR

In ancient skulls of adults it is common to find incisal edges of front teeth worn away, and cusps of posterior teeth worn down or eliminated. In some elderly people the same effect is seen at the present day. In all of these it is obvious that the original form of the teeth has been altered, but one may well question whether such changes should be included in a study of variation in tooth form, although their relevance is easily shown.

The form of unworn teeth, and their arrangement, are the chief factors in establishing the pattern of occlusion; this has a direct bearing on the portions of teeth most subjected to pressure and friction during mastication, and determines where facets of wear will first appear. As time goes on and appreciable amounts of tooth substance are worn away, there are changes in the movements and in their effects, especially if there are no obstructions presented by malocclusions. But where normal inter-digitation of cusps is prevented, as is often the case with present-day teeth, wear becomes irregular in position and degree. Thus form and arrangement largely determine the pattern of wear of this kind.

In our civilized modern communities factors that would otherwise cause excessive wear, chiefly more firm or fibrous texture of foods and more vigorous mastication, are so much reduced that in many cases there is not much loss of tooth substance through wear. But there are other factors to complicate the possibilities of wear—factors sometimes consequent on the need for dental treatment or concerned with artificial prophylaxis or with certain habits—and these may easily produce recognizable effects. These in turn may be related to form and arrangement of teeth, so they cannot be ignored in a study of wear. In human teeth therefore, one may consider wear in terms of variety in relating it to causes. It may also be considered in terms of degree, and in this case Broca's (1879) classification of occlusal attrition with slight modification was found convenient for grading natural wear in native skulls (Taylor, 1962b, p. 175).

In the current study of teeth in the present-day community the question of degree of wear is not so satisfactorily disposed of. While much of it is readily visible to the eye, this is not always so. In the living mouth it is often not apparent as a bulk loss and may be seen merely as a worn facet, and only then if it reflects light. Reflection may not be noticed because of location, curvature of the facet or scattering of light by saliva. An accurate impression and model may overcome some of these difficulties and it is to be noted particularly that the facets are not necessarily confined to the "normal" areas of occlusal contacts or even to occlusal surfaces. With extracted teeth in the dry state, and it is with such that the present study is largely concerned, these facets are easily found by reflection of light. Sometimes it is seen that they have affected the outline of a tooth, perhaps making a cusp appear more acuminate or less so, or a ridge less prominent. This possibility makes observation of facets pertinent to the present study. Moreover they may present evidence as to the normal or abnormal position of teeth in the mouth, and to the presence or absence of adjacent teeth or artificial dentures. Occlusal wear also bears evidence of food toughness, masticatory vigour, habits (such as clenching) and so on. Features which may assist identification of a tooth or individual are especially relevant to this work, and therefore, tooth wear is included.

Earlier work (Taylor, 1962b, 1963a) reported on the nature of wear of teeth in a group of human skulls. Then, after a brief general consideration of wear in animal skulls, a return to the Moriori and Maori skulls showed evidence of excessive loss of tooth substance by wearing away of occlusal surfaces. The probable reasons for such wear were examined and attention drawn to associated conditions such as dislocation. It was shown that explanations presented by other workers were not satisfactory. Some effects not previously reported were described and their cause explained (see also Taylor, 1970c).

In the present study data of wear were obtained not from skulls but from teeth extracted recently by various dentists in the course of daily practice. These teeth present a much greater variety of wear of tooth substance than was found in the skulls, particularly as regards the parts of the teeth involved; but the degree of wear, or the amount of tooth substance worn away, is in the great majority of cases very much less than in the skulls. The present study therefore is quite different, and it goes without saying that conditions under which wear took place in the two groups were as different as the contrast between primitive society and modern European civilization.

The people of those primitive groups did not practise tooth mutilation by any form of filing. They had no leather to soften by chewing, nor pipe stems to hold between their teeth (until the time of contact with Europeans). No operative dentistry or dental prophylaxis was practised, nor any kind of dental appliance used to replace missing teeth. There was no evidence that malocclusion, as so often seen in children now, was present among them. Minor malocclusion resulting from congenitally missing teeth was occasionally present, and local malocclusions were sometimes acquired in later life when teeth were lost following abscesses. In the younger persons however the skeletal remains indicate that jaws and palates were well formed and that periodontal tissues were healthy. Local periodontal pathological effects would of course be associated with the abscessed and dislocated teeth in later years. It seems therefore that tooth wear even to excessive degrees resulted from vigorous masticatory effort, together with some particularly tough and fibrous substances in the diet, along with food contaminants such as sand and ashes, which must have sometimes been present (Taylor, 1975, 1976).

Those contaminants, and tough or fibrous substances in the diet, were virtually absent in the case of the modern civilized persons whose teeth are included in the present study. On the other hand a number of other factors are likely to have been present, in some cases seldom so, in others frequently or habitually. Thus "civilized" teeth (if one may be permitted the use of this convenient term) are frequently subjected to abrasion, not from food contamination but from artificial prophylaxis which involves various surfaces of teeth with no uniformity of results. The chief factors directly concerned are the toothbrush and the dentifrice. Both of these are variable factors in their effects. Firstly, toothbrushes are made in varying degrees of "hardness" according to the diameter of the bristles (whether they be natural bristles, or made of nylon or some other "plastic" substance). Secondly there is considerable variation in the individual "pattern" of using the toothbrush as regards pressure, time and direction of movement. A periodontist in a recent lecture at a dental congress claimed that the dentifrice only, not the toothbrush bristle, was the abrasive factor. But even specialists may err in their conclusions, for the writer has direct personal evidence of the effect of bristles (of medium hardness, lightly used without any dentifrice) as an additional abrasive factor. And moreover this abrasion has resulted from the use of natural bristle only, no brushes of nylon or other plastic having been used. Some people imagine that there is some virtue in using a hard brush (with stiff or thick bristles) and further virtue in using it vigorously. Places of difficult access in the mouth are often missed completely (Taylor, 1971a), while those of easy access often suffer considerable damage to the soft tissue of gums and their attachment. The hard tissues, enamel, cementum and dentine, may be worn away in varying areas and depths. Wear will be greater where an abrasive dentifrice is also used, and of course the abrasive substances and their effects vary considerably. Some degree of softening of tooth surface can result from taking citrus drinks or "soft" drinks frequently and the hard tissues may then be abraded more easily.

Civilized teeth often meet with other abrasive factors as a result of the work of dentists. The placing of fillings may introduce materials of different hardness from tooth substance in places where masticatory movements involve contact with other teeth, or with other fillings. Some of the materials so far used for these purposes have been in the nature of cements (oxyphosphate cements, copper cements, silicate cements, zinc oxide cements), acrylic resins, amalgams, cast alloys and fused porcelain.

Faulty restoration, malocclusions, extractions and prosthetic or orthodontic appliances may lead to, or aggravate, abnormal occlusal contacts during mastication. Another factor arises from occlusal contact under such stresses as clenching or grinding of teeth, known as Bruxism (Wickham, 1968), and this may take place with the mandible in unusual positions such as thrust forward or to one side. The finding of facets of wear in unusual places may establish the existence of such a habit even though the patient may be unaware of it (Every, 1960). Friction from clasps or other removable prosthetic appliances such as bridges and partial dentures is another cause of abrasive wear. It should be emphasized that this is most likely to occur when the appliance is poorly designed or has not been properly maintained and has become unstable. This can easily happen from changes in the supporting teeth or soft tissues, loss of a supporting tooth or loss of part of the appliance such as fracture of a clasp or rest. Where missing teeth have not been replaced by an artificial tooth some remaining teeth are very likely to change position, the change being in the nature of drift, twist or tilt. This is partly the result of changed occlusal stresses and masticatory patterns and is partly the cause of such changes. It is likely to lead to facets of wear in parts of teeth that would otherwise show no such wear.

Thus there is a considerable variety of factors that may lead to signs of wear or abrasion on civilized teeth, even though the amount of tooth substance lost may be much less than that seen in the case of less civilized persons.

There are other factors that may operate in either group, as a result of holding things between teeth, and these may involve little strain or considerable strain on teeth. A well-recognized form of abrasion may follow prolonged holding of a pipe stem between teeth. More severe strains, in view of their concentration in small areas, may follow the habit of biting cotton or holding metal objects such as pins and hair clips between incisors. Typically these produce small ragged chipping of enamel, especially where it has already been worn to a thin edge. Larger chips may be split from teeth already weakened by caries or restorative work, but this kind of trauma, or that caused by removing "crown tops" from bottles with the teeth, is outside the field now being considered. Although wear of teeth from normal mastication is preferably regarded as a natural process, it is readily agreed that some of the factors leading to abrasion or wear of tooth substance may be correctly described as traumatic.

The sites and nature or effects of abrasion are easily demonstrated when actual teeth can be examined and in the present case some thirty-two upper premolars have been selected and mounted. It is difficult to convey an idea of the effects on these teeth with the aid only of words and diagrams, but it must be attempted, at least, for some of them.

In Figure 3-15 *a,b* are shown two teeth with notches at B cervix abraded by toothbrushing. The hard enamel surface has become polished, also the cementum and dentine of the root, and these latter being less resistant to abrasion have become worn away, leaving a large notch. In both teeth there has been destruction of soft tissues and recession, and in tooth *a* the line of attachment at the time of extraction is clearly seen to be much higher up on B side. In tooth *b,* both cusps have been worn down and the dentine exposed. This is second-degree or Stage II wear in the classification of Broca (1879).

Figure 3-15 *c,d* show wear of a tooth that has not been subjected to toothbrushing, at least not "recently" or effectively. It is heavily stained except where subject to food friction during mastication and there is some resultant wear on the enamel of P cusp (first-degree wear). Evidently the owner of this tooth, i.e. the "patient,"

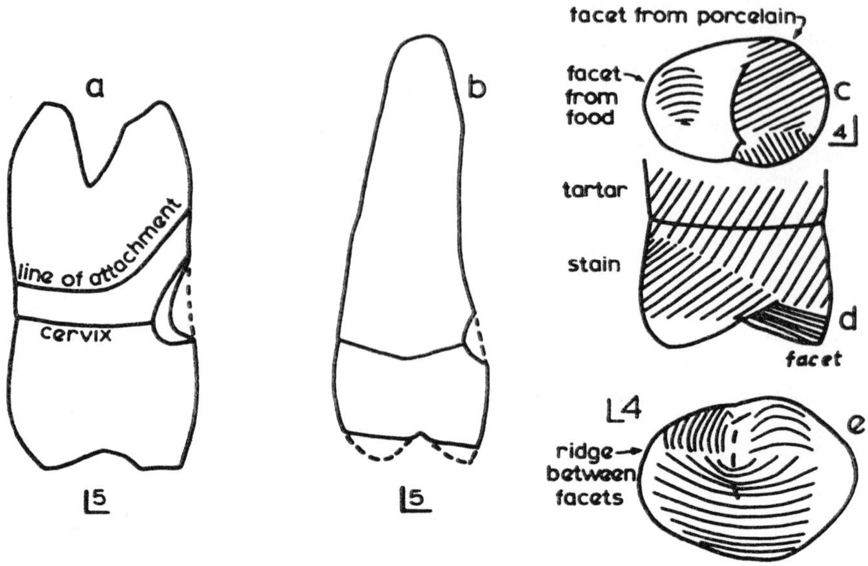

Figure 3-15. Varieties of wear presented in upper premolars.

had acquired lower porcelain artificial teeth, perhaps a partial lower denture. As a result the buccal cusp presents two large facets with the flat glassy surface typical of wear against a porcelain tooth. The ridge-shaped facets suggest that some degree of cusp interference has limited the extent and freedom of movement possible during mastication. In this tooth also there is evidence of deep "pocket" formation and deposition of tartar, particularly on P root.

Tooth *e* in Figure 3-15 presents somewhat similar evidence of restricted movement, particularly in regard to protrusion, for two occlusal facets are inclined to one another with a ridge where they meet, suggesting that occlusal movement was easier in a lateral direction. This kind of wear tends to retain a somewhat cusp-like form.

In Figure 3-16, tooth *a,b* presents this effect in a much greater degree. There is a large distal facet mostly on the buccal cusp and this exposes dentine (dotted

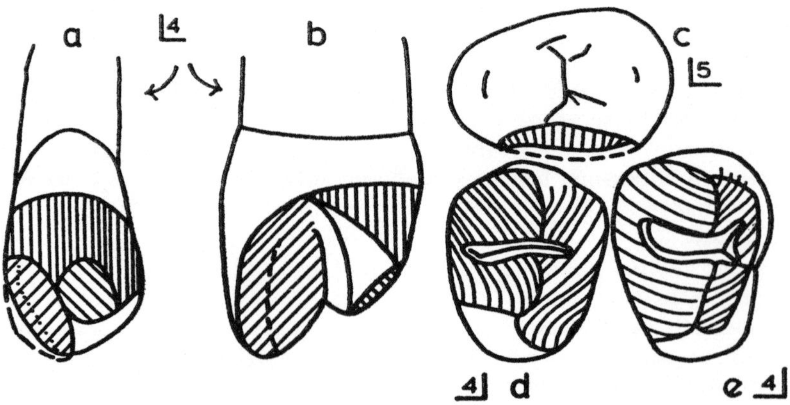

Figure 3-16. Further examples of wear in upper premolars, the shaded areas representing facets of wear.

line) and a smaller facet on the MP of palatal cusp; both these facets are indicated by oblique shading. The vertical shading indicates a large facet, mostly curved around the palatal surface of the tooth, and caused by the up and down movement of an unstable partial upper denture.

The next two groups (not illustrated) are of fully adult (to middle age) teeth presenting mostly second-degree wear, i.e. dentine exposed, that appears to be the result of normal function over a number of years. There is some faceting, but it is not sharply defined and the evidence is that mastication was not vigorous and that the diet contained a small amount of fibre. This is deduced from the fact that enamel is mostly polished or free from stain in the areas that would be subjected to friction if any fibre were present. The presence of stain in some occlusal grooves suggests that toothbrushing if practised was inclined to be desultory and little more than a gesture. That these teeth remained free from caries evidently owed nothing to artificial prophylaxis. One of these teeth presents an abrasion notch at the buccal cervix suggesting that the patient had at some period used a hard brush vigorously and, after doing irreparable damage to both soft and hard tissues, had discontinued the practice. Many teeth in this collection, and many seen *in vivo,* bear testimony to the damage rather than benefit resulting from toothbrushing. This is not surprising in view of the prevalence of badly designed brushes, misleading and bad advertising and lack of instruction or necessary knowledge. It is readily admitted that many more factors are concerned, but this is not the place to digress in that direction (see also Taylor, 1971a).

In an 4⌋ the distal surface shows wear from the clasp of a partial upper denture and the P cusp is worn slightly to a curved facet, highly polished, as is also most of the palatal surface. There has been recession of soft tissues, especially palatal and distal, and there is a rather large cervical cavity on distal, extending to the clasp facet. This region and the whole B and M surface are heavily stained, showing absence of friction. The evidence indicates a preponderance of soft food and failure to brush teeth, even before the denture was made. Another tooth ⌊4 presents somewhat similar evidence of lack of knowledge in the care of teeth and of partial dentures. This particular tooth, in spite of second-degree wear on occlusal, is heavily stained as far as a line of subgingival calculus nearly half-way up the root. Much of the M contour has been lost by abrasion, so that instead of a marginal ridge there is a large concave polished facet extending on to the buccal shoulder of the cusp.

In Figure 3-16 *c* an ⌊5 presents a large facet like a slice removed from occlusal at distal and extending almost to the cervix. The surface of the facet suggests that it has been abraded by almost vertical movements rather than lateral. In the same Figure 3-16, teeth *d* and *e* are each 4⌋ and each presents two very large facets which extend over the occlusal surface on to B and P. The facets are oblique to one another and meet to form a ridge running in a general B-P direction. In spite of extensive loss of tooth substance each cusp retains its cusp-like profile, especially from the buccal aspect. The pattern of wear indicates that while these teeth were in contact, some movement was possible laterally, but protrusive movements were obstructed.

DISCUSSION OF ASPECTS OF VARIATION

A study of variation in tooth morphology must be specific if it is to be effective. Such a task requires an extensive report and this naturally falls into sections, determined by different kinds of teeth, incisors, canines, premolars and molars. But there are aspects of variation that apply to most kinds of teeth, and it was convenient to consider some of them while dealing with premolars.

One of these aspects is the relation between tooth size and sex. In the absence of precise data it is reasonable to expect that tooth length would bear some relation to a person's stature, or that thickness or robustness of a tooth may be in harmony with physical type. But it is obvious that the normal range of variation in these characters is extensive in each sex, and that although the modes are different there is an overlap, or portion of normal range, that is common to the appropriate graph for each sex. In the collection on which this study is based there are many premolars with data relating to sex, physical type and age at time of tooth extraction, and from these have been selected examples to illustrate this aspect of variation. It was easily shown that one cannot reliably sex a tooth from its size in general or length in particular. Further, there was no evidence in the other characters observed to suggest that there may be visibly discernible sex characters in teeth.

The same extracted premolars in most cases presented incomplete roots and were ideally suited for observation of formation of roots and pulp canals. As these show so much variety in upper premolars on account of the many degrees of grooving of roots or division into root branches, with or without division of pulp canals in single-rooted teeth, these characters were readily demonstrated and it was possible to describe or classify patterns in the variation observed.

The shapes of pulp cavities or root canals were studied in relation to root division. Mature teeth were sectioned longitudinally and transversely while immature teeth were used to show the transverse outlines at various stages of root formation. These could be grouped into four main varieties according to the degree of grooving or division of the root, but division of the pulp cavity into separate canals was much more difficult to classify. The place of bifurcation of the pulp cavity into canals varied considerably, from a rather early stage of root formation to a much later one. This point of division could not be determined by observing the presence or depth or width of grooves on the root, but showed considerable variation in position even in single-rooted upper premolars. Indeed, in most such teeth one cannot determine by external examination whether the root contains more than one canal. The possibility of two canals being present is greater when the tooth is known to be a first premolar, but separate canals may rejoin near the apex and present a common foramen.

There are degrees of division of pulp cavity into canals in that the canal portions may still be joined by a narrow bridge of tissue. Perhaps the only certainty in this respect is the obvious one that where there are root branches there is also division of pulp cavity into canals. This must follow from the manner of root formation, but it is conceivable that occlusion of a root canal may occur in one root branch earlier than in another in the same tooth.

Although this study excludes gross anomalies it may sometimes be difficult to decide fairly whether a particular character is anomalous or still within the range of normality. Some characters may therefore be presented as unusual or uncommon, and with the variety of form presented by roots, cusps, ridges and grooves in upper premolars attention was drawn to a number of unusual features in these teeth.

While variation in tooth morphology obviously refers to the form of the tooth as developed *in situ*, it has been considered relevant to acknowledge that morphology may quite normally be altered by wear. Since wear and other acquired characters may provide data useful in dentistry, anthropology and in forensic work, they are important in this study. They certainly have a place in the consideration of aspects of variation. Perhaps also, because of the position of premolars in the mouth, these teeth present a considerable variety of acquired characters, including those related to artificial prophylaxis such as abrasions from faulty toothbrushing habits, or places where stain persists because the areas are "sheltered" from brushing friction.

The manner in which wear alters the form of some upper premolar teeth was shown and some of the causes and effects were referred to. The possible importance of observing small facets of wear in locations indicating unusual mandibular positions was noted. A distinction was drawn between these facets and those which indicate some irregularity in the position of a tooth in the jaw. As with teeth other than upper premolars, a great variety of effects of wear were observed. These varied from patches of stain, or of polishing of certain areas, to actual loss of tooth substance. Ability to evaluate this evidence may enable the dentist to assist his patient to obtain better results from home care of teeth. It may also provide useful information for the forensic odontologist.

VARIATION AS AN AID TO IDENTIFICATION

The two upper premolars have so much in common that one tooth cannot be studied or described without frequent reference to the other. Although there are characters, or aspects of a character, that tend to be exclusive to one tooth, it is important to emphasize the tendency rather than claim exclusiveness. For example, $\underline{4}$ tends to have two roots and $\underline{5}$ to have one root, but in many cases $\underline{4}$ has a single root without even an obvious groove to suggest its tendency to be two-rooted. Similarly, $\underline{5}$ may have two roots, though in such cases its adjacent $\underline{4}$ will almost certainly have a divided root also. Thus an isolated premolar cannot with any certainty be assumed to be $\underline{5}$ merely because its root is single. It was therefore convenient to study the two upper premolars together, rather than separately. Comparisons were made and tendencies mentioned, and sometimes presented almost as generalizations, but one should keep in mind the proverb about rules and exceptions, for variation is so extensive that an emphatic generalization would be foolish. The writer has the notion that the exception usually exists, even though it may not have been recognized in his own experience.

A comment on terminology: Through common usage it is acceptable to refer to a single-rooted, a two-rooted, or a multirooted tooth. This is convenient, and often serves the purpose of the moment, but there are many teeth where such terms are not suitable, either because of degrees of division or because of the attempt to classify the variations noted. Some earlier writers have used expressions such as "the tooth has two fangs," or "the root divides into two fangs." The present writer does not find this helpful, so he has used such terms as root "trunk" and root "branches." Again, he describes a root as having a "tendency to divide," or having a groove "suggesting" division. The part forming the base of the groove may be very thin and be described as the "bridge" between the roots, or as "joining" the roots (although it is obvious that during root formation these parts were never separated). Admittedly these are loose terms for scientific work. This is a study where there are as many variations as there are specimens, and precise description is impossible; if such were attempted the result would be ponderous, complicated and probably incomprehensible. The best that can be hoped for is to convey ideas which facilitate comparisons of form. The study therefore lays no claim to be quantitative, but in a sense it is qualitative in its comparisons. Beyond this we cannot go, for it seems that the differences are the result of so many "variable factors" that their numbers are legion, and we would quail before them.

Black's 1901 descriptions are comprehensive and his illustrations, in spite of subsequent progress in the printer's art and craft, can still be rated as excellent. It is necessary, however, to suggest additions or amendments in some cases. For example, Black divides the term "root" into "body or main portion, apex or terminal end of a root; and the neck. . . ." It is necessary in a divided root to distinguish between the part before the furcation or division, and the parts beyond the furcation, hence the terms root "trunk" and root "branches" respectively.

Again, Black says "a tooth is also marked . . . by the junction of the enamel with the cementum. The latter, which forms a visible line encircling the tooth, is called the gingival line." The present writer prefers to call this the *cervical* line (or cervix), using the term gingival line for the position of the free margin of the gingiva. In his view, therefore, the cervical line on any tooth is definitely fixed, whereas the gingival line may be in whole or in part on crown or root, according to the age of the person and the effect of traumatic or pathological factors.

Differentiation, First and Second Premolar (4, 5)

The reader has been reminded that both upper premolars have much in common, and it has been shown that the range of variation for the two teeth "overlaps" so much that it may be difficult to determine whether an isolated tooth is a first or second premolar. This may be so even though the whole tooth is examined and is undamaged by decay, wear or fracture. But if we have one of each how may we distinguish between them?

To facilitate differentiation let us assume that we have before us a first and second premolar, and that we know they are both from the same person. Comparing roots, if 4 is not bifurcated or 5 is not single, then the tendency towards division or the degree of division would be greater in 4. Comparing crowns, 4 would be larger, with its buccal cusp larger and longer than the palatal. The cusps of 5 are more even in length and there is less contrast in their size (Fig. 2-29). Of the four proximal cervical areas three would tend to be convex or flattened, and one to be concave, namely the mesial of 4 (Fig. 2-30).

Viewed from occlusal there is more contrast in M and D outlines of 4, M tending to straightness more than M of 5. On 4 also there is likely to be a small fissure across the M marginal ridge in line with central groove. In this occlusal view the junction of the M marginal ridge more nearly makes an angle with the shoulder of B cusp than does 5, or than with P cusp of either tooth (Fig. 2-30). We should be able also to find out whether these two premolars are from the same side of the mouth or not.

Differentiation, L and R

To determine whether a tooth is L or R, one must first find the B and P. This should be easy as B is less convex, and is also larger than P, especially in 4. From occlusal, the outline is more oval than elliptical and the minor axis is nearer to B. Looking at palatal aspect, the asymmetry of P cusp should be obvious, with its tip nearer to mesial. If the tooth is 4, further confirmation of M may be found in concavity at M cervix. If the root is single it may have a proximal longitudinal groove. If on one surface, this is likely to be mesial; if on both proximal surfaces, the groove tends to be more prominent, wider or deeper on the mesial. Another guide may be found in the root, for it tends to bend to D, but this is not as reliable as the crown features, and they should take precedence as determinants.

As an aid to placing any tooth L or R, familiarity with the occlusal view of a complete dental arch is recommended. The picture may be modified to show deciduous or permanent teeth *in situ;* or teeth in transverse section at any level, to show pulp cavities, or cervical outlines, or root number and outlines, or socket outlines. A diagram for upper jaw socket outlines of permanent teeth is shown in Figure 2-28. It is not necessary always to refer to a real diagram. It is sufficient to have a mental picture, and it is easy to visualize the tooth in question being placed in the presumably correct position or socket, and its known features checked for that position. For example, if a known $\underline{4}$ is placed in $\lfloor 4$ socket and its cervical concavity then falls to D, it does not "fit," and must be $4\rfloor$. A corresponding diagram for identification of lower teeth is easily visualized and it will of course, face the observer as a U-shape. This method has been found easy to work with, and it has the advantage of conforming to the graphic symbols for identifying teeth as upper or lower, left or right. Others, however, may prefer to identify a tooth by orientation as for their own mouth and then convert to the symbol.

Limitations in Identification

For any upper premolar tooth (the positive identification of which could assist forensically) the following questions could be asked:

1. Is it a human tooth?
2. What class of tooth is it?
3. Is it an upper or lower?
4. Is it a first or second?
5. Is it from left or right side?
6. To what race did the person belong?
7. What was the person's age?
8. Was the person male or female?
9. How long is it since death took place?
10. Is it a "civilized" tooth or not?
11. What was the cause of death?
12. Was the person in good health at time of death?

If other remains including a human skull have been recovered, some further questions might be asked, such as the following:

13. Could this tooth have belonged to that skull?

Before suggesting how far one might reasonably expect to answer the questions, certain qualifications or limitations should be mentioned. Are the answers to be given merely from a naked eye, visual examination? Are laboratory facilities available for microscopy, with or without sectioning? The confidence with which some of the above questions may be answered may depend on a number of factors, so that considerable discussion might be given to the matter. It is intended here merely to give an indication of what might be expected, and to suggest other factors that could be relevant. Some answers could probably be given even if the tooth is not complete.

Partly as a result of the present study of upper premolars, and partly from the wider knowledge possessed by any student of the human dentition, the following comments concerning the above-listed questions are offered:

1. The "humanity" of the tooth should not be difficult to determine. The locality and circumstances of its finding could conceivably have a bearing on possible confusion, and these factors could come into some of the other questions.

2. A premolar stands a very good chance of positive identification.

3, 4 and 5. The present study presents evidence that would facilitate these determinations.

6. One would be foolish to answer this question with any confidence. Although measurements are available for some racial groups, variation usually has a considerable range and the stature of the individual also comes into this question. A dentist with local knowledge of a community (or a student of teeth of a particular racial group) might reasonably say, "I have seen teeth very like this one in such a group," or, "I do not think I would find a tooth like this in people or skulls of that particular group."

7. If the tooth roots were incompletely formed the juvenile nature should be recognizable, and a reasonable estimate of age might be suggested. If the tooth were adult a number of factors might suggest whether the person were a young adult, middle-aged or elderly. Such features as wear, stains, tartar and level of gingival at-

tachment would be helpful. If a section were made, further information could be obtained from the thickness of cementum and the length of translucent root (Miles, 1963). The size of the pulp cavity as regards formation of secondary dentine may also indicate age but not precisely.

8. This study has shown that not even the size of a tooth may be relied on to indicate the probable sex of the person.

9. It seems most unlikely that an isolated tooth can give useful information on this, other than a general surmise based on the circumstances of its finding. This question has a link with the following.

10. A tooth that shows evidence of "dentistry" might provide evidence suggesting where and when the work was done. If a filling were present, its material and evidence of techniques involved may provide some useful information. Absence of evidence of treatment does not necessarily testify that the person was not a member of our present society, and so on.

11. The tooth alone may present evidence of trauma, and support evidence deduced from other skeletal or body material.

12 and 13. The tooth alone may present evidence of local oral pathology through presence of tartar and signs indicating gingival recession. Evidence of other pathology such as hypoplastic enamel may provide useful information such as (a), confirmation of occurrence of an exanthematous illness at an age consistent with medical records, and (b) the probability that an acute abscess of a deciduous molar occurred at a particular age. Of these two examples (a) would probably assist determination whether or not the tooth could have belonged to a known dentition, and (b) similarly in circumstances where detailed records were available.

Examination Procedure

A procedure will now be suggested for the examination of one of these teeth, and how the data concerning it may be obtained.

Identification as a premolar should be almost certain. Occasionally a lower second premolar, an aberrant molar tooth or a supplemental or supernumerary upper premolar may be hard to distinguish from an unusual variation in an upper premolar.

In spite of the wide variation in root forms, the root should give useful information, especially if the root is grooved or actually bifid for part of its length.

Having surmised that the tooth may be an upper premolar some features should be checked:

(a) From occlusal, does it have an oval outline that may distinguish the wider B side?
(b) From occlusal, do marginal ridges form angles at the shoulders of B cusp?
(c) From proximal, can the difference in cusp heights, or B and P convexity, help determine B from P? (P cusp appreciably shorter; it probably equals $\underline{4}$).
(d) Is one proximal cervix less convex than the other, or actually concave, i.e. it equals M of $\underline{4}$?
(e) On this proximal, is the marginal ridge crossed by a tiny fissure or groove? "Yes" equals M.
(f) From palatal, does P cusp tip appear nearer to one proximal than to the other? Cusp tip is nearer M.
(g) Ends of occlusal groove usually turn more obviously to B than to P.
(h) Is the root grooved longitudinally? Is it grooved on both proximal surfaces? The shallow groove on one side only is most likely on M.

Curvature of root has so many variations that although it may indicate probabilities in identification these should not be given too much weight if they conflict with "strong probabilities" arising from other features.

If the root is bifid, or if the pulp divides into two canals even in a single-rooted tooth, it is most likely 4, but this does not necessarily follow. The possibility of it being 5 should be considered, especially if other checks indicate 5 characters.

Thus an upper premolar stands a very good chance of positive identification. There is a good chance that it can be identified as 4 or 5; also a good chance that it can be identified as left or right.

If the tooth is damaged (decayed, filled, crown worn down, crown or root fractured), there may still be sufficient characters to enable identification to come very close to certainty.

Features of forensic value determined microscopically or by other means should also be checked as far as possible if doubt of identification remains, or where additional information is desirable.

In summary, therefore, upper premolars present a number of characters that may help to identify an isolated tooth as an upper premolar. Other characters may enable one to differentiate between a first and a second, and between a left and right upper premolar. There are yet other characters that are of little value by themselves for such differentiation. Their presence in varying degrees, or the association of some with others, may still contribute useful information where comparison is possible with other teeth in a particular dentition, for some of these characters may be recognizable also in other teeth of the same dentition. Such characters include those of overall size, proportionate size in dimensions of length and breadth, acumination of cusps, convexity of outline or of surface areas, number or complexity of main and subsidiary grooves and their depth, smoothness of enamel, colour and so on, whether they are characters of crown only or of roots or of both. These may be regarded as hereditary and congenital characters, which have been built into the tooth. Among these there may be evidence of pathology such as hypoplasia, associated with exanthemata.

In addition, it should be noted whether the tooth presents further characters that have been acquired as a result of environmental or local conditions in the mouth. The presence and nature of stains and their distribution upon the tooth which may bear witness to certain masticatory and prophylactic "patterns"; the nature and degree of polishing or wear which may do likewise; the presence, type, amount and location of deposits of tartar bearing witness to gingival and oral pathology—these also, together with the hereditary characters, tend to be consistent throughout a dentition. Some other characters such as the hypoplasia of enamel of a permanent tooth associated with an abscessed deciduous tooth, a dilaceration of a root or a fracture of a crown, may have a more local significance. From those that tend to be more general, one should be able to say that a particular tooth could, or could not, have formed part of the same dentition as another isolated tooth, or group of teeth.

Morphological Aspects of Dental Variation

Because upper premolars may have one, two or three roots and there are more characters to observe in crown and root, they give more scope for observing variation than do anterior teeth. The molars with more cusps and root branches than the premolars present an even more complex group for study, but with premolars one may make a fairly detailed analysis without the description becoming unwieldy.

The theme of this study is variation. If this key word must be elaborated we may add the phrase "between fairly well-defined limits." The limits are thus defined because we have excluded gross anomalies in any of the categories of incisors, canines, premolars and molars, and it is only among anomalies that we find teeth that cannot fairly readily be identified by some feature and placed in one of those categories. In lower premolars the range in crown form is considerable, but the great majority of upper premolars have two well-defined cusps; and it is the root or roots that present so much variety. From the upper premolars in this collection a selection of approximately 500 have been mounted and labelled on seventy-three cards. In the sixty-eight figures of Chapters 2 and 3 some 440 diagrams or outlines present 354 outlines from actual teeth. It has been amply demonstrated that there is no such tooth as a "typical" upper premolar, particularly as regards the root, and therefore we cannot have a standard or type specimen for our comparisons. The survey covered a much wider field than the collection mentioned above and observed such differences as general and special characters and related these to particular kinds of teeth. The nature of some variations could be assumed and looked for, and in due course examples were found.

General characters include those related to the individual's physique, such as body build and stature, but those associated with anatomy of adjacent structures might also be regarded as special characters. So also in the case of characters associated with differentiation between left and right, or upper and lower teeth, and it was shown how either crown or root, or both, may contribute to differentiation. The study sought variations in crown and root separately, and also in relation to one another.

In the case of the root of upper premolars the list of obvious and of suspected and possible variations suggested the following questions or lines for study:

I. In single-rooted teeth: overall length; length of root relative to crown size; thickness of root in general;

Does the notion of a root axis assist description? change in root thickness, or taper of root;

This change may be gradual from near cervix, or it may be more abrupt from some other point between cervix and apex;

This taper may be as viewed from B or P, or quite differently, from proximal.

Does taper from one aspect imply similar taper from the other, or, may taper be observed in one aspect and not in the other?

Relations between taper and shape of apex: shape of apex—sharp point, blunt and rounded, squared.

Root curves or bends: involving whole root or part of root.

Is it reasonable to distinguish between gradual and abrupt bends?

Is a slight degree of bend or curve truly a change in direction of root axis?

Could it be a visual impression produced by uneven taper in the outlines?

Is curvature in only one, and in one particular direction?

Does the root curve in more than one direction?

If yes, does this mean:

(a) curved when seen from different directions?

(b) curved in more than one direction in a single view?

Can bends in root, abrupt or gradual, be related to proximity of certain anatomical features?

If so, why are such bends not always present?

Grooves in root of single-rooted tooth: Where are the grooves found and are they more likely on one surface than another?

Is depth of groove related to bifurcation of root?

Is depth of groove related to bifurcation of pulp cavity?

Is any particular groove always present?

In what way do grooves vary in width and depth along their length?

Are grooves related to whole length, or any part of root length?

II. In teeth with furcated roots: Is division associated with some constantly present feature in single-rooted teeth?

Is there any regular pattern of root division such as:

(a) the arrangement of root branches;
(b) the position of furcation;
(c) association of root dimension with a particular type of root (thick generally, thick or wide in a particular dimension)?

Is division found in a strongly tapering root?

Root curve or bend: Can the root trunk bend before furcation?

When there are two root branches, placed B and P,

(a) Does either tend always to bend in a certain direction?
(b) Do they diverge or converge or remain parallel?
(c) Are these directions judged by outlines of tapering root branches?
(d) Are they judged by directions of axes of root branches?
(e) Are divergences, etc., capable of measurement, or are they subjective impressions?
(f) Is it possible to describe variations in the outline of the cleft between root branches, such as U- or V-shaped, wide or narrow, long or short, etc.?

The study of grooves could not be completed in single-rooted teeth. While these had presented grooves on M and D surfaces, a groove was also found on the B surface. Sometimes it was so deep that the root from buccal was divided into M and D parts but remained single with no bifurcation involving P root (Figs. 3-8 *e* and 3-10, II *e*). In bifurcated roots the B root was sometimes grooved on its P aspect, but this palatal groove was not found to be closely associated with division of the B pulp canal into two canals. Such division appeared more intimately associated with the longer B groove on B aspect of the root, especially when the groove was deep. One tooth presented a separate MB root branch with the P and DB elements fused, as is not uncommon in upper molars.

As there are so many characters of a tooth root for observation, in their degree of development, in their relation to other characters and in the nature of their variation, too much attention might be given to the subject. But it was thought desirable to convey an idea of the complexity of the study, so that while showing the impossibility of precise description a means was sought to present information concerning those characters. The original conception of relating curved outlines of teeth to diagrams consisting mostly of straight lines and geometrical shapes, and then reducing the tooth outline to a diagram of straight lines, had been developed by the writer in the early 1930s as a method of teaching dental anatomy to student nurses of the New Zealand School Dental Service. It was found to be a great help to them in an appreciation of tooth form. Its principles were applied in 1937 to prove that the Piltdown dentition as restored was not acceptable and the soundness of this criticism was confirmed many years later (see Appendix 6). In the present study the method has been extended to enable variations in root shape to be classified and presented according to a formula. From a formula expressed in words it is possible to draw an outline resembling an outline view of the tooth concerned. Those who have studied teeth closely enough to appreciate the extent of variation will realize how useful this ability could be in some forensic problems.

The study of tooth crowns was much facilitated by applying similar principles and methods. A list of characters and features prepared for checking included the following:

(a) Outlines—in proximal view; crown dimensions, and position or level of greatest B P dimension; height of crown and length of cusps; form of cusps; crown axis at right angles to cervix, and its relation to axis from B cusp tip; curvature of B and P outlines; curvature of cervical lines, M and D.

(b) B cusp from buccal aspect; curvature of proximal outlines and position of "shoulders"; length and acumination of cusp.

(c) P cusp; length and acumination; asymmetry from P aspect.

(d) Occlusal—asymmetry of oval outline; position of axes; relation of occlusal surface to occlusal view; position of cusp tips; ridges, triangular, marginal, buccal; grooves, central, accessory and buccal ("developmental").

(e) Fosse angle and relation to marginal ridges.

It is easy to think of other variations, or other factors likely to be concerned in variation. These could be as follows: (a) enamel, its smoothness or roughness in the nature of "imbrication" lines; (b) enamel, its shade, translucency, and presence of more opaque spots; (c) grooves or fissures starting in enamel and extending to root, as found on lingual of some upper incisors; (d) characters of comparison, related to adjacent teeth; (e) characters of comparison, related to a particular ethnic group; (f) characters that sometimes might be called submicroscopic, and sometimes might be suggestive of pathology, function or trauma, such as spots, scratches and fractures; (g) wear and all its varieties of type and degree; (h) acquired characters such as stains and accretions.

The above lists are incomplete and do not exhaust the aspects of variation that may be observed with the naked eye, and without the further aids of sections, microscopes, or other equipment for tests whose nature is physical, optical or chemical, etc. They do, however, establish the great range of characters that may be used to describe a particular tooth and to distinguish it from others of the same kind.

Some features were found in only a few teeth, and often there arose the problem of degree and subjective judgment. In some ways the collection providing data for this study was not ideal, but the thought arises that even in this computer age a final analysis of any group can only have a moderate degree of exactitude and a limited application.

Discussion and Summary

Normal upper premolars should be easily recognizable as such, especially if crown and root are complete. If one were handed two such teeth and given the information that (a) they were from the same person and (b) they were a first and second premolar, it should not be difficult to differentiate between them. It would not be so easy to determine whether they were both from the same side of the mouth, or to which side they belonged.

If neither (a) nor (b) were known, it could be difficult to identify them as first or second, or as left or right upper premolars. If either tooth were incomplete, so that morphological characters had been lost or altered by fracture, wear, decay or restoration, identification could be very difficult. But identification might be important forensically, so that any character which may assist in this (even to showing that a certain tooth could or could not have formed part of the same dentition as other known teeth) should be examined. This has been a main objective in the present study, but it is relevant to consider others that may have been achieved at the same time.

Among these are the applications to the practice of dentistry. Apart from the obvious advantage of awareness of possible anatomical variations before teeth are extracted, there are implications for conservative dentistry. These bear on the chances of success with various procedures, according to the skill of the operator and the cooperative ability of the patient. The degree of convexity of tooth surfaces is one factor that bears on the site for cavity margins and the fitting of matrices. But before this stage the same curvature has been facilitating or limiting the efficiency of regular home care of teeth, and this has a bearing on the initiation of caries and on gingival health. Prior to this consideration the same factor of curvature also affects the efficiency of mastication. This of course is linked with such things as good occlusion or malocclusion, choice of type of food, nutrition and tissue tone. Thus the variations of tooth form may have some part in determining whether it is easy or difficult to maintain good oral health and, therefore, good general health also. This evidence can assist in explaining why some people fail to achieve certain results in oral health in spite of being conscientious, and why others who are apparently careless appear to be blessed by the gods beyond what they deserve. And further, with regard to the roots themselves, variations in their morphology and in the form of pulp cavities are relevant to orthodontic and endodontic procedures respectively. Knowledge of the nature and range of variation, therefore, has wide application in the various fields of general and specialized practice. It is important not only to student and practitioner, but also to the lay individual, who is entitled to have the knowledge applied to his benefit through the profession concerned.

Dental anthropology has long recognized the importance of teeth in archaeology, and teeth may also contribute much to genetic studies. Forensic odontology is now of increasing importance. In these days when mass air crashes and other disasters are unfortunately more frequent, identification of victims is often a matter of urgency, and dental parts, even to the extent of just two or three teeth, may be among the few recognizable portions of a mutilated or incinerated human body. Familiarity with tooth morphology and tooth variation may therefore contribute materially to identification of victims. That such identification would be facilitated by, and sometimes dependent upon, adequate record-keeping by dentists points to its own moral. The present study contributes to the knowledge necessary for this field.

It was not the purpose of this work to add yet another description of the human teeth to those given in various books on dental anatomy. Such descriptions may have been sufficient for certain purposes but they fail to cover adequately the variations from what is presented as, for example, a typical central incisor, upper canine, first premolar and so on. Perhaps the main obstacle has been the cost of publication, but the fact remains that those descriptions of so-called typical teeth and generalizations about variation are neither scientifically acceptable nor sufficient. In references to variations, or range of variation in the present work, gross abnormalities of form are ignored. Although of interest, these cases are of minor importance except to the persons immediately concerned, and they are adequately described in case reports and preserved in odontological collections. The purpose here has been to present as good an idea of variation as difficulties of publication might permit, but a real appreciation of variation can best be gained by study of many thousands of teeth both extracted and *in situ,* over a long period. This is in fact the source of data here presented.

The present material from which data were obtained (except for a relatively few specimens) lacks records of sex, of age and of race, due to the manner of its collection. Even if it had been possible to preserve such information the handling of the material, already a frightening task for one person through its many sortings and other "processing," would not have been feasible. And what has been lost thereby? Sufficient information was readily obtained to confirm that sex is by no means a major determinant of size of teeth. If sex were responsible in some way for variation in form of human teeth it would surely have been reported long ago, and this does not ignore the possibility that sex may influence differences observed in mean dimensions. Age is no doubt responsible in some cases for thickening a root by cementosis or shortening it by resorption (and for wearing away of crown substance), but the author has tried to recognize and exclude such cases from the study of variation. On the other hand such teeth do have a place in the purpose of the study.

With regard to race as a factor in variation of tooth form the question is not of great importance here. It has been dealt with by other workers and such characters as shovel-shaped incisors have been studied (Moorrees, 1957). Quantitative studies have reported differences in size as well as the range of size variation in certain racial groups.

In an earlier publication I have shown that even with a standardized technique, accurate measurements and statistical analysis, the results of such work on skeletal material may have limited significance (Taylor, 1962a). In the case of teeth, attention was drawn to additional variable factors that confuse results. It was shown that some kind of graphical representation in addition to statistics is greatly to be desired, and that indices do not convey an idea of form, nor does a variation of some degrees in an index appear to have much comprehensible significance. Comparison between groups by measurement and indices seemed to have little to justify deductions that are made. Unfortunately this is still commonly the pattern of research but more attention should be given to variable factors and to the fact of wide variability.

It may be asked why this study is qualitative and in no sense quantitative. The reply may well be another question and enquire what information is desired, and why. Mensural programmes may have limited applicability according to the subject of study. With teeth the feasibility of securing maximum dimensions is accepted, but that is about all. Proportionate dimensions of crown and root would demand exactitude in defining landmarks, and in orientation of tooth and measuring device, as well as ability to treat each tooth in the same way. That this is impossible is found by studying variation in teeth. Somewhat similar limitations apply to measurements of a group of teeth *in situ,* but arch curvature and loss of tooth substance by interproximal wear are major complications if comparisons are desired. For individual teeth, occlusal wear, even if strictly at right angles to tooth axis, is sufficient to render measurements useless, and even tenths of a millimeter are important in such short distances. Very restricted usefulness has been found for the limited measurements so far made of tooth dimensions, and they will depreciate even further in value when the nature of variation receives more attention.

Root division and division of pulp cavity into canals are of special interest and practical importance in certain operative procedures, but what plan of mensuration could produce useful results? Is the investigator to seek furcations or apices, and how can he find acceptable landmarks in the presence of curves, bends and divergences? How is one to decide whether a tooth has a branched root when it is a "borderline" case? Surely grooves and pulp canals are involved here, along with sections and microscopes? Where is one to draw the line? The more categories one has, the less useful are the results; the fewer the categories, the less specific each one becomes.

When it comes to studying proportion it has been easy to show by observing variations but without precise measurements that, for example, (a) crowns and roots are largely independent except for the sharing of common proportions at the cervix; or (b) the degree of taper seen in a root in, say, buccal view is independent of its taper in proximal view; or (c) root thickness in either dimension is independent of root length.

It is popular to devise indices to indicate proportions, but it is clear that indices concerning tooth roots would convey nothing useful. Moreover, an index of such small measurements as root thickness would not only be subject to wide error, but would be different for a particular tooth, according to where the measurements were taken. Thus a statistical presentation regarding variation in tooth form must be highly suspect and therefore almost useless.

The above evaluation of mensural studies of teeth amounts to devaluation, especially as far as comparisons are concerned, and the writer believes that the present study adds emphasis to this conclusion. But what can be said of the qualitative analysis that has been presented? We feel that it has led to conclusions that are useful and informative, even if they relate in some cases to what have been reasonable assumptions hitherto. Among these findings for upper premolars may be listed the following:

Constants. These are the presence of two fairly well defined cusps. It is exceptional for the buccal cusp to be smaller than the palatal cusp. Only one exception was found in the many teeth examined.

Root Form. It is by no means constant. In either the first or second premolar the root may be single, or divided into two or three branches. The degree of division tends to differ in the two teeth in the same person, being greater in the first premolar. This tooth tends to be more obviously grooved if single, or divided for more of its length than its second premolar.

Identification as First or Second. A concavity at mesial cervix is nearly always present in the first premolar. It varies much in depth and may be recognizable only by comparison with thc distal, which is invariably convex in a normally developed tooth. The difference in cusp sizes is greater in the first premolar, the buccal cusp being both wider (seen from occlusal) and longer. In the second premolar the buccal cusp is wider but not so noticeably longer than the palatal cusp. There is appreciable variation in the degree of difference in length, so that both cusps may appear almost equal in length, even in some first premolars. The palatal cusp is usually asymmetrical, with its cusp tip nearer to mesial, especially in first premolars. This feature assists in placing the tooth as left or right.

Root Division. This is much more common into buccal and palatal branches, so that if there are three roots, furcation into B and P is the first division. The second division takes place in the buccal root, and it has not been found in palatal. The division of buccal root with palatal still joined to both buccal branches, or to distobuccal, has been found.

When there are two roots they tend to be approximately equal in length and thickness; when there are two buccal roots they tend to be equal in size, but each shorter and more slender than the palatal root.

The groove on proximal of a single-rooted tooth tends to be more obvious and deeper on mesial.

Grooves were not found on palatal roots but they were sometimes present on B or P, or on both of these aspects of a buccal root.

Root Thickness. Whether a root is single or divided it may be slender, medium or thick. This may apply to the outline from proximal and from B or P aspect, but it may differ in the two views; e.g. it may be slender from B and more robust from proximal viewpoint. The root decreases in thickness from cervix to apex (root taper) and does not increase in this direction in a normally developed tooth, or in the absence of pathological increase in cementum. The rate of taper may increase and this may show more on one side of an outline than on the other, giving a false appearance of root curve.

The Root Apex. This, in a single-rooted tooth, may appear square, rounded or pointed, with varying degrees of taper. Where a root tends to furcate at a late stage the variety possible in apical form and direction is still very considerable.

Root Curves or Bends. There is a very great variety, thus:

(a) In single roots the curve may involve part of, or the whole root. If part only, the curve may be slight or abrupt and may be directed to M, D, B or P, or to any point between these. If the whole root is involved, it may present a slight curve or even a long sweeping curve, and this variety tends to bend mostly towards distal. If the curve is abrupt it may reasonably be associated with close proximity to the maxillary or nasal sinus, and some such curves are demonstrably so associated. A few cases of abrupt or considerable bends may have a traumatic origin through dislocation of an incomplete premolar during extraction of a deciduous molar.

(b) In bifid roots—with a short cleft, the two small root branches may be parallel and straight, or bend in almost any direction; if not parallel they may diverge or converge; with a long cleft, the two long branches (as with short) may be parallel and straight, or bend in almost any direction, or they may diverge at an angle from point of bifurcation and then be straight or curved. And further, in the case of a long cleft, the branches if not parallel may diverge or converge, or (since more length is available for variation) they may diverge and then converge. (Examples of all of these were found, but there was no case where the root branches first converged and then diverged). Or, the two-root branches may curve independently; each branch may curve in more than one direction, i.e. the apical portion may present a different direction of bend, and this may apply to each branch or to only one of them.

(c) In a trifid root (one palatal root and a divided buccal root); with a short B cleft, the B branches may be parallel and straight, or bent. If not parallel they may diverge, or bend independently. If there is a longer B cleft, the two buccal branches may be straight and parallel, or slightly divergent; they may present more than one bend, or may diverge and then converge.

Whether the cleft between buccal branches is short or long, these branches may bend independently. (In the case of a trifid root there is no reason to believe that the relation between P root and the divided B root would not be found to vary in all ways as for a two-rooted tooth. The analysis is terminated before it tends to become mathematical, with permutations and combinations!)

This great range of possible variations in root form arises largely from the fact that the root may or may not divide and that the length of the root gives ample scope for bends, for variation in furcation positions and for variations in direction of bend for the root trunk and its branches.

THE CROWN. There is much less scope for variation in the crown in that manner in spite of presenting probably more features for study than does the root. From the crown alone it is usually possible to identify the tooth as an upper premolar, and to distinguish first from second premolars and left from right. As the formation of two cusps, neither more nor less, is perhaps the most constant character, these identifications and distinctions depend on the ways in which the cusps can vary, with the asymmetries that result. Although B and P views give rather similar outlines, the additional details seen in P view make this more useful for identification because of asymmetry in the palatal cusp whereby its cusp tip is nearer to mesial. The other two main views, occlusal and proximal, are also helpful. Occlusal view, by its oval outline, indicates buccal side near the minor axis; the more angular mesial shoulder of buccal cusp and less convex mesial outline also assist in identifying mesial and distal. The fine fissure crossing the mesial marginal ridge may be seen in this view, especially in a first premolar. Proximal views are best for comparing cusp heights, buccal and palatal convexities, and for noting whether the cervical region is less convex, or actually concave on one of them. These various features assist identification as left or right and as first or second premolars. Fosse angles seen in these views do not assist this aspect of identification, but if clinically appraised they may well assist optimal location of cavity margins. Similarly, variations in cusp acumination do not assist identification of teeth but provide a kind of "family resemblance" through all teeth in a particular dentition.

Although invariably present, the two cusps may be so nearly equal in length or height that any difference is not apparent. If one cusp is longer it should be the buccal cusp, and, if it is much longer, the tooth is likely to be a first premolar. Cusps may vary in thickness according to difference in distance from B or P in occlusal and proximal views, or according to thickness of triangular ridges. The B cusp is usually thicker as regards triangular ridges, perhaps more so when longer. A wide fosse angle may indicate greater separation of cusps or reduction of triangular ridges.

In occlusal view the fissures or grooves may be deep or shallow. If they are deep the subsidiary fissures may be terminal pits at mesial and distal ends of the central fissure. The subsidiary fissures or grooves tend to pass more obviously towards B than towards P cusps. If there is a small fissure passing over a marginal ridge it is likely to be the mesial marginal ridge, and it is seldom seen on a second premolar.

Conclusion

It has been established that the range of variation in upper premolars is very considerable. The details of variation have been classified and described. Their relation to effective prophylaxis, natural and artificial, has been indicated. Where details of form should be noted by the operator, or their effect allowed for, these factors have been indicated or explained and their importance to the "patient" has been noted.

There is no need to stress the importance of an awareness of variation and of its details in dental anthropology, and it is believed that this study will be useful also in forensic work. In these respects the aim has been to show whether and how an upper premolar may be positively identified, and therefore a procedure for examination of a tooth has been suggested.

Although there are some characters, or combinations of characters, or degrees of their development that may seem to be present more often than others, it must be emphasized that there is no selection from these that could define a "typical" upper premolar, either first or second. The many thousands of teeth examined have presented so much variation that it is obvious that the term "typical" as applied to a tooth is not justified. This conviction applies not only to upper premolars, but to any individual tooth in the human dentition.

Chapter 4

Mandibular Incisors

SOME LOWER CENTRAL incisors closely resemble some lateral incisors so that, given an isolated lower incisor, one may be unable to determine which it is (Fig. 4-4 *f*). It may be almost as difficult to decide whether it is left or right. But this does not mean that all lower incisors are very much alike, for within the "lower incisors" group there is a considerable range of variation in every obvious feature. These include length and breadth dimensions when comparing one tooth with another, or length and breadth dimensions separately of crown and root in relation to one another. No gross disharmonies between crown and root were found. Other characters that vary are the curvature or straightness of outlines, degree of taper, roundness of incisal angles, prominence of cingulum, presence of incisal tubercles, "twist" between root and crown and the great variety of root that may be presented by a single-rooted tooth as regards bends or curves and the shape of the apex.

All these are dealt with here. Other features that will be noted are related to developmental and environmental conditions involving the enamel surface and the loss of tooth substance by various kinds of wear, both functional and otherwise. As in previous chapters, opportunity will be taken to relate certain observations to the clinical practice of dentistry. Some characters or features may assist identification of a particular tooth, or enable some deduction to be made concerning the relation of a tooth to others in the same dentition, or may be related to physical characters or habits of the person to whom a tooth belonged.

As before, the text is based on observation of a very great number of teeth, including a collection of extracted teeth. Although these have been reduced to small groups selected especially to illustrate the observations and statements made, they still amount to a considerable number. In the case of lower incisors alone there are 246 teeth mounted on thirty-six cards, and any one of these teeth is referred to by its number in series M and position on that card. Of those selected for illustration in the accompanying figures, line drawings were made with the aid of a camera lucida specially adapted for the purpose. The scale shown in a figure applies to each outline in that figure.

The real differences between lower centrals and laterals are best found, not by comparing a number of known centrals with a number of known laterals, but by comparing centrals with their own laterals in a number of dentitions. Such groups are presented in the collection on cards M1, M2 and M3, and two of these groups are seen in Figure 4-1. At once it is obvious that there is a main difference as compared with the findings presented by upper incisors, for the lower central is narrower M-D than its lateral, and is a smaller tooth in other dimensions also. The most noticeable difference is in the maximal width of crown M-D (Fig. 4-1 *b,c* and *d,e*). The width labio-lingually at cervix is not so obviously different. In length measurements the incisal to labial cervix distance is very similar. The differences, such as there are, always show the lateral as larger. Total length, or root length from labial cervix to apex, may be almost identical; but sometimes they may be appreciably greater in the lateral, especially when there is a curved root, and this is invariably to the distal. Apical curves to labial are common in each tooth.

Comparison of overall size in maxillary

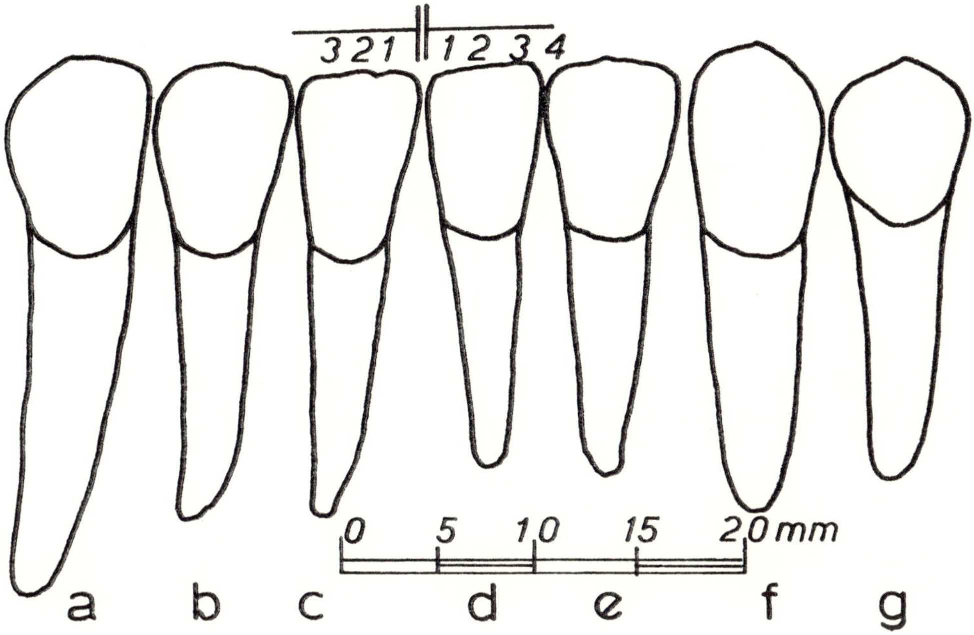

Figure 4-1. Mandibular central incisors compared with their own laterals and canines. *a,b,c,* right-side teeth from one person. *d-g,* from another person, enabling comparison of incisors with their own cuspid and first premolar. (See also Figs. 4-14 and 4-15.)

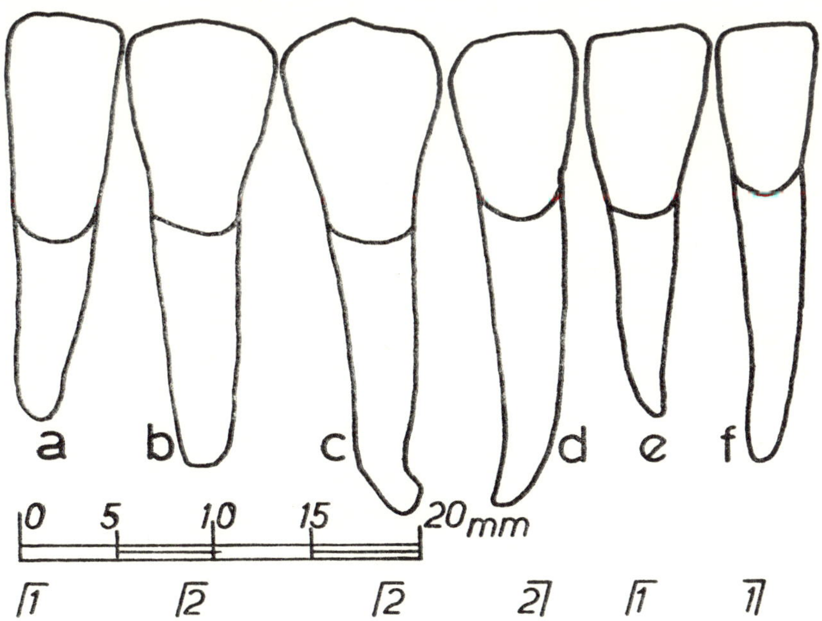

Figure 4-2. Central and lateral incisors from different persons, indicating the wide range of form and relative dimensions of crown and root that are found in these teeth, in labial view.

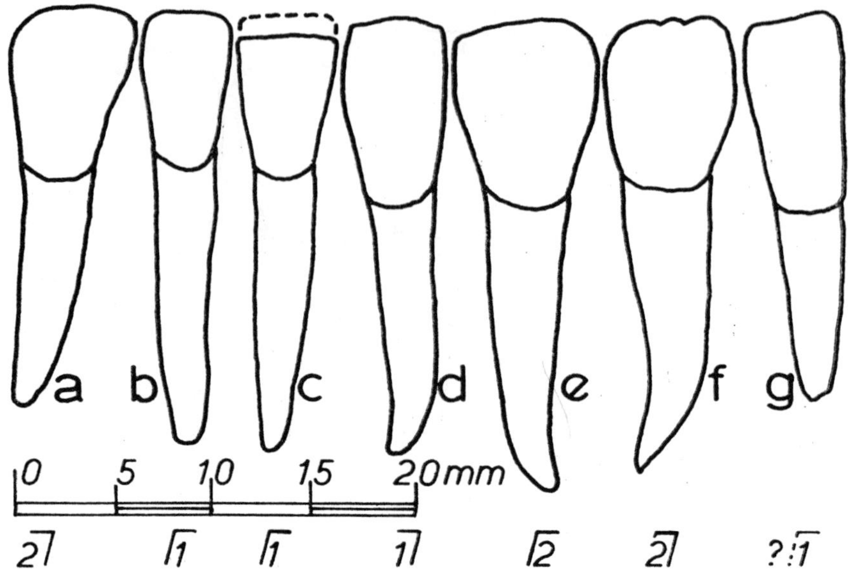

Figure 4-3. Further examples of variation in mandibular incisors, as in Figure 4-2. Tooth *c* has lost crown height through wear of second degree.

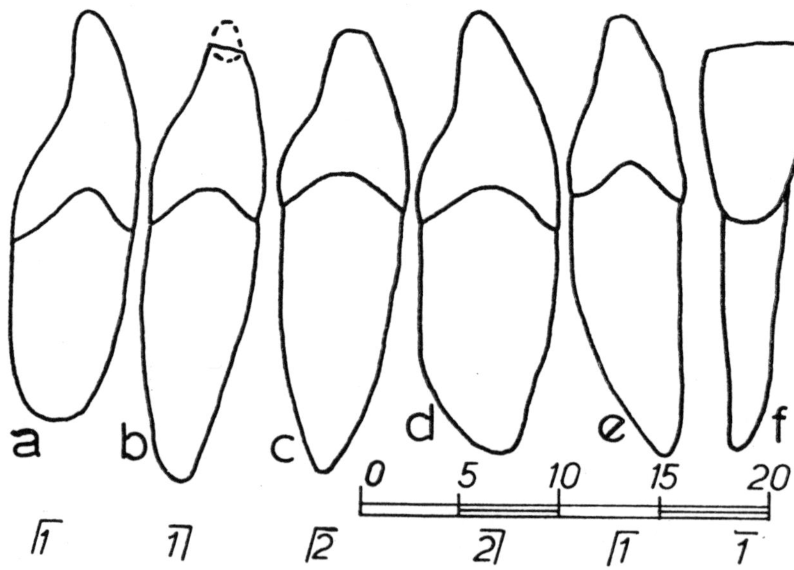

Figure 4-4. *a-e,* proximal outlines of lower incisors showing some of the variations found in root form, in apices, and in crown/root proportions. *f* (and Fig. 4-3 *g*). Sometimes a tooth is almost bilaterally symmetrical and identification as a left or right tooth may be difficult.

incisors showed that large laterals may exceed the size of small centrals, and the size ranges of lower incisors also overlap. Because large lower centrals may be bigger than small laterals, and because of the greater difficulty of distinguishing between lower incisors than in the case of uppers, much of the discussion in this chapter will relate not to centrals and laterals separately, but collectively to "lower incisors."

Thus Figures 4-2 and 4-3 show lower incisors from different persons, and they present considerable variety in form and dimensions. Length of crown in relation to width of crown, or to length of root, obviously are not constant ratios; it would be pointless to attempt a mathematical or statistical description of these differences. Lower incisors therefore, like the upper teeth already studied, call for a qualitative analysis of variation.

THE CROWN OF LOWER INCISORS

Some characters in which these teeth vary have been briefly mentioned. The most easily recognized differences are in the dimensions and shapes when seen from labial, and even an untrained observer may remark that a certain person's teeth are large or small, or long or narrow or wide, and so on. When extracted teeth are examined, and both crown and root may be studied from various aspects, we may appreciate how much wider is the field in which variation can and does occur. Thus, in Figure 4-2, teeth *a* and *f* have similarities in shape of crown though not in size. The wider tooth *a* presents a less convex cervical line. Although both roots are fairly straight, they present contrasts in actual length and in thickness, the shorter root being actually wider. Again, in regard to length, the short tooth has a crown that is actually a long crown, so that its root length is very short relative to crown length. With tooth *f* the reverse is the case.

In proximal view other dimensions and characters invite comparison. Tooth *a* now seen as Figure 4-4 *a* is no longer a wide crown compared with its length, and it may be described as having a long, relatively thin blade that curves over towards lingual with a peaked cervical line. The root presents little taper and the apex is blunt and rounded. The other tooth (Fig. 4-2 *f*) is seen in proximal view in Figure 4-4 *b*, and in this view presents a long fine tapering apex, a more rounded cervical line, and a blade that is more sturdy relative to its size. Differences in the cervical line are apparent in other teeth (*c,d,e* of this Fig. 4-4). They also present variety in curvature and taper of root outline and the position and sharpness of apex associated with these variations. The outline of tooth *e* is not common, though there were a number of this kind in the collection. In this profile it presents a rather straight outline on labial almost from incisal edge to apex, with an arc from apex to lingual cervix. The tooth axis in this view is much nearer to labial, and this is a character found in the great majority of upper incisors and canines. The much more common labial profile in lower anterior teeth presents a more or less continuous arc from incisal to apex, or at least to the apical region (Figs. 4-4 *c,d;* 4-5 *e*).

In upper incisors it is usual to find the distal incisal angle noticeably more rounded than the mesial, especially in the lateral. A similar difference between incisal angles and between central and lateral is found in lower teeth, but the first part of the above statement must be modified, for many lower incisors must be excluded. These are, in general, those incisors which have rather straight sides, especially those tending to be more nearly parallel-sided. Teeth with more flare, such as that in Figure 4-3 *a,* more often present rounded angles and the differences between M and D angles that have been mentioned. More such cases in laterals are in Figures 4-5 and 4-3 *e,f.*

Tubercles on Incisal Edges

Incisal tubercles are more commonly seen in lower teeth and may be prominent

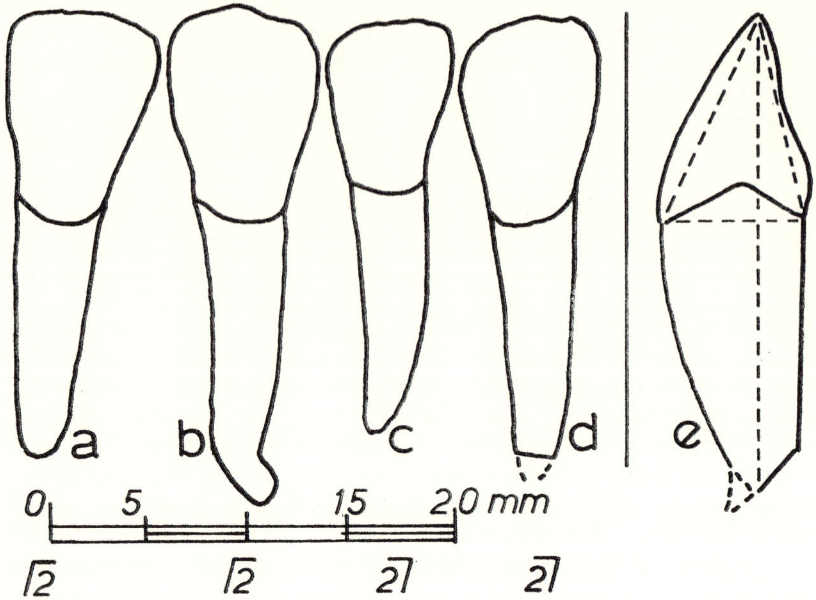

Figure 4-5. *a-d,* differences in curvature and divergence of crown outlines in a labial view—some nearly straight and some concavo-convex or S-curved. *e,* diagram indicating relation of basic form, or main outline, to tooth axis line.

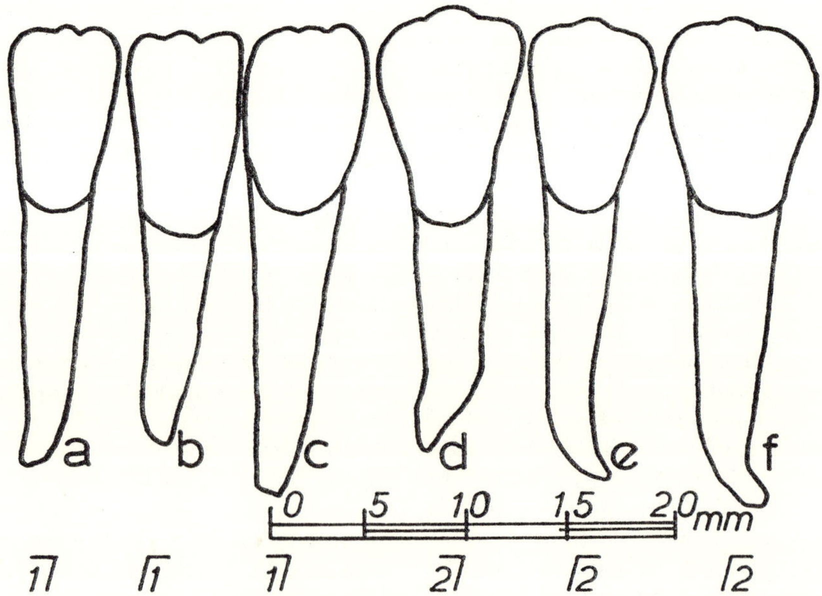

Figure 4-6. Incisal tubercles on mandibular centrals and laterals. Differences in relative width and height of tubercles.

in both centrals and laterals. Where the teeth have flared sides and rounded angles in labial view, more often in laterals than in centrals, the tubercles may be obviously unequal in size. In these the middle tubercle is most likely to be smallest and the distal tubercle largest. An apparent exception to this is in Figure 4-5 *b*, but it may be that the criteria for comparing the size of tubercles are not sound, or that more characters in tubercles must be recognized. One basis for comparison is that of width.

Between these developmental tubercles there are usually developmental grooves extending a short distance down labial and lingual surfaces. If the two notches are evenly spaced we may say that the tubercles are equal in size, but where the developmental grooves can be traced for any distance they tend to converge but not actually to meet. This means that the central lobe of the crown appears to be the smallest, and it is then easy to find the middle tubercle to be the smallest, if size is judged by relative width in labial view. Sometimes the tubercles are not equal in height, and the highest tubercle may be the middle one, as in the tooth last mentioned (Fig. 4-5 *b*).

In Figure 4-6 *a,b,c* are seen lower centrals with tubercles of equal height and sometimes nearly equal width. In the same figure, *d,e,f* are teeth with tubercles of unequal height and unequal width. Two are lateral incisors and one is doubtful. In each case the middle tubercle is the highest, but there was no evidence to suggest that this variation is more common in lateral incisors. The impression was gained, however, that it was more common in teeth with greater convexity of outline. These are usually teeth with relatively wider crowns, and it is the distal tubercle that tends to be the widest.

Another variation in which both central and lateral lower incisors are concerned may be described as fusion of tubercles; it may be an even or an uneven fusion, and each may occur in any degree. Thus a newly-erupted incisor that presents a smooth incisal edge with no interruption of line in the positions where tubercles usually meet could be a case of complete fusion of lobes at the earliest stage of crown formation. Alternatively it may be described as failure of the tooth bud to differentiate into lobes that would lead to formation of tubercles, and this appears a better explanation. The notion of fusion, which seems to imply at least some degree of previous differentiation and then a reversal of that differentiation, is preferred here merely because it facilitates description.

Decreasing degrees of even fusion, therefore, would result in more noticeable tubercles. Each of the three tubercles would be individually distinct and they would be approximately equal in size. It has been shown that size tends to be judged by two main characters in labial view, namely width and height, but for the moment it is felt inadvisable to com-

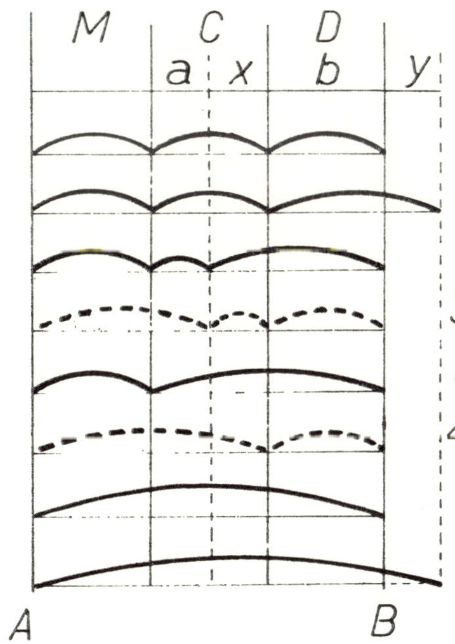

Figure 4-7. Diagram presenting an analysis of variations in relative width of tubercles on lower incisors.

plicate the analysis further by following these characters separately. The term "uneven fusion" is used for those cases where the three tubercles are not individually distinct or approximately equal in size, particularly as regards width. The middle tubercle often appears to be the narrowest when it is not the highest, and these cases may even be found in teeth with greater convexity and prominently rounded distal angles (Fig. 4-3 *f*). The mesial tubercle appears to be the most stable in regard to retaining its individuality and width. The middle and distal tubercles are those most obviously subject to variation in size. With the middle tubercle this includes both height and width. There appears to be little relation between these characters, for while it seems less likely at the one time to be both higher and narrower than the mesial tubercle, this can occur (Fig. 4-6 *d, e,f*).

Variation in width of the middle tubercle appears to be often associated with variation in width of the distal tubercle. The association may be described by saying that the distal tubercle may be increased in width by fusion with the middle tubercle or with part of it; or by fusion with a hypothetical factor that may be added to the distal to give a more rounded angle; but not by fusion with both of these.

The possible "patterns" in which these variations apparently take place may be represented diagrammatically as in Figure 4-7. The diagram may be described as follows: The dimension A B represents the incisal edge of an average lower central or lateral incisor. The headings M, C and D refer to mesial, central and distal tubercles. The subdivision of C into *a* and *x* enables representation of those cases where D is increased in width apparently at the expense of part of C, as in variety No. 3 of the diagram. The portion *y* beyond D indicates that the distal tubercle may apparently be increased without including or fusing with part of C, as in No. 2. In variety No. 4, C and D are fused, and in No. 5 all three tubercles are fused without apparent increase in the total width of the

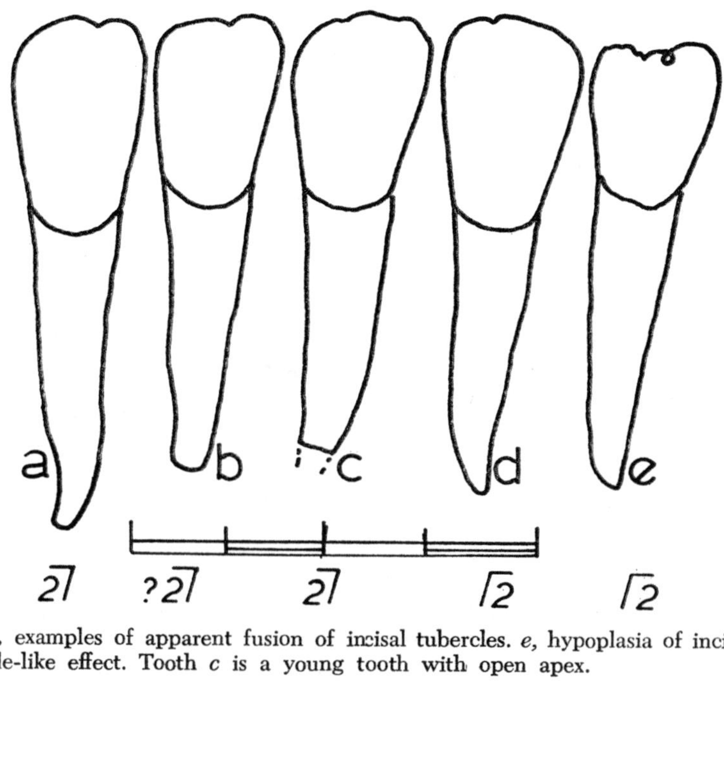

Figure 4-8. *a-d,* examples of apparent fusion of incisal tubercles. *e,* hypoplasia of incisal enamel leading to a tubercle-like effect. Tooth *c* is a young tooth with open apex.

tooth. Variety No. 6 represents a larger version of No. 5, which may include an element such as *y*, or merely a larger tooth within the normal range of variation in width. In Figure 4-8 *a* is a tooth of variety 4; Figure 4-8 *d* is variety No. 4 in a wider tooth where fusion has taken place so early that there is only a trace of the notch representing the limit of the mesial tubercle.

In lower incisors it seems that the mesial tubercle has the strongest tendency to retain its identity, but in upper incisors the impression given was that the distal tubercle was more likely to persist. These are, however, no more than impressions gained from a relatively few specimens. It may be that a definite study of such tubercles, as suggested earlier, would confirm or dispose of the notion of "dominance" in incisal tubercles. If tubercle M were increased at the expense of part of C (or of the whole of C), the patterns resulting would be the reverse of 3 and 4 and would appear as the hypothetical varieties shown by broken lines in 3a and 4a. No specimens of these were found in the present collection. This lends weight to the notion that tubercle M has the greater tendency to be discrete.

IDENTIFICATION AS LEFT OR RIGHT INCISORS

Both the crown and the root may present characters that will assist identification, but in straight-sided teeth, or teeth where the incisal edge has been worn evenly, differentiation may be very difficult, especially in the case of one isolated tooth (Figs. 4-3 *g* and 4-4 *f*). When there is a group of teeth from one patient it should be possible to distinguish central and lateral incisors by size. When a pair of centrals or laterals is examined one of them may provide a clue to identification, even if the other by itself does not. This is possible because left and right teeth may present visible differences so that one is not a true "mirror image" of the other. These differences may arise during formation or later through function, so that a character which could assist identification may be removed (as by wear, injury or decay) from one of the teeth and not from the other. Differences arising during formation may be seen best in roots (curve, apex and length), and those differences that may be lost from one and not the other are likely to be in the crown, such as loss of the more rounded distal angle of the crown.

Curves in roots of lower incisors are nearly always to the distal. In centrals the curve is most often merely a small bend near the apex, but in the longer-rooted lateral incisor there may be a greater length of root involved in a more sweeping gentle curve. The lateral, like the central, may have no more than a distal turning of the apex, or no bend at all in its apparently straight root as seen from the labial.

There is, however, an additional feature of the root, not strongly marked, that may enable one to distinguish a left tooth from a right. This is a longitudinal groove, usually quite shallow, but it does vary. It may be found on both mesial and distal surfaces, but in these cases it tends to be a little more obvious on distal. If it is found on only one surface, this is almost certain to be distal. Thus, even though crown and apex are missing, it should be possible to determine a left root from a right, for there should be no difficulty in distinguishing between the thicker buccal aspect and the thinner lingual aspect of the root.

PROXIMAL PROFILE

The proximal profile has been discussed elsewhere in relation to occlusion. In lower incisors it was shown that the labial profile is frequently in the form of an arc from the incisal edge to apex, except for a small apical bend to labial (Fig. 4-9 *a,b*). This has the effect of bringing the crown axis nearer to lingual cervix and is the reverse of that found in upper incisors. It also facilitates the overlap of incisal edges while maintaining a near vertical relation-

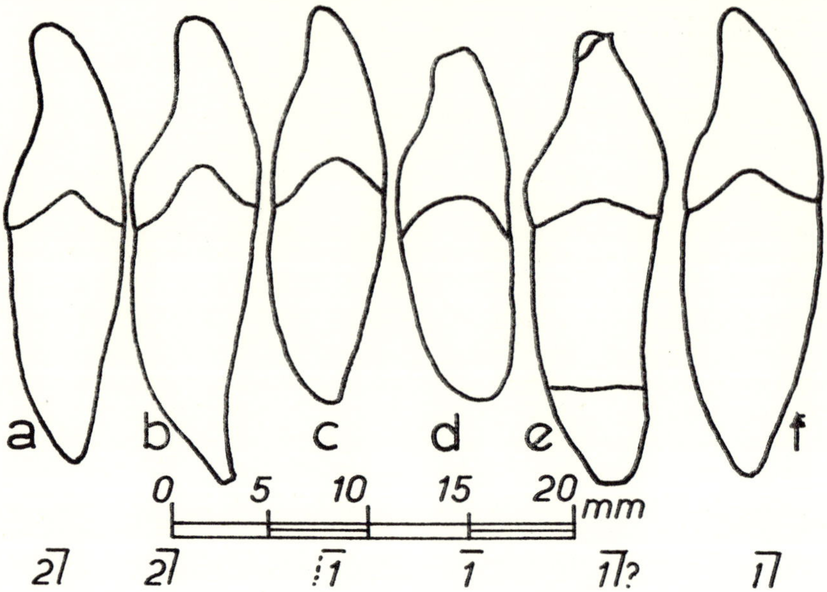

Figure 4-9. Proximal views of mandibular incisors showing variation in arc-like labial profile of crown, root or both. Variation shown also in shape of root and apex and in cervical line. *e,* see also Figure 4-18 *e.*

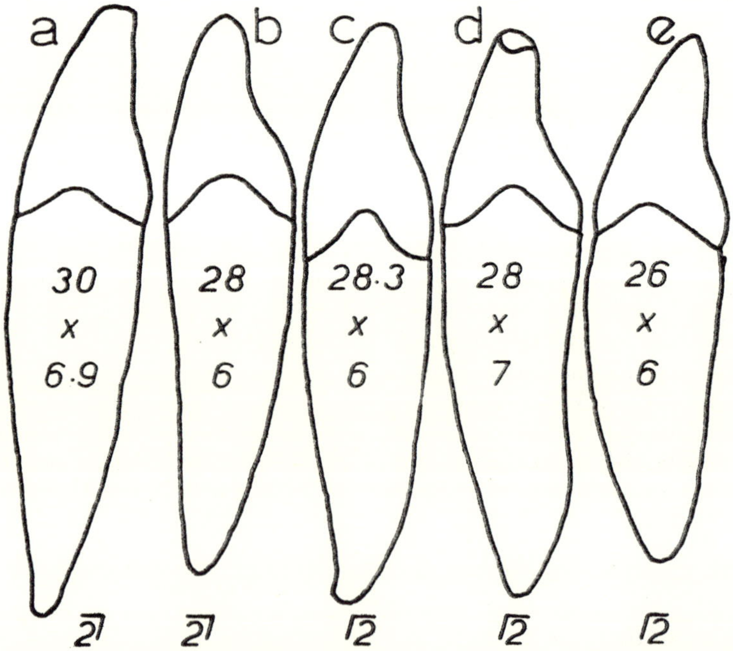

Figure 4-10. Proximal profiles of lower lateral incisors with maximal dimensions in mm. Note variations in crown length and width, in relation to total length, and differences in cervical lines.

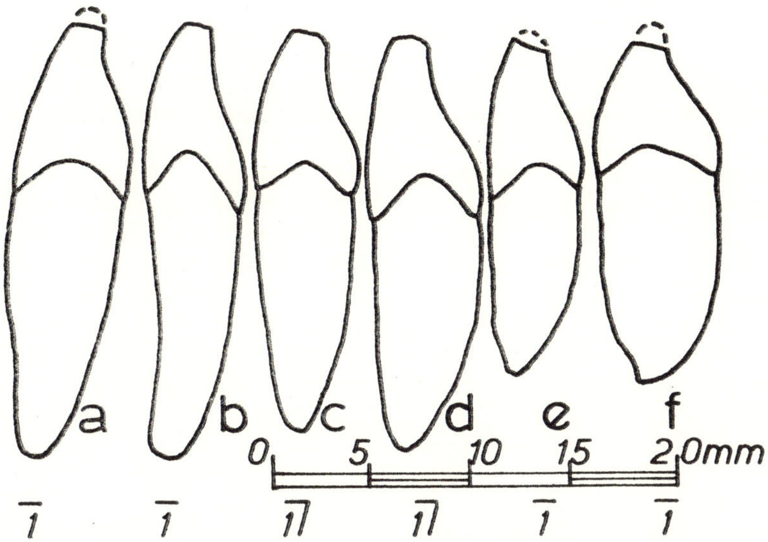

Figure 4-11. Proximal profiles of mandibular central incisors showing much variation in length and breadth proportions in crown and root, and in cervical lines, as in Figure 4-10.

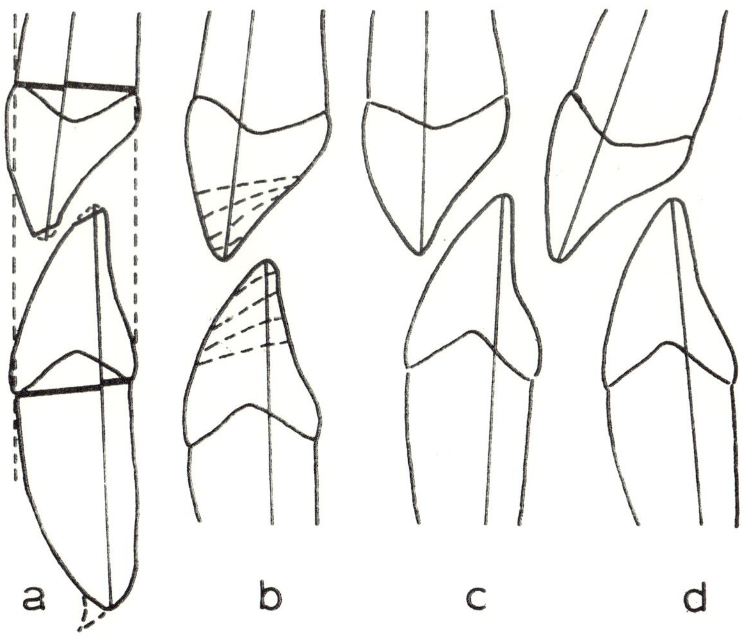

Figure 4-12. Diagrams of anterior teeth. *a*, the near vertical relation of cervices of teeth in upper and lower arches. With this relation overlap is associated with differences in the position of tooth (or crown) axes in upper and lower teeth, the axis being nearer to lingual in the lower. *a,b*, the "levelling" of the facet of wear as the "edge-to-edge" bite develops. *c,d*, relative directions of axes in upper and lower teeth may vary without much alteration in overlap or in the pattern of wear later acquired.

ship of crowns as judged by their cervices (Taylor, 1937b). It was shown there that another factor in this relationship is the inclination of axes of incisor teeth to one another (without approaching the procumbent position of some animal incisors) (Figs. 4-12 *c,d*). This vertical relationship of crowns, therefore, may be found even in those cases where the labial arc is much less convex.

The presence of the labial arc or its absence was shown not to depend on tooth length (Figs. 4-9 *c,d,f;* 4-10 *a,b*). It does have some relation, as would be expected, to the labial-lingual dimension. Thus a tooth that is relatively narrow in this dimension tends to have less convexity of arc (Figs. 4-10 *b,c,d;* 4-11 *a-e*); by contrast, the wider tooth tends to be more convex (Fig. 4-9 *a,b,c,f*).

LENGTH OF INCISORS

Lower incisors present a considerable variation in overall size. Long teeth are shown in Figure 4-10. The length of these teeth, taken by caliper between incisal border and apex, ranges from 26 mm to 30 mm, as shown thereon. The widths, labial to lingual at cervix, are also given. Again the difficulties associated with tooth measurements arise. Must the total length of tooth always be a straight-line measurement between incisal edge and apex, or should it follow a surface around the bends or curves seen in labial or proximal view? Clearly the only convenient measurement is a straight line as made between caliper points. It is equally obvious that a tooth with much curve is not fairly measured in this way, but why should it be excluded because of this quite normal character? Tooth *c* in Figure 4-10 is approximately 30 mm long when measured along its curve to distal (Fig. 4-18 *b*). Tooth *a* in Figure 4-18 gives measurements of approximately 24.3 and 26.0 mm by the two methods. This is but one example of the many difficulties and variable factors that should make one suspicious of conclusions based on measurements of teeth. It is evident, as already stated, that the relatively narrow tooth tends to have a less convex arc in its labial profile, and that the line of arc is often upset by small apical bends to labial. It is relevant at this stage to refer again briefly to root bends, although they will be studied later.

The visual effect of a curved, bent or tapered root may apparently cancel out the arc. The effect, in a small tooth, is shown in Figure 4-9 *d*, and in a longer tooth in Figure 4-9 *e*. If the root portion of the profile is ignored, and the axis of the crown only is examined, the arc is often restored. Also it moves the crown axis nearer to the lingual side and this has been shown to be a very common character of lower incisors. This can be seen in the diagram Figure 4-5 *e*, and in the outlines in Figure 4-9 *d,e*.

Tooth wear is another factor that affects the crown profile, and it is normally present in some degree, except in very young teeth. Early stages of wear in the presence of incisal overlap result in a facet extending on to the labial surface of the lower incisor, and this tends to increase the convexity of the profile arc while at the same time it decreases crown height. It constitutes an important objection to measurements of tooth length. Progressive changes in the pattern of wear as the edge-to-edge bite is acquired are shown in Figure 4-12. This diagram was prepared for the author's Piltdown paper, which showed that the Smith-Woodward restoration was not acceptable (Taylor, 1937b).

It will be shown later how and why there is much variation in evidence of wear in anterior teeth, and particularly in modern teeth, but at present the concern is with the relation of wear to the labial profile. With a small amount of wear it may not be obvious that the blade of an incisor has been shortened and its profile convexity altered. In the teeth used in the figures slight losses in tooth length through wear, or through chipping of the incisal edge, have sometimes been indicated by a broken line.

It was easier to demonstrate variations

in profile curves by reference first to teeth that were long rather than short. In a group of short teeth it is easy to recognize variation in other characters than length, but because of the small distances it is not so easy to show variations in relative lengths of crown and root. Length measurements for this are taken between mesial edge and apex, i.e. maximal length. When length of root or crown is desired it is taken from labial cervix to apex or incisal edge. It is admitted that there are objections to using these landmarks. Thus (a) the measurements from cervix are not quite parallel to the overall measurement of tooth length; (b) root length might just as fairly be made between apex and proximal cervix; (c) because of the undulating nature of the cervix, the crown and root "overlap" and some point within the overlap should perhaps be selected. We have shown, at least in upper canines, that the undulations of the cervical line are different on mesial and distal (Fig. 1-29). It is impossible to select a satisfactory landmark for termini of these measurements, and in such short distances fractions of a millimeter are important. As the measurements are stepped around the labial arc we have been discussing, crown plus root length are together greater than the chord length between incisal edge and apex. If either crown or root length were measured to labial cervix and the other obtained from chord length by subtraction, the result would be less than its true measurement. Bends and curves in apices and roots are further variables that complicate the procedure. At best, therefore, the measurements can be only approximate, but the termini chosen are convenient, and at least the crown length is accessible also for teeth *in situ.*

With these difficulties and objections in mind, the following figures are merely an aid to visual appreciation of variation in relative lengths of crown and root. In Figure 4-2 the approximate percentage lengths of crown to root (teeth *a-f*) are respectively 104.8, 91.7, 74.2, 63.3, 90.9, 64.3 In Figure 4-6, in teeth *a,b,c* the percentages are 73.1, 100.0 and 75.0 respectively.

WIDTH OF CROWNS

Variation in crown width, M-D, is readily observed, but it must be remembered that it is normal for centrals to be narrower and shorter than laterals. Unless there is certainty over the identity of lower incisors therefore, observed differences in these dimensions may be normal, rather than reflect variation, but illustrations given here are confined to known specimens. In Figure 4-13 are shown seven lower central incisors. Apart from size as regards length and width (and length and thickness of roots), it is apparent that there is variation in proportions of length of crown related to its width. There is also variation in straightness or convexity of crown outlines.

In Figures 4-14 and 4-15 are shown a further six centrals but this time each is shown with its own lateral. In addition to the comparisons made in Figure 4-14, it is possible in these two figures to see the consistently larger size of the lateral, and the manner in which it shares characters of form, characters which would be recognizable in other teeth of each dentition represented. In the case of Figure 4-15 *a,b,* the two teeth are held together by a piece of alveolar bone fractured at the time of extraction. This not only preserves the exact relation which the teeth bore to one another, but facilitates examination of the relation of the inter-dental alveolar crest to the cervical outline. Both teeth are worn on the incisal edge, *b* only slightly and *a* well into dentine. Both have carious cavities. In Figure 4-14 there is slight wear on teeth *e,f* but negligible wear on other teeth in the two figures.

Figures 4-16 and 4-17 present lateral incisors. There is considerable variety in all characters, length and breadth of crown and of root, length in proportion to breadth in crown and root, straightness or convexity of outlines and shapes of apices

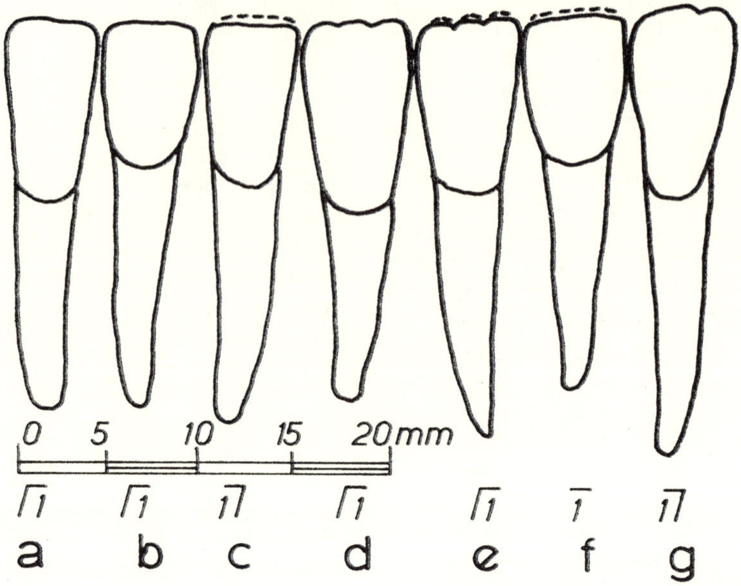

Figure 4-13. Mandibular central incisors in labial view. Variations in overall measurements of length and width, in crown dimensions in relation to root and in curvature of crown outlines. Teeth *c,e,f* present light wear of incisal edges.

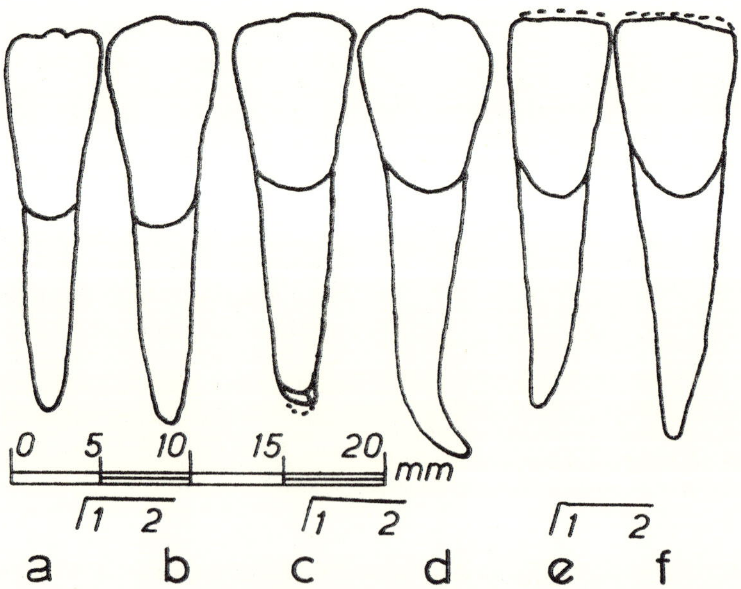

Figure 4-14. Mandibular incisors, centrals with their adjacent laterals, enabling the recognition of characters such as proportion, curvature and tubercles which are personal or common to teeth through the dentition of a particular person. Differences characteristic of a central in relation to its lateral, such as size and incisal angles, are also well distinguished. Teeth *e,f* present light incisal wear.

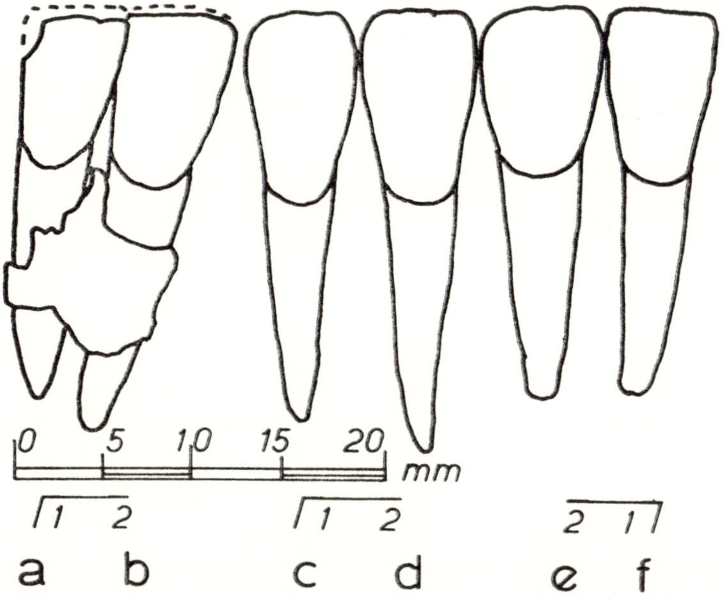

Figure 4-15. Further examples as in Figure 4-14. Teeth *a,b* are still held in their exact anatomical relationship by a portion of alveolar bone which fractured when the teeth were dislodged; whether this resulted partly from trauma or from operational accident is not known. The missing incisal angle is a restoration cavity, and tooth *a* has chipped incisal enamel and longitudinal fracture lines. The chipping does not appear to be "recent," and both teeth present cervical abrasion from dental forceps.

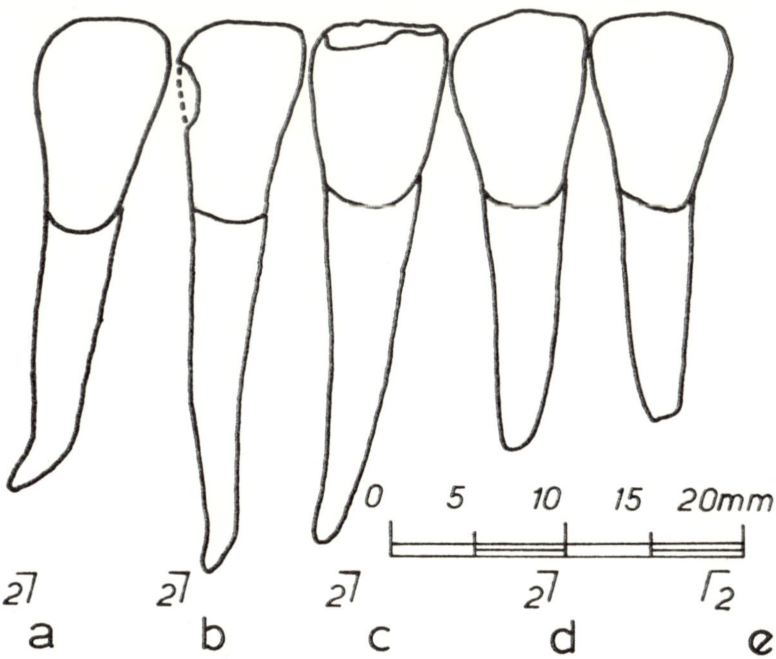

Figure 4-16. Mandibular lateral incisors in labial view presenting variety in root length and root bends. *a,* abrupt apical bend; *b,* abrupt apical bend plus abrupt bend at mid-root; *c,* gradual bend involving whole root; *d,e,* effect of slight curve of whole root to distal, apparently produced by taper of root.

as regards sharpness and curvature. Proximal views of the same teeth would present variation in other characters, and some of these teeth do in fact appear in other figures, e.g. Figure 4-10 *a,b,e*.

ROOT CURVATURE

In lower incisors the root in most cases is straight in line with the crown axis, when viewed from labial, though it is common to find a slight bend to distal in the apical portion. This small curve is not so commonly found in the central, but when it is present it is usually even more noticeable in the lateral (Figs. 4-1, 4-2, 4-3, 4-5, 4-6, 4-15, 4-16, 4-17).

Curves involving a large part of the root when seen from labial, or showing a considerable degree of curvature, are much less common, but they do occur. The examples shown are in long teeth. Figure 4-18 *a, b,c* are from three persons.

As with other teeth in the dentition, curves are not necessarily in one direction only, but for illustration it is not feasible to draw a tooth from more than two viewpoints, labial or lingual on the one hand, and proximal on the other. Figure 4-18 *c,d* shows one such tooth in which the curve or bend has affected about half the root and commences more abruptly than in *a* and *b*. Bends that start abruptly, as is commonly found in upper teeth, are much less common in lower anteriors. In uppers the close proximity of tooth roots to maxillary sinuses and the nasal cavity probably accounts for most such abrupt or excessive changes in root direction, but there are no such structures associated with roots of lower anterior teeth. In these teeth it is reasonable to assume that tooth movements are a likely cause, and they are subject to injury from blows. Evidence of such injury may be seen as fractured enamel or a piece of tooth broken off, or dilaceration in the root. Less severe injuries may leave no readily recognizable sign; among minor injuries might be included movements in orthodontic treatment, movements made too rapidly or over a considerable distance

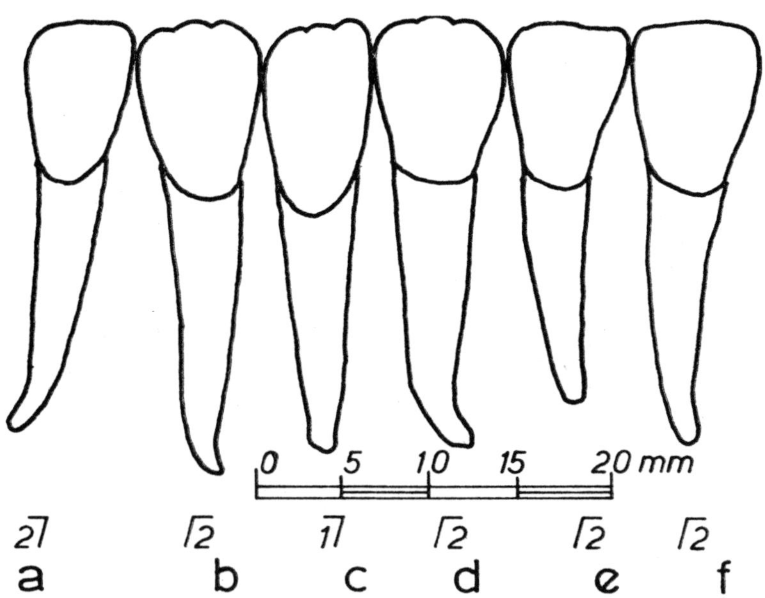

Figure 4-17. Mandibular incisors presenting in their roots further varieties of the kind noted in Figure 4-16; for example, tooth *a* presents in this view a straight mesially tapered root with an abrupt apical bend. The crowns show much variety in shape, curvature and taper.

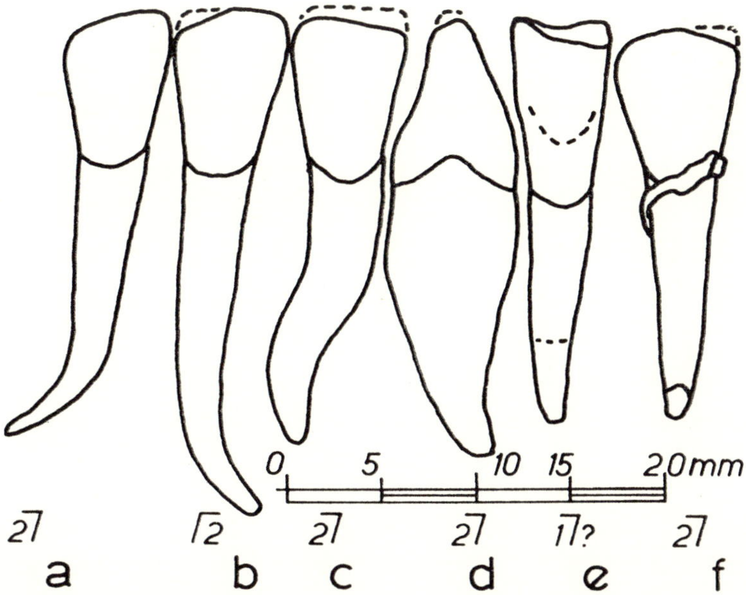

Figure 4-18. Mandibular incisors. *a,b,c,* greater curves, or curves involving much of the root. *c,d,* two views of one tooth presenting an S-bend seen from labial, also taper and labial curvature when viewed from proximal. *e,* a tooth which has suffered trauma during the period of root formation (see also Figure 4-9 *e*). *f,* uncommon wear of labial surface (see p. 153). Incisal wear is indicated on *b,c,d,f*.

or arc of rotation. In the writer's student days it was taught that anterior teeth in lingual occlusion could be aligned immediately by dislocation and splinting to a labial arch, and it is likely that an incomplete root would later present evidence of such an insult. It would be of interest to know the life history of many of the teeth which present irregular and curved roots.

With regard to accidental injury mentioned above, the tooth shown in Figure 4-9 *e* is of interest. The slight change of root direction in the apical third is so abrupt that there is a light but definite line across the root surface. Development would have reached this point at eight to nine years of age. Part of the incisal edge is missing, but not through wear. It is quite obvious that the tooth has received a blow which has broken off some enamel and produced fracture lines in the vicinity of the break. Some of the most prominent sharp edges have been made smooth by function (not by a dentist), showing that the fracture took place long before the tooth was extracted. The surface of fracture is seen in Figure 4-18 *e* in lingual view. Even before a developing crown has been fully calcified it may be grossly disturbed by a blow, and yet tooth formation may continue to the completion of a normal root (Taylor, 1970a).

There are many factors that may be involved in an injury, such as the type of cause (electrical, chemical, a blow, etc.). A blow may vary in direction, it may be light or heavy, from a small or large object which may be hard or resilient, and which may make contact with areas of varying size, and so on. In the case of injuries to teeth, many more factors may be involved and may concern the age of the person, stage of dentition, amount of support by bone and other teeth, resistance of the tooth itself by virtue of its bulk and hardness, or, they may relate to the morphologi-

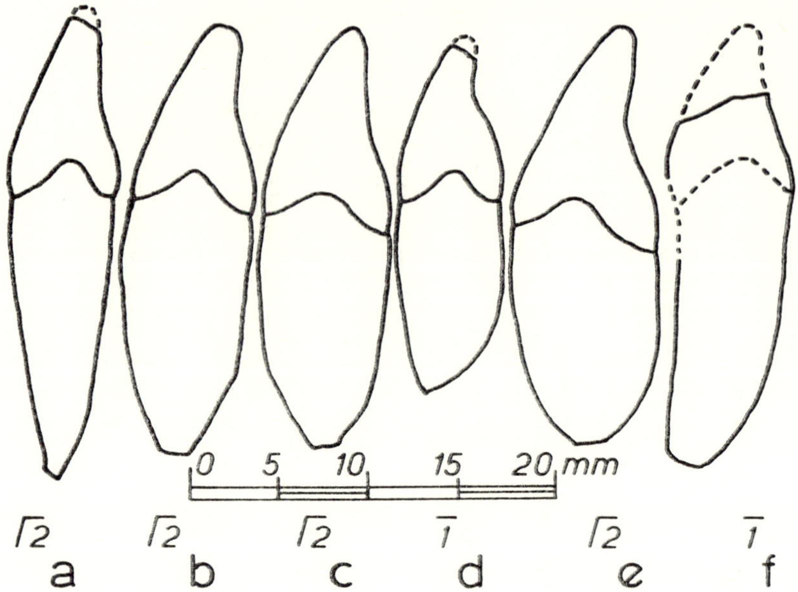

Figure 4-19. Bucco-lingual root width and taper in mandibular incisors. *a,* taper commencing at the cervix. *b,c,d,* a root may have its greatest dimension at some level other than the cervix, but this is unusual in healthy teeth. *e,* incisor with relatively long crown and short, very wide root. *f,* lower incisor with sickle-shaped root curving to labial and no buccal arc in the root profile.

cal differences such as the blade of an incisor crown or a cusp tip, or a slender or robust tooth. Thus the potential for variety in injuries to teeth is very great, and even in adjacent teeth the effects may be quite different. The author recalls a case involving two upper central incisors in a girl aged fourteen years where in one tooth the blow removed the blade portion completely. In the other tooth there was no visible crack in the crown, but excess mobility and X-ray confirmed the presence of a transverse fracture of the root in its middle third. Just a few teeth in a fragment of jaw bone may present evidence of trauma occurring some years before death (Taylor, 1971c).

Even a brief reference to causes and effects of injuries to teeth should not overlook defects in formation of teeth, for the effects are entirely relevant to the main theme. In this way faults in nutrition, metabolic upsets, local pathology in adjacent teeth, or systemic illness, may produce irreversible changes in the various hard tissues recognizable in their micro-structure, or even to the naked eye as a hypoplasia (Taylor, 1972a). Other effects more particularly related to cultural factors have been described in earlier chapters as regards "civilized" teeth, and also in various papers dealing with skeletal material of Polynesians (Taylor, 1962b, c, 1963a, 1970c, 1971b, c, 1972b, 1975, 1976). These show that recognition of the various injuries, through their effects in teeth, can provide data of special interest and of forensic value.

In spite of the fact that so many lower incisors present a labial profile in the form of an arc, the root axis evidently does not bend or curve to the lingual, although the tooth in Figure 4-10 *d* has a trace of such bending. In proximal view, if the axis is not virtually straight, it bends or curves to labial, particularly in the apical region.

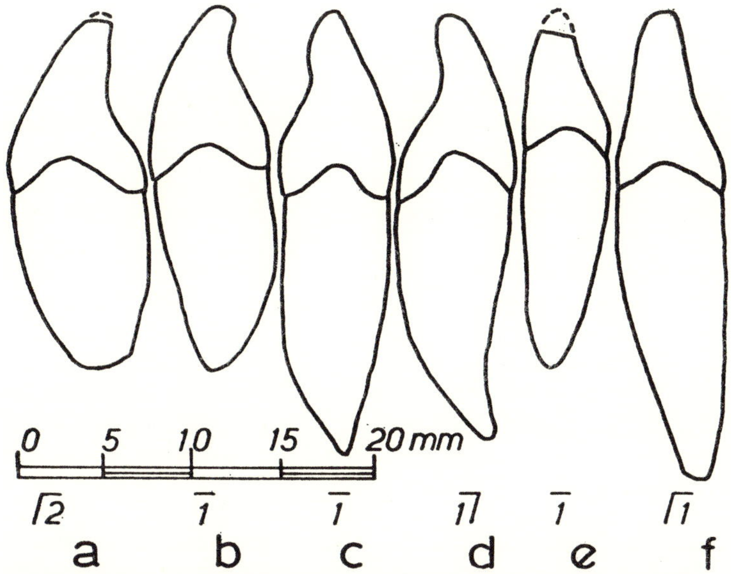

Figure 4-20. Proximal profiles of mandibular incisors showing further variations in roots, from the short wide root of tooth *a* (also Fig. 4-19 *e*) to the long, narrow tapering root of *f*.

This can be seen in the many teeth in the figures. The reason for lack of lingual curves may be seen by reference to a mandible. The relation of the tooth root to the lingual surface of the bone does not normally allow space for lingual curvature, and this applies for both short- and longer-rooted teeth.

But where, in a case of crowded lower incisors, one tooth erupts lingually, it would tend to develop an axial curve of the style illustrated in the tooth just mentioned. This tooth does indeed present other features which support such explanation of its unusual axial curve. There is a mesial curve and a twist (anticlockwise, of over 30°) in the root. There is a high proximal facet on M only. On the incisal edge, one facet on M half is obliquely grooved by protrusive movements. Another facet, indicated in the figure, has removed the D angle by occluding with a different tooth. The stain pattern also is consistent with eruption and function in a crowded and rotated malposition as described.

ROOT WIDTH AND APEX, PROXIMAL VIEW

In the great majority of lower incisor roots the taper is hardly perceptible for an appreciable distance below the cervix, when viewed from proximal (Figs. 4-4, 4-9, 4-10 *a,c,d,e*). In a few cases the change in width is apparent from the cervix (Figs. 4-10 *b*, 4-19 *a*). In very few teeth is the root at its widest dimension elsewhere than at the cervix, but such cases do occur (Fig. 4-19 *b,d*). It is emphasized that these are not cases where the root dimension may have been increased by a pathological deposit of cementum.

Apart from these general comments it may be said that root taper has a very great variety of form. For analytical purposes the root in this proximal view has a cervical base, and a labial and a lingual profile which meet to form the apex. The cervical base, or labio-lingual width, has been shown to bear no constant proportional relation to the length of the root, so that at one extreme there is a relatively short wide root, and at the other a relatively long narrow root (Fig. 4-20 *a,f*). From one extreme to the other, through every intermediate proportion in length and width, there is an almost infinite potential for variation. This may be emphasized through a series of diagrams which consider the proximal view of the root in relation to a triangle. The cervical base is the base of the triangle, and the labial and lingual profiles are the other sides of the triangle.

Thus in Figure 4-21 there are ten diagrams. Each diagram shows how one character may vary or how two characters may be combined:

a, taper even on both sides, point apex; basically an isosceles triangle varying in length but on same width base.

b, as in *a,* basically an isosceles triangle, but of equal lengths although on bases of different widths. Combinations of *a* and *b* could describe a long wide or narrow root, or a short root, both of similar shape.

c, taper uneven on the two sides, point apex; basically a scalene triangle. Of the same base width, and of the same lengths, there may be such triangles as ABF, ACF, ADF, AEF. In this diagram, the first and last are similar but reversed; the second and third are similar but reversed. The intermediate varieties are commonly found but not the extremes. As with varieties *a* and *b,* so also *c* may vary in lengths and widths and sizes.

d, this introduces another character, the truncated triangle as ABEJ, ACEJ, ADEJ, ACGJ, ADFJ and so on. Thus this character, a blunt apex, may be combined with the isosceles or scalene, or long or short, or narrow or wide base, or narrow or wide apex,

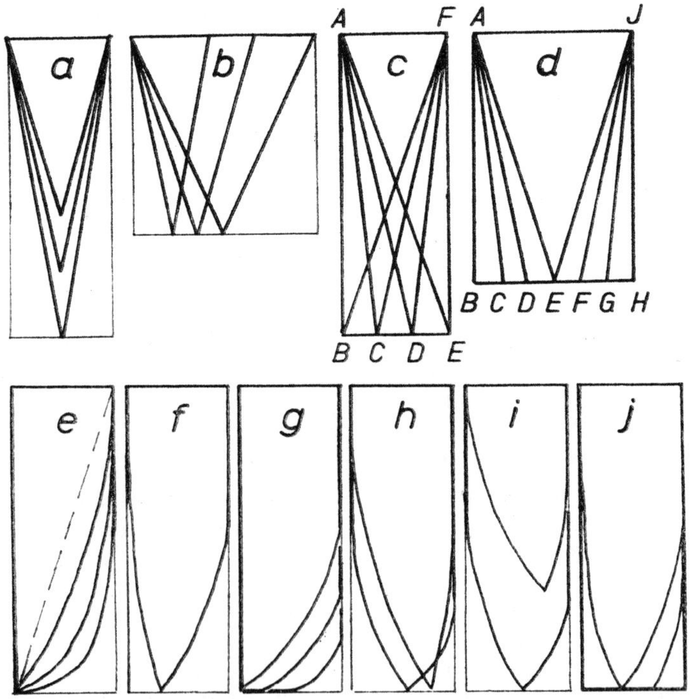

Figure 4-21. Diagrammatic analysis of variations in mandibular incisor roots viewed from proximal. The diagrams indicate variation in a single character and the combination of variable characters.

or one of any of these except incompatibles. An incompatible combination would be a narrow base with a wider apex, for there must not be overall divergence from base to apex.

All these diagrams, *a-d* have used straight lines to represent root profiles. While profiles in teeth do often approach straight lines, at least in part, there is usually some degree of curvature. The next character to be considered is curvature.

e, this diagram illustrates degrees of curvature with length and base of root remaining constant. Approximately it is a series of arcs of different radius on the same length chord. To maintain the idea of taper it is approximately correct, and certainly convenient, to say that the degrees of curvature are limited by the requirement that the curves must fall within the two sides of a rectangle representing length and width of root, and the diagonal or the long side of the rectangle be approximately the chord of the arcs. The rectangle may vary in length and breadth.

f, this diagram shows how degrees of curvature may be combined where the apex is a point between the angles of the rectangle.

g, in this diagram variation in lengths of curvature is shown.

h, different lengths of curvature and different degrees of curvature are combined to produce roots of similar width and similar length but different shape.

i, different lengths of curvature and different degrees of curvature are combined to produce roots of similar width but different length and, of course, of different shape. Variation in width is also relevant here but for simplicity will be referred to below.

j, this diagram introduces the character of a truncated or blunt apex which may be combined with any of the variations indicated in diagrams *e-i*.

Diagrams *e-j* inclusive are all of the same width. In some cases variation in length of curve or length of root has been mentioned, but it will be realized that in each case variation in width also is a possible character for combination.

As the zero degree of curvature in this analysis is a straight line, it is not difficult to find root profiles which have one profile line related to one of the diagrams *a-d*, and the other to a feature from diagrams *e-j*. Variations in degree of curvature may occur in a profile line and may affect varying amounts of the length of these lines, so that this further factor must be recognized. It greatly increases the possibilities for variation in tooth form. In tooth roots the effects of this in various combinations are seen as curves or bends.

Figure 4-22 *a,d* is a group of diagrams which illustrates a few of the simplest variations of root curve in single-rooted teeth such as lower incisors (proximal views), and in all cases the root curves to labial as the apex is approached. For simplicity each diagram shows the root consisting of cervical, middle and apical thirds. These are indicated by chords representing arcs which make up the curved profiles of the roots, generally convex on lingual and concave labially. Each root is represented in relation to a rectangle, the top of which is the linguo-labial width at cervix, and the length of the rectangle is the root length (as in Fig. 4-21).

In diagrams *a* and *c* root taper in the cervical third is mostly on the labial side; in *b* and *d* it is on the lingual side. In the first two mentioned the root axis thus appears more erect and remains within the rectangle at the apex, whereas it falls outside in *b* and *d*. The actual amount of curvature is the same in each root. In *a* and *b* the apex shape is similar, but the second apex falls outside the rectangle. Root *c* has a fine apex within the rectan-

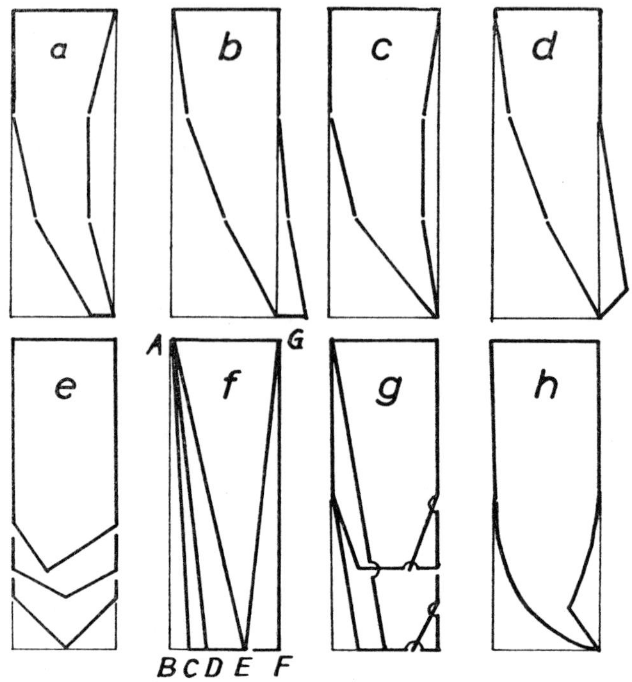

Figure 4-22. Diagrammatic analysis of root characters in proximal views of mandibular incisors. *a-d*, bends in the root axis. *e-h*, analysis of variation in shape of apex.

gle. Root *d* has a thick but pointed apex, quite different from the shape in *a* and *b*. Brief attention, therefore, may be given to shapes of root apex.

The terms fine, thick, truncated, pointed, sharp, blunt, squared, rounded, etc., have all been used to describe apices. These terms are not scientifically definitive for our purpose; however, because of the difficulty of describing apices accurately, and since the above terms are simple and convenient, it is proposed to use them. An indication of variation in apices is attempted in the diagrammatic analysis of Figure 4-22 *e-h:*

e, these three apices are blunt points. They are formed by short, marked tapering at the apex, where taper in the rest of the root is much less. They may be even (symmetrical), or uneven, and may be associated with roots of different length and different thickness. It is understood, of course, that the apical angles in these diagrams represent arcs of varying radius in actual teeth.

f, bluntness of apex arising from taper of the whole, or a large portion of the root. A number of apices of different width, even and uneven, are represented in this diagram: ABEG, ACFG, ADFG, AEFG, ACEG, ADEG. (By analogy with Fig. 4-21 *c,* the basic rectangle here is ABFG, and the points on the apical line are BCDEF.)

g, this diagram presents some eight possible variations of apex, even and uneven, in short and long roots, and they combine both *a* and *b* characters of taper of apex and taper of root, on one or both sides of the root profile.

h, this diagram represents the fine apex offset from the tooth axis, or root axis, by a bend or curve in the apical third of the root. In the present collection such apices curved to labial.

These diagrams in Figures 4-21 and 4-22 have attempted to analyze the elements involved in variation of root form as seen from proximal. They indicate ways in which such elements may be combined to produce the infinite variety in form and size seen in human lower incisors.

ROOT TAPER, IN LABIAL VIEW

In the figures already presented there are many examples of differences in root thickness and taper as seen from labial.

In its simplest form taper is represented by a triangle, expressing the relation between cervical width and the distance of the apex. This is also the case with proximal views, and the possibilities for many variations on the simple basic triangle have been shown. With labial views the variations are less complex and at first sight appear to be simplified by the more obvious relation of root to crown, in that the crown also presents two rather similar outlines convergent in the same direction as the root. Thus the root outlines more or less continue the convergence established from incisal edge to cervix.

Examination of a number of teeth shows that it is necessary to use the qualification "more or less." While in many cases the outline continues smoothly from crown to root without perceptible change in direction, there are many more in which this does not apply. In the first group the outlines of the whole tooth often do conform closely to a triangle (Fig. 4-14 *e,f*), or to a triangle with a truncated apex (Figs. 4-2 *a*, 4-3 g, 4-6 *c*, and 4-13 *a*); but the triangle may be distorted by a root curve or bend in the apical part (Figs. 4-14 *d*, and 4-16 *a*). The second group includes (i) teeth with more convexity of outline (Figs. 4-15 *c,e*, and 4-17 *a,c*); (ii) teeth tending to have parallel sides in the incisal half of the crown followed by a concavity in outline in the lower part of the crown Figs. 4-2 *b,c*, 4-3 *b,d,f*, 4-5 *c*, and 4-17 *d*); (iii) teeth with converging sides and relatively wide in the incisal region (Figs. 4-1 *b*, 4-5 *a*, 4-6 *d,e,f*, 4-16 *d,e*, 4-17 *e* and 4-23 *a,b,c*).

The taper may appear to involve the two sides of the root unevenly in that the taper seems to be on one side only, giving the effect of a slight bend of the root away from the tapered side. This could be described the other way round by saying that a slight bend of the whole root to one side obscures the taper on that side and makes the root appear to taper only from the opposite side. Examples are shown in Figures 4-1 *c*, 4-3 *a*, 4-13 *e*, and 4-23 *a,b,c*. It is worth pointing out that in each of these it is the mesial side that appears tapered. As the tendency of lower incisor roots to bend to distal rather than to mesial has already been noted, this uneven taper might prove to be a useful character when damage to a tooth crown by wear, fracture or caries complicates identification as left or right tooth.

CERVICAL LINES

As with maxillary incisors and canines in Chapter 1, a study was made here also of the curvature seen in cervical lines when teeth are viewed from mesial and distal. In lower incisors very considerable variation was found, as may be seen in the many outlines recorded in the figures.

In these proximal views the cervical line is like a simple wave, passing from a trough at labial up to crest, and curving down to another trough at lingual. Essentially there are three curves, the middle part, including the crest of the wave, being convex upwards (or incisally). The labial and lingual curves are concave upwards. When studying variation in form one is not concerned with the overall length of the wave, or more specifically with the distance in a straight line between the terminals representing labial and lingual, for this is largely related to tooth size. The concern is rather with the height of the wave to relative length, and with the distance taken up by the middle curve in proportion to the two terminal curves. In Figures 4-4 *c* and 4-9 *d* the middle curve is the only part visible, but in Figures 4-9 *b* and 4-10 *c* it involves only about one-third of the visible cervical line. The contrasts here may be described simply as large and small middle curves.

In Figure 4-11 *a,b* are seen two teeth with large middle curves, but quite different from one another. In tooth *a* the curve is almost arc-like, and moreover is a relatively short arc of a large circle. The crest of the curve in tooth *b* is by contrast a larger arc of a much smaller circle, so that the whole middle curve tends to be angular in *b* and more rounded in *a*. This character is found to be even more rounded, or more angular in some cases. These teeth are almost identical in crown length, but slightly different in width in this view. It appears, therefore, that a middle curve may be large and rounded or large and angular independently of the size of the tooth.

Small middle curves are seen in Figures 4-4 *e*, 4-9 *a,f*, 4-10 *c,d*, 4-19 *a,b,d,e* and 4-24 *a*. These include more laterals than centrals; the last is a mesial and the others distal, except 4-19 *d* which is uncertain. There are among them a variety of teeth, long and short teeth, slender and broad teeth. Without a more extensive study and without a more precise classification of cervical lines and their curves, it may be permissible only to note a tendency for small middle curves to be unrelated to length or width of tooth.

The middle curve has been described as including the crest of the wave-like shape of the cervical line in proximal view, and as being rounded or angular, and large or small. These adjectives of size have referred to the proportion of the line taken up by the middle curve, rather than to the height of the wave crest. These middle curves are now looked at and described as low or high. Low curves are seen in Figures 4-4 *c,d*, 4-9 *e*, 4-10 *a*, 4-11 *f* and 4-24 *aa,bb,cc*. High curves are shown in Figures 4-4 *a,e*,

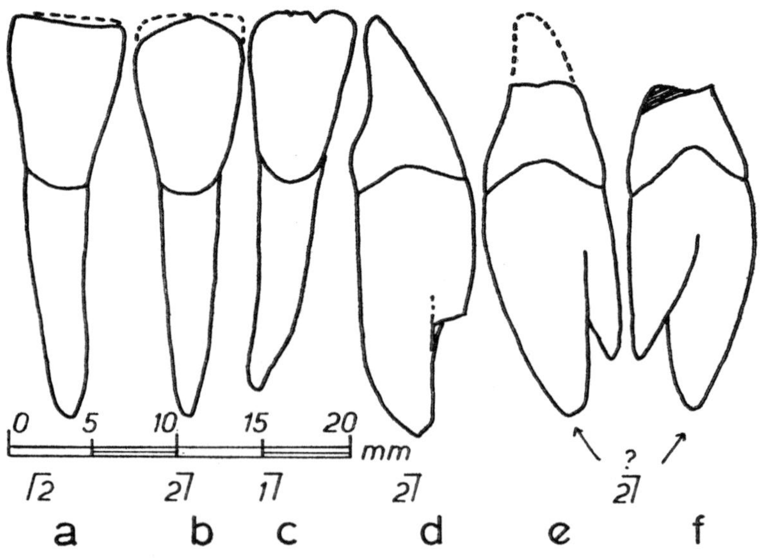

Figure 4-23. Mandibular incisors. *a,b,c*, labial outlines relating crown taper and root taper. There is light incisal wear, and on tooth *b* this has produced a somewhat cusp-like appearance. *d*, a "two-rooted" lateral incisor with labial branch lost by fracture at time of extraction. *e,f*, proximal views of a "two-rooted" incisor with a greatly worn-down crown.

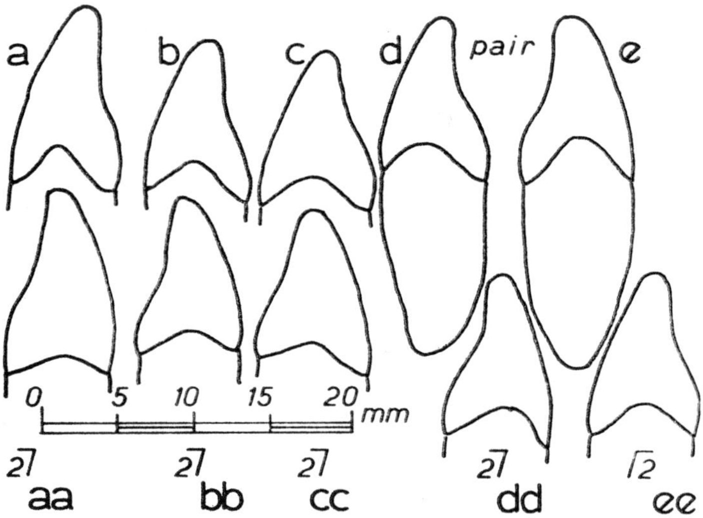

Figure 4-24. Mandibular incisors showing variation in curvature of cervical lines. Top row, mesial views. Bottom row, distal views of the same teeth. Teeth *d,e* are a pair from the same person.

4-9 *b*, 4-10 *c*, 4-11 *b* and 4-24 *a*. Comparison of these shows that a high curve is not the same as a small curve or an angular curve. Again, it is seen that high curves and low curves are formed in teeth independently of differences in size and in proportions of length and width.

Another way of studying cervical curves is by comparing mesial and distal in particular teeth. This is done in Figure 4-24, where *a,b,c* are three lower right lateral incisors and *d,e* are a pair of laterals from one person. The top tracings are mesial views and the lower tracings are the distal views of the same teeth. Thus *aa* is the distal of tooth *a*, and so on. The crowns vary in length and width, and the middle curves also vary in height and size. In general it may be said of this group that the middle curves tend to be lower on distals, but the striking difference in tooth *a* is not seen in the other specimens. It is interesting to observe that in the paired teeth the cervical curves are by no means similar, or mirror images one with the other.

These observations of cervical curves in lower incisors may be summarized by saying that there is great variation in shape and height. There are angular and rounded curves, and the middle curves vary from small to those comprising the whole proximal view. In many the curves tend to be lower on distal but this is not always obvious. In upper canines the curve was much more noticeably wide and lower on distals and it was noted that there is a considerable difference in the width of teeth and of alveolar ridge on each side of the canine. In lowers the situation is different, for in many cases the lateral is not much narrower, and the first premolar about the same width, when compared with their canine.

In the fully erupted and healthy incisor the periodontal attachment follows the shape of the cervical line. A tooth with a high crest in the cervical line, or a small middle curve or an angular curve, might well be associated with a narrow alveolar ridge. A low curve with large rounded middle curve and less obvious crest would appropriately be associated with a wide ridge. But the width of ridge is partly an expression of the amount of basal bone, and this is important in orthodontic prognosis. The cervical line is established before the tooth has erupted and its shape might therefore be regarded as a forecast of the nature of basal bone and alveolar ridge that might be expected in normal development. Unfortunately the orthodontist is not able to examine this feature except in the few occasions when a tooth is extracted. At this stage any such observations as he may make are likely to come too late to be helpful.

Cervical lines, like many other morphological characters of teeth, are unsatisfactory features for study. In the present study the apparent landmarks used as termini are arbitrary points, not anatomical points, but they are convenient and enable some kind of study to be made. Similarly the division of the line into labial, middle and lingual curves, and the relative extent of these, is arbitrary and a similar excuse is offered for their use. There is little in dental morphology that can be measured satisfactorily, and therefore comparisons on a quantitative basis must be highly suspect. Because of this it is all the more worthwhile to attempt analysis of characters and their variation qualitatively. As for cervical lines, the author has not found a report of any previous study but has acquired a familiarity and knowledge concerning them that enables information to be presented. In the case of lower incisors it has been established that there is a considerable range of variation, and the nature of the variation has been described. It has been shown that the differences do not enable distinction to be made between a central and a lateral incisor, or between mesial and distal in either, but they do in some cases indicate a probability as to which sides are mesial and distal. This could be helpful in identification of a root fragment when the crown has been damaged. The significance of variation in this character has not been established. Some variation is related to differences in surface curvature in different teeth, and some is related to orientation of the tooth and the viewpoint of the observer. Problems arising from the latter will receive further attention in the next section. The present section has been concerned with a character where it has been difficult enough to describe what is found without offering more than a suggestion as to explanation, and this applies widely in the field of biological and physical sciences. Much knowledge has been acquired concerning what happens, but why these things happen is another question altogether.

CROWN-ROOT TWIST

In a transverse section of the cervical half of the root of a lower incisor the outline is usually a much flattened oval with the minor axis nearer the labial side. The flattened sides may even present a shallow groove, particularly on the distal (as mentioned earlier), so that a straight edge placed across the root will make contact in two places, as with line CD in Figure 4-25 *a*. Because of the basically oval outline this straight edge is not parallel to line AB, which is the major axis of the oval, and the two lines diverge slightly towards labial. Viewed from incisal, the incisal edge is often approximately at right angles to that major axis.

If, therefore, the tooth is oriented in proximal view so that one looks along the incisal edge or blade of the crown, the proximal aspect of the root will be approximately vertical to the line of vision. This is the orientation aimed at for tracing proximal outlines with the camera lucida, and presented in this study. But in a number of lower incisors, apparently all being laterals, it is not possible (when the root was at right angles to the line of vision) to look along the incisal edge and see only the proximal surface of the blade of the crown. Viewed from mesial, part of the lingual surface was seen (Fig. 4-26 *a-e*), viewed from distal, part of the labial surface was visible (Fig. 4-26 *f*). Viewed from incisal, the incisal edge was noticeably oblique to the major axis of the root section (Fig. 4-25 *b* and 4-26 *aa-ff*).

This character has been called "crown-root twist," and in all cases it was the distal angle of the blade that was nearer to lingual. This is a character, therefore, that may be used to distinguish mesial from distal, and so also to distinguish a left from a right tooth. Moreover, as the teeth in which twist was easiest to recognize appeared to be lateral incisors, this may be a character assisting the differentiation between centrals and laterals. This, however, was not definitely established because of the difficulty of positive identification of some narrow teeth with rather straight-sided crowns and roots that were almost straight-sided in labial view.

It may be contended that since (i) twist appears to be confined to lateral incisors, (ii) it is noticeable best in the wider teeth, and (iii) wider laterals tend to have more rounded distal angles, therefore twist may be an optical effect of bringing the incisal edge lower on the distal. This possibility as an explanation of the visible character of twist is easily disposed of. Because of the slope of the labial surface, an incisal edge extending further down on this surface would approach labial when viewed from incisal. But twist brings the distal part of the incisal edge nearer to lingual and away from labial. Twist, therefore, is not an optical effect but is established as a real character.

Demonstration of twist by means of tracings with the camera lucida presented several small problems. The first was the impossibility of precise determination of the major axis of the root section already mentioned. It was necessary, therefore, to orient each tooth by the side of its root; the distal was chosen in the belief that the shallow groove usually present there would enable a positive two-point contact to be made between this surface and a straight edge. The edge of the specimen table of the camera lucida was arranged to cross the field of view where desired. A small piece of soft wax was placed on the side of the root and the tooth pressed against the edge until two-point contact was established. The soft wax permitted slight adjustment until it seemed that the long axis of the tooth was coincident with the centre line of the camera lenses.

In Figure 4-25 *b* the root section oval and the lines AB and CD are as in diagram *a*, the line EF being at right angles to the straight edge CD. The broken line repre-

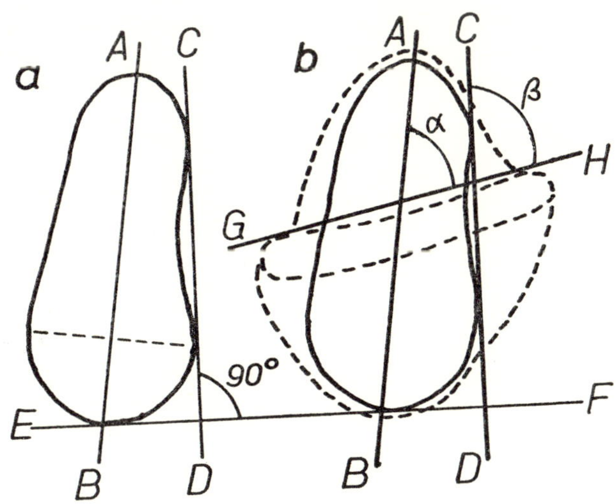

Figure 4-25. Diagrams relating to mandibular lateral incisors. *a*, transverse section of root near cervix. *b*, "crown-root twist."

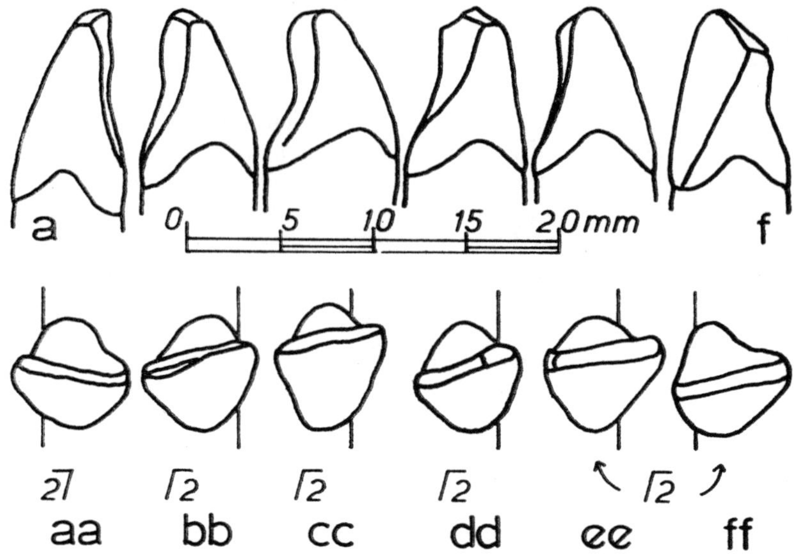

Figure 4-26. Crown-root twist in mandibular lateral incisors. *a-e,* mesial views. *f,* distal view of tooth *e.* Bottom row, incisal views of the same teeth as above. *aa-ee,* lined up by distal cervix; *ff,* by mesial cervix.

sents the outline of the occlusal view of the tooth in relation to the root oval. The line GH represents the direction of the incisal edge, and the true angle of twist is 90 degrees minus angle α. The angle β (which is greater than angle α by the amount of divergence of AB from CD) is the angle represented in the tracings for teeth *bb, cc, dd, ee* of Figure 4-26. As the first tooth shown is from right side the tracings *a* and *aa* appear to be reversed.

The last two sets of tracings, *e, f* and *ee, ff,* are of one tooth in which the whole root curves to distal. Tracing *f* is from distal, and for *ff* the tooth was oriented by its mesial surface. The slight difference in the resulting angles of twist is related to the amount of ovalness as distinct from ellipticity in the root section.

For the upper tracings *a-f* in Figure 4-26 the teeth were placed on a small piece of wax on the specimen table of the camera lucida and adjusted until the major axis of the root section was apparently parallel with the specimen table. In other words, one endeavoured by one's judgment to obtain what may be described as a true proximal view of the part concerned and observe the effect of twist in the blade portion of the crown.

Attention might be drawn to the apparent difference in width and smaller size of the distal surface compared with mesial surface in the tooth represented by tracings *e* and *f*. No significance is attached to this difference, which is more apparent than real and results from the difficulty of differentiation between proximal and lingual or labial surfaces on account of curvature. The practice adopted was to scribe with the side of pencil lead along the apparent position and trace the line so obtained. This character of crown twist is noted briefly by Black (1901).

ROOT DIVISION IN LOWER INCISORS

Although root division is sometimes found in lower canines it is much less common in lower incisors. Figure 4-23 *d,e,f* shows two such cases in lateral incisors. The root branches are labial and lingual, as in canines, and in both these cases the labial branch is much finer than the lingual. In *d* the fine root branch has broken at the bifurcation and appears to have curved to distal. In *e*, although it is intact, the fine labial root is much shorter than the major root branch. This tooth is much shortened by stage III wear of the crown, exposing secondary dentine.

It is of interest to compare the proximal profiles of these teeth. In *d*, as is so often the case with lower anterior teeth, the tooth axis is nearer the lingual, and the labial profile from incisal is a large arc which includes the greater part of the root. The lingual root profile is parallel to the tooth axis except for the apical curve to labial. In tooth *e* the reverse is found; the lingual root profile is arc-like from cervix to apex and the labial profile is more nearly straight. The blade of the crown is lost by third-degree wear exposing secondary dentine, but there is sufficient remaining to show that the crown was more "erect" than in tooth *d*. There is some doubt as to whether tooth *e* is a lateral incisor or canine. Viewed from mesial, its minor root is seen to arise as almost equal in bulk to the lingual root, as judged by the root groove. In both teeth, root-crown twist is apparent.

HYPOPLASIA OF ENAMEL

There were a number of lower incisors presenting hypoplasia of enamel in the teeth of the present collection. These cases presented either a number of pits in enamel (related horizontally to one another according to the stage of enamel deposition when the exanthematous or other illness occurred), or as a shallow groove around the tooth. Most of these were found in the incisal half of the crown, and some involved the incisal edge. Attention has already been drawn to one such case where the pits were so placed as to produce an effect not unlike incisal tubercles or mamelons (Fig. 4-8 *e*).

When enamel hypoplasia occurs at an early age such as in the first year of life, the evidence of damage to enamel may easily be lost through wear. Some cases were found where this stage had almost been reached and the presence of hypoplasia might easily have been overlooked but for the presence of stain in the slight irregularities of enamel still remaining. It is to be noted that these cases present less resistance to wear, so that reduction of the incisal edge more easily occurs.

WEAR IN LOWER INCISORS

Loss of tooth substance through function must be considered normal, but there are a number of factors that produce wear, some of which are unusual if not abnormal, and some are fairly regarded as pathological. As lower incisors usually fit slightly behind the uppers through the differing directions of the blades of their crowns, the effects of wear are often more easily seen on lowers through involving their labial surfaces as well as incisal edges.

Most wear is the result of friction, but sometimes the effects are intensified or otherwise modified by a reduction in the hardness of the dental tissues rendering them more easily worn. One such factor has just been mentioned above in enamel hypoplasia. Another is a chemical effect. This may result from unusual habits or food factors, or from the production of acid within the mouth from certain kinds of food debris. Allied to this is the loss of substance producing the so-called erosion cavities, but it is common knowledge that in some types of dental caries an early stage involves decalcification and weakening of the enamel surface. Friction may be associated with such cavities in anterior teeth, particularly in the cervical regions.

Friction may be of many kinds. It may occur between tooth surfaces in a normal or in an abnormal manner. It may occur between tooth surfaces and food substances of various kinds, and these may contain natural substances or contaminants which are abrasive in varying degree. Anterior teeth are more involved than any others in artificial prophylaxis, and this introduces a host of possible factors. Where prosthetic dentistry is involved more factors may be introduced, not the least of which in their effects are partial dentures or other removable appliances which may be pressed upon or moved against tooth tissues. Tooth wear has been discussed in earlier chapters and in other papers (Taylor, 1962b, c, 1963a, 1971b, 1972b, 1975, 1976).

The variety of wear caused by unnatural substances, which has been responsible sometimes for visible effects with the minimal loss of tooth substance, is that associated with prophylaxis and may amount to no more than a polish of enamel. It leaves on the tooth a demonstration both of the effectiveness and of the limitations of this procedure. Dental areas that are "sheltered" from the person's particular individual pattern of prophylaxis may be heavily stained, encrusted with tartar or actively carious. Examination of the polished surface or worn facet by means of a low-power lens will often clearly show fine scratch lines, and indicate whether the abrasion is associated mostly with a habitual directional pattern of movement of toothbrush, etc.

Sometimes this kind of wear is associated with rounded and polished notches in the labial surface of the root at the cervix. These notches result from the fact that the cementum and dentine are more readily worn away than where dentine is covered with enamel, thin though the enamel may be in this region. The notches are, of course, associated with recession or loss of gingival attachment. Whether the loss of attachment precedes abrasive action or is caused by it may sometimes be doubtful, but in many cases the technique and equipment used in prophylaxis are probably the cause of damage to both soft and hard tissues. The difference in the notches on the two sides of the mouth, particularly if the canines or premolars are involved also, may follow a recognizable pattern. The author has been able to interest a new patient in better prophylaxis by remarking at his first dental examination that he was evidently left-handed.

Wear from the incisal edge that results in shortening of the crown is very common and is normal in man. Small amounts of loss have been indicated by broken lines in some of the outlines figured. Appreciable loss often renders a tooth unsuitable for illustration of certain morphological characters. The majority of the teeth used to illustrate this book are adult and unworn, and in that respect are not "normal." They are normal, however, in regard to their morphological formation and morphological variation, and in regard to the lack of wear that is most often associated with modern dietary and eating habits as distinct from those of earlier or more primitive cultures.

Appreciable and even excessive loss of tooth substance is by no means absent in a modern community. Persons with appreciable wear are often relatively free from dental pain, at least for a much longer period than many other people, and form a minority of patients seen in dental practice. Among those is the occasional case where teeth are worn to fourth degree. This signifies that almost the whole of the crown has been worn away, but the tooth may have remained vital through the effective plugging or occlusion of the former pulp cavity by secondary dentine. This was the condition often found in old Maori and Moriori skulls (Taylor, 1962b, c, 1963a, 1970c, 1975, 1976). All stages between this and first degree, where only incisal enamel has been worn, are found, and there are several features of the worn "occlusal" surface or facet that may be noted. Wear is often more advanced on the labial than on the lingual surface, i.e. the facet tends to incline labially, at least in the earlier stages. This is the reverse of the condition found in the upper incisors and arises because of the normal overlap of the blades of the incisor crowns (Fig. 4-12). The sequence of changes from incisor overlap to the acquiring of the edge-to-edge bite was demonstrated by the author in 1937 in the same paper from which the diagrams of Figure 4-12 are taken

(Taylor, 1937b). The facet tends to lose this inclination and become level as the edge-to-edge bite is acquired and maintained. Although the term "edge-to-edge" has been long established and accepted, it is not a good term, because what is acquired is not edge-to-edge but surface-to-surface. The incisors acquire occlusal surfaces which are in occlusal relationship in the same manner as those of the posterior teeth.

The facet surface may be simple or compound, and small or large, but these descriptions cannot be precisely defined, for examination of many teeth shows that a very great variety is presented. Thus analysis is complicated by irregularities in shape of teeth themselves and by differences in their size and arrangement. For example, should a facet be judged "large" by its area or by the amount of tooth substance lost? And how could one determine which has resulted in the greater loss of tissue, a "shallow" wearing over a larger area or a deep wearing over a small area? Again, is the wearing away of nearly the whole crown of a small tooth like a lower incisor to be regarded as a larger facet than the mere reaching of dentine by the wearing of several cusps on a posterior tooth? A different method of classification, by tissues or regions of the tooth involved, has much to commend it for convenience, and the author made use of and modified Broca's (1879) classification in an earlier work (Taylor, 1962c, p. 175). Even Broca's classification has its difficulties. Not only may a number of different degrees, or stages, of wear be found in the same dentition, but even in the case of a single tooth the wear may be presented in a number of forms. Thus facets may vary in curvature and extent, and in their general slope in relation to tooth axis, with further complication arising in the presence of local irregularities in the arrangement and occlusion of the teeth. Examples are common in the present collection, but in the Moriori and Maori skulls already reported they were often outstanding features of the dentition. In some cases they were shown to be related to habits apparently peculiar to those ethnic groups (Taylor, 1963a, 1970c, 1971b, 1972b, 1975, 1976).

The teeth in the collection forming the basis of the present study are from a modern civilized community. The variety of patterns or facets of wear shown therein may be greater (though usually less extreme in degree) than those likely to be present in the teeth of a primitive community. There are several reasons for this. (a) In the primitive group (except for particular chewing habits) there is less variety in food. Moriori and Maori diet frequently compelled vigorous mastication (Taylor, 1934, 1962c, 1963a, 1975, 1976). Some other Polynesian groups present very little wear of teeth (Taylor, 1971b, 1975, 1976). Thus there is a general pattern within the group such as much wear or little wear. (b) Modern groups with much refined food may have little wear from mastication. Within these groups malocclusion is common and some teeth get no wear. Other teeth are required to bear excessive strains and may show excessive or unusual wear. (c) In modern groups dental diseases, particularly decay, are more common and teeth are often extracted. Gaps caused in this way result in malocclusion and malfunction, with effects often similar to those listed in (b). (d) In modern persons it has been shown that abnormal habits of clenching and teeth grinding (often indulged in unknowingly) produce facets of wear in unusual situations on teeth (Every, 1960). (e) Incisal and occlusal facets are often produced by dental restorations and appliances—restorations using materials of varying hardness, and appliances similarly, such as metallic "occlusal rests" and porcelain artificial teeth. (f) Incisal, occlusal (and other) surfaces are subject to wear during artificial prophylaxis, both by toothbrush bristles and by abrasives in a dentifrice. (g) Habits must be included as involved in wear of incisor teeth. Clay pipes are an occasional novelty in modern communities but pipe-smoking is so common that pipe stems of various materials are still a cause of wear. In women, the widespread use of metallic hairclips, and the habit of holding them temporarily in the mouth while hands are in use, introduced another variety of wear. This, however, like the biting of cotton while sewing, tends to produce an irregular fine chipping of the brittle enamel edges. It is different from the smoother but greater wear of incisors, "probably due to working leather thongs or threads between the teeth," found in old skulls from Spitsbergen (Christiansson et al. 1967).

Having indicated some reasons for variety in facets of wear it is obvious that analysis, description, and classification of facets, and the amount of wear they represent, are very complicated. Returning to the adjectives simple, compound, small and large, it is found that the addition of two more, shallow and deep, will make it possible to give a fair description of many facets and their differences.

A simple facet is one that appears to be caused by one kind of movement (possibly against more than one tooth) without presenting a ridge or angular change in direction of the facet. It may be shallow or deep, and small or large. A shallow and small facet of this kind is one that may glint as the tooth, or the light directed on to it, is moved. A large and deep facet is often seen on each incisor where an edge-to-edge bite is well established and much of the tooth worn away. The facet may be straight or curved on its surface but the curve will suggest movement in one axis of direction. In an animal a good example of a large, deep, curved simple facet is produced in a boar's tusk by the movement that sharpens the tusk against the upper "grinder." (This facet is sometimes made blunt at the tip through use as a tool, perhaps in scratching.) In human incisors in a well-established edge-to-edge bite the facet surface is often convex, but still "simple." The facet may be concave or cupped, as a result of the relatively less resistant dentine being worn more easily than enamel by a proportion of tougher foods in the diet.

A compound facet has at least two distinct portions, with a fairly easily distinguishable ridge or groove, straight or curved, between the parts. It may arise through contact with different teeth, or different parts of teeth, during the movement that produces the facet. It may arise from the extension of two or more facets until they meet. It may be deeper or larger or more convex or concave in one part than in the other part. One part may be caused by contact with an object or material different from that which causes another part of the facet. Thus teeth may wear against one another to produce a simple facet, or the latter may become compound, perhaps through wear from an appliance that is unstable or through wear from faulty toothbrushing habits or abrasives used therewith. A compound facet may extend far from what is reasonably called an incisal or occlusal facet.

The adjectives small and large are here used to indicate the relative size of areas of the tooth surface involved. Thus a large facet on a small tooth is not precisely differentiated from an equal area on a larger tooth. Whether the latter is also called a large facet may depend on the observer.

The adjectives deep and shallow similarly are not precisely differentiated but are so convenient that it is reasonable to use them. A facet that was almost entirely confined to enamel would not be called deep, and a facet that exposed secondary dentine or the pulp cavity would be called very deep. These terms, deep and shallow, therefore tend to correspond to the stages or degrees of such classifications as Broca's, but it is felt that the need for something more than a classification based on depth has been amply demonstrated.

ILLUSTRATIONS OF WEAR, ABRASION AND TRAUMA

A few examples of wear and facets may be illustrated by drawings.

In Figure 4-23 *b*, and more so in Figure

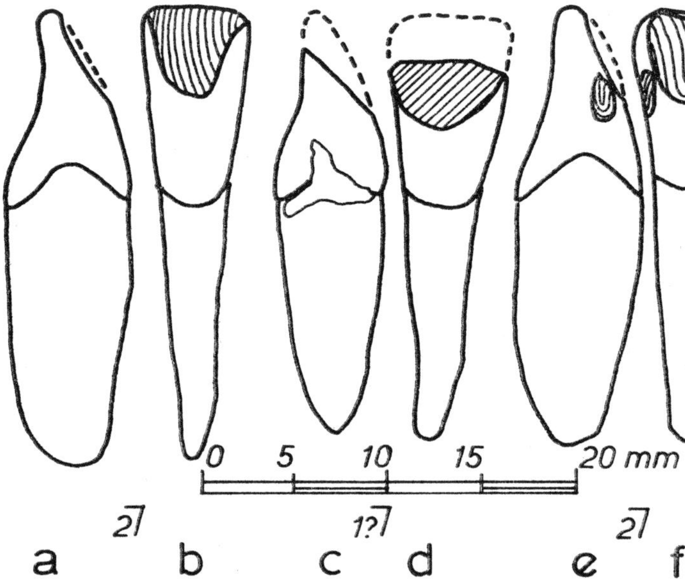

Figure 4-27. Facets of wear in mandibular incisors.

4-28 *e*, both angles have been worn and the teeth have acquired a cusp effect somewhat like a canine. The approximate original outline of the crown has been indicated by a broken line, and in the second tooth the stippled line indicates that the compound facet extends further on the lingual side. This latter is unusual in a lower incisor and, together with the very unusual cusp-like effect, indicates that the tooth was in a position of malocclusion. Tooth *e,f* in Figure 4-23 presents a large deep simple facet which is "level" and indicates a well-established edge-to-edge bite.

Figure 4-27 presents proximal and labial views of three lower incisors. All indicate a deep overbite and present large, simple facets. Tooth *c,d* is worn obliquely to second degree. The facets on the other two teeth are shallow and concave.

The tooth in Figure 4-28 *b* is a small incisor with a large, simple facet and third-degree wear. The facet is even and slopes a little to lingual instead of the more usual labial slope. It is likely that in this case the long axis of the upper or lower incisor was inclined forwards. The other specimens in this figure present the following:

a, the tooth shows a large compound facet, labially inclined and cupped, or concave, with the dentine worn more deeply. There is also a shallow notch at the cervix worn by toothbrushing.

c, this tooth had evidently received a blow which had split a large flake obliquely from the tooth, possibly through striking against the upper tooth. The tooth had remained in use and the sharp edges of the fracture became smooth. The appearance is of unusual "up and down" wear.

d, this is another tooth presenting evidence of severe trauma, although at first sight it looks like a large, simple facet and third degree wear. The crown has been broken off transversely and the surface has become almost smooth. There is secondary dentine, and apparently also a minute exposure of pulp cavity. The person was evidently not young at the time of the injury, which is of a kind likely

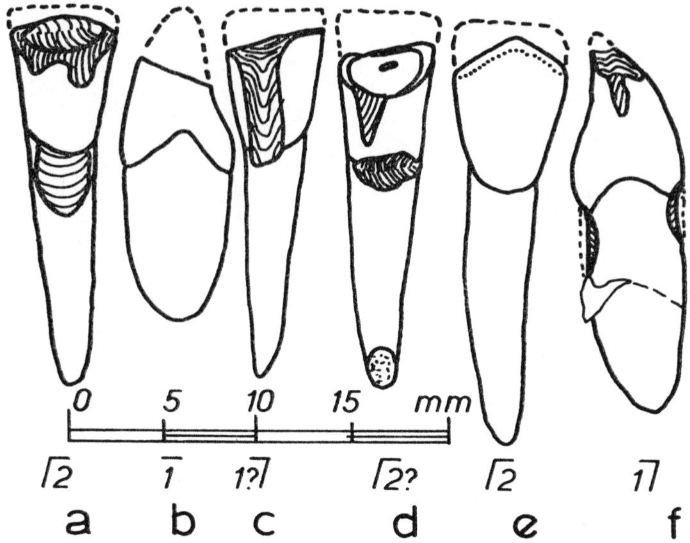

Figure 4-28. Loss of tooth substance in mandibular incisors. Recognition of wear and fracture, and possible forensic value of interpretation. In tooth *d* the dotted area at apex indicates pathologically eroded cementum, and in tooth *e* the dotted line indicates that wear is oblique also from labial to lingual, being deeper on the lingual side.

to be caused by direct contact with a foreign body. Thc small arca of roughening at the apex indicates that the pulp may have died following the injury and a chronic abscess then led to resorption of cementum. There is a cervical notch from toothbrushing (similar to that in tooth *a*). The shallow labial facet extending from the fracture almost to the cervix on labial enamel joins sharply with fractured enamel. Thus it is probably part of a larger facet, formed before the fracture by a deep overbite. One assumes that such wear ceased with the injury, which may well have involved the upper tooth also.

e, this tooth has already been described on p. 151.

f, this tooth presents five facets of wear or abrasion, each of the four shown having arisen from a different cause. There is a normal incisal facet from second degree wear. A polished notch on labial cervix has been caused by abrasion in toothbrushing; the cervical half of the root is exposed, and it is polished on labial. Recession of soft tissue attachments had reached a similar low level on the lingual surface, where a small part of a deposit of tartar is still adhering to the root. From this tartar, extending upwards to the cervix, is a long, shallow area where the root has been abraded by the bar of an unstable and latterly ill-fitting partial denture which had settled as conditions changed. There are two small proximal facets, one each on mesial and distal, in the incisal region. These have been worn by movement of the teeth during mastication, partly because of "pushing" by the unstable denture and partly on account of the reduced bony support of the teeth. Heavy stain on the lingual surface of the crown bears further testimony to the inefficiency of the person's toothbrushing technique.

In Figure 4-18 *f* is shown a tooth which presents an uncommon kind of wear confined to the labial surface. The lingual and proximal surfaces are rather heavily stained and there has been a lingual mass of salivary calculus. Subgingival calculus at labial cervix extends through both proximal surfaces to the lingual surface of the root, and there is a carious cavity between this calculus and the cervical line on the distal surface.

The labial surface is polished from incisal edge to cervix but does not present a facet with the usual defined outline and polished surface highly reflective to light. As with a convex mirror, the source of light is reflected as a reduced virtual image from differing points as the mirror is moved. In this case, however, there is no mirror-like polish, but rather a sheen, and the image is distorted and not sharply defined. The appearance is quite different from a facet worn on it by an opposing tooth, quite different also from the toothbrushing facet which tends to have horizontal markings and deeper abrasion at the cervix. In this case the cervix evidently was still covered by subgingival tartar and soft tissue when the tooth was extracted. The dull polish, therefore, is not from attrition, or food abrasion, or a dental appliance or from toothbrushing. Nor is it produced by chemical solution of enamel.

This particular variety of abrasion may be produced by a form of oral prophylaxis that does not employ a toothbrush. A fine, mildly abrasive substance used as a dentifrice is applied to labial surfaces of anterior teeth, usually by a piece of cloth wrapped around the finger. Obviously it has a very limited area of effectiveness, but this seems to be acceptable since the areas cleaned are the parts that show. Much of the movement is up and down, and examination of this tooth discloses microscopic scratches in every direction over the surface concerned as well as in an up and down direction.

In Figure 4-29 the last two outlines *f* and *g* are of one of two central incisors presenting similar evidence of trauma at an early age. At approximately three years of age the crowns of central permanent incisors are partly formed and the roots of deciduous incisors have been fully formed and shortening by absorption has hardly commenced. These deciduous roots, therefore, are in close relationship with the developing crowns of their permanent successors. It seems likely that at this age in the specimen the child received a blow, or "bump," which struck the lower deciduous incisors. The blow was transmitted through their roots and moved the developing crowns in their crypts. These partly displaced crowns remained in this position, but as the enamel and dentine forming tissues were not much damaged, further formation of the crown and root proceeded normally. The tooth duly erupted and functioned, but it bears permanent evidence of the injury in the form of displacement of the incisal portion of the crown and hypoplasia of the enamel, visible externally as a broken line of depressions around the crown. Some effects of more severe injury to incisor crowns at approximately the same age have been reported elsewhere (Taylor, 1970a).

The first five sets of outlines in Figure 4-29 are labial view outlines together with proximal outlines of each root from cervix to apex. The teeth on examination are so similar in form and condition that they seem to be from the one person. To determine whether there is a supplemental tooth additional to the normal four incisors, or whether one is in fact from another person, is an exercise in applied dental anatomy. In this case it will be shown that consideration of the minor morphological and acquired characters described in this book apparently solves the puzzle. Without these it may well be impossible to make a decision from visual examination alone. The problem may be presented as follows.

In Figure 4-29 the teeth have been arranged as presented, on the basis of width of crown and total length of root, because

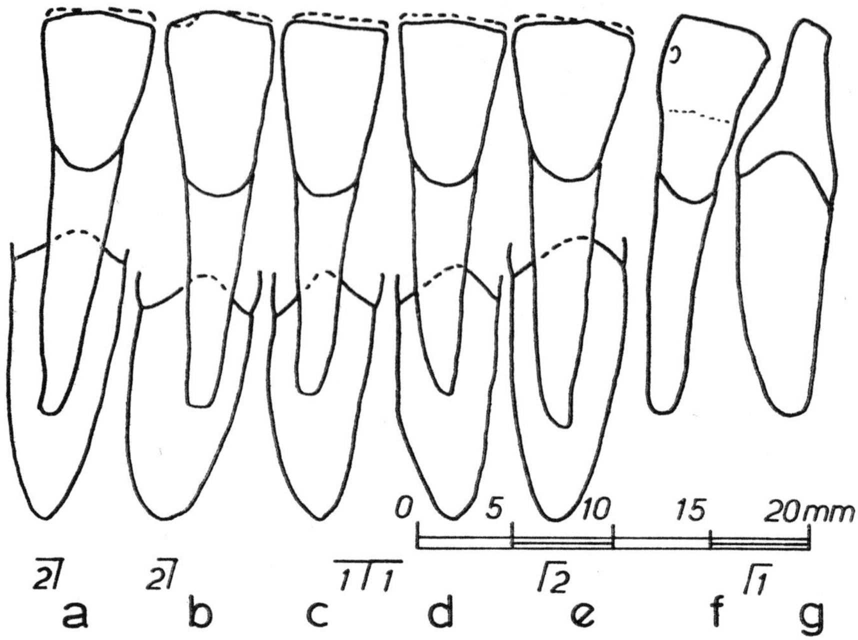

Figure 4-29. *a-e,* five mandibular incisors, apparently from one person, examined as a forensic exercise. The lower outlines are proximal profiles of the root of each tooth. *f,g,* unusual labial and proximal profiles of a mandibular central incisor, one of a pair showing evidence of trauma and pathology.

c,d seem to be a pair of centrals and *e* appears to be a left lateral. Teeth *a,b* could both be right laterals. All teeth are clean and of the same "colour," both crown and root. Some have a slight calculus deposit. All have very light incisal wear, least on *b* where it is noticeably rounded on to labial aspect. In the others the facets are flat but sometimes compound.

Crown *b* is over 1 mm longer than *a* or *e*. Crown *c* is narrowest, and *d,e* are almost equal in length to cervix. Crown *a* is almost as wide as *e*, and *b* is narrower than either, so that there is appreciable difference in the proportions of crown *b* compared with *a* and *e*. In total length *a* and *e* are equal, and *c* is slightly shorter. Shallow root grooves are recognizable on distals of *a,b,e,* particularly on *b*. Cervical lines are almost identical on *a,e* but a little more rounded on *b*. Cervical widths labial to lingual are identical on *a,b,e*. In this view the apex of *b* is widest or bluntest; all others are consistently more pointed.

There is no salivary calculus on *a* or *b*, but the light proximal calculus on *c,d,e* shows that these teeth obviously belong together. There is a small distal cavity on *b*, and this is the only tooth with caries. On labial surfaces the imbrication lines appear to be very similar on *b,c,* but in the other three teeth they are less evident and the surfaces are more polished.

In spite of the many characters which at first sight might suggest that all five teeth are from one mouth, the minor morphological and acquired characters indicate that this is unlikely. Tooth *b* is shown to differ so much that it is almost certainly not supplemental but from a different person. If the teeth were sectioned and examined for such microscopic features as incremental lines, secondary dentine and apical anatomy, more information would be obtained, but the value of observing the characters herein described has been shown (Cameron and Sims, 1973, pp. 28-29).

SUMMARY AND DISCUSSION

In the introduction to the nature of variation reference was made to the possibility of confusing central and lateral incisors when there is only one tooth to identify, and also to the wide range of variation presented by lower incisors. It will be realized, of course, that the variation occurs between persons rather than between teeth in a particular dentition. Thus one does not expect to find a narrow lateral and a wide lateral in the same patient, but even this very obvious disharmony may apparently be present in some cases of twin formations where the anlage of the twin included the completely fused germ of the supernumerary (Herbst and Apffelstaedt, 1930). Similarly, it is not expected that a short-rooted tooth will be found on one side of the mouth and a long-rooted tooth will pair with it on the other side. Variable characters of formation such as slenderness, robustness, length, breadth and convexity of outline tend to be found in all the teeth of a particular individual.

Formative characters for which it is easy to recognize the appropriateness of their presence throughout a dentition are those which are obviously in harmony with other physical or anatomical characters of the individual. Thus a big and heavy-boned person should reasonably have large teeth with thick strong roots, and a tall thin person teeth with long fine roots, or a shorter person having broad features and having also short wide incisors would present dental variations as between these individuals. Each of these varieties of tooth form is accepted as being within the normal range, equally with the more obvious physical differences between the individual people concerned.

There are other characters, fixed at the time of formation of the tooth, which are much more difficult to associate with general bodily features. Such characters clearly arise from the genetic make-up of an individual for they are easily recognized in most teeth of a dentition, though least of all in the group of anterior teeth with which this chapter is primarily concerned. The characters referred to are such as the following: (a) prominent cusps with clearly defined grooves and fissures; (b) deep narrow fissures or shallow, wide occlusal grooves; (c) many subsidiary grooves, fissures or pits; (d) rounded cusps and few grooves or fissures; (e) early or late furcation of roots; (f) divergent, or hardly diverging root branches; (g) sloping or erect cusps and associated convexity or flatness of crown surfaces, and so on.

Variations in dimension, absolute and relative, and in form, were described and demonstrated graphically, and in this latter respect the outlines speak for themselves. It is clear that there is no hypothetical average tooth that will fairly permit comparison between groups, but it is tempting to compare some measurements between individual teeth or their outlines, and this enhances an appreciation of the nature and range of variation. Thus length and breadth measurements (length overall, or separately for crown and root), or the proportions of these to one another, may be compared. Difficulties in deciding landmarks are shown to relate in part to these differing proportions, and in part to differences in contour and convexity. For example a short "stumpy" tooth may have different convexity in the outline of apex, or cervix or crown outline. But this does not always follow, for small and large teeth are sometimes near replicas of one another in form if not in size.

Figures 4-2 and 4-3 were used to illustrate the variety of dimension that may be found in the same kind of tooth among different persons. These show variation mostly in length and width of crowns in relation to root length, and length of crown in relation to its width. It is clear that in neither respect are these dimensions related to one another in any particular ratio. It would be pointless, therefore, to make any attempt to express such relationships mathematically, even if it were possible to establish satisfactory landmarks for accurate measurements of such small distances. But this is not the only objection to attempts at measurement, as may be shown by reference to two other characters, namely length and shape.

LENGTH MEASUREMENTS. For total length, presumably this would be between perpendiculars, but how are the perpendiculars to be established? Are crown lengths to be measured parallel to the perpendicular, and how can the cervical landmark be established and accessible if length must be taken from a proximal surface? If length is measured on a labial surface it will ignore labial curvature, and ignore the lingual cingulum, and both these conditions would be unacceptable.

CROWN SHAPE. This does not bear a constant relationship to any geometrical figure, regular or irregular. Even if shape in proximal view were ignored, how could shape in labial view be established by measurement? Some teeth "tend" to be straight-sided and these sides may tend to be parallel or divergent. They may be parallel in the incisal half and divergent in the cervical half with varying degrees of curvature as seen in Figures 4-2 and 4-3. How could measurement, or any ratio, convey a notion of these varying outlines? We have seen that linear dimensions of teeth are not even related to their bulk. Statements claiming that teeth in a particular group are wider (or longer, etc.) than those of another group are not scientifically acceptable as standards of comparison if they ignore demonstrably variable factors, and we believe that very similar variation can be found in any ethnic group. Statistical methods and standard deviations also ignore form in the way we have described, but as variation in form is shown to be an inherent quality, it must not be ignored. Things have to be accepted as they are, and this analysis of form enables one to see the nature of variation and to describe it.

Within the limits of basic form, the characters have been sought out that may be subject to variation, and the obvious ones are concerned with dimension, bulk and curvature. Also important was the search for less obvious characters, their analysis and description and an assessment of their consistency and usefulness in aspects of identity. Identity concerns the individual tooth, its relation to other teeth in the dentition both of the species and of the individual, and it also has a bearing on the identity of the person concerned. From these implications it is easy to see that the information gained has importance in several directions. Tooth morphology and tooth arrangement and function concern the individual person, for they have the effect of physical as well as anatomical factors. These physical factors have a bearing on a person's susceptibility to dental decay, to periodontal disease and to other morbid conditions of the dental and associated tissues. Insofar as the dentist is aware of the significance of these factors so will he be able better to advise his patient. And not only so, for some of these characters have a bearing on the difficulty of operative procedures and the prognosis of the likely effectiveness of services rendered. Some mouths are either easy or difficult to maintain in a high degree of oral health, and some teeth are either easy or difficult for the operator to place therein an effective restoration (Taylor, 1971a).

Information concerning variation in tooth form has always been important to the physical anthropologist, and finally, variation and its implications have an obvious importance in forensic studies. The dental scientist increasingly provides important data and deductions, not only in criminal but also in civil cases. Disasters involving air crashes and fire have sometimes left nothing but dental evidence towards identification of victims.

Reference was made above to "the limits of basic form." This was intended to refer to such characters of lower incisors as (a) the crown having a wedge-like form with a flattened blade extending from incisal edge to the crown body, or wedge base, in the cervical region; (b) the root being single and flattened throughout; (c) the crown flattened from the incisal edge through the blade but in a direction almost at right angles to the flattening of the root; and the base of the wedge (or crown body) also flattened but on mesial and distal in order to fit the root at the cervix; (d) the labio-lingual dimension of the root being seldom greater at any other level than at the cervix whence it decreases, or at some point is seen to taper, towards the apex; (e) in proximal view the labial outline of the crown being arc-like or convex and the lingual concave except at the cingulum; (f) the incisal edge being approximately at right angles to the long axis of the tooth when seen from labial; (g) the long axis of tooth, or crown, when seen from proximal tending to be nearer to lingual than to labial.

These features may be illustrated and easily modelled if a small length of soft wax, shaped as a blunt-ended spindle or near cylinder, is pressed between finger and thumb of each hand. Those of each hand should be in contact in an inter-digitating relationship. Slight variations in pinching pressure and in bending of axis will easily reproduce from this basic form a near replica of most of the variations of crown and root proportions, of crown and root profiles and of root curvature that have been described in this study.

Conclusions, and characters that have been described, are as follows:

1. With some isolated lower incisors it may not be possible to say definitely whether they are centrals or laterals, or from left or right side, especially if there is appreciable wear on the incisal region. These teeth usually have straight roots and are apparently bilaterally symmetrical.
2. With some of these doubtful specimens, observation of minor characters will establish a strong probability regarding identity and/or right or left side.
3. Minor characters may be present in varying degree. Thus the shallow groove on a lower incisor may be present on each side of the root in both central and lateral, or so shallow as to be negligible or actually absent. If recognizable, this is most likely to be on distal surfaces, or more so on the lateral than the central. It can therefore aid identification, as between central or lateral, and left or right. This character is useful when more than one incisor from one set is present, or when crowns are missing.
4. Although lower incisors are amongst the simplest teeth in the dentition in that they have a single flattened root and a flattened crown with no cusps or grooves, yet they present many characters for examination and comparison and many possibilities for variation. Examination, listing and analysis of these have been included in this study.
5. Variation in overall dimensions, so that there are large teeth and small teeth, has long been obvious, and such has been illustrated here, but attention has also been drawn to morphological variation largely concerned with proportions.
6. Within total length of tooth, proportions of crown length to root length vary.
7. Widths labio-lingually vary in relation to both of the above.
8. Widths mesial to distal (M-D) at incisal and at cervix bear no constant relation to one another, so crown dimensions are largely independent of root dimensions except that both must be identical at the cervix.
9. Crown widths M-D at incisal and cervix are related to such characters as straight-sided and tapering-sided crowns, or narrow and wide crowns, but these variations may occur independently of convexity of outline or of surface. Thus, in labial view, a tapering crown may have rather straight, or more convex outlines, or these outlines may have an S-shaped

character (Figs. 4-2 *b,c,* 4-3 *f*). The outline may be partly parallel-sided and partly tapering (Fig. 4-3 *e*).

10. The incisal edge may be almost straight, or so curved that the expression "width at incisal edge" has no meaning (Fig. 4-2 *c* and Fig. 4-8 *c*). These emphasize the wide variation in curvature at the incisal "angles," so that the dimension becomes "maximal width" and it is usually near to the incisal "edge."
11. Cervical lines in labial view vary considerably in convexity rootwards, but this is not entirely related to the apparent M-D dimension of the cervix (Figs. 4-3 *f,g,* 4-6 *c* and 4-13 *g*).
12. Cervical lines in proximal view showed very considerable variation (Figs. 4-19, 4-24 and many others). There does not appear to be a consistent difference between M and D cervical lines in lower incisors as was noted in upper canines.
13. Crown length is neither an anatomical nor a scientific measurement because there are no consistent anatomical landmarks as termini, and because it might be taken in several different ways. The direction of the measurement will vary according to the method and according to the curvature of the particular tooth, and in such short distances tenths of a millimeter are almost units percent. The most convenient measurement, since it may also be made on living teeth, is from labial cervix to incisal edge.
14. In proximal view the incisal edge is nearer to lingual than to labial in the great majority of lower incisors.
15. In proximal view similarly the tooth axis (especially if small apical curves are ignored) is nearer to lingual.
16. Tubercles on incisal edges vary considerably in degree of development. There was evidence suggesting tendencies for a particular tubercle to be "dominant" in that its position could most often be recognized, and for "fusion" of two tubercles to involve the same two.
17. The mesial tubercle appears to be the most stable in regard to retaining its individuality and width (but in upper incisors the distal tubercle was more often recognizable).
18. The middle tubercle in lower incisors appeared to be the narrowest when it was also the lowest of the tubercles.
19. The middle tubercle tended to be the highest when tubercles were of similar width, or when it was the widest tubercle.
20. In lower incisors root curvature is nearly always to the distal.
21. In central incisors a very small bend close to the apex may sometimes be to mesial.
22. Root taper, especially in lower centrals, was shown to involve the mesial outline more than the distal (in labial view), and to be a character of value in identification of teeth.
23. The different position of tooth axis in upper and lower teeth was shown to permit a near vertical relationship of cervices while providing for overlapping of the blades of upper and lower incisors.
24. The change from overlap to "edge-to-edge" was shown to follow from normal crown wear without alteration of tooth position.
25. Root curvature was analyzed in detail. It could sometimes be described as an optical effect of the difference in taper between opposite profile lines.
26. Root curvature in proximal view is to the labial and occurs in the apical part of the root.
27. Root curvature in labial view occasionally involves the whole root, but in the majority of cases is in the apical half or third, and directed towards distal.
28. Root curvature may arise from trauma which causes displacement of a developing tooth. There may be coronal evidence of trauma and the root may show a rather abrupt (though "prob-

ably" slight) change in direction. The position of this visible evidence of trauma indicates how much of the tooth was formed at the time of injury. As the progress of tooth development in relation to physiological age is known, one can state approximately the child's age at the time of injury. Such estimates are often confirmed by a parent's recollection of the occasion.

29. In proximal view the variation of root form is considerable. Either outline, but much more often the labial outline, may present an arc-like contour with sometimes a small apical counterbend to labial. The arc may continue a similar curve of the labial outline of the crown.
30. In proximal view the lingual outline often runs nearly parallel to the tooth axis for the greater part of its length, but sometimes it is arc-like instead of (or occasionally as well as) the labial outline.
31. Taper may commence at any point below the cervix, on either outline, and continue until near the apex. Thus apices may be formed that are sharp or blunt, rounded or squared, as were illustrated in many diagrams and actual contours.
32. It was found in a number of lower lateral incisors that in incisal, i.e. "occlusal," view the incisal edge was not at right angles to the sides, or to the major axis, of the root. This character was called "crown-root twist" and was shown to bring the incisal edge invariably nearer to lingual in its distal part. In these teeth a proximal view with the crown blade in profile required the tooth root to be slightly twisted on its long axis, but it made no appreciable difference to the root outline.
33. Crown-root twist is a character that is sometimes of great assistance in identification of a tooth as left or right. The character has not been clearly recognized so far in lower incisors known to be centrals.
34. The very uncommon condition of root division in lower incisors was illustrated with two examples. In both of these the minor root branch was on the labial side, but the proximal profile of the two teeth was very different as regards root detail.
35. Modification of crown form by illness or injury during the period of tooth formation was illustrated.
36. Modification of tooth form after formation and eruption was illustrated by evidence of fracture and of wear.
37. A number of different kinds of wear, abrasion and erosion were described and their effects on teeth illustrated.
38. The kinds of wear were more numerous, and the variety of their effects were more widespread (though seldom so severe) than in another ethnic group which was earlier reported on by the writer (Taylor, 1962b, c, 1963a).

For the data in the present study 246 teeth were selected from many more lower incisors in the collection of extracted teeth, and were mounted on thirty-six cards with the series indicator "M." For illustration twenty-nine figures have been presented containing 193 outlines and diagrams of which 158 have been traced with a camera lucida from actual teeth.

While demonstrating the great variation in tooth form and in actual size in the teeth comprising the collection on which this study is based, opportunity was taken to comment on the long-established custom of sorting and comparing ethnic groups by the statistics of metrical procedures. Such methods employ arbitrary measurements, process them statistically and impute definitive values to them. The morphology and mass of a tooth prevent the establishment of precise landmarks as measuring points. Variation has been shown to void the comparative value of measurements made on teeth and to preclude the prospect of finding any tooth that could be regarded as typical of its group. As no teeth conform to regular geometrical figures, and since teeth show variation in actual and relative maximal dimensions, and in the positions of these "axes" for measurement, no such measurements nor combination of measurements, nor indices however cunningly devised, can convey a notion of the morphology of a hypothetical average tooth. Even if they could, it is a fact that no such tooth could represent the intricate display of variations that express normality in nature. That must surely render useless the comparisons deduced from such quantitative methods.

Thus, by a somewhat different route, the writer has reached the same conclusion as in an earlier study (Taylor, 1962a). In a monograph concerning the form and orientation of the bony palate in the skull, one of the objectives was to assess the value of a metrical study in physical anthropology. At that time the cult of craniometry had been long established, but, in the course of the study, previously accepted procedures were tested and found wanting. Some of their defects were as follows: (a) techniques were inadequately described to permit exact duplication by another worker on similar material in a different ethnic group; (b) anatomical landmarks as termini for measurements were not precisely defined; (c) where measurements or landmarks were described, the information was insufficient to cover normal anatomical variation; and (d) orientation of the skull was largely ignored and thus a further variable factor and source of error was present.

These difficulties were overcome and the results were shown both by accurate contours and by graphs, and also were expressed statistically. The range of variation expressed statistically was also illustrated graphically and by superpositions of contours in various ways. Coefficients of variability were related to the measure under consideration and evaluated. Indices were examined and modified. Palate outlines were shown with their indices and compared, and the failure of indices to convey any idea of contour, much less a comparison of contours, was demonstrated. Thus was achieved the following: (1) an evaluation of conventional methods in craniometry; (2) an accurate technique, which was also demonstrated; (3) an evaluation of metrical methods for recording material; (4) an intensive record of skeletal material in an extinct ethnic group; (5) demonstration of the scope and limitations of a combination of metrical and graphical methods in anatomical description; (6) an assessment of the significance and the uselessness of statistics when divorced from awareness of method.

The nature and extent of variation must be recognized and analyzed. In spite of the suspicion which must surround any efforts to measure some aspects of variation, the fact of its normality must be accepted. As more is learned of the genetic patterns from which variations arise, perhaps there will be less tendency to regard some ethnic groups of our day as genetically stabilized over long periods, or to seek relationship to other groups by such flimsy yardsticks as cephalic and other indices. The study material of former populations may well represent no more than a stage in the changing pattern of genetic make-up, no more final than the possibilities for variation in genetic patterns that appear to be operating at the present time. Surely the variety that has been revealed in the present dental study indicates that teeth provide one of the most stable records of arrangements that are possible in this perpetual change. Surely also, one must be impressed by the basic harmony revealed in the vast majority of individuals in the presence of an apparently infinite number of variable factors.

Chapter 5

Mandibular Canines

THE MANDIBULAR or lower canine presents a wide range of variation in a number of characters. It is usually single-rooted, but not uncommonly the root bifurcates, giving what is called a double-rooted, a two-rooted or bifid-rooted canine tooth. For descriptive purposes it is reasonable to make from this character a major division. The single-rooted tooth will be presented first.

SIZE

Evaluation of size may be expressed in quantitative terms for many objects, but in the case of teeth it has been seen that measurements cannot be made satisfactorily. Moreover, the usual adjectives relating to size cannot be used to convey precise images or ideas concerning them, so that those words become vague abstractions. Concepts of size therefore are predominantly relative, and as they are inseparable here from concepts also of form, they call for some visible or graphic demonstration to establish them.

The reasons for the particular methods used in this study, unusual as they may be, may have already been outlined without establishing the soundness of their foundations in point of fact. It is appropriate to demonstrate that soundness by examination of what is involved in studying size, for it could serve as an introduction to the characters and difficulties concerned in an analysis of variation.

A quantitative study could include measurements of weight, volume, girth and dimension. For a relatively small and irregular object such as a canine tooth, weight might at first sight appear a useful quality for examination since it could be readily and accurately determined, but it is easily seen that the results would be of little use for comparison with other canine teeth, chiefly because of the nature of a tooth.

Thus weight is not directly proportional to volume, partly because density varies as between teeth, and partly because it varies in a particular tooth at different times for a number of reasons. Not only does the tooth consist of tissues of different densities, but also these tissues vary in their proportions to one another in a particular tooth, and as between similar teeth in different individuals. A tooth consists essentially of dentine, enamel, cementum, pulp cavity and pulp. Secondary dentine which forms normally may be regarded as a fourth hard tissue and its increase causes a corresponding reduction in size of the pulp cavity. The pulp loses bulk and weight as it dries out in an extracted tooth, and the same tooth may have adherent periodontal tissue. Tooth wear inevitably means loss of hard tissues in varying amount and this may in part be offset by formation of secondary dentine. Pathological conditions may lead to increase in weight from cementosis, from formation of pulp stones or calcification of varying portions of pulp tissue as distinct from formation of secondary dentine. Root resorption, deposits of stain or calculus, and dental caries all have some effect on weight, as does also the change of density through hyalinization of tooth roots in an ageing individual. As these many factors of varying effect are not measurable it is evident that weighing can serve no precise or useful purpose in comparisons of teeth. Bulk could be determined simply by displacement, but this would still not permit accurate comparisons, for some of the above variable factors, although still operative, would have to be ignored.

Some idea of variation in size may be obtained by approximate measurements of length and width, but it has already been shown that such measurements are open to serious objections. Landmarks, for example, cannot be accurately defined, robustness is ignored and such results as are obtained are invalid for comparisons because of complexities of root curvature. Again one finds that analysis of variation cannot be made satisfactorily by quantitative studies, and it must be approached qualitatively. Visual presentation by means of accurate outlines and diagrams therefore appears to be the best way to show how a particular kind of tooth retains its morphological individuality in spite of diversification of detail associated with variation in its many minor characters.

To describe the size and form of teeth represented by the outlines we may simply use the adjectives large, small, long, short, wide, narrow, etc., and qualify these by adding such words as slender or robust for the whole tooth. Further details are given for the crown and root in relation to one another, or separately as regards cusp or blade of crown, sharpness or bluntness of apex, or curvature of root.

Thus in Figure 5-1, *a,b,* and *d* are large teeth and the others are small. Tooth *a* is robust and *d* is slender. Both were almost the same in length before *a* was shortened by second degree wear, but *d* is appreciably shorter from apex to proximal cervix. All three have almost straight roots, but *b* shows a greater curvature in arc-like proximal profile; its tooth axis is nearer to lingual and its cusp blade is inclined to lingual.

Of the smaller teeth, *g,h* and *i* are short but *g* is robust and *k* and *l* are slender; *g*

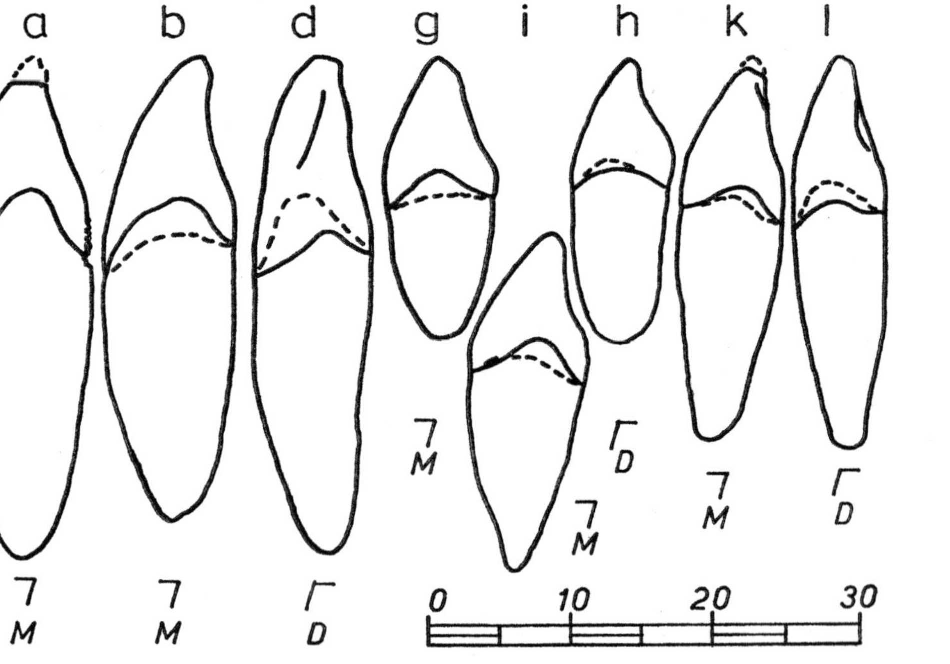

Figure 5-1. Variation in size of lower canines as regards length overall, length in relation to proximal width and proportionate length of crown and root. Teeth *a,k* are worn away at cusp tip. Tooth *a* has been damaged at cervix during extraction. For explanation of additional cervical lines (M or D in broken line) see Figure 5-29 and page 196.

is shorter than *h* or *i* but has a larger crown than either of them. Tooth *i* has a shorter crown and shorter root than *k* or *l*, but in labio-lingual diameter at cervix it exceeds them both. Again, therefore, the same kind of tooth shows much variation in all dimensions, and in crown-root proportions, as between persons. This is to be expected, even more so when there are no data of stature, sex, or body type of the individuals concerned. (The consideration of tooth width, Figure 5-8, is also relevant to tooth size.)

LEFT OR RIGHT

As with most kinds of human teeth, most lower canines are bilaterally asymmetrical in outline when viewed from buccal or lingual, and also from occlusal. This applies particularly to crown form, and it means that as between left and right teeth from one person there is a considerable degree of bilateral symmetry, or that one is almost the mirror image of the other. This facilitates distinction between left and right teeth, and also determination of the side to which an isolated tooth belonged. The characters concerned in this are very similar to those described for the upper canine, and any differences that arise are those chiefly used to distinguish between an upper and a lower canine tooth. These are that the lower is more slender than its upper, it is narrower and more straight-sided in buccal view, the cusp occupies less of the crown length, its tip (and also the tooth axis) is nearer to the lingual side, and the minor axis of the cervical transverse section "oval" is relatively shorter.

In Figure 5-2, teeth *a,b* are a pair, *c,d* are left teeth and *e,f* from right side. Below each tooth is the outline of its occlusal view.

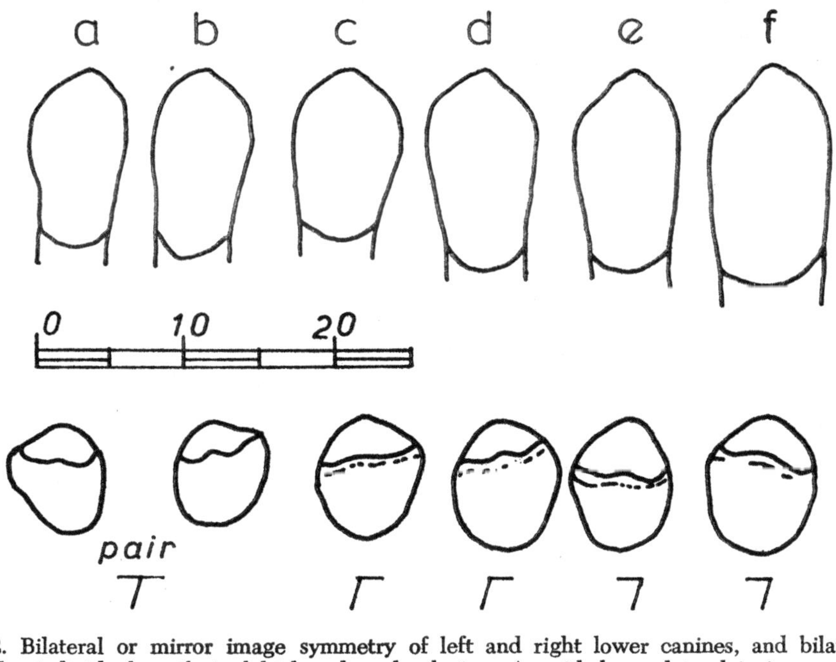

Figure 5-2. Bilateral or mirror image symmetry of left and right lower canines, and bilateral asymmetry of the individual tooth in labial and occlusal view. As with lower lateral incisors, some degree of crown-root twist may often be observed in the occlusal view. These characters assist in identification of isolated teeth as left or right. The occlusal view is of the tooth shown above it. Teeth *a,b* are from one person.

In *a,b* the mirror image likeness of left and right is easily seen. The mesial slopes of cusps are shorter and higher than the longer, more sloping and more rounded distal slopes. In occlusal view there is a distinct resemblance to the character described as crown-root twist in lower lateral incisors. In this pair, the small cusp-tip tubercle on lingual is unusually prominent, but labial grooves are not.

In outlines *c-f* the bilateral asymmetry of the individual tooth in respect of characters just mentioned is well shown. In none of these teeth is the cusp ridge outline altered by wear, yet all are different, and one could not readily make the mistake of grouping any two of them as a pair. Apart from differences in apical form and stain or polish on enamel, crown *a* is smoothly rounded, while *b* has prominent labial and lingual grooves which accentuate the central developmental lobe as a ridge and indent the outlines of the cusp ridges. Tooth *e* has a long narrow crown which is a little shorter than *d*, and it has quite a prominent and asymmetrical cusp, but no labial or lingual grooves or ridges. Tooth *f*, of similar total length to *d* but shorter than *c* or *e*, is a sturdy tooth with a much larger crown than others in this figure. The crown is straight-sided and very wide M-D at cervix, lacks noticeable grooves or ridges, yet has a prominent cusp with relatively straight ridge outlines. One could expect this tooth to have been associated with upper centrals of a long square type and that all teeth in that particular dentition would present features of this same "tooth family" character.

It should be added that both *e* and *f* have a slight root curve which is directed mesially, as this is unusual.

ROOT

Root Grooves

The single-rooted variety only is considered at this stage. On card N 6 of the author's collection (not figured) there are three lower canine teeth. All have rather sturdy roots, straight and of almost identical length and of medium bluntness as regards the apices. The proportion of crown to root is about the same in each; *a* and *c* have quite prominent cusps, but in spite of some wear, tooth *b* evidently had a rather blunt cusp (although it had the finest or least blunt apex of the three teeth). The crown of *a* is quite slender as seen from labial; *b* is sturdy and much thicker at M-D cervix; and *c* is intermediate in these respects. But there are noticeable differences between the roots in regard to grooves. Tooth *a* is deeply grooved on M and D, *b* is lightly grooved on both sides and *c* has no trace of either groove, and its labio-lingual dimension at cervix is noticeably less than in the others. Tooth *b* may have two root canals reuniting before the apex, but *a* must have two separate canals throughout its root length, terminating in two fine foramina close together. This deep grooving could be regarded as an intermediate stage between a single and a divided root. A study of canal "irregularities" in mandibular incisors (Laws, 1971) is of interest in this respect.

Root Curvature

Root curvature is most conveniently studied in labial (or lingual) and proximal view, although, as with other teeth already described, there are many examples of curves that cannot be properly shown in either of these. They may curve in an intermediate direction entirely, or curve in slightly different directions in different parts of the root. Unevenness of taper of the root, and thinning of the root towards the apex, may give an impression of bending or curving, or increase such impression when some degree of curvature obviously does exist.

Starting with labial views in Figure 5-3, tooth *a* has a considerable curve to distal, and it evenly involves the whole root. This tooth has a small lingual facet of wear indicating malocclusion which could have contributed to the curvature as the tooth erupted into position. Tooth *b* has a very

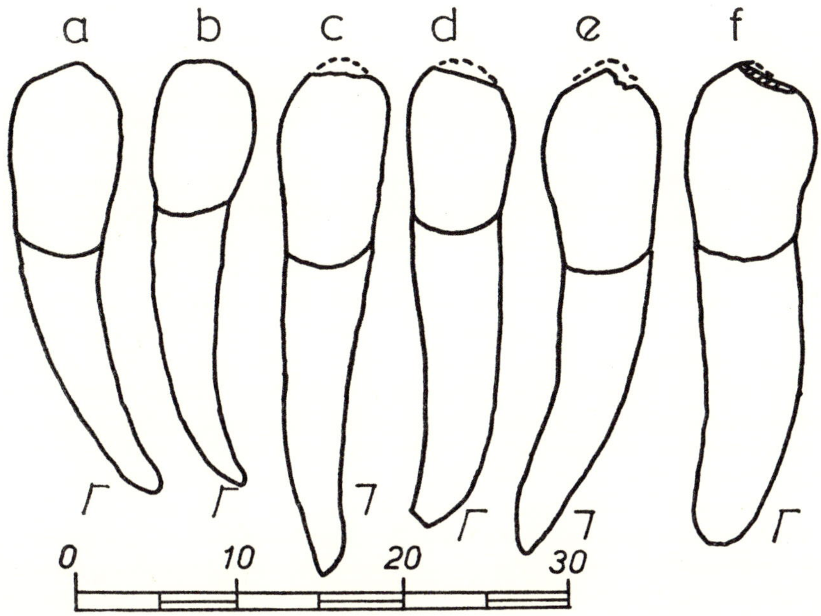

Figure 5-3. Root curves in lower canines. In a few cases the curve is mesial, as in *c* and *d*. See text for details of root grooves and cusps in these teeth. In proximal view of tooth *e* (Fig. 5-9 *b*) the root is seen to curve also to labial.

similar curvature but its labial facet and stain line show that occlusion and position were normal. The large teeth *c* and *d* are somewhat similar except that in these the curve involves only the apical half of the root; but these teeth are noteworthy in that in both cases the curve is to mesial, which is much less common than curvature to distal. Tooth *e* again is a large tooth with the apical half of the root involved in change of direction; in this case the change is more abrupt and may be called a bend rather than a curve. There is an additional feature, for the root tip curves strongly to labial, ending in a fine apex shown in proximal view in Figure 5-9 *b*.

In Figure 5-4 are shown lower canines in which there is variation in proportionate length of crown and root and the figure also presents an analysis of slight differences in direction of root axis from crown axis, or of parts of the root axis in regard to the rest of the root and crown. Tooth *a* has a slight difference in direction of axes of crown and root, and in this case one is doubtful whether it should be described as a bend, or as an appearance of bend given by taper in the root. Tooth *b* gives no such illusion, for there is an obvious bend arising at about the junction of cervical and middle thirds of the root. Tooth *c* is less easy to describe but the cervical half of the root has a slight bend first to distal then to mesial, and the rest of the root bends to distal. The shorter tooth *d* has a large crown which is in line with most of the root, the apical fourth of which curves sharply to mesial. These four teeth are from the left and the remaining two, *e* and *f*, are from the right side. In each case there is a long crown with a straight root except for the apex which turns to distal in *e* and to mesial in *f*.

A study of root curvature in proximal view shows more variety than in labial view. In addition to the relative length of crown and root (which has been seen already as a principal factor when viewing from labial) there appear to be perhaps three other characters important to the proximal view. These are the greater width of cervix, variety in the labial arc which is present in so many lower canines and incisors, and details of the apical region. These latter may increase or reduce either the chord or the radius of the arc (or even largely cancel the arc-like labial outline); they may give an impression of root curve to labial (or occasionally to lingual) or merely by the details that make for a sharp, blunt, round or square apex this apical region may largely determine the apparent character of the whole root.

With regard to the lower incisors the frequent apical curve to labial could reasonably be explained or accounted for by study of the bone surface morphology as regards alveolar ridge and mandibular body in this region. The root of the canine, as well as extending further into the basal bone, is less intimately related to the chin in many cases, and this may in part account for differences in apical morphology between lower incisors and canines.

In Figure 5-5 are shown six lower canines, five viewed from distal. Tooth *b* is the only one here which has a definite root curve to lingual, although even here there is a suggestion of reversing this at the extreme tip of the apex. The root of tooth *a* resembles *b* in the greater part of its length but its apical region turns definitely to labial, and in both of these teeth the apex is rather blunt. In *c* the apex is almost pointed, and the root could be described as straight and as having a fairly even taper labially and lingually from cervix to apex. It is rather a short tooth overall, and the shortness is mainly in the root. Teeth *d* and *e* are much more sturdy, larger and longer both in crown and root; *d* has a thick blunt apex, and this character is present in an extreme form in *e*, and gives the root a truncated appearance, although there is no visible evidence of pa-

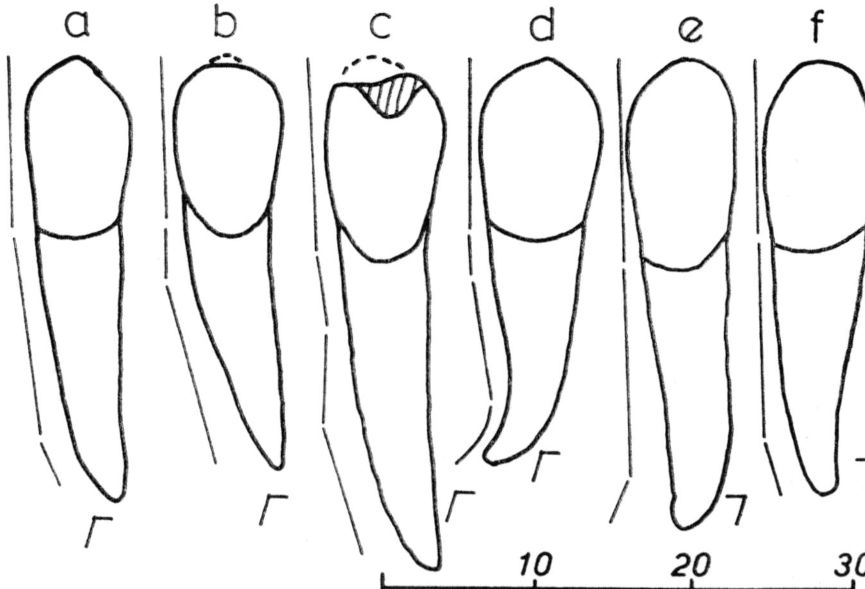

Figure 5-4. Variation in proportionate length of crown and root. Differences in direction of axes of root and crown, or of parts of the root axis from axis of remainder of root, and crown, are shown in the broken straight lines alongside each outline. Cusp wear on *c* extends to labial as shown in shaded area.

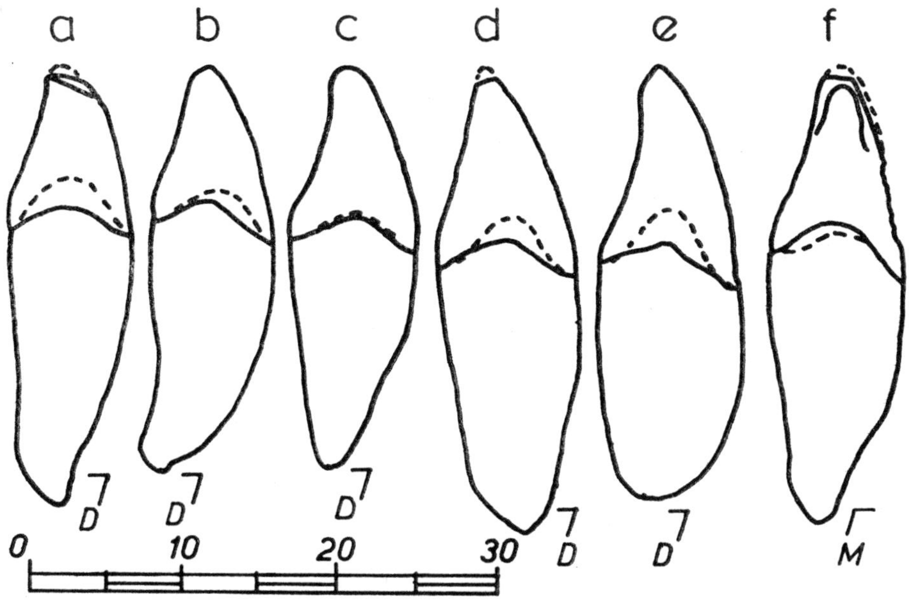

Figure 5-5. Proximal views of lower canines showing variation in curvature of root, or of one of the root profiles, or of the apical part of the root. The labial surface of *f* has a large area of hypoplastic enamel, and a facet of wear extends to meet it.

thology. In labial view this blunt apex turns slightly but definitely to mesial. Tooth *f* presents an outline that differs considerably from the other five in this figure. It is a sturdy tooth but not long overall. The crown however is long. It has a facet of wear extending from cusp tip nearly half-way to labial cervix, and just beyond this there is a slight concavity in labial outline, corresponding to a labial area which, under low power magnification, looks like mild hypoplasia of enamel. Such a confined area of defective enamel could easily have been associated with injury to the tooth's deciduous predecessor at an early age, say between approximately five and six and one-half years (Taylor, 1970a, 1971d). The morphological character for which this tooth has been included here, however, is the rather abrupt change in labio-lingual dimension as the apex is approached. The reduction of root width is confined to the labial half of the root.

Curvatures seen in proximal profile are involved also when considering the position of the crown on the root. This is referred to below in the text relating to Figure 5-9. There are further considerations also of apical form in the text for Figure 5-10.

Root Length

It has been shown that root length is not a definite dimension that can be measured. Among the variables and characters that frustrate the search for acceptable anatomical landmarks are the undulating cervical outline, curves and bends in the root, and the variations in apical morphology. Herein essentially are the qualities that contribute to a concept of the overall characteristics of a tooth. To these might be added the general impression of sturdiness (or otherwise) and the apparent proportions of crown and root length.

Data concerning these may be obtained by examination of buccal and proximal outlines in the figures. Most of these outlines show also some other particular character, but those in Figure 5-6 are chosen here firstly for overall length and proportions of crown to root.

Teeth *a* and *b* are both rather long teeth with straight and strong roots, and *c*, while a little shorter, has a heavier root and a crown that has much rounder outlines. The crown has almost a transverse groove at about the junction of middle and cervical thirds. This is confined to mesio-labial surface and has a smooth enamel surface, but between it and the cervix is an area of hypoplastic enamel. This has been made more rough by damage during extraction but the lingual cervical enamel is normal and undamaged. It appears that this tooth also has suffered trauma very similar in nature and effects and at about the same stage of development as has just been indicated for tooth *f* of Figure 5-5.

Other large teeth are seen in Figures 5-3 *c* and 5-4 *e,f;* small teeth in Figure 5-1 *g,h,i,k,l* are small in that they are slim although their roots are relatively long for the size of their crowns.

CUSP

The cusp in lower canines varies considerably in form, and this is borne out by the teeth figured. The impression gained regarding acumination is that it is affected by two main characters, namely the angle at which cusp ridges meet and the straightness or curvature of the ridges. Another factor involved is the tendency of the crown to have straight or rounded sides and to be broad or narrow.

Some of these differences in cusp form may be seen in the outlines already presented. The mirror image differences of Figure 5-2 *a,b* are those as between left and right in a pair from the same individual. Teeth *c,d* of the same figure show differences associated with ridges or grooves in the labial surface, and *e,f* present a similar degree of acumination in teeth of contrasting widths. In Figure 5-3 the cusp tips of some teeth have been slightly modified as indicated, and this applies also for Figure 5-4 *b,c* and 5-5 *a*. This last tooth is a good example of a straight-

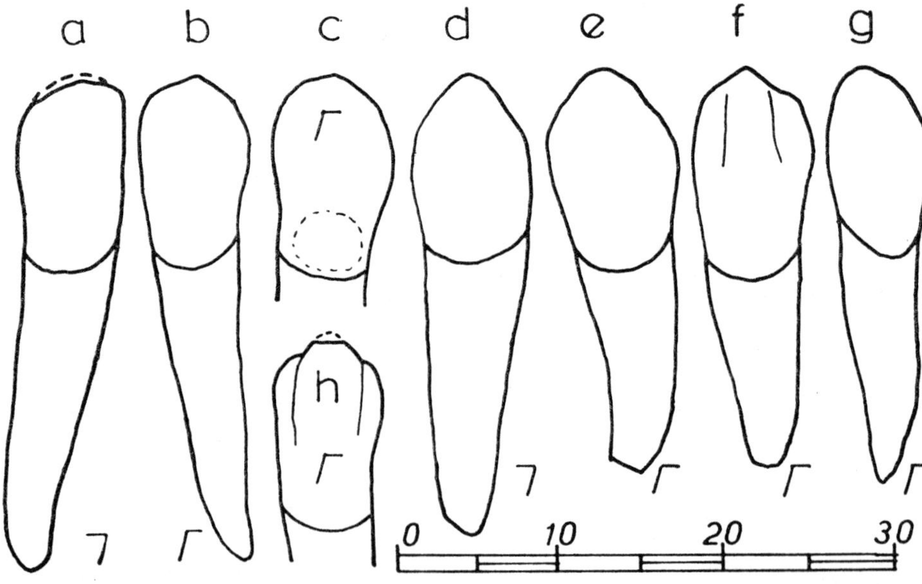

Figure 5-6. Crown of lower canines. Variation in acumination of cusp, in cervical width and in divergence or curvature of M and D profiles in labial view. Tooth *c* has an area of hypoplastic enamel which has been damaged during extraction of the tooth. Tooth *e* is a young tooth with an incomplete apex. See also Figures 5-9 *d* and 5-31 *l* concerning tooth *h*.

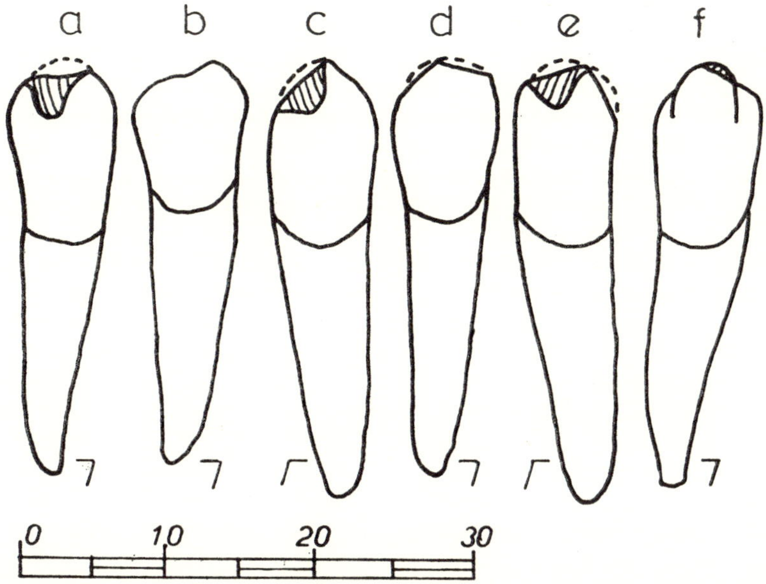

Figure 5-7. Crowns of lower canines in labial view. Further examples of characters shown in previous figure, and modification of cusp outline by wear.

sided tooth, as also are *d* and *f*. Figure 5-6 *b* shows a tooth slightly curved on M and with marked curvature on D. Uncommon degrees or forms of acumination are shown in Figure 5-6 *d* and g. These illustrations are sufficient to show that the cusp outline in labial view may be approximately an obtuse angle, a right angle, acute angle or so curved or flattened that there is no recognizable angle. Further comment on cusp form is made in the text relating to Figures 5-11 and 5-12.

Cusp Modification

It has been mentioned that the form of a cusp may be modified by wear, and the examples just mentioned had involved very little loss of tooth substance from the tip or the shoulders of the cusp. Wear extending to labial surfaces (as is normal for lower canines) does not call for other than brief mention here. Such a facet of wear is illustrated in Figure 5-7 *a* and the probable former cusp outline indicated. But tooth *b* shows modification from a different cause. This tooth never had a cusp. There is no central facet to show that the cusp has been worn away, and no sign of fractured enamel to indicate trauma. But there is roughened and somewhat pitted enamel in this region. This is a hypoplasia of enamel and one infers that it was associated with some severe illness. According to the tables of dental development given by Schour and Massler (1944), the illness probably occurred during the second half of the infant's first year of life.

In Figure 5-7 *c* the facet is confined to the mesial ridge and the labial surface of the cusp. It is a curved facet and its effect has been to increase the natural acumination of the cusp. Tooth *d* has rounded outlines except for the cusp which is definitely acuminate with straight shoulder ridges meeting at an obtuse angle. Close inspection shows that these straight outlines have been acquired by a slight degree of enamel wear and that it is confined to these ridges. The modification here is slight and could easily be overlooked, but it does alter the "family" character of the tooth in a way that could have significance when checking "affinities" among isolated teeth relating to identification of remains. In the same figure tooth *e* is very straight-sided and also has retained the appearance of a cusp, but the wear is greater and not symmetrical. From the mesial ridge a facet extends to labial surface, but the distal ridge is more deeply worn and has no such associated labial facet. It is a much more sturdy tooth than *b* and the root tends towards the hyaline character; there is calculus and stain and evidence of alveolar recession. None of these is present in *b* where the root is pale and dense and the labial enamel polished. Although well aware of the foolishness of diagnosis from so few data, one could easily imagine youthful femininity surrounding tooth *d*, and middle-aged masculinity for *e*.

In lower canines, as in incisors, there may be seen shallow labial grooves associated with, or without, small indentations of the cusp slopes. These no doubt represent the counterpart of mamelons and developmental lobes in incisors. With canines the central lobe is the longest and largest (and the mesial one the narrowest) so that the canine tends to have a labial ridge which is nearer to mesial. This ridge has been mentioned in connection with the bilateral asymmetry of an individual canine, and the bilateral symmetry (or mirror image effect) as between left and right. As for the labial ridges and developmental grooves and mamelons, an example was given in Figure 5-2 *d*. Another such tooth, this time modified by slight wear of the cusp tip, is in Figure 5-7 *f*.

CROWN SHAPE AND TOOTH WIDTH

Tooth width is concerned mainly with curvature of outline and width at cervix, or the association of the crown with a slender or more robust root. It will be considered first from labial and then from proximal viewpoints. Length of root and its shape undoubtedly contribute to the impression as to whether a tooth is wide or narrow, particularly in proximal view.

In labial view it is the proportions of length of crown to its width to which we wish to give greater attention. As the cusp is a dominant feature of the crown, outlines already given for the cusp serve also to illustrate crown outlines and proportions.

In Figure 5-2, teeth *a,b* are a pair of medium length teeth with relatively long slender crowns and moderately curved outlines. Tooth *c* has a relatively wider crown with more curvature in outlines and very marked convexity of labial surface. Teeth *d* and *e*, like *a,b*, have moderate curvature and are also slender or rather narrow for length of crown. Tooth *f* contrasts strongly with these, for although of approximately the same overall length, it is a sturdy tooth with a much wider crown, having slightly tapering straight sides and wide at the cervix. One would expect this to be associated with large upper central incisors of the long square type described in Chapter 1.

In Figure 5-3, teeth *c,d* have medium-width crowns of mixed type, unlike the square tooth just mentioned, but relatively wide at cervix, while the crown of *e* is quite large with well-curved distal outline. Tooth *a* of Figure 5-4 has a much smaller crown, but it is also straight on mesial and very rounded on distal. Tooth *d* has a large crown and a relatively short and sturdy, but deeply grooved, root with a wide cervix and a very convex labial surface in the crown. Teeth *e,f* both have large long crowns with rather straight sides, especially *f* which is wide at the cervix.

Figure 5-6 presents considerable variety of crown shape and the manner in which these teeth differ from those already described is easily appreciated, and the same applies to those in Figure 5-7. With reference particularly to M and D outlines (instead of to cusp length or acumination) it is clear that these outlines may both be straight, one straight and one (distal) curved, or both curved; there may be little or a considerable degree of taper, and the cervical line may be wide and "flattened" or narrow and strongly convex.

Proximal Width and Profile

As with labial views, the outlines already used present considerable variety. From Figures 5-1 and 5-5 it will be appreciated that in general the proximal outline form is not greatly dependent on the overall length of the tooth but rather on the relative lengths of crown and root and the relation of cervical width to those lengths. Another character to be noted is the relation of crown axis and root axis to the whole tooth axis. When visualizing these it is easier to form a fair judgment if minor, but often very noticeable, bends in the apical region are ignored (Fig. 4-5 *e*).

Further examples in Figure 5-8 show: *a,b,* two large teeth which are both wide although *b* has a relatively short root; *c,* a slender tooth with narrow cervix but a long root; *d,* a small tooth with relatively wide cervical width from proximal; *e,* a relatively large crown with very short wide root and acuminate apex; *f,g,* two teeth very similar in cervical width and crown length, but *f* with a curved fine-bladed crown contrasting with a straighter thick-bladed crown in *d,* and also contrasting root profile curvatures (although each has a straight root and pointed apex).

Position of Crown on Root

Teeth have just been referred to as having curved or straight crown blades and curved or straight root profiles. These concepts are closely related to those discussed in such terms as axis of crown or root or of the whole tooth, and arcs to which profile contours, usually the labial ones of crown and root, seem often to conform. If these terms are acceptable in describing

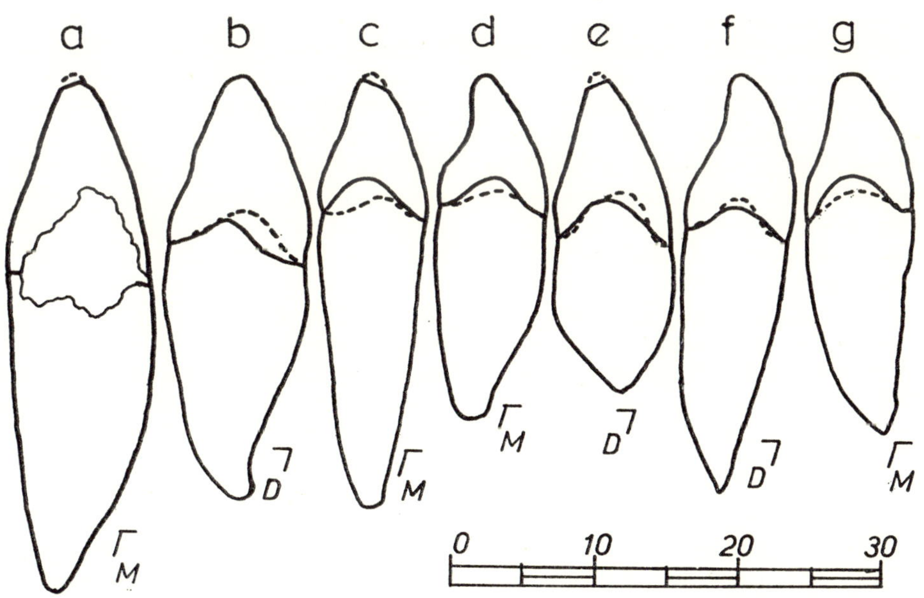

Figure 5-8. Proximal outlines of lower canines showing variation in cervical width, and in root length and profile curvature. (See also Figs. 5-1, 5-5, 5-9 and 5-10.) Extraction of the large tooth *a* was evidently complicated by the position of adjacent teeth, for it has had to be drilled away (as outlined) to clear the obstruction.

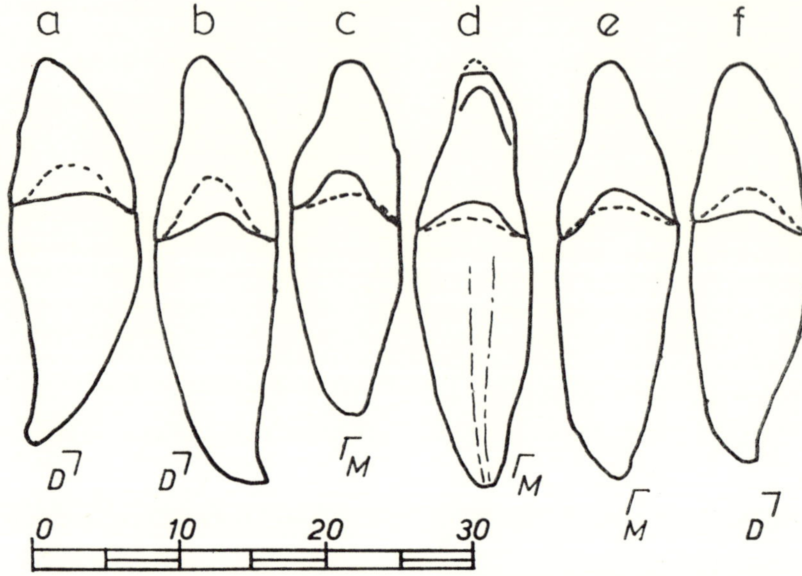

Figure 5-9. Proximal outlines of lower canines showing variation in profile curvature, in position of tooth axis and in position of crown on root. Tooth *b* is seen from labial in Figure 5-3 *e*. Tooth *d* has a long groove on each side of the root suggesting bifidity of pulp cavity without branching of the root.

morphological variations there should be no difficulty in accepting some other terms that assist in describing crown-root form and relations, such as straight, erect or bent crowns as regards their position on the root, and such indefinite terms as fine, pointed, rounded and square or blunt to describe apices. Of course these are terms of convenience for description, and what would be more correct would be to describe the position of the root on the crown. It must be acknowledged also that genetic influences must largely determine crown morphology, but that root form is more likely to be influenced by additional nutritional, functional and anatomical factors.

Figures 5-1, 5-5 and 5-8 indicate the wide range of variation seen in these characters. A commonly seen and perhaps uncomplicated relation between form of crown and root is not unlike that of 5-1 *b* or 5-8 *f* in which the arc-like labial curve of crown or root is easily recognized and the crown is set fairly "straight" on a straight root (apart from minor apical curves).

An extreme example of labial curve in both crown and root is seen in Figure 5-9 *a*. The next two, *c* and *d*, present almost the opposite extreme in which there is very little labial curvature in either root or crown, and the crown is set erect and near the labial, instead of nearer the lingual, as is most commonly found in lower incisors and canines. Tooth *b*, in which the root curve is in this view much like an upper, is seen in labial view to curve strongly also to distal (Fig. 5-3 *e*). In tooth *e* there is no recognizable labial arc in crown or root, but the crown appears to lean towards lingual, and the tooth axis is certainly nearer that side. Tooth *f* presents a labial arc in crown and in root but this is not continuous. The lingual root outline is almost straight and vertical and, except at the apex, the labial root arc provides the whole appearance of root taper in this view.

The position of the crown on the root is involved also when considering curvatures in proximal profile. This was referred to above in the text relating to

Figure 5-5. At that time also there was some reference incidentally to the form of the apex.

APEX

When considering root curves and bends it was inevitable that comments should be made concerning the form of the apex of the root. Although much variation in apical form as regards sharpness or bluntness, etc., may readily be seen in labial views of teeth, the variation is often better appreciated from proximal views. Many such differences are seen in Figures 5-1, 5-5, 5-8 and 5-9. In the last three figures the apical variations are mostly associated with bends in the root or differences in curvature between labial and lingual profiles. In Figure 5-1 most of the roots are "straight" or they taper evenly, and this is true also of the outlines of roots in Figure 5-10.

Teeth *b, d* are both rather small teeth from right side in which the root tapers evenly to a fine apex. Tooth *a* is even smaller and from the right side with even taper, but it has a much more blunt apex. Tooth *c* is a large and long left tooth with an extremely fine sharp apex and even taper. Teeth *e,f* are right and left, both large. Tooth *f* is wider both from proximal and labial than *e,* and each has a very blunt rounded apex, one directed slightly to lingual and the other to labial.

CROWN

At this point another look will be taken at variations in the form of the crown of the lower canine. It is useful to view it from occlusal, from proximal and from labial, and all these aspects have already received attention for particular purposes. In Figure 5-2 the occlusal views were to show "crown-root twist" and other characters of asymmetry that assist in identifying a tooth as left or right. In considering the position of the crown on the root, the crown axis and curvature of profiles were examined in proximal view. In all outlines in proximal view there was seen to be much variety in form of cervical line.

In labial view the outline has two principal components, cusp form and curvature of M and D outlines. These are close-

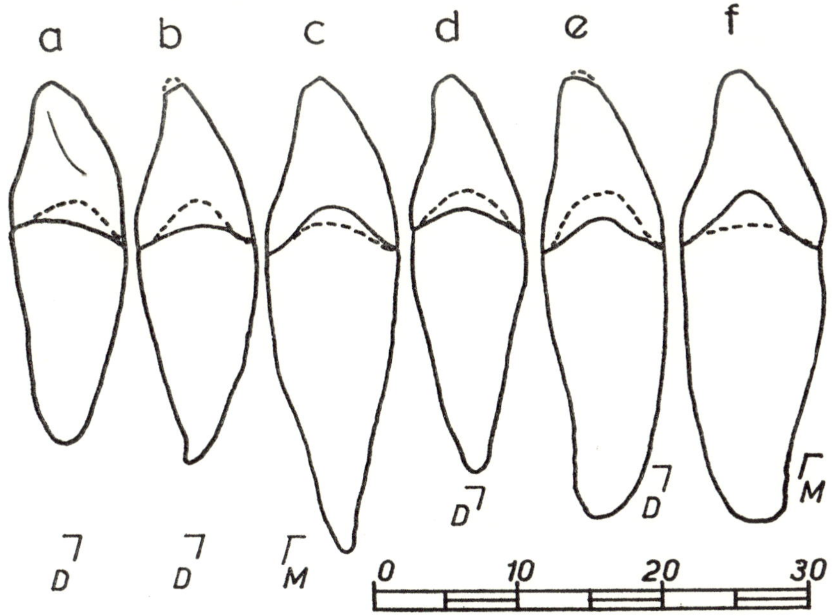

Figure 5-10. Proximal outlines of lower canines showing variation in cervical outline, and of apex in teeth that have roots of relative straightness or even taper.

ly interrelated, for a long or acuminate cusp often dominates the shape and reduces the length of M and D outlines, or the two parts may merge so gradually that they lose any semblance of separate identity. Also, the straightness or curvature of M and D outlines, and their degree of convergence, is closely related to the cervical width of the tooth in this view.

All these features have received attention in Figures 5-2, 5-3, 5-6 and 5-7, particularly in the last two. It is proposed now to give further examples of variation in crown form. While the characters of actual size and of cusp form are necessarily included, attention at present is directed chiefly to M, D and cervical outlines.

In Figure 5-11 the crowns vary in actual size and in proportions of length to width, but they all have straight sides M and D which are nearly parallel, a little more divergent in *f* and a little rounded in *g*. All except *c* tend to have robust roots, all are of the long square type and rather wide at the cervix. In *a,b,c* the two-sloped form of a cusp has been maintained by wear from both slopes, more on the distal slopes of *a,c,* but it is still wear of enamel only. In *d,e* the cusp form has been lost by wear from the tips, and wear has just reached dentine. Teeth *f,g* have retained the original form of the cusp with negligible wear. Tooth *f* has calculus and deep stain on proximal and lingual surfaces, but a high polish and no stain on labial surface and these differences indicate that the person concerned may have practised regular artificial prophylaxis but only for the sake of appearance. The fact that this sound tooth had to be extracted suggests that teeth "that did not show" had been neglected until a "clearance" was necessary for the fitting of artificial dentures.

Figure 5-12 continues the study of crown shape and presents examples of divergence or curvature, or both, in M and D outlines, again using teeth ranging from large *(a,d)* to small overall *(b,c),* and from those with broad thick roots *(a)* to relatively slender roots with a fine apex and nar-

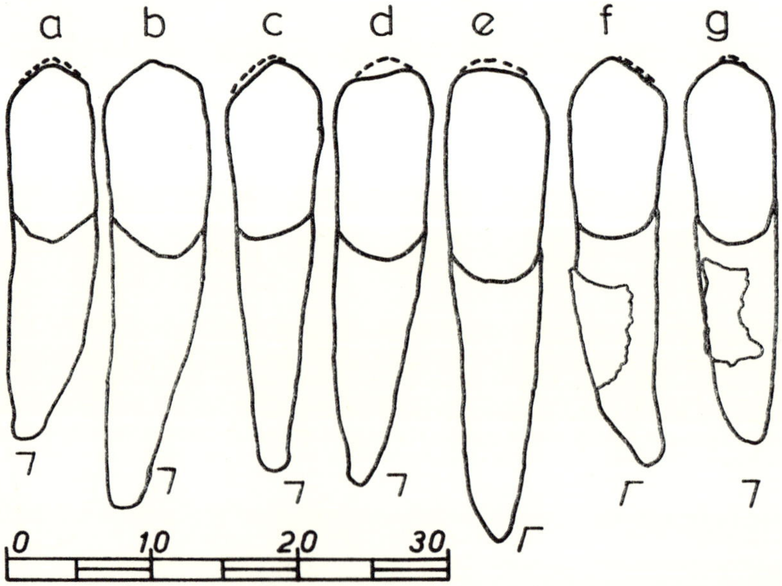

Figure 5-11. Labial outlines of lower canines showing M and D profiles nearly straight and nearly parallel, and cervical outlines. Compare and contrast with Figure 5-6. In *f,g,* fractured portions of the thin labial plate of alveolar bone are adherent to the roots.

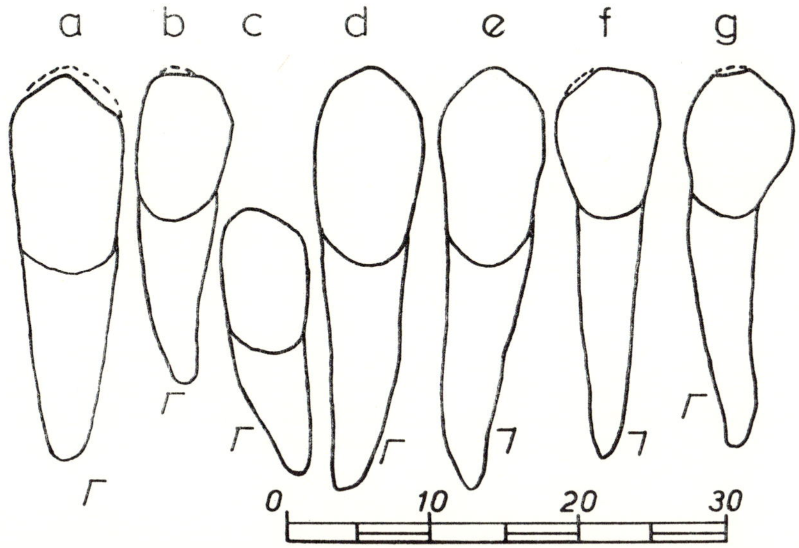

Figure 5-12. By contrast with Figure 5-11, these lower canines present more divergence and curvature in M and D profiles.

row cervical width *(f)*. Teeth *d*-*g* and tooth *c* of Figure 5-6 have had negligible alteration to original cusp form through wear. The last three teeth mentioned are noteworthy for the degrees of curvature in their outlines and surfaces. Another look at teeth *a* or *d* of Figure 5-11 and their contrasts in comparison with Figure 5-12 *g* will emphasize the range of morphological variation presented in "teeth of a kind."

With these figures we may now extend the observations made concerning cusps on p. 168. The form of the cusp consists essentially of two slopes which often meet at a recognizable angle to form the cusp tip. The slopes may meet M and D outlines at angles or curves, but it is usually acceptable to refer to the "shoulders" of the cusp, as with teeth already studied. The "slopes" seen in labial view may also be called the M and D ridges of the cusp.

It is noted that these ridges may be approximately of the same length (Fig. 5-6 *d*, *e*) but usually the D ridge is longer (Fig. 5-6 *f*). One ridge may be almost horizontal and the other sloped steeply (Fig. 5-4 *b*,*e*, *f*) and either M or D may be the horizontal or steep ridge. The ridges may be very unequal in length (many examples) although this may be sometimes a subjective interpretation involving continuity of cusp ridge into cusp shoulder. The D cusp shoulder may have an even curve (Figs. 5-3 *b*, 5-4 *c* and 5-6 *b*) or may be "segmented," lowering the point of contact with a vertical tangent (Figs. 5-6 *c* and 5-12 *d*,*f*). The ridges may be of approximately equal inclination where cusp acumination is noticeable and there are many such examples of this, as there are also of rounded or flattened cusps. The almost flattened cusp may be regarded as one where both ridges are near horizontal, and such a tooth when extracted and examined on its own may suggest an unusually robust lower incisor.

These remarks apply of course to unworn teeth. The variety of "slopes" or flattenings produced by wear is infinite and is determined by many factors. Some of the factors are of course such things as individual habits and variations in occlusal relationships and movements. Others are closely related to the "family characters" of a dentition whereby they tend to have acuminate or flattened cusps and straight or rounded contours; in other words the variations that are the subject of this study.

WEAR

Like other teeth the lower canine is subject to wear. As with other anterior teeth, the causes are more varied and the effects more easily seen than in posterior teeth. But there are additional factors which may contribute to differences in the effects of wear seen in this tooth as compared with those in incisors or upper canines. Thus it is the largest and strongest of lower anteriors, it normally occludes with the mesial slope of the upper canine, and it may have a more acuminate cusp. It is active in function whereas the upper is passive, and it may form an angle in the arcade as facial surfaces pass from the labial to the buccal regions.

For reasons which might in part be morphological and physical, the lower incisors and canines are less subject to tooth decay and are often retained as attachments and support for prosthetic appliances. But if proper maintenance and attention are not forthcoming, the appliance becomes unstable because of changes in its environment of living tissues. The appliance through its instability becomes an active factor in further changes, some of which involve the teeth. Among these are various kinds of wear found on these teeth.

Because the anterior teeth are readily visible and easily accessible by contrast with posterior teeth, they are usually given most attention during artificial prophylaxis or home care. But even in anterior teeth some parts are relatively inaccessible and hard to see so that labial surfaces receive most attention and various visible signs testify to the differences in treatment of these and lingual surfaces. Where normal incisal overlap is present the differences are reduced in the case of upper anterior teeth and increased in lowers. The differences relate largely to the tendency of enamel to be relatively stain free and polished where subject to friction, and to have adherent stain and calculus in the regions that are relatively sheltered from friction.

Most such friction comes from function, i.e. from mastication of food, from friction between food and tooth and from friction between tooth surfaces. This is normal. Abnormal friction of various kinds takes place during artificial prophylaxis, from substances held between teeth (such as a pipe stem) and from movements of a prosthetic appliance. These last two are sometimes called abrasion. Whatever the distinctions in terminology, the essential fact is that tooth substance is removed in varying amount from regions of teeth that vary in position and extent. From these variations it is usually possible to determine the causal factor or factors. Thus minimal loss of substance from labial surfaces leaving a polished enamel surface suggests artificial prophylaxis as the main factor. Polished notches at labial cervices indicate more vigorous prophylaxis or that it has involved a habitual pattern of movement with insufficient regard for the real objective or of the abrasive quality of equipment used. Evidence of an associated recession of periodontal attachments or of alveolar bone is common in such cases.

Conversely, deposits of stain or of calculus in sheltered areas indicate that friction from fibrous food during mastication, or from prophylactic activities, did not reach these areas. Carious cavities or facets of wear of such size, shape or location as are commonly associated with prosthetic appliances (and their supports) of faulty design may all provide the observer with data regarding habits or conditions that were present in the mouth prior to, or at the time of, extraction of the tooth or the death of the individual concerned.

Other evidence that may indicate pathological or traumatic experiences has been referred to in earlier chapters and its possible forensic significance indicated. While

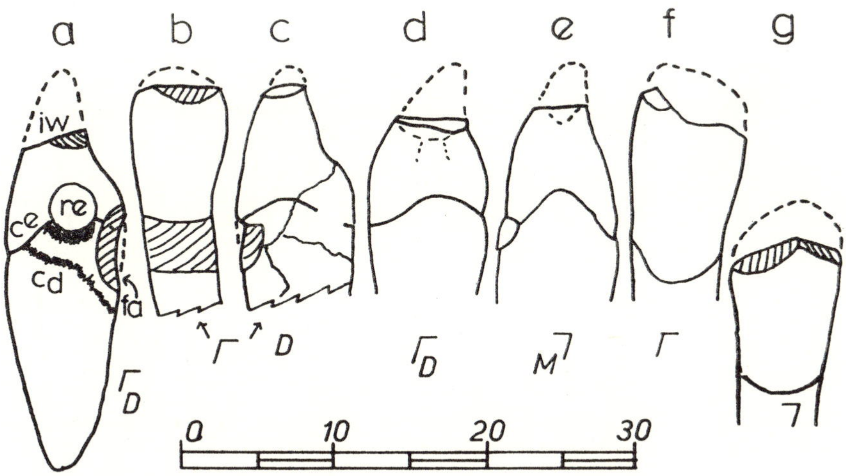

Figure 5-13. Wear in lower canines—a variety of effects (in various regions of the teeth) which are the results of a variety of causes.

the range of such "clues" seems to be greater in a modern civilized community, much information can also be obtained from archaeological material. A fragment from the chin region of an ancient Tongan provided such a case (Taylor, 1971c).

Figure 5-13 shows a variety of effects of wear in various regions of the teeth and these effects have arisen from a variety of causes as follows:

Tooth *a:* iw, incisal wear of third degree resulting from normal function; ce, cervical line; cd, calculus deposit marking recessional line of periodontal attachment; re, old amalgam restoration with recurrent decay; fa, facet of abrasion from bar of unstable partial denture.

Tooth *b,c:* Two views of a tooth with a very high polish of labial surface extending beyond cervix to root where the soft tissue attachment has receded as a result of trauma from toothbrushing; outline *c* shows how the less resistant root has been abraded to a notch at cervix. A calculus deposit and deep stain adhere to proximal and lingual surfaces.

Teeth *d* and *e:* Severe incisal wear and cupping of dentine beyond the level of enamel wear.

Teeth *f* and *g:* Normal incisal wear has been modified by restricted mandibular movements during occlusion and/or by holding a foreign substance such as a pipe stem. Fine scratches on *f* suggest only labio-lingual movement against the abrading surface. In *g* the facets are polished and have smoothly rounded edges. There is no cupping.

In Figure 5-14 there are further examples of teeth that have been modified by wear or otherwise. In some the results are unusual, and it is useful to show how the causes or unusual conditions may be deduced from clues presented. These are as follows:

Tooth *a:* Unusual wear with several indefinite facets almost confined to mesial aspect of labial surface, one of these facets exposing dentine almost as far as the cervix. The surface involved is highly polished. There is an irregular area of root abrasion below the labial cervix, and a fragment of very thin alveolar bone extending on to the proximal surface. This is a region where, normally, alveolar bone is much thicker

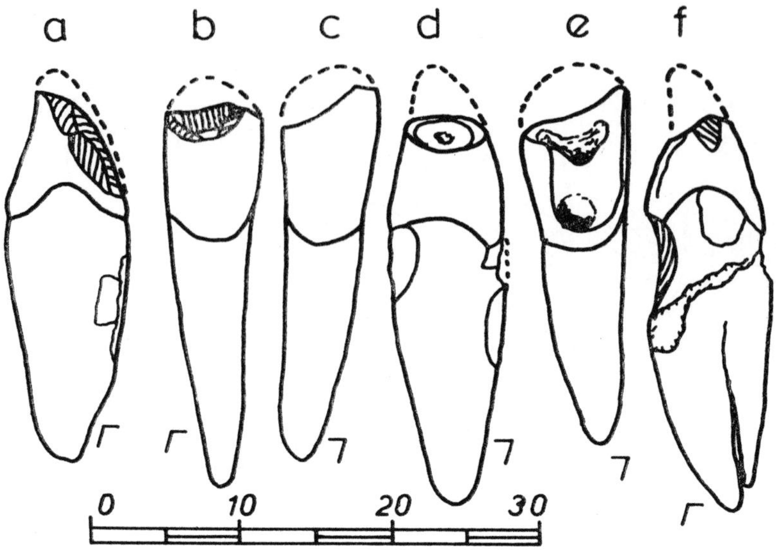

Figure 5-14. Lower canines that present clues to the manner of their modification by wear or otherwise. See page 185 with special reference to tooth *f*.

and forms part of the inter-dental septum and tooth socket. The presence of such thin bone (as would be found normally below the labial cervix) in this unusual position indicates a local irregularity in position, a torsiversion or twisting of the tooth on its long axis. The mesio-labial portion of the crown was therefore forming the prominent angle of the dental arch and received the brunt of friction from occlusion and from toothbrushing. In these circumstances the disto-labial aspect of the crown would be sheltered from friction, and that this was the case is shown by stain which has remained in this sheltered position. The roughly abraded area of root alongside the thin piece of bone already mentioned has resulted from "slipping" of the dental forceps during extraction of the tooth.

Tooth *b:* Incisal wear on this tooth has extended much further on labial than on lingual surface, and this condition as well as cupping of dentine is not uncommon. But in this case the "facet" extends in the form of a deep V on to labial surface. The lingual enamel wall of the facet does not have the usual "straight" surface of enamel bordering a facet of wear, but is irregular. One might well expect such an upstanding enamel edge to be easily damaged by chipping, and the irregularity considered as normal in these circumstances. In this case however the irregularity is not jagged but has been worn smooth by use, instead of suffering chipping by use. It may be suggested therefore that the cusp was fractured obliquely some considerable time before the tooth was extracted.

Tooth *c:* The major curved facet in this tooth shows no cupping and is very smooth with rather sharp enamel edges. Under low magnification there are fine scratches, almost without exception passing from labial to lingual. It could reasonably be assumed that the first premolar and corresponding upper teeth would also have shown similar curved facets of wear, and that collectively they would bear testimony to the habitual holding of a pipe stem in that position.

Tooth *d:* This is a sturdy tooth with third degree incisal wear suggesting that it was part of a "strong" dentition with edge-to-edge bite and labial stain almost to the edge of the facet. There is no evidence that toothbrushing was practised. Below the lingual cervix there is loss of tissue (not unlike the facet seen in Fig. 5-13 *a*), but in this case it is rough and irregular as if a small flake has been split off from the root surface. This probably did occur during extraction, since there is typical forceps damage below the labial cervix also. Further support for this explanation comes from the writer's conviction through experience that this would have been a difficult tooth to extract.

Tooth *e:* At first sight this appears to be a much worn tooth that presents carious cavities near the labial cervix and in the pulp chamber. Enamel edges and exposed dentine show definite signs of wear. But the form or contours suggest that the wear was secondary to exposure of dentine, which could have resulted from severe trauma and breaking off of much of the crown. Treatment had proceeded at least as far as the placing of a root filling, but if any restoration had been added, this had long since been lost leaving an open cavity which had become carious. Decay had also commenced on the external labial surface.

Tooth *f* of this figure will be described later (p. 185).

In Figure 5-15 lower canines present further clues as to what may have happened during the periods of development of the tooth, or of its functional life, and at the time of its extraction. Thus in tooth *a* the whole of the cusp region is grossly defective but the rest of the tooth is normal. The defect has nothing to do with wear (of which there is the slightest trace where shown). It could be described as a dentine cusp devoid of enamel on labial and lingual, but with some abnormally thin enamel towards the shoulders of the cusp. The enamel edge is irregular but smoothly rounded, and there was then formed a band of apparently normal enamel. This band, nearly 2 mm wide and of full thickness, appears to have been followed again by normal enamel which may be slightly thinner or of different density, for there is a visible difference where the two portions meet. The defect in this tooth is severe hypoplasia of enamel, probably of exanthematous origin and occurring during the first year of life.

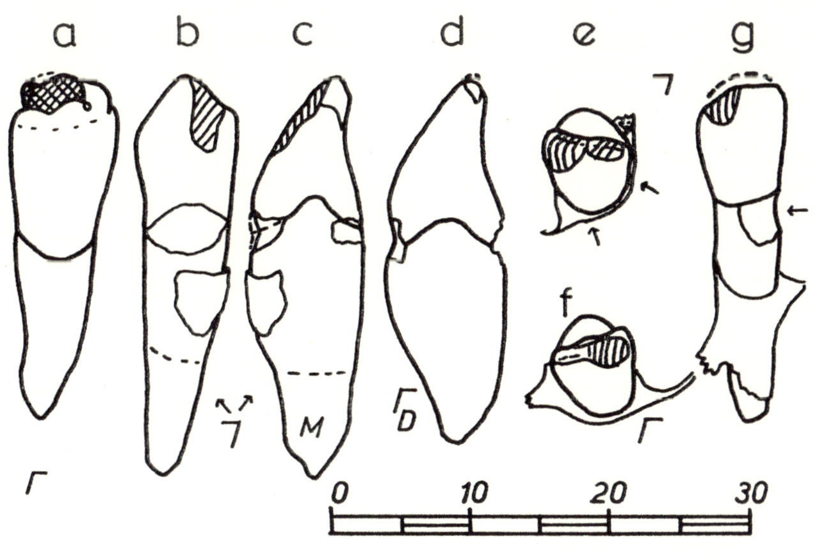

Figure 5-15. Lower canines showing further examples of pathology, or of damage during extraction.

The tooth shown in two outlines in Figure 5-15 *b,c* has several features of interest. The labial surface has become highly polished from toothbrushing and the cusp tip has no wear, but there is a facet on the mesio-labial, extending from cusp tip approximately half-way to cervix, so that there certainly was a deep overbite. There is a deep notch at labial cervix involving cervical enamel. This notch is unusual in appearance, for although carious it does not appear to be the result entirely of dental decay, and its margins are partly covered by calculus. It is suggested that initially a notch was formed by faulty and vigorous toothbrushing (as in Fig. 5-13 *b, c*), and that this became so sensitive that the cervical area was then avoided during toothbrushing. As a result of this "neglect" and in the presence of suitable conditions the abraded and now sheltered area became carious and in due course calculus was deposited here as well as on adjacent teeth. This area and another at lingual cervix have been treated with silver nitrate.

There are two other features of this tooth which are of interest. There is a small fragment of thin alveolar bone representing the outer wall of the tooth socket which has come away with the tooth when extracted, but this is of no special significance here. The more noteworthy feature is the sudden narrowing of the lower part of the root, best seen in *c*. This might well indicate that the tooth received a blow soon after eruption in late childhood or early adolescence (Schour and Massler, 1944). The blow did not cause a fracture but evidently was sufficient to affect subsequent completion of the root, and this may represent a mild case of dilaceration. This diagnosis is tentative, because no section was made to allow the part to be examined microscopically.

The tooth in Figure 5-15 *d* shows severe damage during extraction. The factors that could be involved are: poorly fitting forceps blades, sharp blades, and movement of the blades during the operation. Movement of the blades implies an insufficiently firm hold on the instrument, possibly combined with a tooth firmly attached in its socket. These factors are not mutually exclusive and could operate in varying degree. The basic cause of the damage obviously was movement of the forceps blades. One may well question the skill of the operator and suspect that he was as relieved as the patient when the tooth was eventually removed without fracture.

The occlusal views *e* and *f* show lower canines with attached portions of alveolar bone which fractured during extraction. They serve here to extend the information obtainable from the teeth and yet to show how the information may differ between them. In tooth *e* a labial cervical notch has been worn and polished with toothbrushing, but, as indicated by arrows, the notch is well rounded to the mesial aspect of the tooth, suggesting that the tooth was rotated in its socket. That this was in fact the position is confirmed by the attached bone, which shows the relation of the tooth to labial plate and inter-dental septa of alveolar bone. The labial view of the tooth is shown in g.

The left canine *f* is shown by the adhering alveolar bone to have been in normal position in relation to adjacent teeth. Comparison of these teeth indicates that tooth *e* was rotated approximately 45° from its normal position.

LOWER CANINES WITH BIFID ROOTS

The character of bifidity in these teeth is not uncommon, but attempts to measure its incidence or to analyze its nature soon prove frustrating. The following figures show numerous examples that are obviously bifid, but also others (like some in Figure 5-19) which make one despair of defining a bifid-rooted lower canine. On the other hand there are teeth like that shown in Figure 5-9 *d* which do not present any visible bifidity. This tooth has a groove on both proximal surfaces of the root, extending from apex almost to cervix in each, and there must surely be two canals for most of the root length. It could be

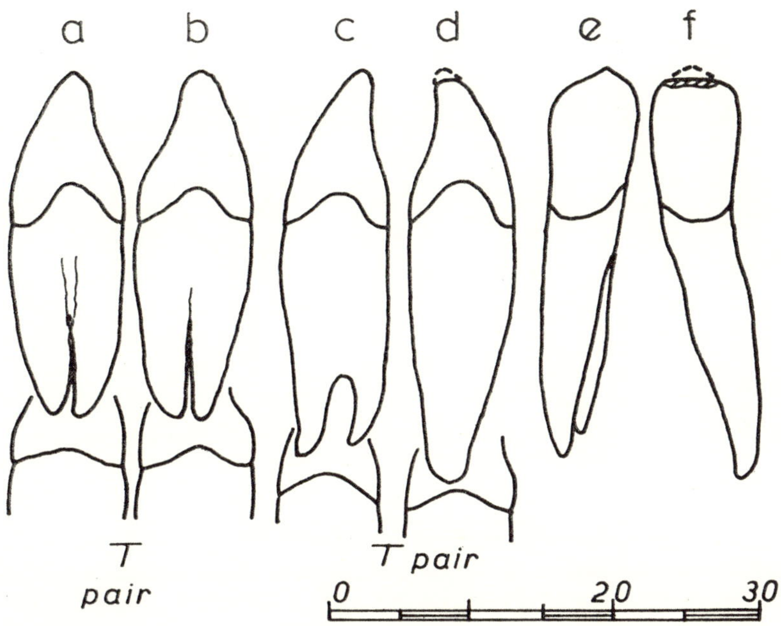

Figure 5-16. Bifidity in lower canines. *a,b,* a pair showing a high degree of symmetry as regards mirror images of left and right. *c-f,* another pair seen from mesial and from labial, and in these lower canines there is obvious asymmetry. The full outlines, *a-d,* are mesial views and below each of these is drawn the cervical outline as seen from distal. The cervical arch is higher and steeper on mesial than on distal.

reasonably claimed that such a tooth is more truly bifid than a tooth with a miniature root tag. There has to be some kind of limitation established as a criterion somewhere; and in this study visible bifidity, however small the cleft or second branch, was the only qualification for a root to be called bifid. The two branches are placed labially and lingually as with upper premolars, but differences in size as regards thickness, or in actual or relative lengths of the two branches (which was uncommon in premolars), are characterized in lower canines by great variety.

One can readily accept the notion of a major and minor root or branch, but whether the distinction should be based on a visible impression of relative bulk or of length may be largely a subjective decision. Thus in Figures 5-17 *f* and 5-22 *e* the lingual root is longer but more slender than the labial root. Again, are such separate or adherent "tags" as in Figures 5-18 *c* and 5-19 *d,e* to be accepted as constituting a bifid root? It is not practicable always to section such a tooth and seek a pulp cavity in these cases. It was not done in this study, but under low power magnification one could not deny that a fine apical foramen could be present. These cases therefore were classed as bifid-rooted teeth.

The tooth shown in Figure 5-18 *c* shows well the difficulty of defining a bifid-rooted tooth, and the caution necessary in making generalized statements about them. For example, while it appears that the two root branches are always placed labially and lingually, in this case the minor root tag tends to arise from the disto-lingual aspect of the major branch. This tendency is made more obvious by the curve of the main root to M while the tag curves to disto-lingual. Again, the main root branch has grooves both M and D, but the apical region is missing, evidently broken during extraction. The fracture surface shows

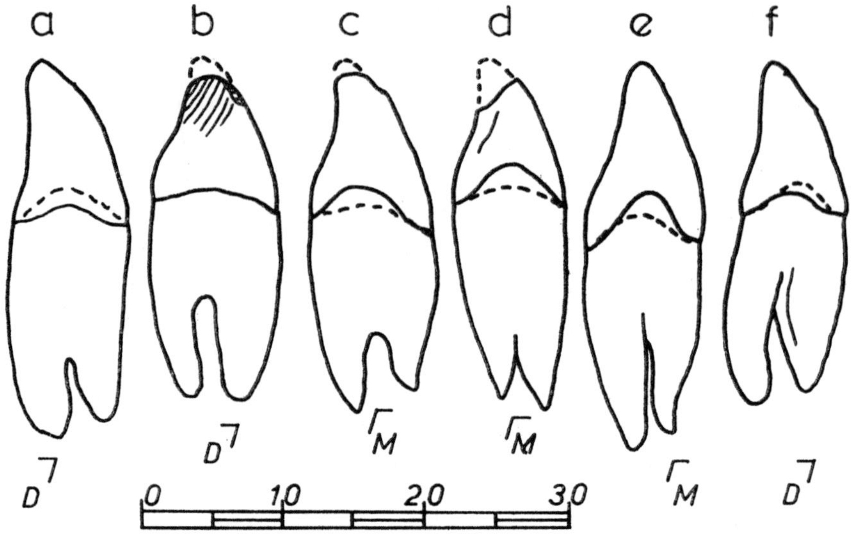

Figure 5-17. Bifidity in lower canine. Variety in root branches, short or long, straight or curved, cleft parallel or V-shape, apices sharp or blunt, etc. In tooth *c* the mesial cervical region is mutilated by caries.

two pulp canals, so that with the canal of the minor root tag this tooth presents three canals. Thus the root has been classified as bifid because of the root tag, but apart from this the pulp cavity presents bifidity in the major branch. There must be a number of lower canines that present such bifidity of pulp cavity in roots that have been classed as single because they are not visibly branched, although grooving is apparent.

From the collection of extracted teeth forming the present study, bifid-rooted canines were separated from single-rooted, and from such bifid-rooted teeth 131 were selected for mounting on twenty-six cards to form Series "O." In the following sixteen figures there are 102 outlines relating to those mounted teeth, and thirteen diagrams. For the reported study of single-rooted lower canines the fifteen figures contain 105 outlines relating to 154 teeth on thirty-seven cards comprising Series "N."

The study of bifid teeth did not disclose any character in which they did not vary in the same ways as single-rooted teeth. Those characters included size of teeth overall, and in proportions of root and crown, features of asymmetry that distinguish left and right teeth, convexity of contours of crown generally or of cusp in particular, proportions of length and breadth of crown and its relation to the root. For the root itself there are the usual observations relating to size, length and sturdiness, curvature and taper of profiles, curvature in root axis, slenderness, sharpness or bluntness of apices and so on. However, the reporting of these is condensed, and attention is focussed mainly on the characters of bifidity and the relation of their variation to differences between bifid and single roots.

Relative Size of Root Branches

In upper premolars there was a strong tendency for the branches in bifid roots to be similar in thickness and length, and for the apices also to be similar in fineness, bluntness or sharpness. In bifid canine roots this latter similarity was apparent when the size of the two branches, either short or long, was similar. In other cases, however, where the terms major and minor could be applied to the root branches, this was not so; the difference in apices inevitably became greater as the differences in size of branches increased. The extreme of difference was reached in such teeth as those referred to already as having the minor root in the form of a small tag (Figs. 5-19 and 5-18 *c*).

In some cases the designation of root branches as equal or as major and minor is difficult, because the difference is so little. Another problem has been referred to, namely whether sturdiness (thickness) or length should decide the matter, and it is also questionable whether the presence of a small tag should (as it did in this study) qualify a root to be called bifid. It is inevitable that the classification of some teeth must be subjective. Such qualifications and difficulties should therefore be kept in mind regarding percentages given here.

In the present study relative length was the deciding factor when grading major and minor root branches, but neither the width nor the length of the cleft between the branches was considered in grading. On this basis, of 179 lower canines with bifid roots 117 (65.3 percent) had roots of equal size. Teeth with the major root on labial side totalled forty-nine (27.4 percent), while the major root on lingual side occurred in thirteen teeth (7.2 percent). On that count there was no attempt to separate left from right teeth, and as explained elsewhere it is not known which teeth in the collection are from males and which from females, except in a few cases. Bearing in mind the many characters of variation in bifidity that have been ignored in this count, it may be said that in two out of three cases the root branches were equal, and that of those with unequal root branches just over three out of four had the major root branch on the labial side.

It was not possible to measure the degree of similarity between left and right lower canines as regards the incidence or form of bifidity in roots, although there is reason to believe it is high. Figure 5-16 *a,b* shows a pair of such teeth presenting only minor differences. It is known however that in some cases there is considerable difference, and such a pair is shown from mesial in Fig. 5-16 *c,d* and from labial in *e,f* of the same figure. This asymmetrical pair were among ten anterior teeth extracted from an adult female. The upper canines also differed appreciably in their roots.

In Figure 5-17 are shown six bifid roots in which bifidity differs in a number of ways such as length of branches, length of cleft, width of cleft, shape or sharpness of apices, straightness or curvature at apex. Thus in *a,b* there are blunt apices; branches are unequal in length in *a*, equal in *b; a* has a medium length rather narrow cleft and *b* has a very long wide parallel-sided cleft. In the next two teeth with much finer and sharper apices, in *c* the branches are unequal in length and the cleft rather long and wide, but in *d* the cleft is short and wide, and branches are straight in both teeth. In *d* the root narrows towards the apex in contrast to the root of *a* (and the considerable differences in crown shape and proportion to root may also be noted in *a,d*). Comparing *e,f*, each has a longer branch on lingual; in *e* it is the major root in all respects, but in *f* the shorter root is wider. In *e* both roots curve to labial, and each apex is fine and sharp, but in *f* the lingual root is curved and has a blunt apex while the labial branch is straight and has a sharp apex.

For Figure 5-18 six teeth have been selected to show variation in lingual and labial profiles of bifid roots. In *a,b,* in spite of a broken off branch in each, it is seen that *a* has a straight lingual and curved labial contour, but in *b* the labial is straight and the lingual is curved. Tooth *c* is bifid because of a very short and fine tag curving to distal from lingual near the incomplete apex, while the main root, which narrows sharply in the apical half, bends to mesial in this part. In *d* the root

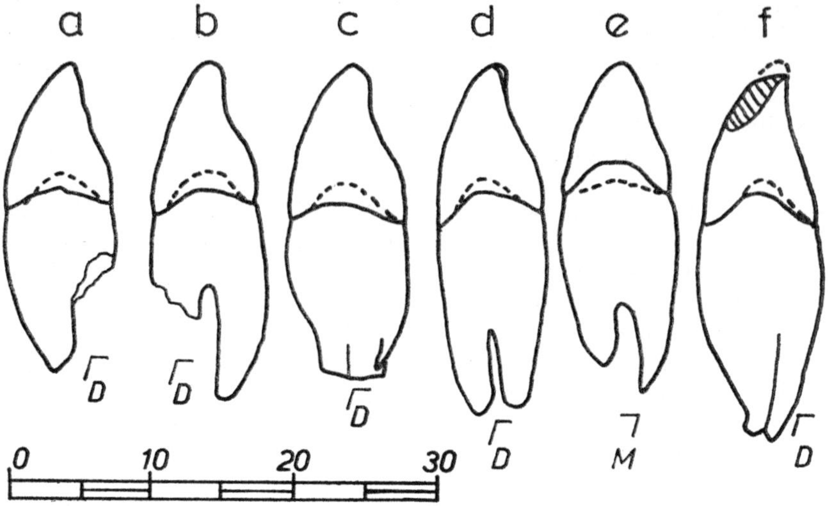

Figure 5-18. Bifidity of root. Further variation in characters of cleft and branches, and in profiles of whole root. In the first three teeth there have been root fractures, lingual branch of *a*, labial branch of *b* and apex of the main branch of *c*. It is noteworthy that this main branch is grooved on both sides and presents two pulp canals.

profiles are both rather straight and nearly parallel while in *e* both are arc-like. In *d* the cleft is long and narrow and each apex thick and rounded, but *e* has a wide U-shaped cleft with sharp apices of unequal length. In tooth *f* again both profiles are arc-like, but instead of a U-shaped cleft the root branches are in contact ex-

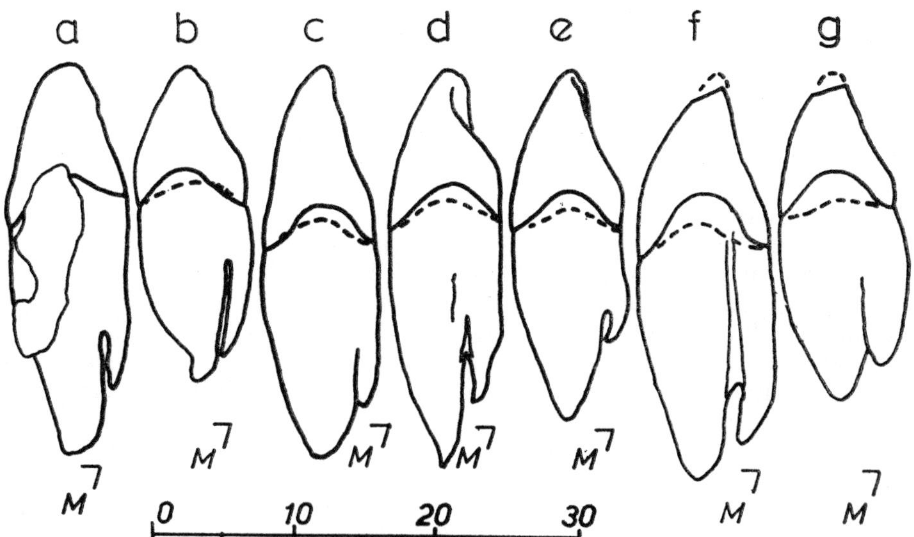

Figure 5-19. Variation in bifidity of canine roots, continued, introducing the further character of inequality in size or bulk of root branches. In this figure the major branch is on labial side, as was the case in over 27 percent of bifid roots. The area outlined on tooth *a* represents an adhering mass of calculus. Concerning tooth *d*, see also Fig. 5-31 *n*.

cept at the extreme tip where there are two fine curved apices.

Inequalities in size of root branches have been referred to above. It was shown that efforts at quantitative analysis of bifidity are confounded by the number of varying characters, not the least of which involve the definition of bifidity itself and of classes for enumeration. In Figure 5-19 were illustrated some extreme examples, and in the three subsequent figures more common characters of variation, rather than the extremes, are presented from proximal view. The description of further complications arising from other views is deferred.

Thus in Figure 5-20 are shown teeth *a-e* with short or long clefts, narrow or wide clefts, and grooves that are short and wide *(c,e)* or long and narrow as in *a* where the minor root is separated from the major root for barely half of its well-defined length. These teeth (except *f*) were all among the approximately 7 percent of bifid-rooted lower canines in which the major branch was on the lingual side. In *d,e* the root branches are approximately equal in length, but in *a,b,c* the major root is appreciably longer. In all of these except *c* the major root is also visibly thicker or wider than the minor.

Amongst the bifid roots with the major branch on lingual is a tooth which illustrates the data of a forensic nature that could sometimes assist towards identification of a person. This tooth (Fig. 5-14 *f*) has been shown with others presenting varieties of wear or evidence of pathology or trauma. In this case, apart from interest related to bifidity, the following may be noted: The person concerned had worn a partial denture for a long time, during which it had become ill-fitting and had "settled" so that the lingual bar of the denture came to bear on soft tissue below the cervix. This, in association with inevitable chronic periodontitis and deposition of calculus, had resulted in movement of the denture and abrasion of tooth crown and root. There is root caries on mesial, just below the cervix, and this appears to have become only slowly progressive if not actually arrested, and it probably was not painful.

Above the carious area is a small proximal facet that was probably reduced in

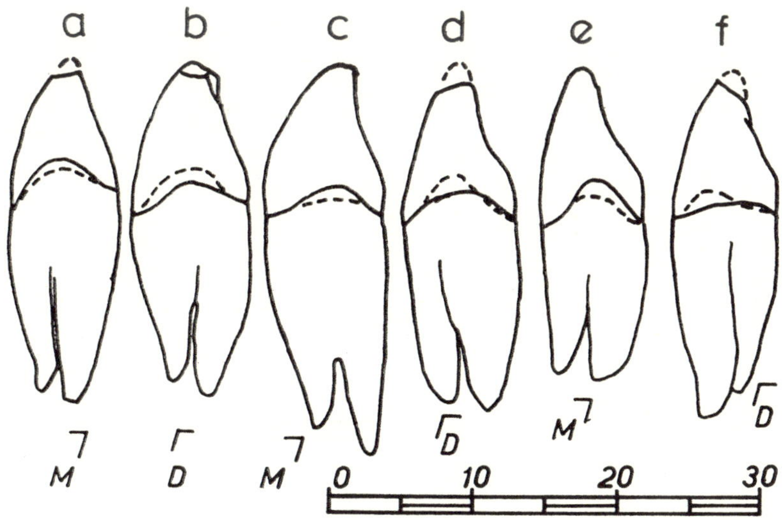

Figure 5-20. *a-e*, bifid canine roots with the major branch on lingual as in over 7 percent of bifid roots examined. Note also variations in cleft, groove and apices. *f*, a bifid root in which the groove is long, the cleft very narrow, the branches unequal in length, and labial branch is twisted to D.

area by occlusal wear and this is now dull and partly covered with stain, so that conditions must have changed after the period in which it was receiving friction from the lateral incisor. Similarly the stage III occlusal wear testifies to an edge-to-edge bite, and also to a change in conditions. The main facet is now modified by supplementary minor facets and loss of sharpness on enamel edges. This would be consistent with replacement of upper teeth by an artificial denture and consequent different occlusion and masticatory pattern.

On labial cervix a small piece of root has split off. This, together with the general appearance of the root (which has at some time been subjected to "cleaning" by scraping with a not very sharp blade), suggests that the tooth was not loose at time of extraction. Even without making a section to assist in age determination, one may reasonably assume that this tooth was extracted from a somewhat elderly person who had long worn an ill-fitting partial denture, and probably an upper denture as well. There is no evidence that a toothbrush had been used, and perhaps the person was a casual patient who seldom consulted a dentist.

Root Grooves

While Figure 5-20 *a-e* was mainly concerned with examples of inequality in size of root branches, with special reference to the less common cases of major branch on lingual, attention was drawn also to variation in cleft shape and length, and to grooves related to clefts. In Figures 5-20 *f* and 5-21 attention is given more particularly to grooves. Examples are chosen from roots with branches that are not very different in size as regards length and thickness. There is some variety in length and width of clefts, but these do not seem to bear any particular relation to the width, depth or length of groove. It could be expected that where the cleft is long, the length of cleft plus groove will involve a greater proportion of total root length, and in a general way this is so. But it will be realized that grooves are not readily defined, classified or measured, and therefore this

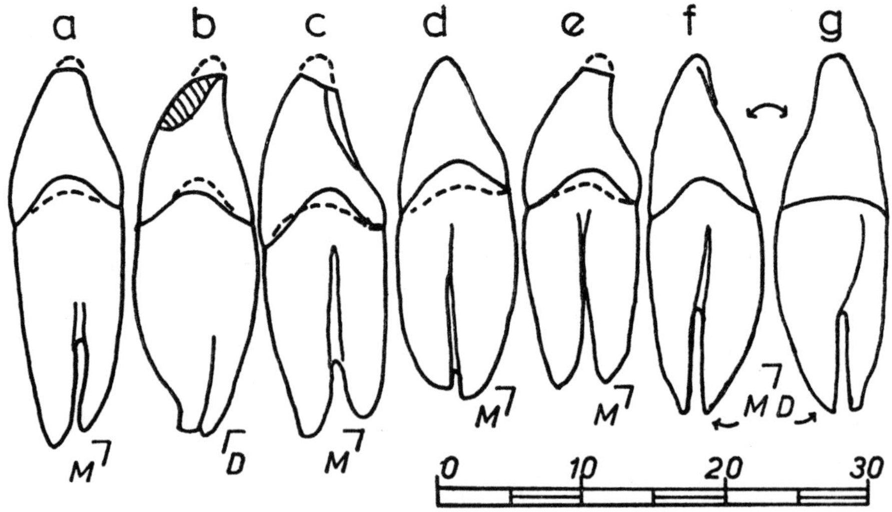

Figure 5-21. Root branches of equal or unequal length, variations in amount of separation and in depth or other characters of groove beyond cleft. *a,b,* shallow grooves, wide cleft in *a*, but in *b* both branches are in contact except for deep grooves on M and D. *d*, very short cleft but long grooves, that on mesial being much deeper. *e*, long, open cleft and long grooves of similar depth on M and D. *f,g,* two views of one tooth in which the cleft and groove are oblique and give a fold effect. As a result the difference between major and minor branch is affected. See also Figure 5-20 *f*.

was not attempted. Description is confined to rather obvious characters that may be described in terms that are simple rather than precise.

In Figure 5-21 *a* and *c* the teeth are approximately equal in length, as are their clefts. Tooth *c* is a much bigger tooth; its cleft is rather wide and the groove is long and shallow, although distinctly deeper on mesial. In *a* the groove is shallow and wide, and even on mesial it is difficult to follow. In *b* where the branches are in contact there is a deep narrow groove instead of a cleft, and beyond this there is a very wide shallow groove on both sides. Tooth *d* has scarcely a cleft at all but it has a long deep groove on each side, much wider on mesial. Tooth *e* has a long cleft and a long deep groove reaching nearly to cervix on both M and D. Two views, M and D, of one tooth are in *f* and *g* respectively. On M there is a very long deep groove with rounded sides making the lingual root the major one. On D the lingual root is much flattened and the long groove passes somewhat obliquely, increasing the apparent difference in width of the two branches. This oblique direction of cleft and groove is very noticeable when the tooth is viewed from the apical end along its long axis. A similar oblique effect in such a view is also found where there is a difference in curvature of the long axes of the two branches. This condition is seen in Figure 5-23 *d,f*. Again, in Figure 5-20 *f* the labial root is twisted to D and the lingual root is more nearly straight. On both M and D surfaces there is a very long, deep, narrow groove.

In Figure 5-22 the study of grooves is continued. Teeth *a,b*, although very similar in overall size, are very different as re-

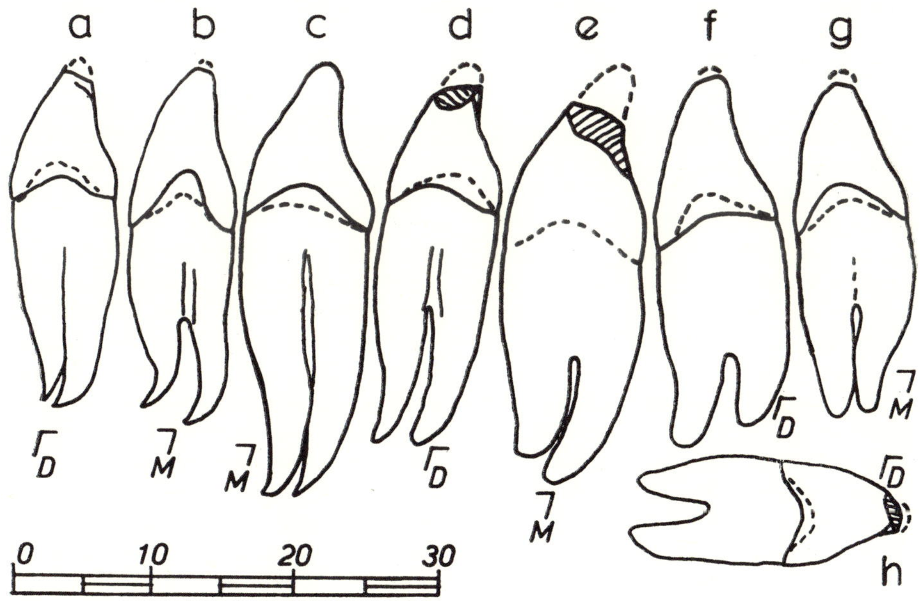

Figure 5-22. Root bifidity in lower canines, showing variation in length and width of cleft relative to tooth size. Variation also in sharpness or separation of apices is similarly unrelated to tooth size. Curvature in one or both root branches is associated with much variation in tooth profiles. ***a,b,*** curvature in apices only, fine sharp apices, with narrow or wide clefts, and both curved to labial. ***c,d,*** curvature involving more of the root with short cleft and long groove, and with long cleft. ***e,*** a sturdy tooth with straight labial major root, but a longer minor lingual root curved throughout its length. ***f,*** bend in labial root diverges sharply from straighter lingual branch. ***g,*** wide bifurcation, then convergence of branches to near contact, then diverging apices. ***h,*** widely spaced branches for such a small tooth, giving almost parallel labial and lingual profiles. See also Figure 5-23.

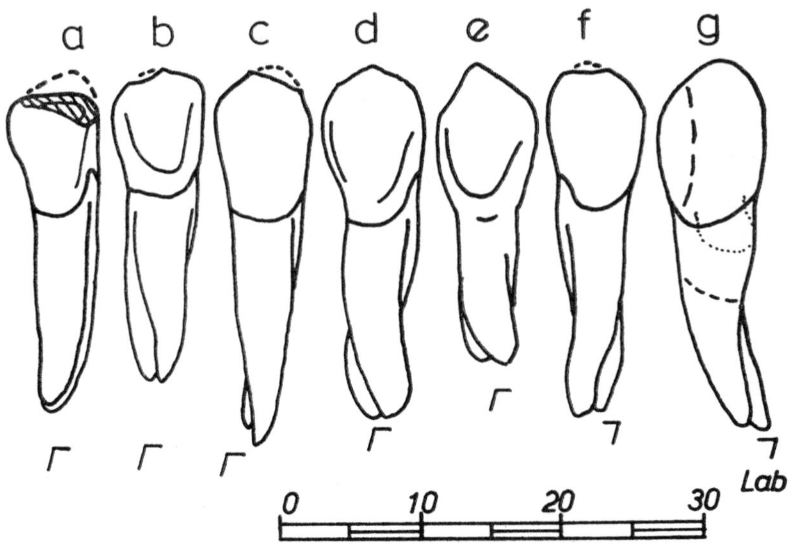

Figure 5-23. Bifid lower canines. Curvature in root trunk and branches, seen from lingual (except g). *a,* curve starts near apex and is similar in each branch. *b-f,* root branches may curve independently of one another, thus one straight and one curved *(c,e)* one curved to M and one to D *(b,d,f).* In *f* the lingual branch after curving to D from furcation has an apical bend to M. Tooth *g* is shown from B as it has major root on lingual as in Figure 5-20 *c.* Long broken lines show stained distolabial area of crown. Dotted area at cervix is highly polished, and short broken lines show limit of attachment of periodontal tissue.

gards clefts, but both have long shallow grooves. Comparing *a* and *c,* although *c* is a much larger tooth, their clefts and apices are very similar in form but the grooves are quite different, being long, deep and narrow in *c.* Teeth *d,e* both have long narrow clefts but *d* has a wide shallow groove and *e* has a long wide deep groove, and these differences apply to M and D surfaces. In *f,g* both have long clefts, but the form of clefts, apices and contours is quite different; yet in each tooth the groove is short, deep and wide. In the small tooth *h* where the cleft is relatively long and wide, the groove is shallow, long and wide. These examples amply demonstrate that the depth, width and relative length of the groove are independent of characters of width and length of the cleft. Further variations in clefts and grooves are indicated in Figure 5-24.

Curvature

The character of curvature of root branches in canines with bifid roots has so far received only brief mention. Figures 5-22 and 5-23 illustrate this character. As with other teeth, deviations from the hypothetical straight long axis of a tooth or root are not confined to any one or more planes through that axis. In bifid roots the two branches may or may not both diverge similarly from that axis. One branch may be affected in more than one direction. Before branching, the pre-branch position of the root trunk may present curvature of its axis as Figure 5-23 *b,f.* A view from labial, lingual or proximal therefore may record the presence of some variety of curvature but cannot show whether, or in what manner, there is curvature involving some other direction as well. Since (as with other roots) the wider part is usually nearer the labial surface, a better idea of curvature as it affects the root branches is seen from lingual, and outlines in Figure 5-23 are drawn in this way in most cases. In tooth g however, as the major root branch is on lingual, the tooth has been depicted from labial.

Outlines in Figure 5-22 have already been discussed in regard to clefts and grooves, but these teeth were selected to show variety also in bends and curves as viewed from proximal. Teeth *a,b* show curvature confined to fine apices, although one tooth has a long cleft. Both apices in each case curve to labial. In *c,d* the curve involves the whole of each branch and part of the root trunk. Again there is a short cleft and a long cleft, and all branches curve to labial. In teeth *e,f,* one branch is almost straight and the other curves to labial. In one it is a long sweeping curve involving all of a long lingual branch; in the other it is more like a sudden bend involving half of a much shorter branch, labial in this case.

In tooth *g* the labial branch is straight, and at the furcation it is well separated from the lingual branch, but this branch then curves almost to make contact and then turns away from the labial branch. In other words an earlier convergence gives place to divergence. In the small tooth *h* the widely separated branches are almost parallel and have a slight but uneven tapering which veers to labial.

Although there is variety in length and width of cleft, the axes of branches of these bifid roots tend mostly to remain parallel rather than diverge.

Figure 5-23 gives a quite different impression of curvature by viewing teeth from lingual (tooth *g* from labial). Tooth *a* has a straight root and the two short branches each bend slightly to distal (and in proximal view slightly to labial also). In *b* both root elements have a double bend, but in *c* the less marked double bend is found only in lingual root while the labial is straight. Tooth *d,* a much more robust tooth than *b,* has also a double bend in labial root while the lingual is straight, except for a slight apical bend to mesial. It was shown above that in these teeth with double bends the first bend commences in the root trunk well before branching of the two elements. The short tooth *e* has a straight labial root and the lingual branch bends to mesial. In tooth *f* the two elements and branches curve independently so that in apical view they appear to be slightly twisted against one another.

In tooth *g* the curvature is different from all the others. It has been mentioned that the outline gives a view from labial, since the major root is lingual. It is a large tooth and the crown shows strongly the ovoid form referred to in Chapter 1. After a short distance of straight root trunk it commences a long sweeping curve to mesial, and this curve is maintained in each root branch.

The distal part of the labial surface is covered with stain but the rest of the labial surface is highly polished, as is part of the root on mesio-labial angle. There is a facet of wear on the mesial ridge of the cusp. These conditions would indicate a state of malocclusion when *in situ,* such that the tooth was twisted or crowded forward in the dental arch. The lingual surface is even more darkly stained than the area already mentioned and both would be protected from masticatory friction, while the position of polished areas shows that toothbrushing was associated with considerable recession of soft-tissue attachment. These indications of friction, and protection from friction, lend support to the belief that there was malocclusion as described. In that case it is highly probable that the root curvature noted was the result of the erupting tooth being forced into the abnormal position described.

Tooth Length

Although variations in root branches, clefts and grooves have received special attention, bifid-rooted lower canines, like those with single roots, present a considerable range in overall size, in length and width, in proportions of crown and root, and in form of crown and of root. Many of these characters may be followed in the outlines already given in Figures 5-16 to

5-23, and further comments upon their variations are illustrated in the later figures.

In Figures 5-24 and 5-25 are shown teeth that vary widely as regards length overall, and particularly in length and width of roots. Figure 5-24 *a,b* shows rather large teeth, but *a* is slender and *b* is robust with a large crown. The root branches are of uneven length with the lingual longer in each, both branches curved to labial in *a* and both straight in *b*. The other teeth are all very short, but the crowns of *c,e* are large, *d* is medium, and only *f* is really a small tooth. In all four the root branches are short, but there is much variety in width of cleft and thickness of apices, which all tend to be straight. Grooves are very long in *a,b*, relatively long in the short teeth *d,e* and short in *c,f*.

In Figure 5-25 *a-e* the outstanding character is length—length of root or length of branches. Teeth *a,b* are relatively slim for length and have long parallel root branches, clefts and grooves. Teeth *c,d* are big robust teeth with parallel root branches (long branches in *c* and relatively short in *d*), and long grooves in each. These are both right teeth seen from mesial. Tooth *e* is a very big left tooth seen from distal. It has relatively short curved branches, a narrow cleft and a long shallow groove. The root trunk, particularly the labial element, makes a long sweeping curve to distal, the apical region reversing the curve but not quite lining up

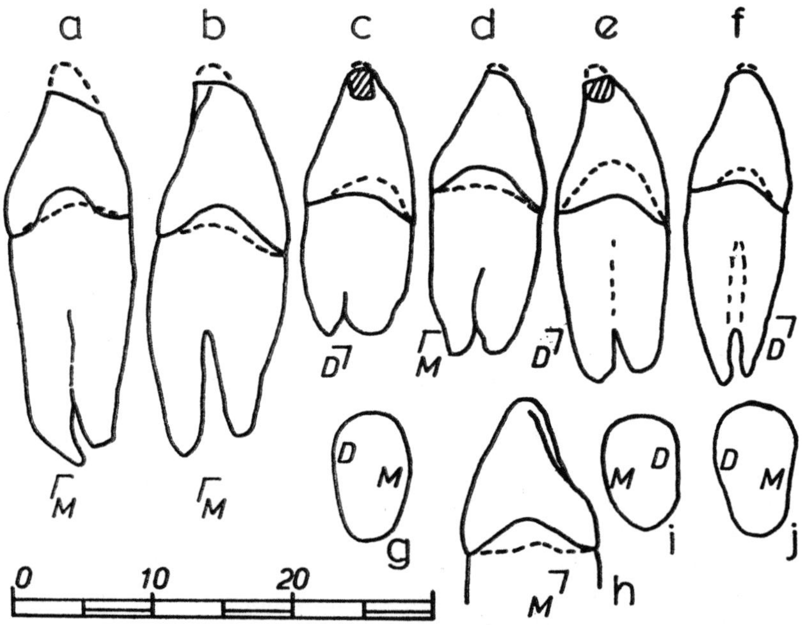

Figure 5-24. Root bifidity in lower canines. *a,b,* long root, long cleft and long groove. Branches of unequal length (shorter lingual in each case), both branches curved in one and both straight in the other. *c-f* short teeth, with variety in groove and cleft and apex. *c,* large crown longer than very short sturdy root, with major branch on labial. *d,* tooth similar in length to *c* but much smaller crown, long groove with short wide cleft and relatively sharp apices. *e,* long groove, short narrow cleft and thick blunt apices. *f,* slender tooth with shallow groove; short narrow parallel cleft with fine branches and sharp apices. *g-j,* the outlines *g,i,j* are of transverse sections of lower canine roots tangential to labial and lingual cervices. Outline *h* is from the same tooth as *g,* a tooth with a very minor lingual root branch. Tooth *i* is single-rooted (Fig. 5-9 *e*), and tooth *j* has a well-developed lingual root branch (Fig. 5-19 *f*).

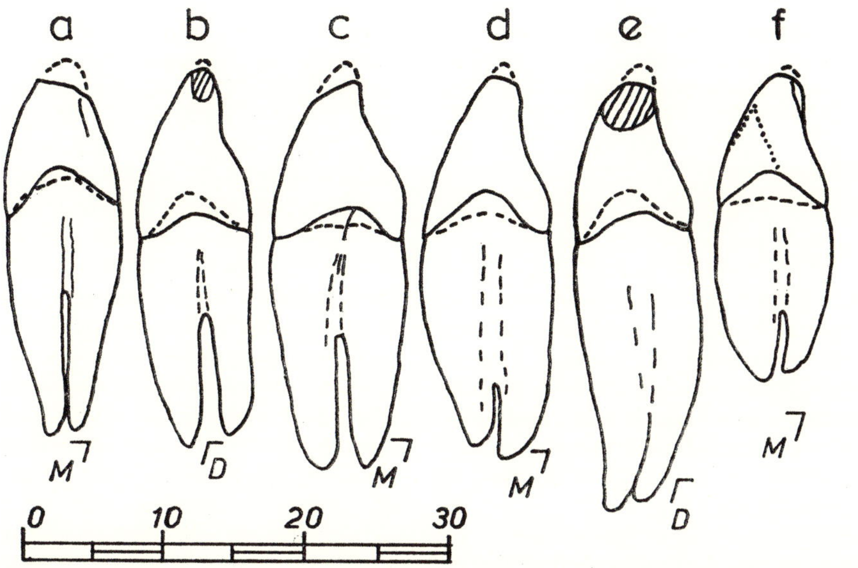

Figure 5-25. Bifidity in lower canine roots. Proportion of root trunk to branches. Variation in amount of separation of branches as distinct from divergence. (See also Fig. 5-20 *f*.) Teeth *b,e* show facets of oblique incisal wear. In tooth *f* the mesio-labial area of the crown in dotted outline was heavily stained showing that the tooth was twisted in malocclusion.

with the lingual element which is relatively straight as seen from lingual.

Tooth *f* of Figure 5-25 is a short sturdy tooth, with relatively long root branches of uneven thickness (major on labial). The cleft is almost parallel-sided, the groove long and shallow and the appearance in this mesial view is of a straight labial and a curved lingual branch. From labial or lingual however it is seen that the whole root, trunk and branches curve to distal. There is a stain line high on mesiolabial angle and a carious cavity on distolingual surface. Like the tooth in Figure 5-23 *g* described above, it is clear that this tooth was in malocclusion (torsiversion), and the curve in its root was probably associated with its eruption to this position.

In most teeth there is an indefinite harmony in size between crown and root, so that one could use the term "normal proportions" when describing these parts of a large or small tooth. Such judgment of course is subjective and comes with extensive experience of handling extracted teeth. There are also teeth where one considers that proportions of crown and root are not harmonious. Of these only a few would be considered to have a small crown in relation to root size, and the greater number are teeth where the root is relatively small in length rather than thickness. In the outlines of teeth presented throughout this work, and not only in this chapter, there are many that have a relatively large crown, or, in other words, a relatively short root.

One is aware that a young tooth with an incomplete root might be described in this way, and that there are pathological processes that increase root thickness by deposition of additional cementum, or reduce root length by absorption. These should be readily recognized by an experienced observer and such cases have been rejected in the present study. A few lower canines with short but bifid roots are shown in Figures 5-24 and 5-26, some from labial and some from proximal. These serve also to show differences in curvature and contour in crowns and roots. Tooth *c* of Figure 5-26 has already been shown in Figure 5-21 *c*.

Cervical Lines

In Chapter 1 the curvature of cervical lines as seen in proximal view was analyzed (p. 6), and these lines were again studied for upper canines (pp. 33, 38). For canines the tracings of both proximal cervical contours were presented separately. One of these was reversed as though seen through a transparent tooth and this facilitated comparison of mesial and distal contours detail by detail, from labial to lingual, in any particular tooth (Fig. 1-29).

Proximal contours have been studied for lower canines also, but presented differently. When a tooth outline is traced from mesial or distal the contour from the opposite proximal view has been added in a broken line labelled M or D. But these broken lines do not represent a "seen-through" contour as in Chapter 1. These broken-line contours have been added by turning the tooth over after tracing the outline of the whole tooth and matching the ends of the new contour to those of the first. In theory the end points are common to each contour, but in this case the labial end of one is matched with the lingual end of the other and vice versa. A number of findings and implications were disclosed by this different method of study of cervical lines, and some will be considered later. For the present some of the more obvious will be reported under three headings—variations in form of M or D contours between teeth, variations between M and D contours in single teeth and an apparently invariable relationship.

Firstly, there is the wide range of variety of form. The middle part of the curve, like a wave or hill, may involve a relatively small, or a much larger, segment of the proximal cervical view (Fig. 5-8 *f,g*). It may be peak-like or more flattened (Figs. 5-9 *a-d*, 5-22 *a,b,c* and 5-24 *a,c,d*). Either of these forms may be high (Figs. 5-22 *b*, 5-24 *e*), or low (Figs. 5-10 *a*, 5-9 *d*). These comparisons are made between corresponding contours, M or D in different teeth, not

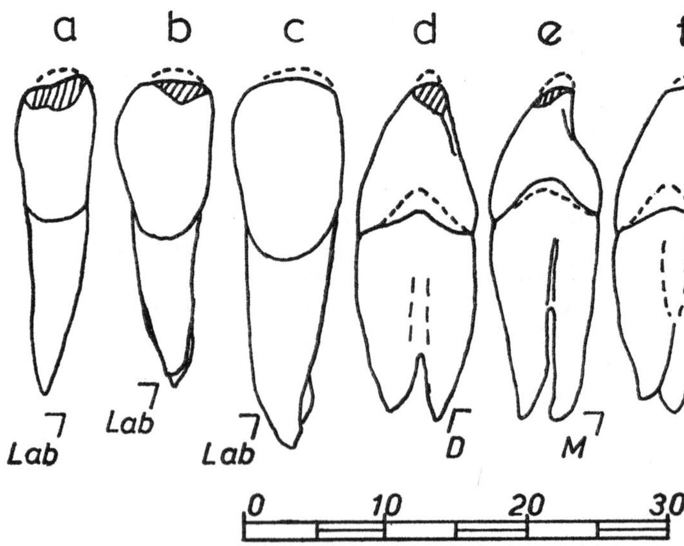

Figure 5-26. Bifidity in lower canine roots. Variation in proportions of crown and root in labial or in proximal views of six teeth.

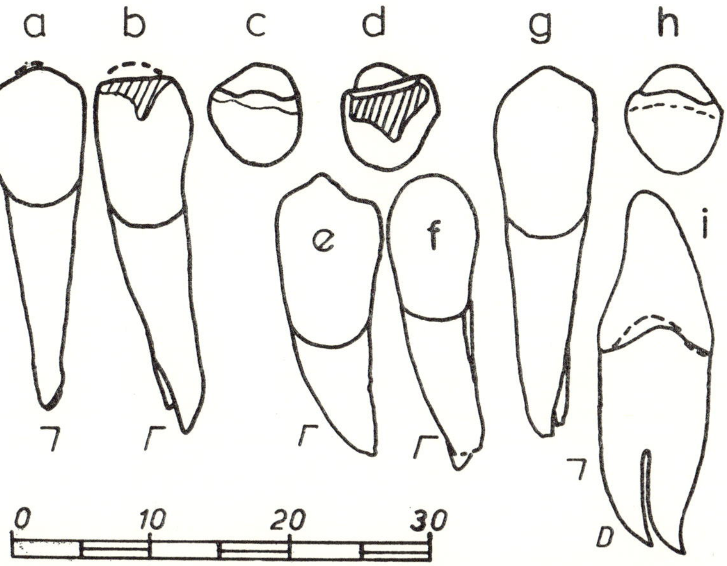

Figure 5-27. Asymmetry of crown in bifid-rooted lower canines. *a,c,* labial and occlusal view of a right canine. *b,d,* similar views of a left canine. *e,f,* left canines of very different character as regards curvature and cusp, and yet each bears characters which enable it to be positively identified as a lower canine from left side. *g,h,i,* three views of a lower canine in which some characters are not clearly presented, with the result that identification as left or right is more difficult than is usual with a complete unbroken tooth.

between M and D contours in any particular tooth.

Secondly, with regard to comparisons of M and D contours in individual teeth, there is variety in several respects. No case was found in which both were identical, but similarity was close in some (Figs. 5-5 *c,* 5-22 *h,* 5-25 *a,* and 5-27 *i*). In those with contrasting curves this occurred in height of peak (Figs. 5-9 *b,* 5-19 *f*), in shape of peak (Figs. 5-9 *c,* 5-20 *d,* 5-21 *c*) and in both height and shape (Figs. 5-5 *d,* 5-9 *a,* 5-10 *b,f,* 5-19 *g,* 5-21 *f,g,* 5-24 *e* and 5-25 *f*).

Thirdly, in one noteworthy respect all teeth examined were consistent. The peak or "hill top" of the mesial contour always rose above the distal contour; in other words, the mesial contour was found to rise higher and more steeply than the distal. This is an important finding since it assists identification of a tooth as left or right. Thus, where either bilateral asymmetry in tooth outlines or other characters that usually assist identification are not very obvious, as in the tooth described below (Fig. 5-27 *g,h,i*), or where these characters have been affected by wear, fracture, decay or dental restoration, comparison of the cervical lines may enable a positive identification to be made.

These differences in proximal cervical outlines in lower canines are like the differences already described for upper canines. In both jaws the tooth distal to the canine is larger and wider than the tooth against its mesial surface. In the canines themselves the mesial surface is more flattened and, especially in the upper, it is wider in the cervical region than is the distal surface proper (Fig. 1-33). The wider or thicker alveolar ridge distal to canines to accommodate roots that are wider than those of lateral incisors may well have a morphological association with the more flattened distal cervical contour of the canines, but this does not assist in explaining why the mesial contour rises higher on the tooth (in lower canines).

If a clue is to be sought amongst morphological characters there are several that may be noted. The mesial angle of the lower canine crown is higher than the distal, and there tends to be a similar difference in levels of contact points. Associated with these is the considerable difference in shape of proximal surfaces of lateral incisor and first premolar which face the two sides of the canine (and the contrast is even greater between their deciduous antecedents). In some dentitions the incisors have a longer crown than the premolar and a higher contact point with the canine, and these features are in harmony with the observed higher crest of the canine's mesial cervical contour.

The other findings and implications referred to above will now be considered. Examination of the outlines presenting both cervical lines shows that in some cases the contours are placed evenly as regards above and below one another, but in most cases this is not so. The nature of the difference now referred to concerns the ends of the contours and the position of the crests in relation to the tooth axis, rather than their shape as peaked or more rounded, or as high or low. These aspects of shape have been considered already. Now it is noted that one or both ends of either contour may tend to flatten out, or they may not (Fig. 5-19, *c* and *d* respectively). Absence of the flattening appearance may affect the same end of each contour, as in Figure 5-21 *c* (where of course the lingual end of the D contour appears at the labial end of the M contour). The other difference noted is that the crests of the contours are often not in vertical relationship and may be on opposite sides of, or at different distances from, the root axis.

These two kinds of variation, namely crest relationship and end-style of contours, may suggest that either or both of two factors account for the differences. Firstly there is the possibility that for drawing the outlines as seen through the camera lucida the tooth had been viewed off-centre, so enabling one to see further around on to labial or lingual surface, and consequently that portion of the cervical line became more flattened out in the drawing. Secondly, if the crests were both nearer to labial or to lingual, the reversing of the broken-line contour (as distinct from a "seen-through" contour) would produce the kind of separation noted. Regarding the suggested off-centre viewing this no doubt was sometimes a factor. In the presence of crown-twist sometimes the tooth was deliberately turned a little to simplify the crown outline, but this had little effect on root outline or cervical contour or crest, which were the main features to be recorded.

Further study of recorded contours and checking against teeth concerned led to the following conclusion: The effects of the two factors just considered did not adequately explain the differences noted and might well be of relatively minor importance.

If time and technique had permitted the presentation of many outlines of transverse sections of teeth at the cervix, it would have been easy to show variation in how far one may see around to labial and lingual cervices. Appreciation of curvature, angularity or flattening will help in understanding why some contours tend to flatten out or otherwise. This character was referred to when describing cervical lines for upper central incisors (p. 7). Good examples in lower canines are seen in Figures 5-9 *e* and 5-19 *f* where one sees (from mesial) further around the lingual end of the cervical line. In the outlines of transverse sections of these teeth (Fig. 5-24 *i* and *j* respectively) it is clear that the labial portion is wider and less convex than the lingual. In Figure 5-24 *g* this difference is less; and correspondingly, the cervical contour of the same tooth, shown in *h*, is almost symmetrical. It was shown in upper incisors

(Figs. 1-13 and 1-14), and also in upper canines (Fig. 1-33), that the transverse section at the cervix is usually more angular at the mesio-labial than at the disto-labial. This also would tend to reduce flattening of the mesial end of the traced cervical contour. The same character does occur in lower canines, but it is less easily recognized because the lower root appears more compressed mesio-distally.

Whether the crest of proximal contours falls on, or away from, the mid-root axis may also be determined from the outlines presented. These may be noted for either M or D contours but not for both in any one tooth, as here presented. In other words, the broken-line contour should be ignored for this purpose. The position of the cusp (in proximal view) in relation to the root axis has been studied here for both upper and lower canines; for the latter it has been found mostly lingual to the root axis, although often close to it and occasionally on the buccal side of it. The relation of cusp and crest to root axis and to one another was examined and it was found that there was considerable variation. If cusp and crest could each be labial to, on the axis, or lingual to it, they could theoretically be related to one another in nine different styles. To simplify the analysis a series of nine diagrams was devised in three groups, each group having three styles (Fig. 5-28). Omitting the two unlikely combinations (where each was on opposite sides of the axis) the outlines already drawn were examined for examples of the remaining seven varieties.

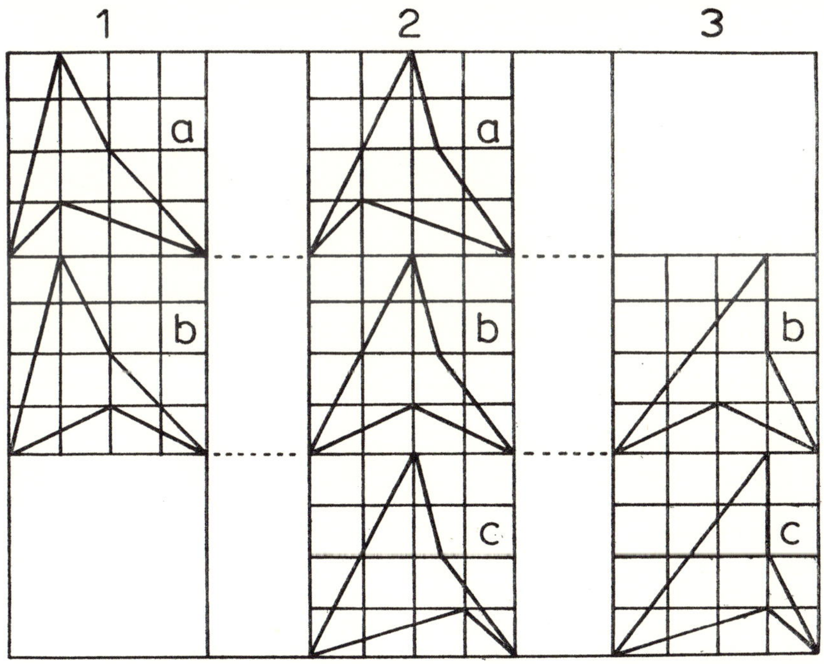

Figure 5-28. Diagrams representing proximal outlines of crowns of lower canines. These have been designed to show variations in relationship of cusp tip and cervical crest to the central root axis, and to one another. Group 1, cusp tip nearer labial, which is uncommon in lowers (but common in upper canines). Group 2, cusp tip in line of root axis. Group 3, cusp tip nearer lingual, which is common in lower canines. Diagram *a* in each group has the cervical crest nearer to labial; in *b* the crest is in the root axis and in *c* it is nearer to the lingual. It is unlikely that the hypothetical association of crest and cusp on opposite sides of the axis would occur and so there is no 1 *c* or 3 *a* diagram. References to specimens illustrating the other seven varieties are given in Appendix 5.

Examples of these may be recognized in the outlines presented. It is emphasized that these relate only to the full tooth outline and contour of the view as given, and not to the turn-around cervical contour in broken line. A list of examples is given in Appendix 5, the letters M or D indicating whether the example is from mesial or distal view.

It would be expected that for lower canines the most common relationships would be found in style *b* of groups 2 and 3, and it is seen that examples of these two styles were most easily recognized. At the same time it must be remembered that this is a subjective analysis in the presence of a number of variables. Some of the latter are as follows: cusp height and thickness, slight wear of enamel, height, steepness and shape of cervical contour, and the relative heights of labial and lingual cervix (as discussed below). Subjective judgment is further complicated by inability accurately to determine the root axis and the relation of cusp or crest to the axis when not obviously to one side of it.

The fact that the sorting revealed examples of all the varieties assumed to be present, and that most specimens fell in the expected places, clearly justified the exercise, and attention was then given to the effect of another variable that had been observed.

This concerned the relative height, or distance from cusp tip or root apex, of the labial and lingual parts of the cervical outline. These are the ends of the cervical contours presented in the outlines. The difference was not always obvious, but its frequent presence in some degree became apparent while making "turn-around" cervical contours on tooth outlines already drawn. It was often necessary to rotate or swing the drawing paper when lining it up with the turned-around tooth for the fitting of the second cervical contour to the termini of the first. It was revealed that, compared with a "seen-through" second contour, the resulting relationship of contours in the turn-around method was sometimes quite different. It was felt desirable to determine the nature of the differences and whether in spite of them the turn-around method could lead to valid and useful conclusions. It was obvious that there was a displacement which involved separation of the crests of the two contours, at least in their lateral relationships if not also in the vertical.

Examination was to be related to two variables. Firstly it had already been established that cervical crests were found in varied relationship to the root axis and that these may lie on either side of it. Secondly there was the observed difference in level of labial and lingual ends of the cervical contour. While the lingual contour might be found lower than the labial (Fig. 5-9 *e*), in the majority of cases this was not so. In most cases the labial cervix was lower, i.e. further below the cusp tip or nearer to the root apex in lower teeth; in some the difference was slight and in others it was easily recognized. Examples of the latter condition are Figures 5-9 *c*, 5-18 *d;* 5-20 *a,b;* and 5-21 *a,c,d,f,g*.

To assist in understanding the degree and direction of displacement, these two variables were studied in diagrams relating to one or the other. Assuming first that cervices were at the same level, the crests might be related to the root axis in three ways—in the root axis, on the same side of it or on opposite sides. The last was discarded as unlikely to occur. If both were in the root axis the crest of a turn-around contour would again be in that axis. If both were at the same distance to one side the turn-around would separate them horizontally by twice their original distance from the axis.

The next effect considered was that of turn-around when both were on the root axis but labial cervices were lower than lingual. This is represented in Figure 5-29.

In this figure, *a* is the mesial and *b* the distal view of a lower right canine. The visible cervix is drawn in continuous line and the "see-through" cervix in broken line. The base lines DL and L1.D1 are bisected at right angles by the root axis through R and R1. The cusp tip A and A1 falls to the lingual side of that axis; B and B1 are vertically below D and D1 respectively. Let BL and L1.B1 be called the cervical base.

If *b* is superposed on *a*, so that the cervical base of each coincides, we have diagram *c* in which the crest of the distal contour (light continuous line) is displaced labially compared with its "seen-through," or true, relation to the mesial crest. Similarly, if *a* is superposed on *b* as shown in Figure 5-30 *a*, it is seen that the crest of the mesial cervix (heavy continuous line) is displaced to the labial compared with its "seen-through" or true position. It should be noted that if one attempts to determine displacement of both crests relative to one another from a single diagram one might draw the erroneous conclusion that the crests have moved in opposite directions.

The cause of displacement clearly is re-

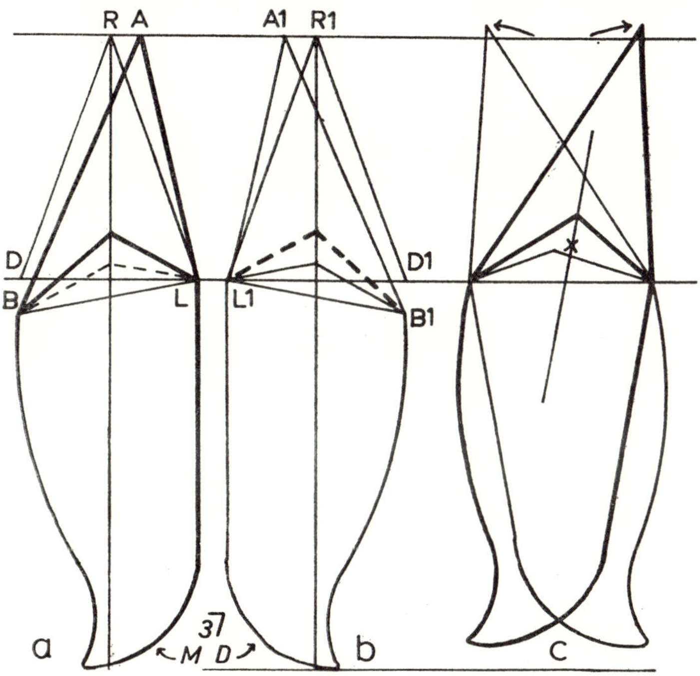

Figure 5-29. Factors involved in lateral displacement of crest of "turned-around" cervices (broken lines) relative to crest of visible cervices (continuous lines) in earlier proximal outlines. The diagram represents a hypothetical lower right canine with cervical crests in the root axis but cusp nearer to lingual and cervix lower on labial. The root axis is at right angles to the line D.D1 which passes through the lingual ends of the cervical contours, which are represented by continuous lines in the appropriate view, and by broken lines for the "seen-through" contour. *a,b,* mesial and distal views respectively. B.B1, buccal ends of cervical contours, which are raised to lie in the line D.L.L1.D1 for the superposition in *c*. The heavier lines in each case refer to the M outline. In *c* the only points common to each outline are the end points of the cervical lines, B on L1 and L on B1; cusp tips move apart as shown by the arrows so that neither they nor the apices will coincide, and root axes intersect. Part of the root axis of the mesial outline is shown. This diagram shows that in a turned-around distal contour placed on a mesial contour (where the tooth style is as in *a,b*) the distal crest is displaced to appear labially of its seen-through, or true, relation to the mesial crest as marked at X.

lated to the rotation or swing of outlines involved in causing the cervical base to coincide at each end of the contour, and in these diagrams the swing has arisen from the labial cervix being lower than the lingual. It would appear to follow that in the few cases where the lingual cervix is lower (as in the outline Fig. 5-9 *e*), comparison of cervical contours by turn-around would displace the crest of the turned-around contour to the lingual of its "seen-through" position. That this is so is shown in the diagram of Figure 5-30 *c*. This diagram is the result of superposition of outlines of the style of Figure 5-30 *b* where the cervix is lower on lingual (contrast with Fig. 5-29 *a*). The crest of the distal cervix has moved towards the lingual of the mesial tooth outline, compared with its "seen-through" or true, position at x. The difference in position of cusp tips and root apices in *a* and *c* of Figure 5-30 arises from the lifting of lingual instead of labial cervicals, reversing the direction of swing in the second case. As each diagram represents a tooth with the cusp the same distance lingually of the root axis, the swing involved in superpositions separates the cusps in the first case and approximates them in the second.

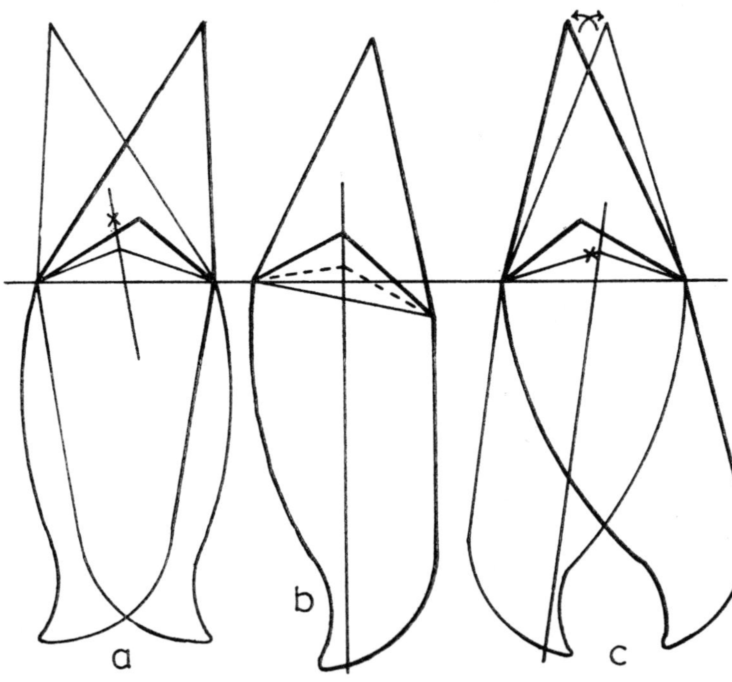

Figure 5-30. Continuation of theme of Figure 5-29. Further effects when lingual cervix is lower than labial cervix. In diagram *a*, the turned-around M contour is placed on the D contour, i.e. *a* of Figure 5-29 is placed on *b* of that figure, to determine the apparent displacement of the mesial crest in its relation to the seen-through, or true, position of that crest on the distal contour. Again the apparent displacement is towards the labial as shown at X. Diagram *b* represents a style of tooth in which the lingual cervix is lower (Fig. 5-9 *e*) by contrast with the much more common lower labial cervix represented in Figure 5-29 *a,b*. Diagram *c* shows a corresponding superposition, turned-around distal contour (lighter line) placed on mesial contour (heavier line). With this style of tooth the distal crest is now displaced lingually from its seen-through or true, position (marked X) in relation to the mesial crest. See text for significance of difference in displacement of crest, and of cusp and apex positions compared with Figures 5-29 *c* and 5-30 *a*. In this case superposition caused the cusp tips to move first towards, and then past one another, as indicated by the arrows.

Thus with regard to crests of cervical contours in turn-around superposition it has been established that they may or may not be displaced from their relative seen-through, or true, positions. Displacement is common and is affected by several factors. These are as follows: (a) position of cusp in relation to root axis; (b) position of crests in relation to root axis; (c) whether the lingual and labial cervices are at different heights, or, in other words, whether the cervical base and root axis intersect at right angles or obliquely, in proximal view. Assuming that mesial and distal crests in any particular tooth bear the same relation to root axis, it has been shown that there may be, as there are examples of, seven different relations possible between (a) and (b) above (1, 2, 3 of Fig. 5-28). It has been shown that there are three different kinds of relationship for (c) namely labial lower, both equal and lingual lower. This is not all, for since many of the styles represented in (a), (b) and (c) are themselves subject to variation in degree, it is evident that variations or differences that may be found are numerous. Moreover it was shown that a cervix that is lower on labial tends to cause labial displacement, and if lower on lingual the displacement tends to be lingual. The amount of such displacement will be affected by degree of difference in level, by (a) and (b) factors as above, and by other factors not investigated here. These last include length of cervical base, actual and relative heights of cervical crests above cervical bases, convexities of cervical arches, tooth surfaces and so on.

Displacements have been considered in respect to lateral or labio-lingual movement, and while difference in height of mesial and distal cervical arches must introduce a factor of vertical displacement, it is believed that this may largely be ignored. Among the sources of error which relate particularly to the present exercise, although it is considered that they have not appreciably affected the results, one has already been mentioned, namely, the slight difference in viewpoint that may arise in an effort to avoid complication of outline in presence of the condition described as "crown-root twist." An example of this is seen in Figure 5-1 *d*. Another arises from differences in convexity or thickness of teeth in the cervical region which affect one's ability to see the "true" termini of a cervical line half way around labial and lingual cervices. Against these difficulties may be set the accuracy of tracings that have resulted from technique, or from modification of a camera lucida to the special requirements of this study. It is probable that some of these findings have previously been noted, as for example the different heights of mesial and distal contours. They are easily seen, where looked for, in the excellent drawings and more recent photographs in textbook or atlas of tooth morphology. But description or analysis has been impracticable hitherto because of the small numbers examined or the limitations of technique. In the present study the number of specimens studied and of outlines presented is very considerable and, combined with the accuracy of technique, has enabled a significant analysis to be made and presented.

This analysis of cervical lines therefore has led to positive conclusions, at least for lower canines: The cervical lines on a particular tooth may almost invariably be distinguished as mesial and distal. The mesial line rises higher and more steeply than the distal. Comparison of cervical lines by turn-around does not alter this difference, but it may by lateral displacement alter the relation of the turn-around crest to that first recorded. The amount of lateral displacement, real or apparent, may be the result of interaction of a number of variable factors, and it is unlikely that the degree of influence of a particular factor in a particular tooth could be determined. Factors involved may be recognized, as also the way in which they tend to cause displacement when acting alone, and in both respects these have been described above. At the same time the description has drawn attention to hitherto unrecognized characters and aspects of variation.

Cusp-Tip Bulb in Lower Canines

In proximal views of lower canines much variation is seen in the contour of the cusp tip. For want of a better term the word "thickness" perhaps indicates the character referred to, but neither sturdiness nor size is being referred to. The feature concerned is rather a thickening on the lingual side of the tip, and it is sometimes in the form of a tubercle or small bulb. In some cases it is continuous with a central ridge passing down the lingual surface of the cusp blade. In other cases again there may be a mesial and distal ridge on the lingual surface, or three ridges on the labial surface, with two separating grooves. In these last cases one is reminded of the conception of lobes and developmental grooves often seen in incisors.

Presence of the lingual ridge and cusp-tip bulb may be recognized in some of the outlines. Among the outlines in figures in this chapter some indication of these characters is recognized in sixteen cases. These are all mesial views. Easier recognition in mesial views is related to the character that has been referred to as crown-root twist. Where the latter character is well developed

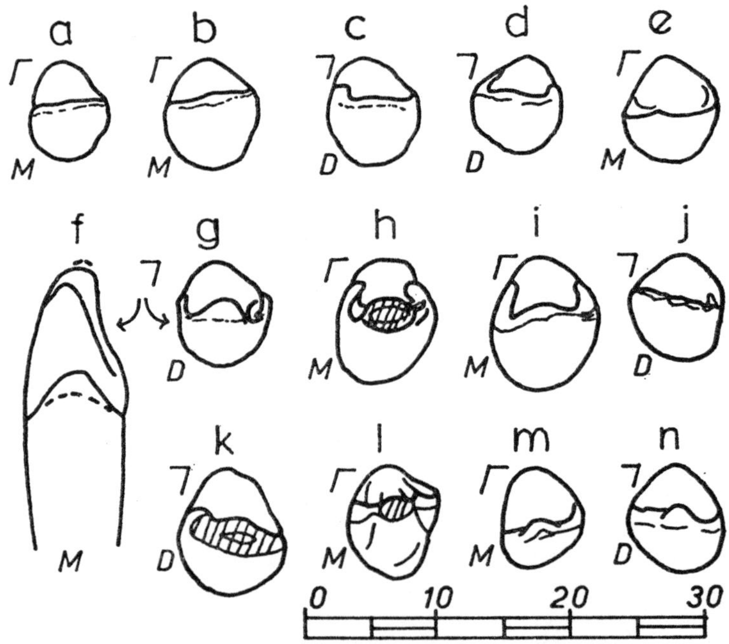

Figure 5-31. Variation in development of the cusp-tip bulb or tubercle; occlusal outlines to supplement proximal outlines in other figures. Top row *(a-e)*, and also *j*, are teeth in which the tubercle is absent although one or both side ridges may be present in some degree. Outlines *f,g* are of the same tooth which is lobed (Fig. 5-7 *f*), but was not figured elsewhere in proximal view. In tooth *h* (Fig. 5-24 *b*) the cusp-tip bulb was well developed, but what remains after wear is partly obscured by the prominent side ridges. In tooth *i* the stronger ridges do obscure the bulb in proximal view (Fig. 5-10 *f*). In *k* there is a ridge on distal only, so that what remains of the bulb after incisal wear is seen in mesial view (Fig. 5-21 *c*). In tooth *l* the lobe-like form somewhat confuses recognition of ridges but the bulb character is also present (Figs. 5-6 *h* and 5-9 *d*.) Tooth *m* has a tubercle rather than a bulb and this is seen in distal view in Figure 5-18 *d*. Tooth *n* has a strongly marked bulb which is seen from mesial in Figure 5-19 *d*.

a small part of the lingual surface of the cusp blade is easily seen in a mesial view. According to the degree of development of the bulb and of the ridge descending from it these features also may appear in such view. Although these are relatively minor details of tooth morphology there is sufficient variation for it to be recorded that in a particular tooth, bulb or ridges are both present or both absent, or that one of them is present, and whether the character is only slightly developed, or more prominent. A similar feature may be found in upper canines.

With regard to lower canines, examples of absence or presence of some of these features in proximal outlines referred to are supplemented by occlusal views in Figure 5-31. Outlines of teeth in which the bulb or tubercle was absent are seen in Figures 5-8 *d*, 5-17 *e*, 5-19 *c*, 5-22 *b*, 5-24 *d* and 5-10 *a*. These are the same teeth respectively as in Figure 5-31 *a-e*, and *j*. The last tooth, seen in distal view in Figure 5-10 *a*, appears therein to have a thick cusp blade. Reference to Figure 5-31 *j*, where there is neither cusp-tip bulb nor lingual ridges, shows that it is not a thick blade. The explanation lies in the greater-than-usual crown-root twist which causes part of the labial surface to be included in the distal view. The large tooth *f* in Figure 5-10 also appears to have no crown-tip bulb, but in occlusal view (Fig. 5-31 *i*) it is seen that the explanation is different from that of the previous case. In the larger tooth the crown-tip bulb is quite well developed but the side ridges are even more so, and these obscure the bulb in proximal view. These two examples serve to emphasize firstly the considerable amount of data that can be recorded about a particular tooth and secondly the misleading impression that may be gained through incomplete information conveyed by a single illustration.

The two teeth represented in Figure 5-31 *f*,*g* and *l* show how proximal and occlusal views are complicated by the lobe-like form presented in some crowns. Further views of these two teeth are given in Figures 5-7 *f* for the first and 5-6 *h* and 5-9 *d* for the second. The last two occlusal views in Figure 5-31 are of the teeth shown in mesial view in Figures 5-18 *d* and 5-19 *d* respectively. The latter tooth has a well developed cusp-tip bulb continuous with a central ridge. The former represents a very small but sharp and well-defined bulb that would be better described as a tubercle. There is no central ridge nor side ridges.

Difficult Identification

Asymmetry of the individual crown of a lower canine which assists in its identification as a left or right tooth, and bilateral symmetry of the mirror image type as between left and right teeth, were illustrated in Figure 5-2. That study is extended by the outlines of bifid-rooted teeth in Figure 5-27. The opportunity has been taken when selecting specimens for illustration to use teeth which also show variation in curvature or contour. It is of interest to note how the basic characters enabling differentiation between M and D or left and right may still be recognized or appreciated in the presence of such wide variation in the contour, morphology or profiles of crown and cusp.

It is said that a rule has an exception, and in this matter the exception may be the tooth in which there is a very low degree of asymmetry. Recognition of asymmetry is made even more difficult when one is asked to identify an isolated tooth rather than discriminate between a known pair. Such a problem case is the tooth drawn in Figure 5-27 g.

In labial view the crown of this tooth closely approaches bilateral symmetry in such characters as proximal profile, position of cusp tip, and length and height of cusp slope. The root tapers evenly and is straight except for a small curve at each apex and a slight twist effect between them. There is a long shallow groove on each side and therefore the root does not assist identification. In proximal views the cervical contours differ and if the crest with greater radius is to be distal the tooth is right side. There are no proximal facets to indicate the height of contacts of adjacent teeth. There is a light stain line indicating a gingival margin well above the cervix on both sides, and no calculus deposits. There is a rather large carious cavity which would be mesial, or mesio-lingual if the tooth is from the right side. The high gingival line, the stain position and the absence of faceting from opposing teeth all suggest that the tooth was extracted from a rather young (adult?) person whose activities as regards mastication and artificial prophylaxis were minimal.

Viewed from occlusal aspect the slight obliquity of the cusp ridges and detectable slight asymmetry of outline combine to suggest again that the tooth is from right side. It may be concluded, therefore, that the tooth is identified as such, but that some doubt remains. While describing the tests undertaken to determine identity of a tooth, characters have been mentioned that may seem to be outside the study of variation, but they provide data of a kind that could be relevant to a more personal question of identification, and that has been mentioned as a main objective in this study.

Summary

Lower canines have presented many characters for examination. It was convenient to make a major division with the character of root bifidity and deal separately with single-rooted and double-rooted teeth, because bifidity added so many features for study. Although this is a character of roots alone, its manifestations varied greatly and while in some cases it was a major feature of a tooth, this was often not so and almost every imaginable gradation down to its presence as a very minor feature was represented. Thus in spite of description under two main headings relating to root form, description of the crown, and indeed much description also involving the root, applies to lower canine teeth as such and without regard to whether root division was present in some degree. In this respect study of the cervical outline, the form and position of its proximal crests, and differences between mesial and distal contours is a good example.

Bilateral asymmetry of individual teeth was shown to resemble that for upper canines and while the differences are less marked in lowers they do enable left and right teeth to be identified, and in conjunction with features characteristic of lowers they assist in distinguishing lower canines from uppers. Root grooves were examined and they showed great variation. Some grooves were obviously related to root division; others were suspected as being so related, but in the absence of knowledge of associated variation of pulp cavities this could not be determined precisely.

As with other anterior teeth, there was much variation in root curvature, both in direction and in degree of curvature and in the proportion of root involved. There were no "sharp" bends of the kind that in uppers might well be associated with closeness to, and morphological variations of, the nasal fossae or maxillary sinuses. The tendency found in uppers for slight curvature of the whole root or of the apical portion to be distally inclined is much less apparent in lower canines. Some cases of curvature involving much of the root of the lower canine might well have resulted from eruption to malocclusion through crowding of adjacent teeth. In some this surmise was supported by facets of wear or presence of stain in unusual positions. The roots of lower canines showed much variation in actual length and in proportion to total tooth length, also as regards thickness or slenderness, in taper and in form of apex.

Although the cusp of canines is often described as less prominent in lowers than in uppers this is an unsatisfactory term, for there is much variety in cusp form in both. The lower canine, on account of its usual occlusal relationship, is probably more subject to change in the cusp tip by wear, but the manner of wear is in its turn subject to various factors. Some of these are the morphology and occlusal relationship of the unworn cusps, and the individual variations in mandibular movements. Much data concerning relationships and movements may be obtained from position and form of facets of wear and of areas of stained or polished enamel or of deposits of calculus.

In lower canines with bifid roots it was shown that the range of variation does not allow a precise definition of bifidity nor, consequently, a meaningful estimate of its occurrence. Other workers however have not only published percentages of the incidence of double-rooted lower canines but offered comparisons between the groups studied. Alexandersen (1963) reported the frequency of double-rooted lower canines using "the number of root-tips irrespective of size of the roots to determine whether a tooth should be considered double-rooted or not." It is agreed that exclusive categories must be postulated in order to obtain percentages, but it is impossible to make the material being examined conform to that method of reporting. Multiplicity of categories is impracticable and therefore percentages of this nature are not acceptable either for descriptive or comparative purposes.

Accurate tracings of cervical lines and of their proximal crests show that in addition to the features mentioned by Alexandersen they present great variety. Factors concerned in this, and comparison of mesial and distal contours, have been dealt with in the present work as thoroughly for single-rooted as for double-rooted lower canines. Similarly Alexandersen's statements concerning the root taper and apical form in double-rooted teeth are easily shown to cover few of the variations herein presented.

It did appear however that examination of the relative sizes of the two branches in bifid roots was justifiable in spite of the difficulty of making a subjective decision on borderline cases, and for what they are worth, percentages have been given for those having the major branch on labial or lingual. A useful character for noting variation in bifid roots was found to be the cleft between them: its width and the parallelism or otherwise of its sides; its length and the nature of grooves associated with it. It was found also that the presence of bifidity, or its nature, were apparently unrelated to the size of tooth or length of root.

Curvature of root branches was examined and, as with two-rooted upper premolars, it was found that similar deviations may be seen in both branches or that one or both may present curvature independently. As with other teeth, it was often impossible to represent curvature satisfactorily in a two-dimensional outline.

Returning to the subject of cervical outlines, these were studied in some detail, and it is believed that the technique adopted and the accuracy of outlines obtained have justified the work involved. As a result the nature of variations and the factors involved in recording and interpretation are now known, and they may contribute useful data in problems of identification.

A small non-metrical character has been called the cusp-tip bulb and it has been described and illustrated with the same accuracy as other morphological features. It has been shown to be relatively prominent in some teeth and absent from others, and, like other characters, it varies considerably in form. Sometimes it is continuous with a central ridge, and sometimes there are lateral ridges. The variations in these ridges, in the bulb itself and in other characters such as crown-root twist, account for the fact that the bulb may be present but not clearly discernible in a proximal view.

Finally the characters that have been noted are considered in relation to a particular tooth. This tooth, although undamaged by trauma, wear, or decay, is not easy at first sight to identify as left or right. It has been shown how some less obvious characters may then assist in positive identification.

Chapter 6

Mandibular Premolars

In the mandible there is a greater range of variation between the first and second premolars than in the maxilla. Whereas in the upper teeth perhaps the most common character of premolars is the presence of two well-developed cusps, this does not apply to lower premolars. For this reason the old name "bicuspid," as applied to premolars, is very often quite unsuitable for a lower premolar, and this obtains for both first and second lower premolar teeth. The first premolar $(\overline{4})$ may have only one cusp and resemble a canine in some features, while the second premolar $(\overline{5})$ may have two well-developed lingual cusps in addition to the buccal cusp, so that it could be described correctly as a tricuspid tooth.

Teeth that are morphologically near either of these extremes must be described separately, but there is much variation between the extremes. Also, some teeth have characters of both teeth. In these cases, especially where there has been wearing of the crown or damage to crown or root by fracture or pathology, it may be impossible to identify an isolated tooth as left or right or as first or second lower premolar. Such teeth therefore can be described only as lower premolars.

In the case of lower incisors it was shown that sometimes it was difficult or impossible to make corresponding identification or distinction as regards central or lateral incisor. With lower premolars there may be more characters for consideration, especially in the crown, and yet one cannot confidently generalize when referring to some of the most obvious characters of these teeth. This has already been mentioned as regards the presence of two cusps, but it applies also to the root. For example it cannot be said that the root is oval or flattened on mesial and distal, because it may be round in cross-section. In many teeth the root has one or more grooves, but sometimes there is no trace of a groove and sometimes there is a deep groove, but oblique in such a way that it resembles a longitudinal fold. Again, it cannot be said that the root is single, for sometimes it is bifid; nor can it be said that the root branches are always placed in a certain way much as M and D or B and L, because they may be either or neither, or rather obliquely divided.

It is clear that lower premolars present wide variation, and their description is difficult and therefore of interest. And again it will be seen that there is no such thing as a premolar that is typical of its group or that may be described by measurement.

Like upper premolars, both lowers are approximately the same length, and are shorter than their adjacent canine. Whereas, in the maxilla, the first premolar is usually larger than the second, this is not so in the mandible, for the second premolar may be the larger tooth (see Fig. 6-1). In the first premolar the anterior portion of the occlusal surface may appear lower than the posterior, especially where the anterior groove is prominent (Fig. 6-5 *h*), but this is not always so because there is so much variation in the occlusal surface. Where the lingual cusp is insignificant and there tends to be a ridge, the posterior portion is lower (Fig. 6-5 *k*). This lower posterior portion is a very common feature of the second premolar which often has a disto-lingual ridge or third cusp in that region.

From the collection, 382 lower premolars were selected and mounted on sixty-seven cards in Groups Q and R. From 308 of

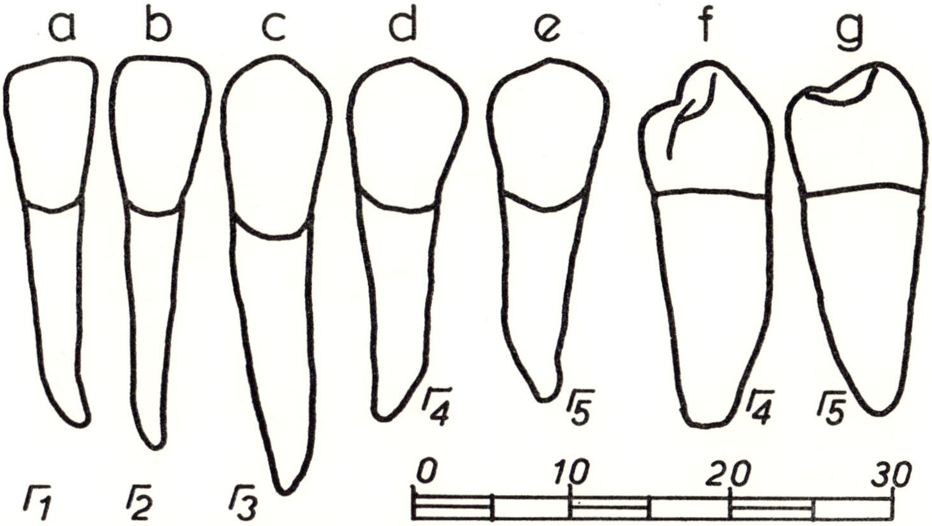

Figure 6-1. The first five teeth in the lower left quadrant. As these are all from one person they show relative sizes. *a-e,* labial views; *f,g,* mesial views of first and second premolars. The mental foramen was probably between the premolar apices in this case.

these teeth there were drawn the 425 outlines and five diagrams in the thirty-nine figures supporting this chapter.

LOWER FIRST PREMOLARS

A human tooth with an oval or partly flattened single root, presenting a major buccal cusp and a minor lingual cusp, is most likely to be a lower first premolar. On the other hand one would not be justified in saying that lower premolars may usually be described in this way, although it would be true in many cases. Like other teeth, lower premolars bear a dimensional relationship to adjacent teeth and the first premolar is shorter than its canine. As between persons, however, there is considerable variation in length of first premolars and it would be expected, as has been assumed with other teeth, that most of these differences are associated with the stature of the individual.

Examples of short and long first premolars are shown in Figure 6-2. Tooth *a* is one of five premolars (four lowers) from one person, and all are approximately the same size and may be called very small. The other small teeth (*b* and *c* are one tooth) show variety both in form and in proportions of root and crown. Teeth *d, e,f* would be best described as long rather than large, for their crowns are not large and the roots are relatively slender for their length. A large tooth (for the ethnic group of the collection) is seen in Figure 6-3 *a.* This is a young tooth with incomplete root and there is no X-ray or other record to indicate the likely length to which it would have grown. Alongside this tooth Figure 6-3 *b* shows the corresponding ⌈4 from the prehistoric jaw of a young Tongan (in which it was noted that the teeth were large) but this crown is smaller than tooth *a.* The root is complete but is not normal, and the abnormality was reported elsewhere (Taylor, 1972a). The Tongan mandible containing this tooth was illustrated in another paper (Taylor, 1971b). When comparing size of teeth it is relevant to consider also the form of crown and root. The crowns of *a* and *b* are similar in that both have a prominent buccal cusp and a small but definite lingual cusp. In buccal view however they are different in that *a*

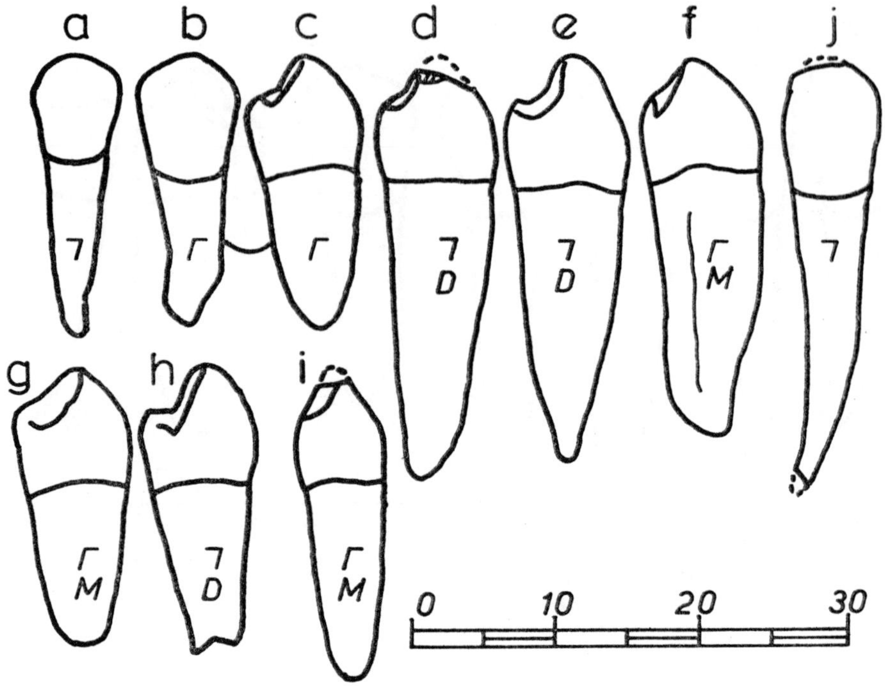

Figure 6-2. Proximal views of short and long first premolars. Tooth *j* measures approximately 29 mm between apex and lightly worn cusp tip.

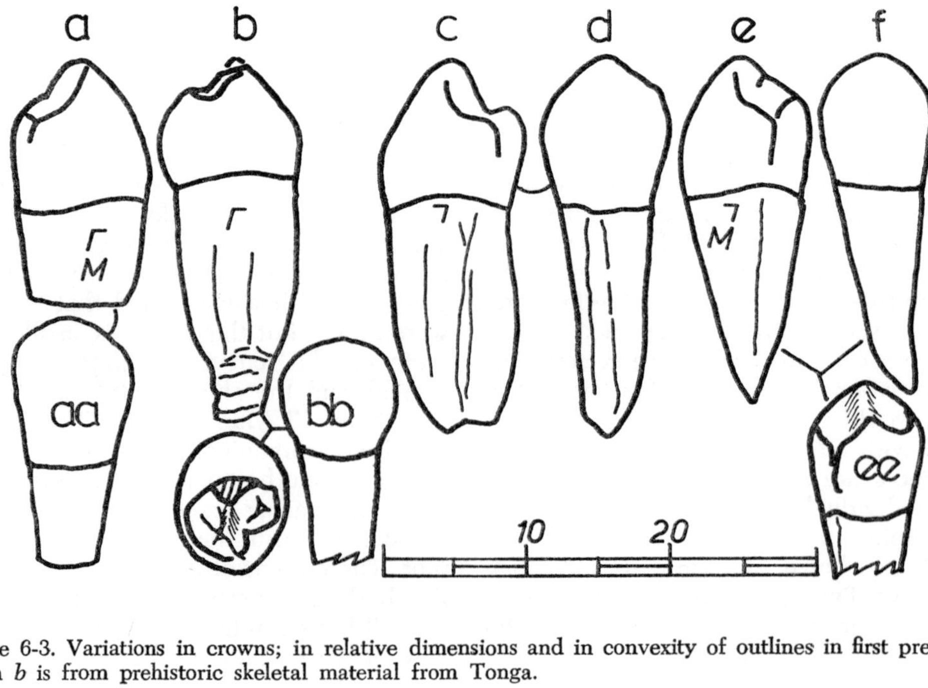

Figure 6-3. Variations in crowns; in relative dimensions and in convexity of outlines in first premolars. Tooth *b* is from prehistoric skeletal material from Tonga.

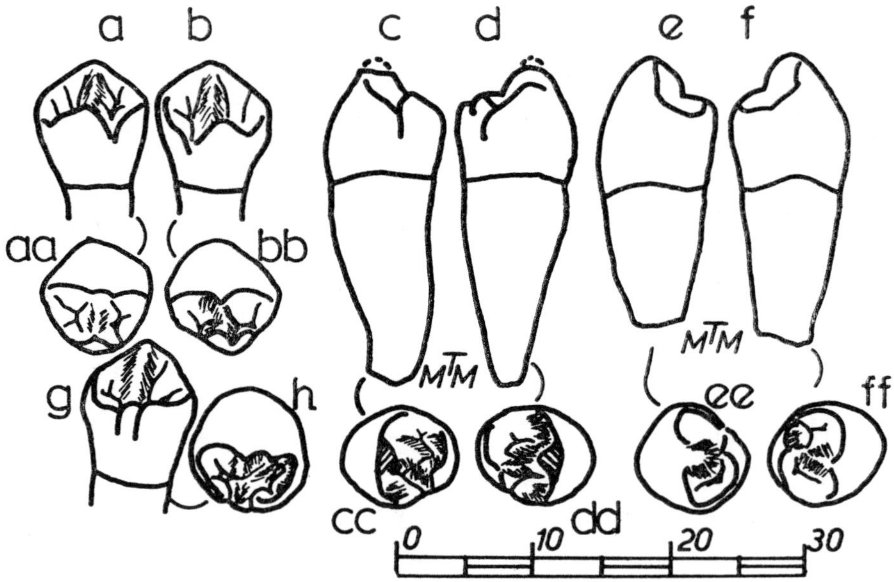

Figure 6-4. Pairs of first premolars showing characters of symmetry and asymmetry useful in identification of teeth.

is relatively long and straight-sided but *b* is short and convex, *aa* and *bb*. The roots of these teeth cannot be compared, for reasons given above.

In the other two teeth in Figure 6-3 (*c, d* and *e,f*) crowns and roots can be compared and are quite different, although both crowns are large. In tooth *c,d* the crown has a relatively prominent lingual cusp and the root is wide in proximal and lingual views; it has a prominent mesial cleft and a buccal groove. The root of *e,f* is relatively short and in both views it tapers to a fine sharp apex. There is a shallow mesial groove. The crown has no lingual cusp but this is replaced by a prominent ridge passing obliquely to join the buccal cusp.

It is not sufficient therefore merely to say that a tooth is large or small. The statement should be qualified by naming the character or region that merits such description. A particular dimension may attract attention, such as length or width, or length or width of crown or root; or the prominent dimension may be notable in one of these parts because of its relation to another. Thus in Figure 6-3 crowns *a* and *b* are large, crown *a* in height and width, and crown *b* in width but relatively short for that width. In tooth *e,f* the crown is large in height and width but the root is relatively small in length and thickness.

LEFT OR RIGHT

Differentiation between a pair of lower first premolars, or identification of a single tooth as left or right, is sometimes a simple matter, and in most cases the exercise is not very demanding. In some cases however it is very difficult so to identify one of these teeth or to distinguish it from a lower second premolar, because certain characters of cusp, ridge, pit or groove in crown or root may not be clearly defined. There is not likely to be difficulty in distinguishing buccal from lingual unless wear has been excessive or features have been involved in pathological conditions. The key to identification lies in ability to recognize asymmetry and associate it with details which are characteristic either of mesial

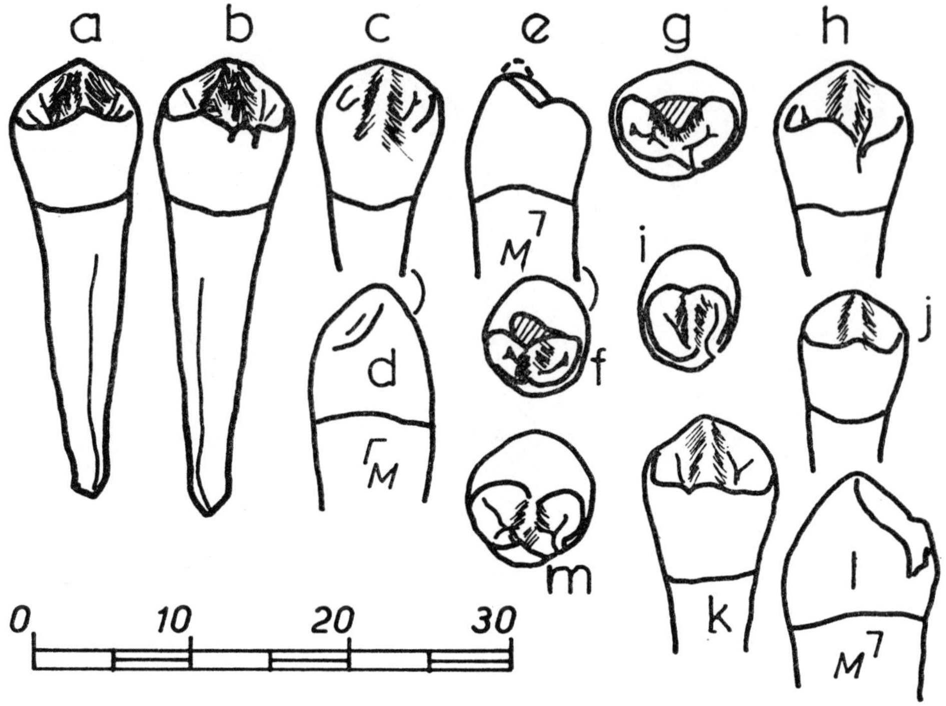

Figure 6-5. Identification of teeth. Variation of characters that identify mesial or distal, using mostly single teeth although *a,b* are a pair from one person. First premolars.

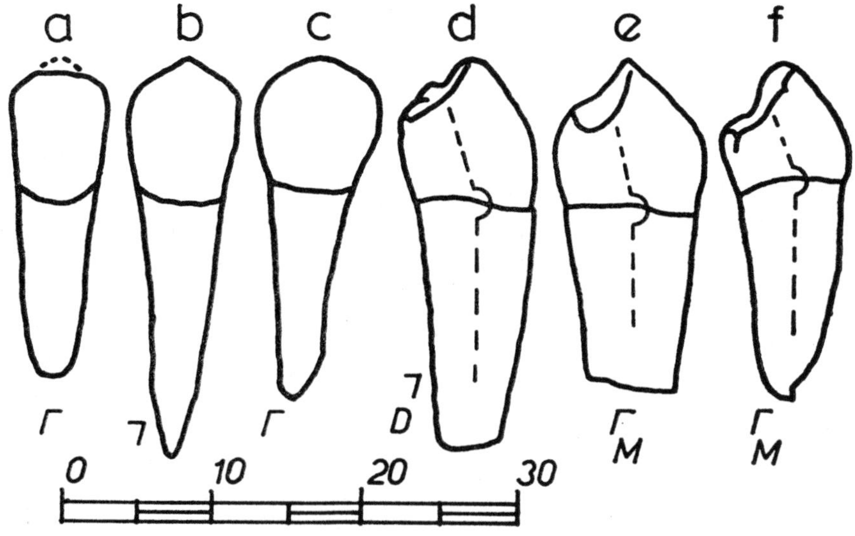

Figure 6-6. Crown contours and crown-root relation in first premolars.

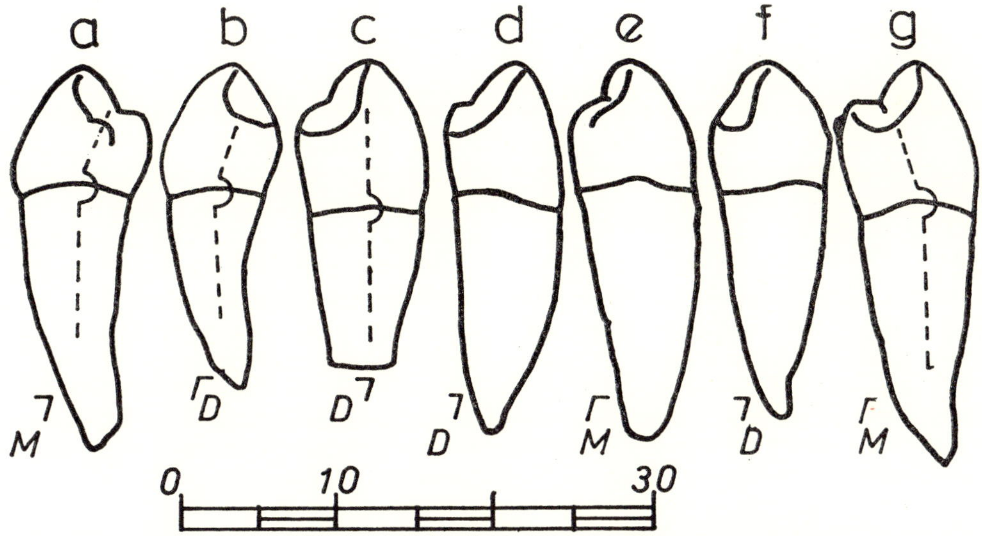

Figure 6-7. Crown contours and crown-root relation in first premolars.

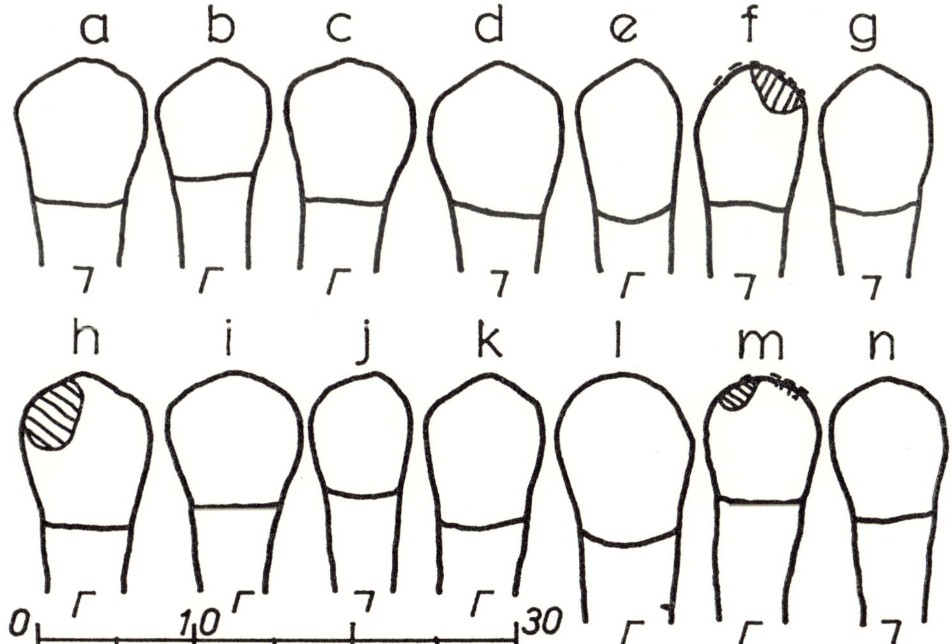

Figure 6-8. Crown outlines and proportions—buccal height to buccal width. First premolars.

or distal surfaces, or of anterior or posterior portions of the occlusal surface. Figures 6-4 and 6-5 employ outlines made from pairs of lower first premolars to show details that may be used for identification of these teeth, and to distinguish between left and right.

CROWN OF FIRST PREMOLARS

Reference to features concerned in identification has already established that there is much variation in these teeth. Description of the nature and range of variation in those and other features embraces aspects of variation that are common to most teeth as well as variation in features that are found only in first premolars.

In buccal view the crown may be straight-sided, with sides almost parallel (Fig. 6-6 *a*) or divergent (Fig. 6-6 *b*); or it may be rounded (Fig. 6-6 *c*). In proximal view it may be rather long and straight (Fig. 6-6 *d*) or shorter and more convex (Fig. 6-6 *e*). In this view also the crown axis may appear to incline to lingual (Figs. 6-6 *f* and 6-7 *a,b*), or be more erect, whether the crown be long or short (Fig. 6-7 *c-f*).

In buccal view the crown may be relatively short and wide (Fig. 6-8 *a-d*), or tall and narrow (Fig. 6-8 *e,f,g*), and in proximal view similar descriptions may apply (Fig. 6-9 *a,b,c,* and *d-g*).

Description of the variations found in occlusal surfaces may be facilitated if the crown of lower premolars be likened to a barrel or base on top of which may be erected various forms to make cusps, ridges and grooves. There is always a more or less prominent or dominant buccal cusp, and in the second premolar there may be two additional cusps. In the first premolar the lingual cusp is always relatively small, but it may be quite prominent (Fig. 6-7 *g*). There is great variety in the triangular ridges that pass from each cusp, reaching towards the other.

These ridges may be prominent and continuous one with the other. If there is a distinct col or depression this serves to make the lingual cusp more distinct (Figs. 6-7 *g* and 6-9 *g*) but there may be no col, or no lingual cusp recognizable as such, as in teeth *c,d* and *e,f* of Figure 6-5, so that the occlusal and lingual surfaces merge into one another. In these cases there may be pits or shallow fissures representing the anterior and posterior portions of the occlusal surface. In some cases the anterior feature is pit-like and the posterior one is

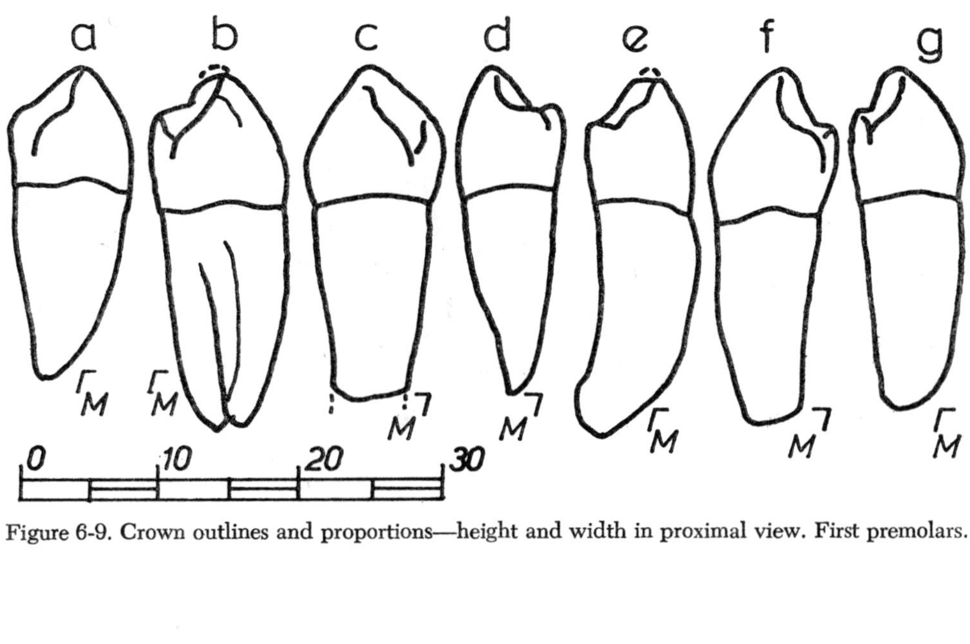

Figure 6-9. Crown outlines and proportions—height and width in proximal view. First premolars.

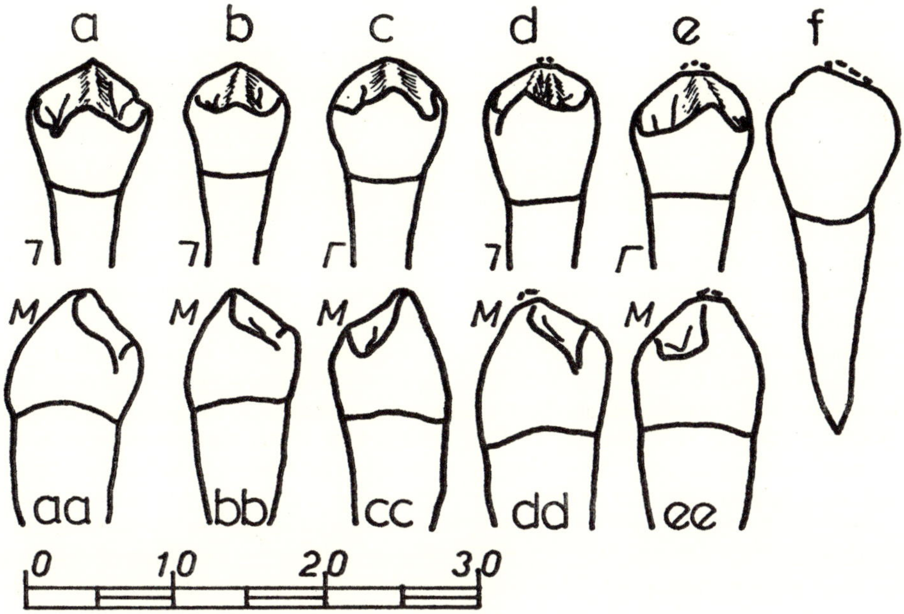

Figure 6-10. Crown variation—cusp height and form in first premolars.

elongated bucco-lingually (Fig. 6-5 *c*). In the less "extreme" cases of merging of lingual cusp with central ridge, the lingual aspect may present a somewhat cusp-like outline (apart from the buccal cusp), although there may not be a truly cusp-like projection on the occlusal surface (Fig. 6-10 *a-e*).

A cusp-like form, in the absence of a lingual cusp, may also arise from variation in grooves rather than in ridges, as will be shown presently. Thus when it is said that a lower first premolar may have no lingual cusp, this does not imply that the tooth is like a canine. There are several modifications of form where absence of a lingual cusp does not hinder recognition of the tooth as a first premolar. Instead of a cusp there may be a lingual ridge very similar to that in some second premolars (Fig. 6-11 *a,b*). There may be, as mentioned above, a prominent transverse or triangular ridge descending from the buccal cusp and, without a deep col or saddle, passing across the tooth to merge with the lingual surface (Figs. 6-5 *c,d*, 6-10 *b*, 6-12 *c*). Another variation, where there is no lingual cusp, is seen where the lingual ridge is not prominent (Figs. 6-11 *d* and 6-14 *i*, same tooth), or is interrupted (Fig. 6-4 *g,h*). A mesial view of the last tooth is seen in Figure 6-9 *f*, and a somewhat similar example is shown in Figure 6-15 *a*.

A true lingual cusp (Figs. 6-7 *g* and 6-11 *f* illustrating the same tooth) is not very common. It is different from the somewhat cusp-like form shown in Figures 6-5 *h,m* and 6-13 *f*, which again relate to one tooth. This cusp-like form might well be called a "pseudo" cusp. It is found where a groove passes through the lingual part of the mesial marginal ridge from the anterior occlusal pit on to the mesial surface. This groove is approximately in line with the "cleft" groove on the mesial surface of the root (Fig. 6-13 *f*). This association is seen in other outlines depicting mesial views of these premolars, and it is the drop in level of the occlusal groove that provides the mesial slope of the lingual "cusp." Another variation may be described as presenting a ML cusp and a DL ridge (Fig. 6-11 *g*). This type is more common in second premolars where it presents further variations from a full lingual ridge to two lingual cusps (Figs. 6-27, 6-28). There is great variety therefore in the relative prominence of cusps, of lingual and transverse ridges, and of pits and grooves and minor ridges between them.

The buccal cusp also varies as regards lateral width, and height and acumination. It always dominates the crown outlines of the tooth when viewed at right angles to its long axis. Many examples are given in the outlines of Figures 6-1 to 6-12. Whether the buccal cusp is considered as short or long depends partly on one's rating of the lingual cusp, and also on the above-mentioned conception of the crown as having a barrel-like base upon which the cusps are placed.

Within that notion, teeth *e,f* of Figure 6-4 have a short base and large buccal cusp, and teeth *d,e* of Figure 6-9 have a long base and short cusps. Tooth *a* of Figure 6-10 has a short base and long wide buccal cusp. Tooth *a* of Figure 6-13 has a large wide base, a large lingual cusp but a relatively small buccal cusp. Very long buccal cusps are shown, with a long base, in Figure 6-13 *b*, and with a medium base, in Figure 6-2 *h*. Both cusps prominent are seen in Figure 6-13 *c*, and neither cusp prominent in a rather large crown in Figure 6-13 *d*.

Acumination of buccal cusp may be examined with respect to proximal outline, or in buccal or lingual view, and for a particular tooth the assessment is not necessarily the same in each view. In proximal view the cusp appears more blunt where the triangular ridge is prominent, as in Figure 6-13 *a,e*. The first of these teeth is slightly worn on the cusp tip but *e* is a young tooth without any wear. More acu-

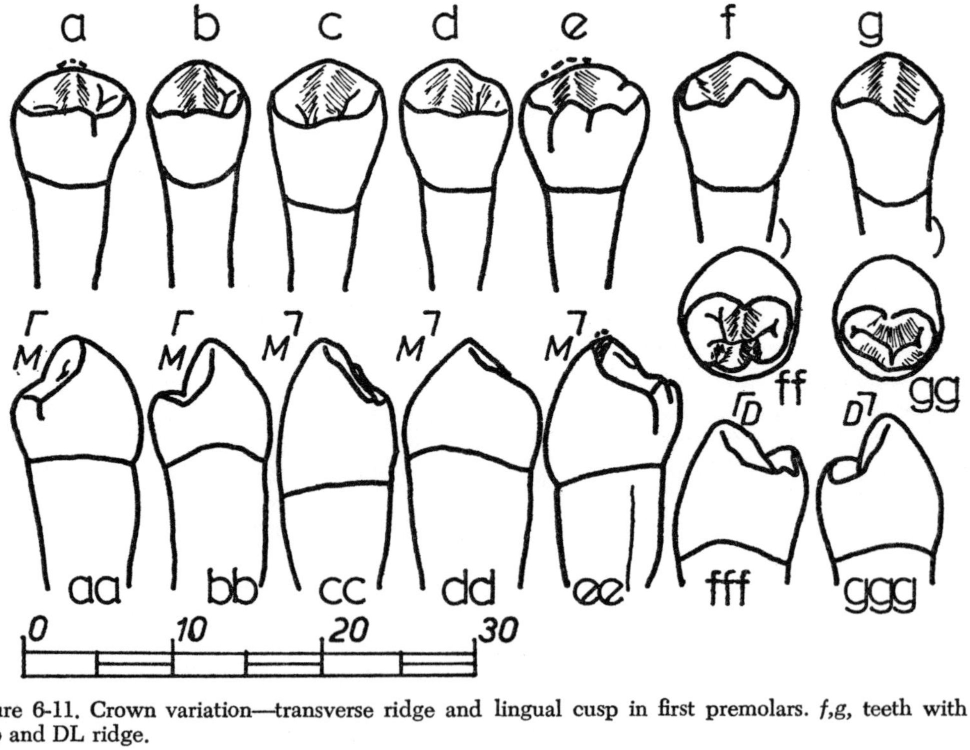

Figure 6-11. Crown variation—transverse ridge and lingual cusp in first premolars. *f,g,* teeth with ML cusp and DL ridge.

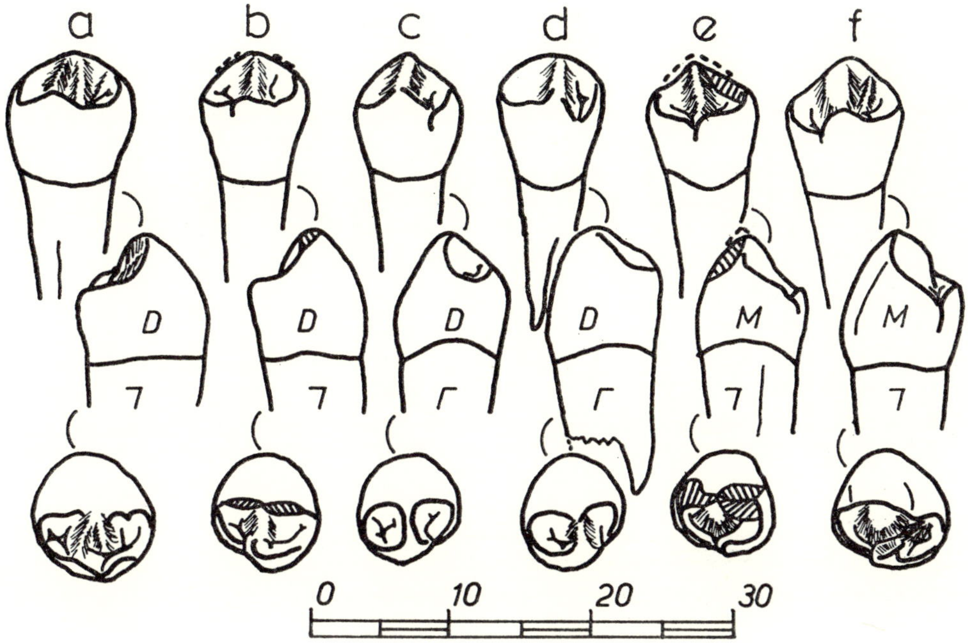

Figure 6-12. Crown variation—transverse and lingual ridge, and absence of lingual cusp in first premolars.

minate teeth are shown in Figure 6-5 *l*, 6-6 *e* and 6-9 *c,f*.

In buccal or lingual view there is not much variation in the angle between the slopes of the cusp, but it does occur. This is illustrated by contrasting outline 6-8 *d* (blunt) with outlines 6-14 *a,b* (more acuminate). All are young teeth, and in the last two mentioned the cusp slopes are more straight; *a* is more obtuse than *b*. This last tooth *b* is the same as outline 6-13 *b* which illustrates a long buccal cusp.

Description of the crown must include variation seen in the outline in occlusal view. Because of the relation of the buccal cusp tip to the tooth axis and the difference in convexity of buccal and lingual outlines in proximal view, the occlusal view of the lower premolar includes part of the buccal surface but none of the lingual surface of the tooth. This is seen in the occlusal outlines in Figures 6-4, 6-5 and 6-12. In these there is recognizable, although often slight, asymmetry in that the greatest B-L diameter is nearer to distal than to mesial.

There is certainly no consistency in the crown proportions M-D and B-L, or in the crown shape in occlusal view, as shown in the many outlines presented here. The term "bucco-lingually compressed" has been applied to the more extreme form shown in Figure 6-31 *g*, which is one of a number of such teeth in the writer's collection.

A similar form of crown in both second premolars of a Japanese boy is figured by Suzuki and Sakai (1960). Using their descriptive term one may cite those cases shown in Figures 6-5 *g*, 6-14 *e,f,g*, and 6-31 *b,e* as less extreme. But one might just as reasonably refer also to mesiodistal compression, as in Figures 6-5 *i* and 6-14 *i,j*. And again there are others that are so asymmetrical as to give the impression that they may have been compressed obliquely as in Figures 6-14 *h* and 6-31 *c,d*, if the term

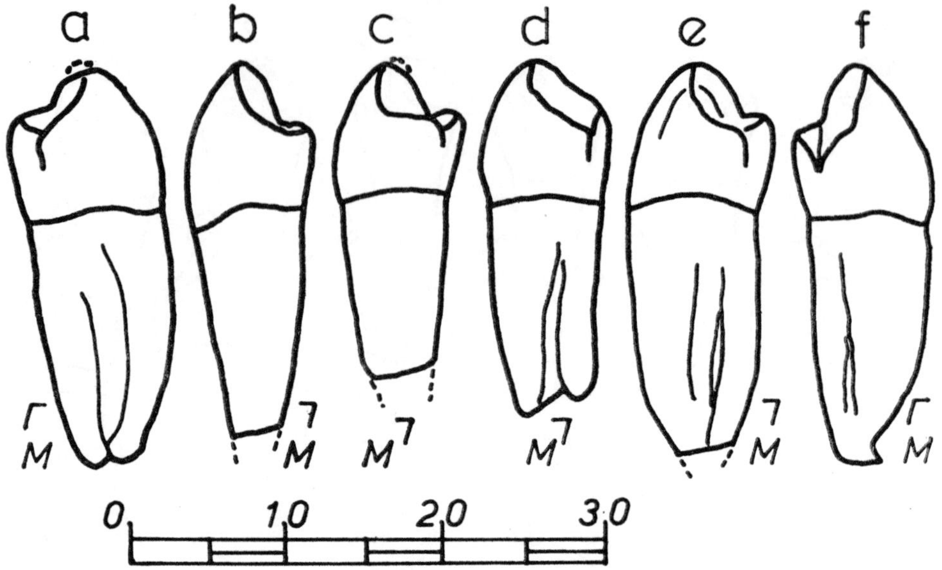

Figure 6-13. Crown and root variation—cleft groove, true lingual cusp and pseudo-cusp in first premolars.

compression is indeed justified at all in describing these teeth.

This variation in lower premolars bears no similarity whatever to that in upper molars, which I have described as compressed, i.e. teeth which are flattened mesiodistally and sometimes distorted, or concave mesially (Figs. 7-2 *e*, 7-5 *g,j*, 7-6 *b,f,k*, 7-18 *e*, 7-19 *d*, 7-20 *c*, 7-24 *d* and 7-34 *b*). In some of these molars the visual impression of compression is strong, perhaps the more so where the DP cusp appears "pushed

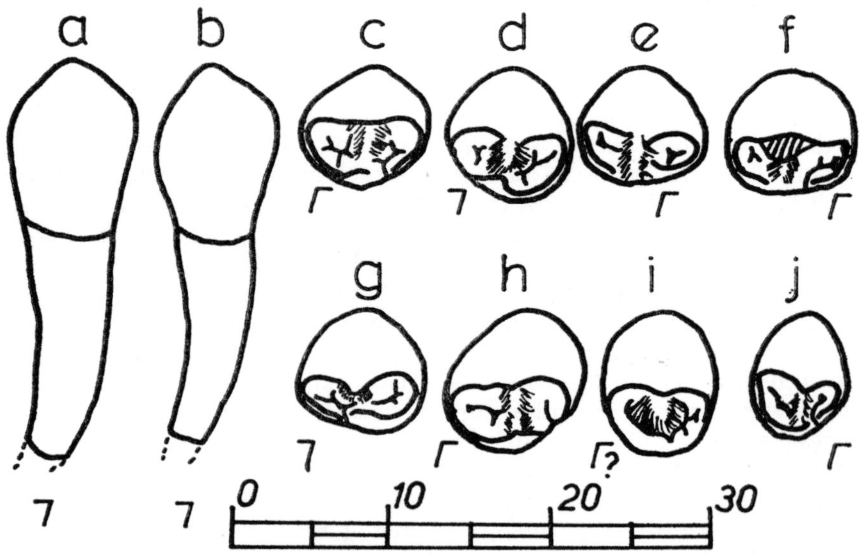

Figure 6-14. Crown variation—cusp acumination. Crown proportions in occlusal view in first premolars.

round" to lie palatally of the larger MP cusp. Moreover, in early development of second and third molars, as will be shown, it is not difficult to imagine anatomical relationships that could produce the compressed effect. In lower premolars there are no such relations.

The majority of lower premolars, however, both first and second, are approximately symmetrical in this view, as will be observed in many of the outlines in Figures 6-14, 6-15, 6-26, 6-27 and 6-28. These, with the asymmetrical, and the so-called "compressed" teeth, therefore form a series as regards variation in these characters. The majority do perhaps tend to be a little greater in the B-L dimension. The selection of some of the more extreme examples from that part of the series where the B-L dimension is shorter than the M-D dimension, and then the assignment of genetic or ethnic significance to their form, would be difficult to justify.

Reference has been made to variety presented as regards prominence of the triangular or transverse ridge which descends from the buccal cusp tip on its lingual, occlusal and proximal outlines already presented. In some views it is apparent that the ridge passes without interruption from buccal to lingual (Figs. 6-3 *e*, 6-5 *l*, 6-6 *d,e*, 6-7 *b,f*, 6-10 *b,c,d*, 6-11 *c* and 6-12 *c,d*). An unusual pattern of continuity is seen in Figure 6-15 *a* where a groove passes to lingual on each side of the ridge. An unusual pattern of discontinuity of the ridge is seen in Figure 6-12 *e* where there is no trace of a lingual cusp, but in its place is a groove which interrupts the lingual ridge. This transverse ridge varies in height and in width and in the distance it extends from buccal towards the lingual side of the tooth. It may be nearly parallel-sided or have divergent sides, sometimes wider at buccal end and sometimes wider towards lingual. In proximal view its contour may be convex, straight or concave. In occlusal view it may be single or have accessory ridges diverging from it or converging towards it in a bucco-lingual direction. In occlusal view also it may pass obliquely towards lingual, or straight across (Fig. 6-15 *b* and *c* respectively). The crest of the ridge may be relatively fine or sharp (Fig. 6-12 *a*), or it may be wide and

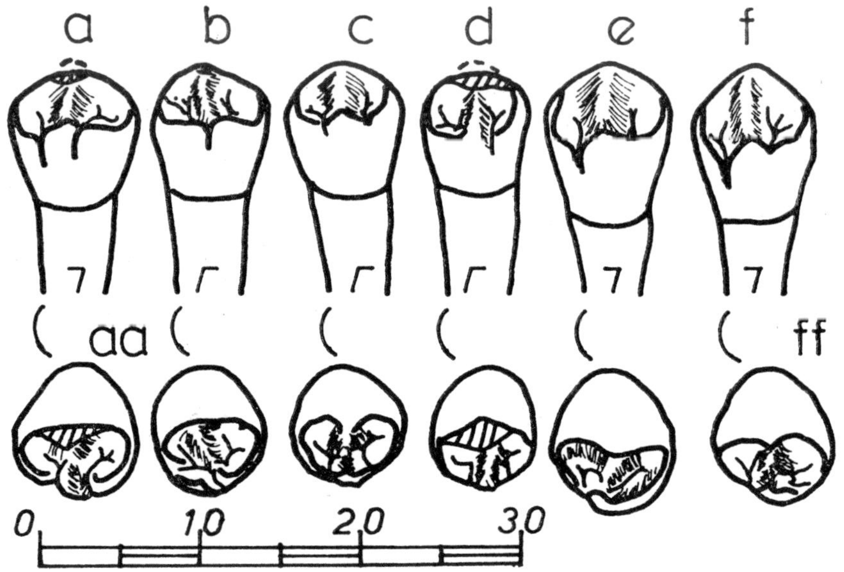

Figure 6-15. Crown variation—lingual ridge and transverse ridge. Lingual and occlusal views in first premolars.

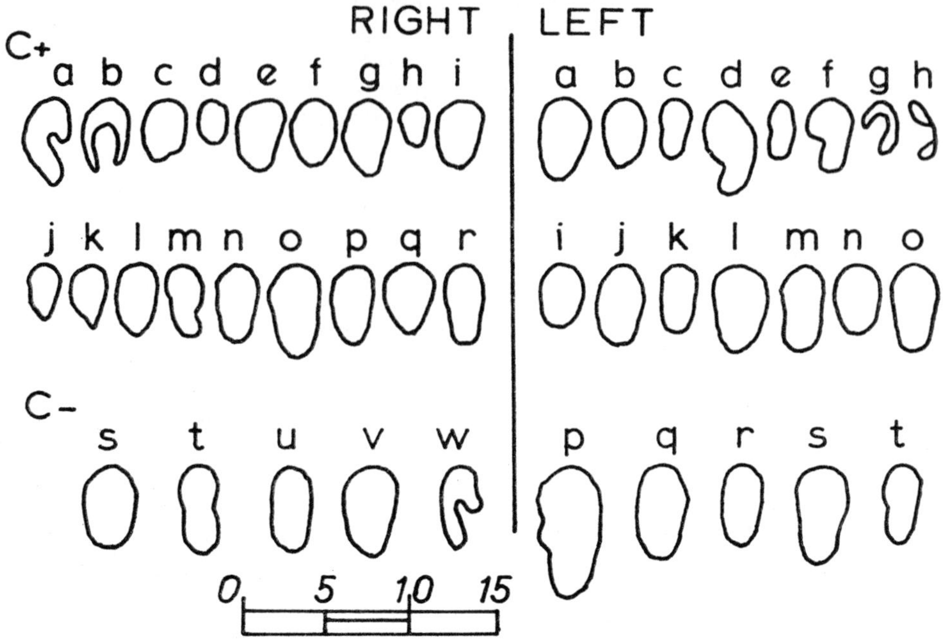

Figure 6-16. Root shape in young teeth. End outlines of incomplete roots in first premolars.

rounded in its cross-section (Fig. 6-15 *c*). Obliquity of the ridge may pass from buccal towards mesial, thus making the anterior portion of the occlusal surface smaller than the posterior portion, as in Figure 6-15 *b*, but this is not always so. The ridge may be virtually absent. If other reasonable variations can be imagined it seems likely that teeth could be found presenting them.

ROOT OF LOWER FIRST PREMOLARS

It has been shown that there is much variation in features of the crown of lower first premolars; also much variation is found in the root. Some of the characters in root variety appear closely related to crown variation, such as the shape in transverse section of the cervix and the relative lengths of mesio-distal and bucco-lingual diameters. In the majority of these teeth the bucco-lingual diameter is the greater, and like other single-rooted teeth the minor diameter is usually nearer to buccal than to lingual. A good idea of the shape of roots in transverse section may be simply obtained by studying the shape of the incompleted roots of young teeth which have been extracted for orthodontic reasons. Some of these are shown in Figure 6-16. These have been presented in two groups according to whether the completed root is longer than the height of the crown from cusp to cervix (C+), or whether it is equal to or less than that height (C–). Difference in size of these outlines bears little relation to the actual size of the tooth but it tends to indicate the extent of root development—the greater the portion of the root that has been formed, the smaller is the outline, as the root tapers on approaching its apex and completion.

In Figure 6-16 some outlines, right and left, are known pairs, i.e. each from the same person. Among these it is of interest to note bilateral asymmetry in several cases. The following are examples (right, then left): *p,m; t,q; w,t*.

Where the crown is longer in its M-D axis, as in Figure 6-14 *c-h,* the transverse

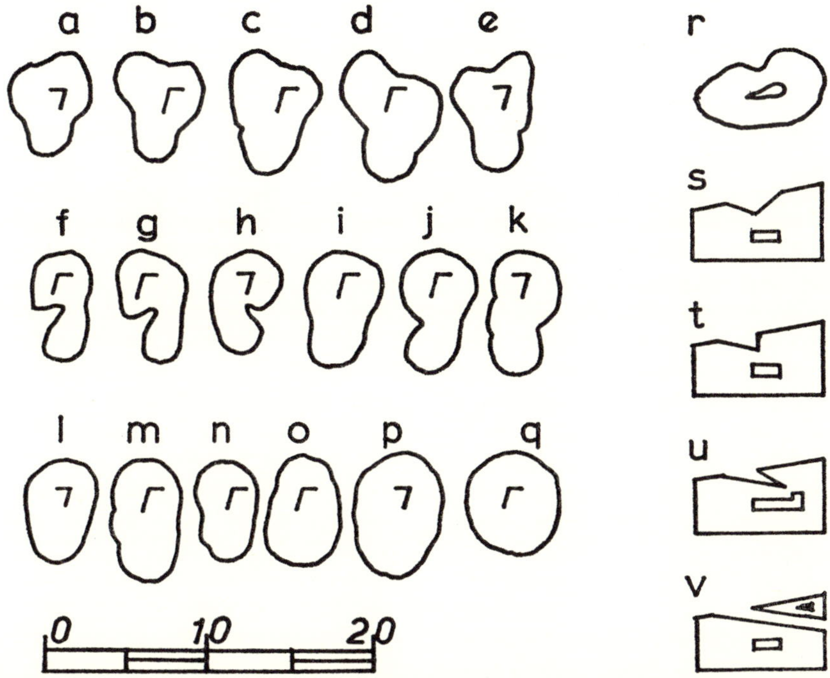

Figure 6-17. The circumferential outlines *a-q* correspond to transverse sections at approximately midway between cervix and apex. Orientation as viewed from root end and with buccal towards top of figure. *a-e*, roots with grooves on M,D and B, suggesting three fused root elements. The MB element is nearer to buccal than the DB element. *f-k*, roots without B groove, and the M or oblique groove more prominent. *l-q*, roots with only shallow grooves or no grooves at all at this level. *r-v*, diagrams illustrating asymmetry of root grooving and root division as the oblique groove on mesial surface varies in depth. *s*, straight-line representation of root lightly grooved as in *r* (hypothetical) or *j* (actual case). *u*, deep oblique groove, as in *f,g,h*. *v*, representing complete bifurcation of root.

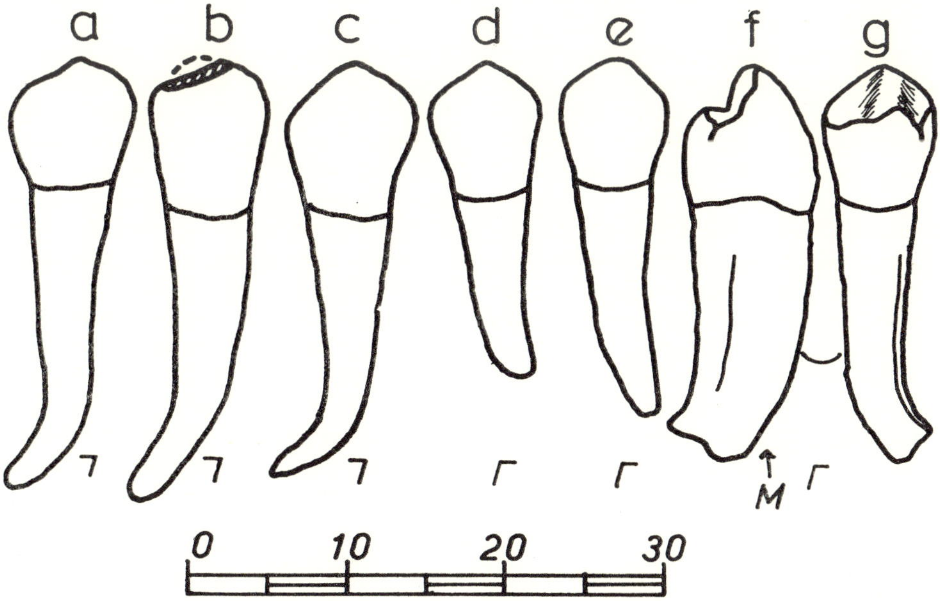

Figure 6-18. Root bends. *a-e*, roots with single bend to distal as seen from buccal. *f,g*, mesial and lingual outlines of a tooth having an abrupt bend to mesial and lingual in the apical region. The apex is flattened and almost bifid and there appears to be an apical foramen on each tip. This region has a twisted appearance.

section of the root does not always follow suit. In teeth *c,d,g,h* of that figure the longer axis at the cervix is B-L. In teeth *e,f* the two axes are approximately equal. In teeth *i,j* the B-L axis is much greater than the M-D axis, as would be expected. This is also the relation of the axes in roots which present a cleft-like groove on the mesial surface. Where there is also a groove on the buccal aspect of the root, the transverse section may be of the style of Figure 6-17 *a-e*. Outlines *a* to *q* in this figure were made by placing a loop of fine copper wire held by artery forceps over the root, approximately half-way between cervix and apex. The loop was made to conform with the tooth surface by a combination of twisting to tighten and burnishing to conform with grooves. The tooth was placed apex upwards under the camera lucida, and a tracing was made of the wire loop *in situ*. Diagrams *r* to *v* relate to variations in depth of the oblique groove and are explained in the legend to the figure.

The roots of these teeth, like others already studied, often present changes in direction of root axis, when viewed from proximal or buccal, and these may be called curves or bends. They may involve a considerable portion of the root, or a shorter portion near the apex. These bends or curves are found in short or long roots and some idea of the variety in which they occur may be gained from the outlines presented in Figures 6-18, 6-19, 6-20 and 6-21.

In Figure 6-18 *a-e*, buccal views show single bends in short and long roots, a long curve in some and a more abrupt change of direction in others. In Figure 6-19 are shown double bends. In teeth *a,b* the bend is first to M and later to D. In the remainder the reverse is the case. In the first five teeth the root tapers to a fine or medium thickness, but tooth *f* has a much thicker root.

Returning to Figure 6-18, outlines *f,g* give two views of an unusual variety of bend, of which there were several examples in the collection. It involves the apical region of the tooth, which is broad and somewhat flattened and has a twisted appearance. In other words the bend cannot properly be shown in a buccal or proximal view. In the absence of any history one can only suggest that these root forms might have been related to a malocclusion where the erupting tooth has been deflected.

In Figure 6-20 there is no particular character of bend common to each tooth, but certain details are worthy of note as possibly indicating some factor responsible for change of direction in root axes. A radiograph of tooth *a* before extraction shows the inferior dental foramen midway between the roots of the premolars, each root curving away from the foramen. Close relation to this structure appears to explain the bend to M in this first premolar. The abrupt bend to M in tooth *b* might well be explained in the same way.

Tooth *c* in this figure was extracted from a subject aged $13\frac{11}{12}$ years because it had been "crowded out" and was in buccal occlusion. The complex curve in its root may well be the result of changed direction of the tooth as it erupted into this position of malocclusion. Tooth *d* presents a root curved to D, but a radiograph before extraction (age $14\frac{4}{12}$ years) shows that it would be more correct to describe the apical portion as erect, and the rest of the root, with the crown, as deflected to D. In the course of eruption the tooth was deflected from the canine, and its crown became partly impacted under the mesial surface of the second premolar.

Outlines *e,f* of Figure 6-20 represent right and left first premolars extracted at ages $12\frac{10}{12}$ and $13\frac{7}{12}$ respectively. Radiograph at the earlier age led to deferment of extraction of the left tooth until it became more accessible. A radiograph at an even younger age had disclosed uneven absorption of roots of deciduous molars on this side of the mouth and deflection of the premolars. It seems likely that this

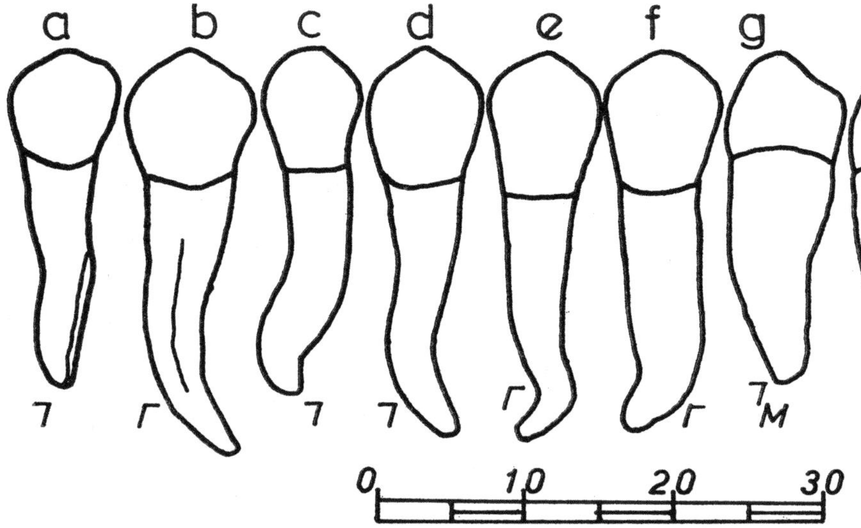

Figure 6-19. Roots with double bend as viewed from buccal. *a,b* bend first to M and then apex to D. *c-f* bend first to D and then apex to M. Tooth *f* has a thick root. *g* and *h* are mesial views of teeth *a* and *c* respectively.

accounts for the root asymmetry in this pair of first premolars. Tooth *g* is one of a pair presenting asymmetry of roots. The root of the left tooth is straight, and the D bend in the right tooth shown was evidently associated with different anatomical relationships in the two teeth. There is no case history with this pair of teeth.

It is not uncommon to find a lower premolar in which the root curves lingually,

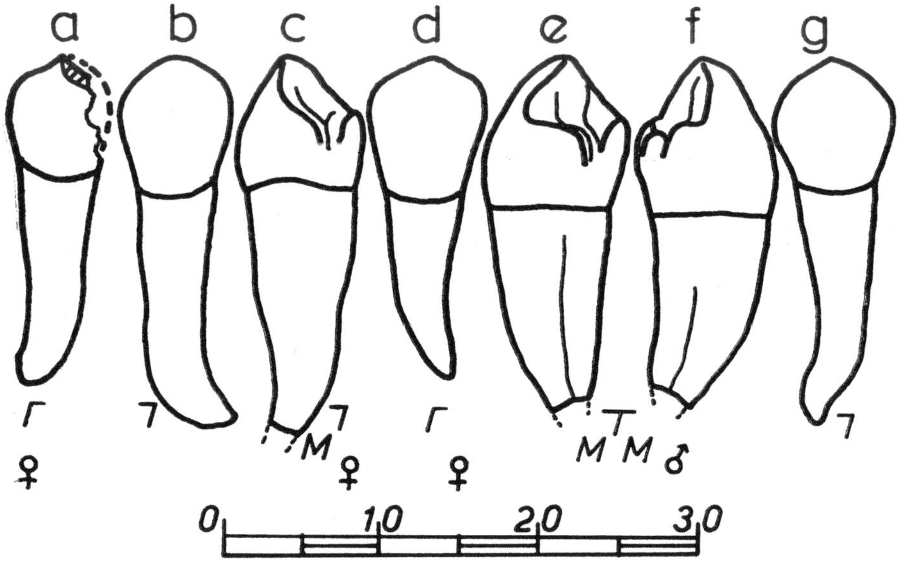

Figure 6-20. Roots with bend related to known malocclusion or radiograph.

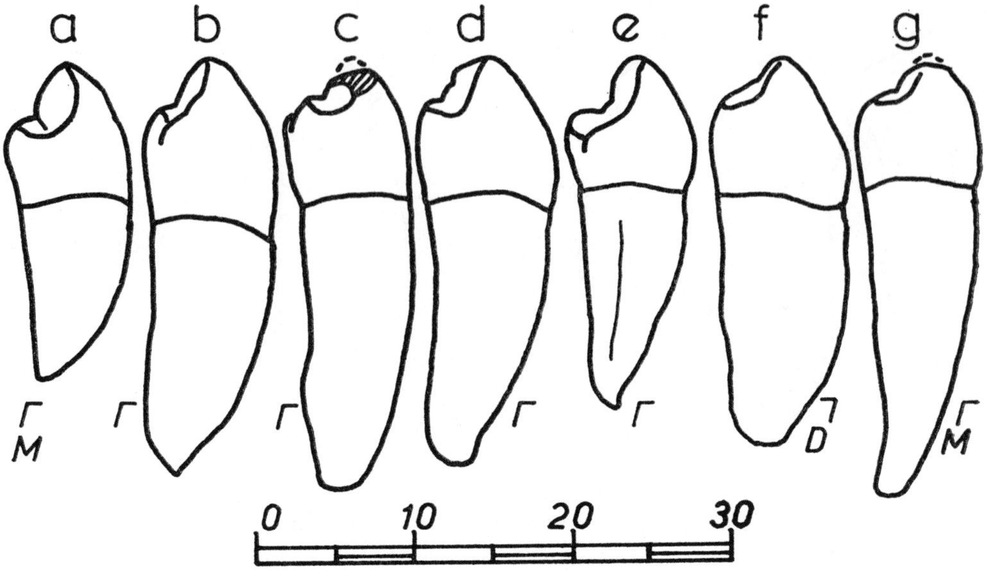

Figure 6-21. Root or root axis apparently curved to lingual in proximal view.

but sometimes the curve is more apparent than real. When in proximal view the root taper is on the buccal side as in Figure 6-21 *e,f*, the root apparently curves to lingual. In Figure 6-9 *e* and Figure 6-21 *a-d* the root axis is bent and the curve to lingual is real. At least some of these cases may well have been associated with malocclusion in which the erupting tooth has been crowded out and deflected lingually—the reverse of the known deflection of the tooth in Figure 6-20 *c*. In the writer's experience he has gained the impression that in such deflections of lower premolars it

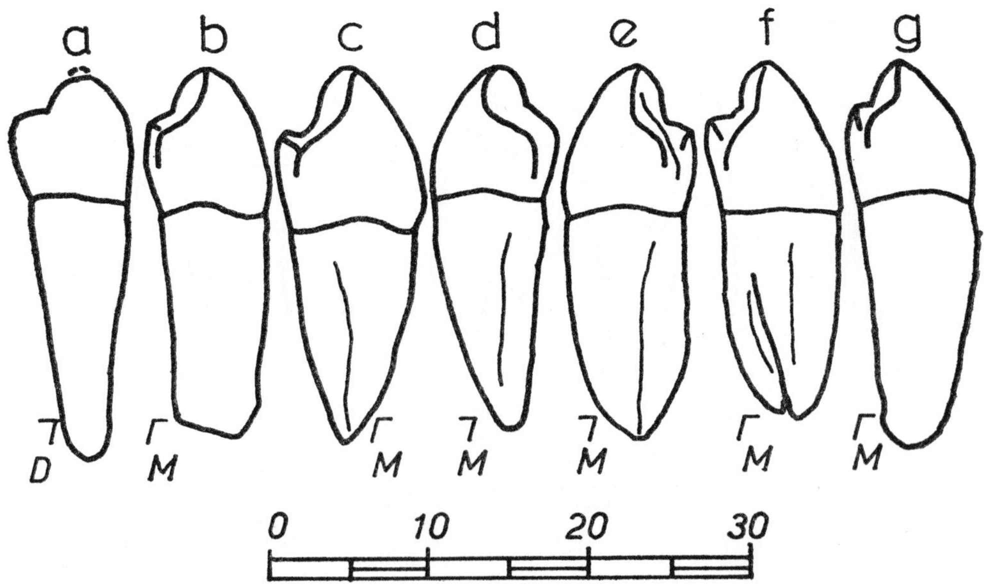

Figure 6-22. Variation in outlines in "straight" roots, in apex and in root groove, from proximal.

is more usual for the first premolar to erupt buccally and the second premolar lingually. Other examples of lingual curves are seen in Figures 6-7 *a,b* and 6-20 *f*.

Roots that are straight rather than curved may present much variety in proximal outline, as in Figure 6-22. Tooth *a* tapers evenly in straight outlines to a rather fine apex, but tooth *b* has a much broader apex. Tooth *c* tapers evenly with curved outlines to a fine apex and tooth *d* tapers unevenly on one outline to give the apparent bend referred to for Figure 6-21 *e,f*. It has a fine apex, but a somewhat similar curvature of outline in *g* is associated with a broad thick apex. Teeth *e,f* have uneven, almost bulbous, root outlines and blunt-pointed apices associated with a cleft-type groove on the mesial surface.

Grooves and Clefts in Roots of Lower First Premolars

This cleft-type groove is relatively common in lower first premolars. It is found in varying degrees of depth from slight to complete penetration or bifidity of the root. In these cases the tooth has a minor branch usually placed mesio-buccally. The separation of roots passes obliquely in this MB direction as also does the cleft when division is not complete. In many of these teeth the cleft is more prominent in approximately the middle third of the root and may be much less obvious in the apical and cervical thirds of the root. It passes in an oblique direction from its apical portion towards the lingual cervix, which however it does not reach. It often appears to be in line with the small groove which frequently interrupts the anterior marginal ridge of the occlusal surface.

This cleft in the mesial surface of first premolar roots serves as a useful identification feature, especially where the crown is damaged by wear or trauma or caries. It is different from the grooves that have been described in other single-rooted teeth. In those teeth the grooves tend to be longitudinal rather than oblique, to be almost

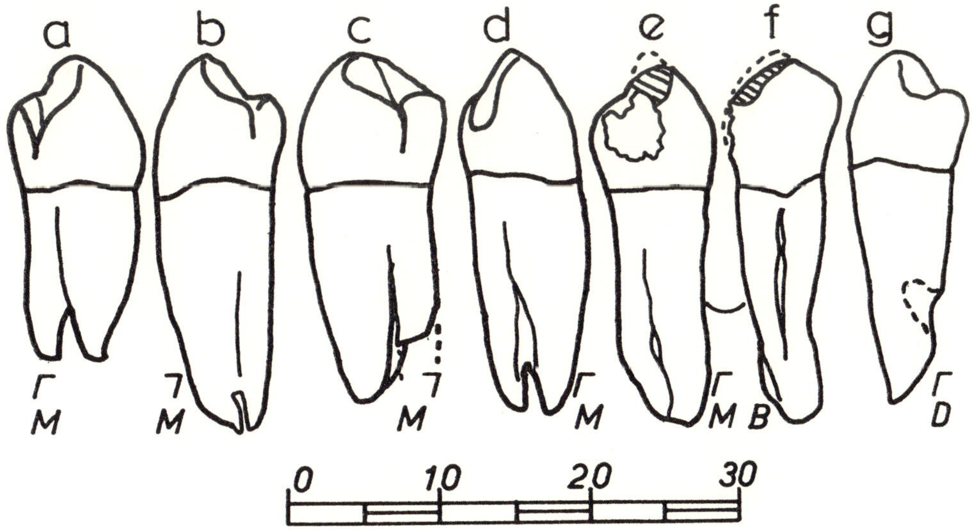

Figure 6-23. Root grooves, and root branching in lower first premolars. *a*, prominent cleft groove, approximately in line with mesial pit groove—the relationship commonly found. The cleft groove here is prominent and the root is branched. There is no buccal groove. *b*, unusual form of bifid apex. Cleft and pit grooves very lightly indicated. *c*, root strongly bifid, and very light buccal groove. *d*, deep and prominent cleft groove, bifid apex, no buccal groove or pit groove. *e,f*, prominent cleft and buccal grooves, but single apex. Caries of mesial surface. *g*, tooth with broad shallow groove passing somewhat spirally from distal surface to lingual.

evenly placed between labial and lingual, and to be approximately symmetrical in transverse section, as in diagram *r* and *s* of Figure 6-17. Diagram *s* is the straight-line version of diagram *r*.

By contrast, the cleft type of groove found in lower first premolars may be represented by diagrams *t,u,v* of Figure 6-17. Diagram *t* shows the asymmetry of the groove compared with *s*, and represents a moderate degree of development of the cleft-type groove. Diagram *u* represents a greater degree, and diagram *v* represents a full cleft and a MB branch of the root. This style of root division appears analogous to that found in the lower premolars of some anthropoids.

Actual division of the root trunk into root branches is uncommon in the lower first premolars but grooves suggesting a tendency to division are common, and they vary in position and style. The cleft-like groove has already received some attention. It may be present with or without the groove in the marginal ridge as has just been mentioned (Figs. 6-13 *a* and 6-12 *a* respectively). That marginal ridge groove may be present with or without the cleft groove (Figs. 6-13 *a*, 6-22 *f* and 6-9 *c,g* respectively). There may be actual bifidity of the root with little or no trace of the cleft groove (Fig. 6-23 *b*, and other teeth on card Q 33 but not figured). The root branches may be relatively long (Fig. 6-23 *c*) or actually short in the presence of a long deep cleft (Fig. 6-23 *d*).

In addition to the cleft groove on the mesial surface there may be grooves in the distal and buccal surfaces. The approximate shape of some of these roots in transverse section is indicated in the freehand end-view drawings of Figure 6-17 *a-e*. Two outlines of the root of Figure 6-17 *b* are shown in Figure 6-23 *e,f*. Some of these roots indicate a tendency to form three root branches, but one which was sectioned had only one pulp canal. That it is possible for lower premolars to present not only three pulp canals but three separate root branches is reported by Armitage (1971). In his case each of the four first premolars had three roots. Goh (1957) de-

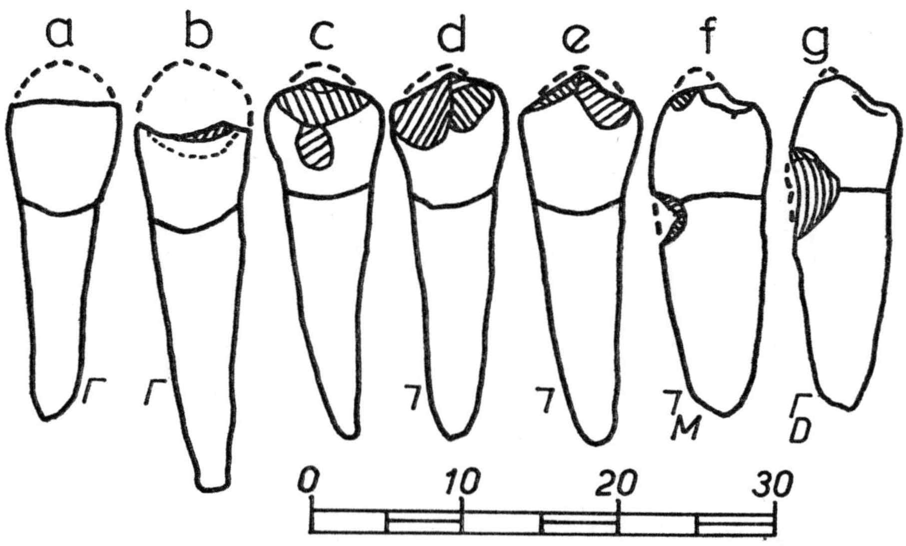

Figure 6-24. Varieties of wear in first premolars. *a*, flat occlusal. *b*, cupped occlusal. *c*, one facet extending down buccal surface. *d*, two buccal facets meeting in a ridge. *e*, two facets involving chiefly the buccal cusp ridges. *f,g*, cervical abrasions from toothbrushing; *f*, a deep sharp notch, and *g*, a wider shallow groove.

scribes grooves and division in roots of lower premolars. Ignoring crowns and many variable characters of roots described herein, he creates a classification of several basic forms, but the classes are filled to overflowing with combinations and variations in development of the characters selected.

A quite different kind of groove is shown in Figure 6-23 *g*. In this tooth a broad shallow groove passes part way around the root in an oblique or spiral manner from the distal surface down to the lingual surface. Below this groove the apical part of the root has a slight bend to buccal and mesial. It is likely that this part of the root was close to the branching of the inferior dental canal to form the mental foramen, but there is no radiograph to confirm this.

WEAR IN FIRST PREMOLARS

As with other teeth already considered, the effects of wear are varied in regard to the degree of loss of tooth substance and to the position and shape of facets produced. Some of these are illustrated in Figure 6-24. In tooth *a* the whole of the buccal cusp has been worn away evenly, leaving a virtually flat level surface or facet. The occlusion in this case would be "edge-to-edge," and the amount of tissue removed would grade this as second-degree wear on Broca's Scale. Tooth *b* presents third-degree wear as defined in the writer's modification of Broca's Scale (Taylor, 1962b) because secondary dentine has been reached. The form of the facet also is different in this tooth for the dentine is deeply cupped below an enamel rim. Wear in this case is approximately even on all surfaces as in the edge-to-edge wear in tooth *a*.

In tooth *c* there is a single but oblique facet which extends lowest on the buccal surface. Wear is early second-degree, since it has just reached dentine, and it was probably worn against one opposing tooth. In tooth *d* it appears that two opposing teeth were involved and that protrusive movements were minimal. The two resulting facets are confined to the buccal surface and they meet in a ridge. Although these facets are relatively large, enamel only is worn and the wear is therefore first-degree. Tooth *e* presents some features of wear similar to tooth *d*. Two facets meet in a ridge maintaining a cusp-like profile. Less enamel has been worn away and there was less overbite, for wear involves cusp ridges rather than buccal surface. The buccal surface, however, has been polished by toothbrushing; but other surfaces present stain; and there is salivary calculus on the mesial surface and at the buccal cervix.

Since buccal surfaces of premolars are readily accessible to the toothbrush, these teeth often present evidence of the abrasion and other traumatic effects of toothbrush bristles, abrasive dentifrices and faulty toothbrushing technique. Two examples are shown in Figure 6-24 *f*,*g*. In each tooth a notch has been worn at the buccal cervix. In tooth *f* the notch is relatively narrow and deep with sharply defined margins. In *g* the notch is much wider and relatively shallow with rounded margins; it extends to the disto-buccal surface of the root. This uneven placing of the notch suggests that the tooth was slightly twisted from normal alignment in the arch. The production of these notches has been associated with injury to the soft tissues and recession of alveolar support in the regions involved.

CERVIX OF FIRST PREMOLARS

On proximal surfaces the cervical line tends to be almost straight or arched slightly towards occlusal. No particular difference was observed in height of arch or in level of cervix that could be useful in distinguishing between mesial and distal as was noted in canines and some incisors.

LOWER SECOND PREMOLARS

The second lower premolar, like the first, presents considerable morphological variation, especially in the crown. While the first often has a rather prominent

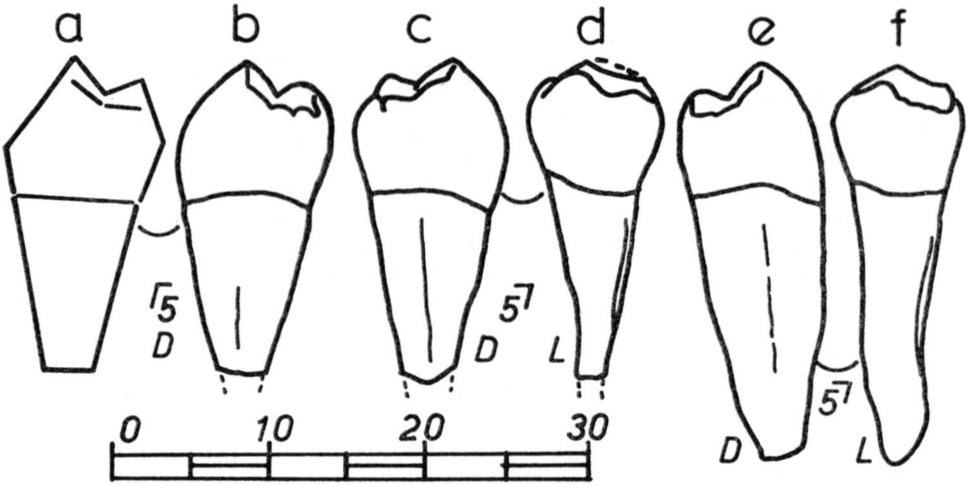

Figure 6-25. Crown contours in second premolars. *a,* the same tooth as *b,* but drawn in straight line diagrammatic form to show different proportions of B and L profiles. *c,d,* distal and lingual views of the tooth that paired with *b*. These are two young teeth with incomplete roots, each having a prominent ML cusp and DL ridge. Each cusp has a prominent transverse or triangular ridge, and these ridges meet at a col which separates the anterior and posterior portions of the occlusal surface. The posterior portion is the larger (Fig. 6-26 *a*), and these asymmetrical features in lingual and occlusal view assist identification of the tooth as left or right. *e,f,* tooth with similar occlusal features but the crown is longer and less convex. The root is thicker and complete. The occlusal is shown in Figure 6-26 *b*.

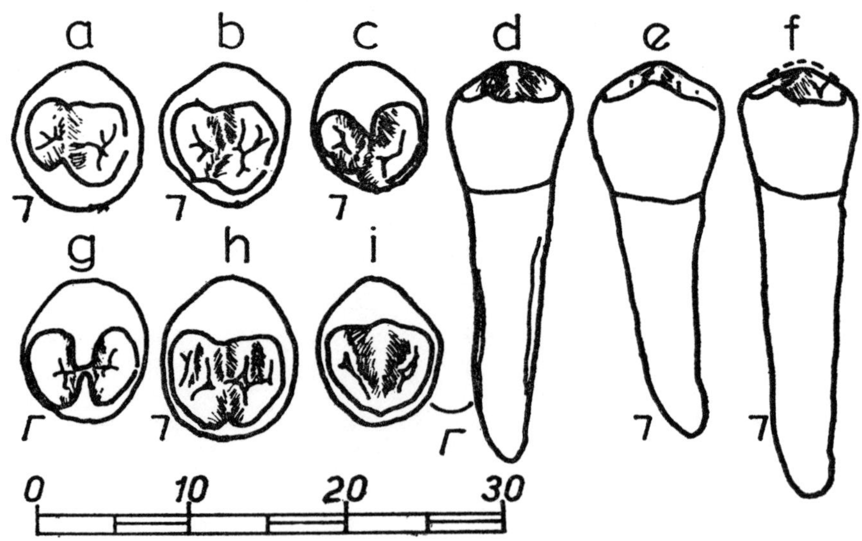

Figure 6-26. Variations in convexity of crown outlines and lingual cusp. Outlines *di* are of one tooth, as also *eh*. Second premolars.

transverse occlusal ridge, and sometimes no trace of a lingual cusp, the second premolar has a less prominent transverse ridge. There is always a recognizable lingual border or limitation to the occlusal surface, whether in the form of ridge or cusp or both, and there may be two well-defined lingual cusps. There is less difference in height between cusp tip and occlusal grooves, since the lingual surface rises higher, and the occlusal surface faces more upward or is less tilted in the second premolar.

If one has both premolars from one person there should be no difficulty in distinguishing between first and second. The range of variation in each tooth "overlaps" in some characters so that in the case of an isolated tooth it is sometimes difficult to determine which it is. The difficulty may more easily arise in teeth that have no "cleft" groove on the root, or that have been modified by wear or caries involving the occlusal surface.

CROWN OF SECOND PREMOLARS

In proximal view, like other lower teeth, the buccal outline is very convex. In premolars this brings the buccal cusp tip close to the line of the root axis and makes the crown appear to lean lingually, although the lingual outline is shorter, less convex and more upright than the buccal. Another way to describe the buccal outline is to say that it presents an obtuse angle at the junction of the cervical and middle thirds. The cervical third follows approximately the line of taper of the root, while the remaining two thirds approach the produced root axis. This character (which is also seen in the first premolar) is shown in the diagram and outline (Fig. 6-25 *a* and *b* respectively).

Outlines *b,c* are distal views of left and right second premolars, in each of which there is a well-formed lingual cusp towards ML and a lingual ridge at DL. The lingual outline of tooth *c* is shown in *d*. These are young teeth with the apex still incomplete. Outlines *e,f* are distal and lingual views of another right second premolar. The crown of this tooth is relatively longer, less bulbous and more erect. Like the previous teeth it has a cusp and ridge on the lingual surface.

The occlusal surfaces of these last two teeth are shown in Figure 6-26 *a,b*. In each there is a transverse or triangular ridge passing between the cusps but interrupted by shallow grooves ascending from anterior and posterior occlusal pits or grooves. This point of interruption usually marks also a change in direction so that the ridge from the lingual cusp (which is nearer the M than D surface) passes obliquely to meet the ridge from B cusp. This obliquity, and the asymmetry whereby the anterior portion of occlusal surface is smaller than the posterior portion, are two of the most useful characters in distinguishing M from D in the tooth, and left teeth from right teeth. Associated with these is the tendency for the larger posterior area to be lower than the anterior portion. In tooth *c* the interruption in the ridge is much less noticeable, but it is still possible to distinguish obliquity in the lingual part and asymmetry of the occlusal areas.

In tooth *g* the ridge is interrupted, but in occlusal view one cannot recognize either obliquity of ridge or asymmetry of area, or difference in level of areas, so that identification is difficult. The lingual cusp is not prominent, but in lingual view the contour is that of a left tooth rather than a right. The pattern of this lingual ridge contour is one of "levels" and is like that of tooth *f* but in reverse, for *f* is from right side.

Tooth *d,i* presents another problem in identification. There is no lingual cusp but there is a prominent transverse ridge which has been completely "annexed" by the buccal cusp. The slight asymmetry in occlusal view would identify this tooth as left side.

Tooth *e,h* has a recognizable cusp. The transverse ridge is interrupted by a deep col, but it is scarcely oblique; the usual asymmetry is not recognizable in occlusal view. A slight difference in occlusal levels and the pattern of ridge in lingual view lead to the conclusion that this is a right tooth. This tooth presents bulbous or concavo-convex contours in B or L profile, very different from those in tooth *f*. This last tooth *f* has a slightly worn buccal cusp, a small lingual cusp, well-defined obliquity in the transverse ridge and differences in occlusal levels. Occlusal asymmetry is apparent, and it is easily and positively identified as from right side.

Analysis of transverse and lingual ridges is continued in Figure 6-27. The young tooth *a,b* has a bulbous crown with a well-developed lingual cusp placed nearly centrally and comprising almost all the lingual contour. There is a prominent transverse or triangular ridge from each cusp, the lingual portion being not appreciably oblique. The two portions of the ridge are separated by a deep col so that there is virtually a continuous groove from anterior to posterior occlusal pits. All cusp ridges and marginal ridges are very rounded and contrast strongly with those of tooth *c*. This tooth has sharply-defined ridges. It also has a prominent lingual cusp, but the two cusp tips are widely spaced so that the occlusal surface "proper" takes up more than usual of the occlusal view of the tooth which is also noteworthy for its straightened outlines. It is strange therefore that the crown of this tooth may be described as short and bulbous in lingual view.

Tooth *d* also has a bulbous crown but in other respects it is very different from the two preceding teeth. It has no lingual cusp but there is a broad and somewhat flattened ridge extending right around the lingual from the two shoulders of the buccal cusp in a horseshoe shape. The crescentic occlusal groove encloses an irregular but prominent transverse ridge descending from the buccal cusp. There is no difficulty in noting asymmetry and difference in height of parts of the occlusal surface and therefore in recognition of the tooth as from the left side.

The ridges in these three teeth *b,c,d,* present a variation in character that may be described as a personal or "family" characteristic of the dentition to which each belonged. In the first the ridges are smoothly rounded. In the second they are relatively prominent and sharp-crested. In the third the ridge is flattened along its

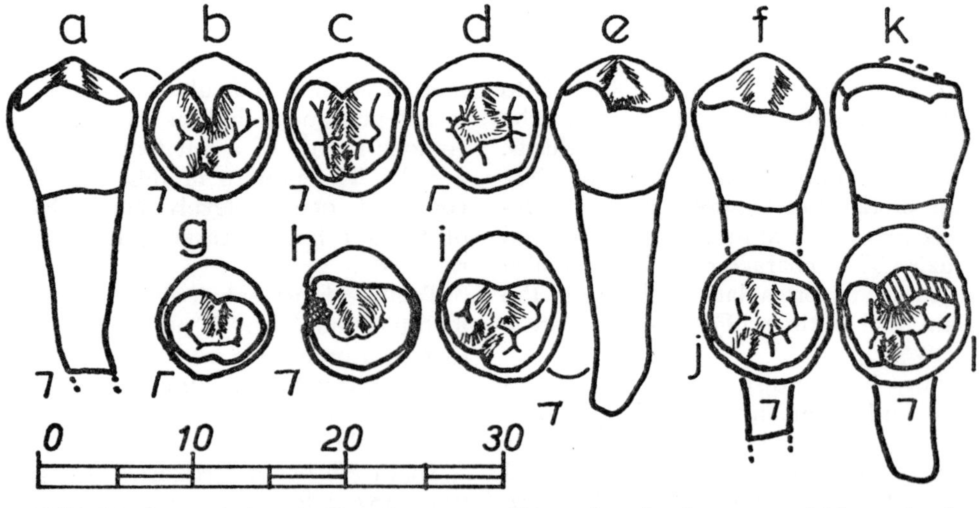

Figure 6-27. Further variations in lingual cusp or ridge and occlusal grooves, which are involved in identification as left or right. Outlines which related to one tooth are *ab,ei,fj,kl*. Second premolars.

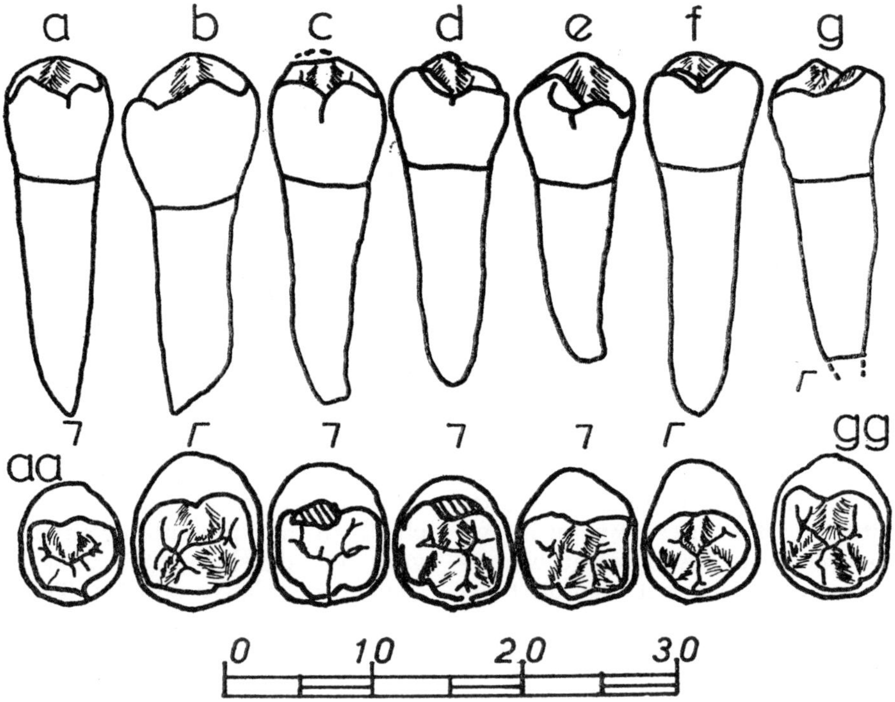

Figure 6-28. The tricuspid crown in second premolars; lingual and occlusal views.

axis so that there is no crest, but it is transversely marked by irregularities that give it a crinkled appearance. Recognition of personal characters in teeth is of importance in deciding whether a particular tooth could or could not belong to the same dentition as other teeth that may be recovered. Ability in such recognition is largely dependent on appreciation of the variations or differences that may be found, and this character of ridges is perhaps a minor one among the many considered in this study.

Figure 6-27 *g,h* depicts two further examples of total absence of lingual cusp or its transverse oblique ridge, and replacement by a crescentic ridge and groove. Tooth *g* has a relatively long root for its small crown, and the buccal transverse ridge is small and flattened. Tooth *h*, by contrast, has a relatively small root and large crown, and the buccal transverse ridge is very prominent. Tooth *g* is clearly from left side, but *h* lacks the diagnostic asymmetry mentioned, and from other features it may be judged as "probably right." Its root has an abrupt but minor bend to buccal.

Teeth *e,i,* and *f,j,* are both from right side. The former has a minor ML cusp and prominent DL ridge. Both its transverse ridges are well-developed and oblique and separated by a deep col, so that there is an anterior pit almost joined to a posterior crescentic groove. Occlusal asymmetry is marked, and the lingual outline *e* is very uneven. In the latter tooth *f* the lingual outline is gently undulating; the almost absent lingual cusp is represented by a low and oblique transverse ridge, and the occlusal groove is crescentic.

Therefore these last two teeth combine, in different proportions, the style of occlusal surfaces found in teeth *b* (with lingual cusp) and *h* (with crescentic groove and ridge and no lingual cusp). Tooth *f,j* has almost the symmetry of *h*. Tooth *e,i* exaggerates the asymmetry of *b* by placing the lingual cusp in ML position, and presenting also a strong DL ridge. A further stage in this variation is the conversion of the DL ridge into a cusp, thus giving the tricuspid variety of lower second premolars.

Tricuspid Crown in Second Premolars

The designation given to this form of crown is not intended to imply that there is a variety of second premolar that is distinct from all others. On the contrary it has just been shown that some teeth which may not even have two distinct cusps do have features of the three-cusp form, and truly tricuspid teeth also present characters of crown and root that identify them as lower premolars. In other words, within the wide variation of second premolars there are many teeth that present features that could be described as tending towards three cusps, as well as those that are clearly tricuspid. It is convenient therefore to adopt the notion of a tricuspid form, with certain characters showing a tendency towards, or away from, this form, as facilitates description.

In most second premolars the buccal cusp with its shoulder ridges is the highest part of the tooth, and the widest part mesio-distally. In some tricuspid teeth the greatest mesio-distal diameter is towards the lingual (Fig. 6-28 *dd*), and the buccal view of such teeth may include a part of the mesial, or more likely part of the distal, surface. In the buccal view of most second premolars however the large buccal cusp is all that is seen, and there is no indication of the variations in detail that may be seen in other views, particularly from lingual and occlusal aspects.

In these views the principal features are cusps, ridges and grooves, and variety arises chiefly in their presence or absence, or degree of development rather than in changes of relative position. This tends to be constant, such as the one cusp that is placed buccally. This cusp varies in length and acumination and its transverse or triangular ridge varies considerably in width, in length, in prominence, and in sharpness or convexity, as was shown for the first premolar. If the lingual cusp is large enough to monopolize the lingual part of

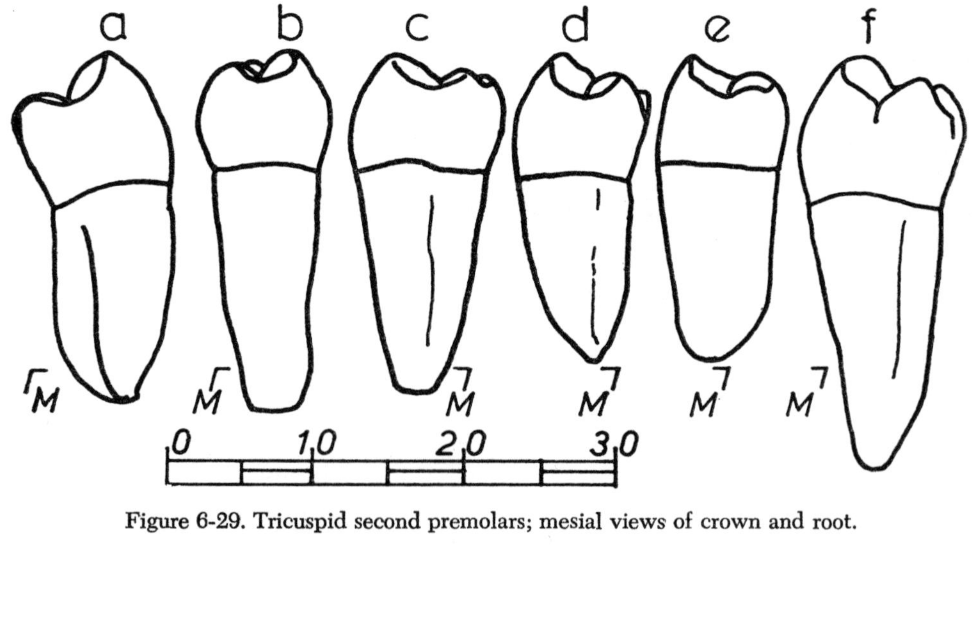

Figure 6-29. Tricuspid second premolars; mesial views of crown and root.

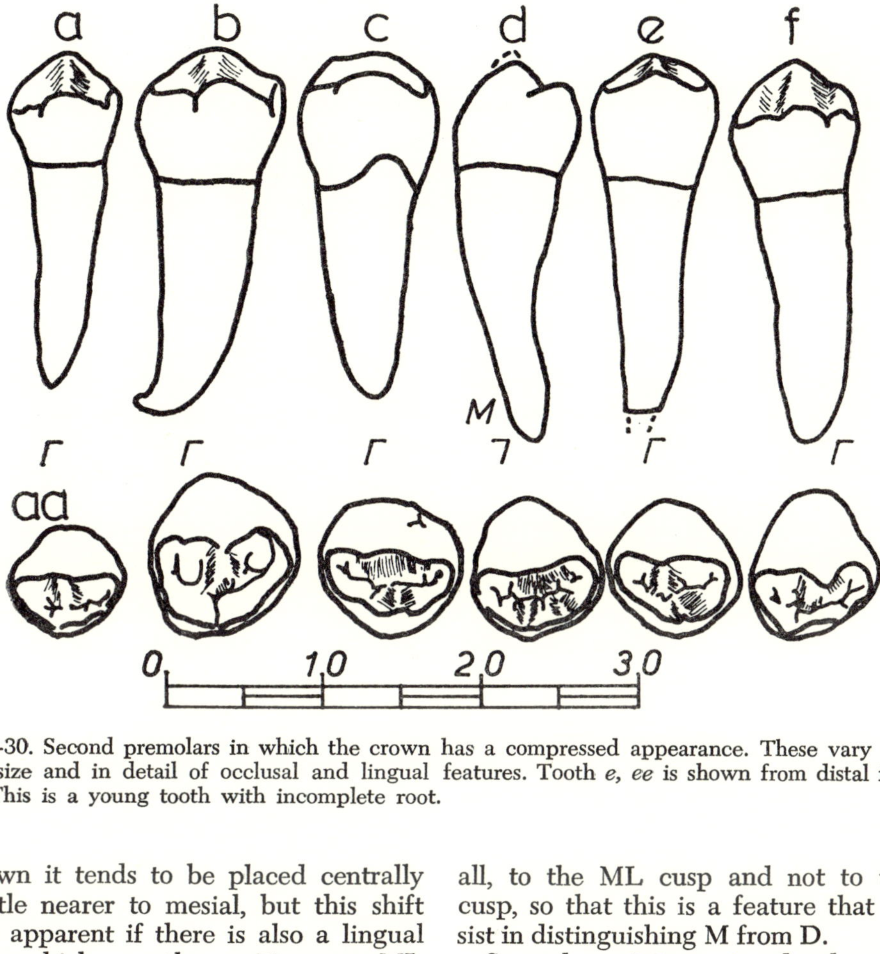

Figure 6-30. Second premolars in which the crown has a compressed appearance. These vary considerably in size and in detail of occlusal and lingual features. Tooth *e, ee* is shown from distal in Figure 6-31 *i*. This is a young tooth with incomplete root.

the crown it tends to be placed centrally or a little nearer to mesial, but this shift is more apparent if there is also a lingual ridge, in which case the positions are ML for the cusp and DL for the ridge. The transverse ridge from the lingual cusp has been shown to be sometimes oblique, passing from the ML position towards the centre of the tooth and often separated from the larger buccal transverse ridge by a V-shaped col (Fig. 6-26 *a,b*).

Where the ML cusp is relatively large this col tends to be replaced by a fissure, but the two transverse ridges may still be readily distinguished (Fig. 6-28 *b*). Where the DL cusp also is prominent it tends to be separated from both other cusps by a fissure. It appears that the transverse ridge from the buccal cusp is connected, if at all, to the ML cusp and not to the DL cusp, so that this is a feature that can assist in distinguishing M from D.

Several variations in development of ML and DL cusps are shown in lingual and occlusal views in Figure 6-28, and in mesial views in Figure 6-29. An indication of the relative sizes of the three cusps may be conveyed by grading them on a three-point scale in order of B, ML and DL cusps respectively. The grading is subjective and cannot be precise, for the further reason that variation occurs in fractional degrees rather than in three units. The grading is rather an overall impression than an assessment of height, thickness and convexity.

In many tricuspid premolars the grading on this basis would be 3-2-1, by which it is intended to imply not that the DL cusp is half as big as the ML cusp, but that it is smaller. In the teeth of Figure 6-28 *a-g*, the suggested gradings are, respectively, 3-2-1, 3-3-1, 3-2-2, 2-2-1, 3-2-1, 2-2-2 and 3-2-1. Tooth *a* is much smaller than tooth *b*, but in each the buccal cusp is graded 3 because it is relatively large. The grading refers only to the relative sizes of cusps in one tooth, and does not compare sizes of a particular cusp as presented by different teeth.

Where the sum of the gradings of the two lingual cusps exceeds that of the buccal cusp, it is likely that the M-D dimension of the crown will be as great on the lingual side as on the buccal (teeth *b,c*). It may be greater on the lingual side, particularly where the buccal cusp is relatively smaller than usual or the lingual cusps are well developed (teeth *d,f*). The rather large tooth *g*, from a girl aged 10 3/12 years, presents a difficulty in grading because the limits of a cusp cannot be defined precisely. The buccal cusp appears rather small but the tooth is wide buccally, for the cusp has unusually prominent shoulders which might almost be called tubercles, and this was a character of other teeth also in this girl's dentition.

In proximal views of tricuspid premolars it is usual to see something of both lingual cusps, but if the DL cusp is small it may not appear in a mesial view (Fig. 6-29 *e*). This tooth was graded 3-2-1. It also has shoulders as just described, but they are not as prominent as those in tooth *g* of Figure 6-28.

Other Variations in Occlusal Form

Some variations in lower second premolars involve the whole crown. They include teeth where the variations in lingual cusp morphology already considered, namely single cusp, lingual ridge, cusp and ridge or two lingual cusps, can all be recognized. In others there may be additional minor cusps, or grooves and ridges, but for convenience in description they may be grouped by one character—in occlusal view the outline is different from the more usual form, particularly as regards the relative lengths of major and minor axes. The most obvious variants in this respect have an M-D axis which is appreciably longer than the B-L axis, so that the crown appears to be distorted by compression from buccal and lingual (Figs. 6-30 and 6-31 *f,g*). Both small and large teeth are involved. See also p. 213.

The small tooth *a* in Figure 6-30 has an uncomplicated occlusal surface with a quite minor cusp and ridge, but the large tooth *b* has two lingual cusps, additional occlusal ridges and grooves, and bulbous outlines. Tooth *c* is appreciably less convex and the buccal surface of the root is flattened and grooved. Tooth *d* has a lingual ridge with occlusal pits and minor ridges, and the slender root bends strongly to lingual. The young tooth *e* has a prominent lingual cusp, transverse ridges, uncomplicated occlusal grooves and a root that is widely elliptical in cross-section, the major axis being B-L. In tooth *f* the "occlusal surface proper" has the compressed appearance but the convexity of buccal surface removes this appearance from the outline of the occlusal view of the tooth. By contrast, tooth *f,g* of Figure 6-31 looks greatly compressed in occlusal view and is noteworthy also for the prominent double bend in its sturdy root. Tooth *h* of Figure 6-31 has a similar and much compressed crown, but the root is noteworthy less for the sharp apical bend than for the wide shallow groove passing from lingual around to mesial surface. It is suggested that this could indicate a close relationship with the branching of the inferior dental canal to form the mental foramen although one would expect this would be placed nearer the apical bend in the root (see also Fig. 6-33 *c,d,e*). The bend previously mentioned in tooth *f* seems more likely to suggest that the tooth was deflected to erupt lingually into malocclusion.

Tooth *a,b* of Figure 6-31 has a relative-

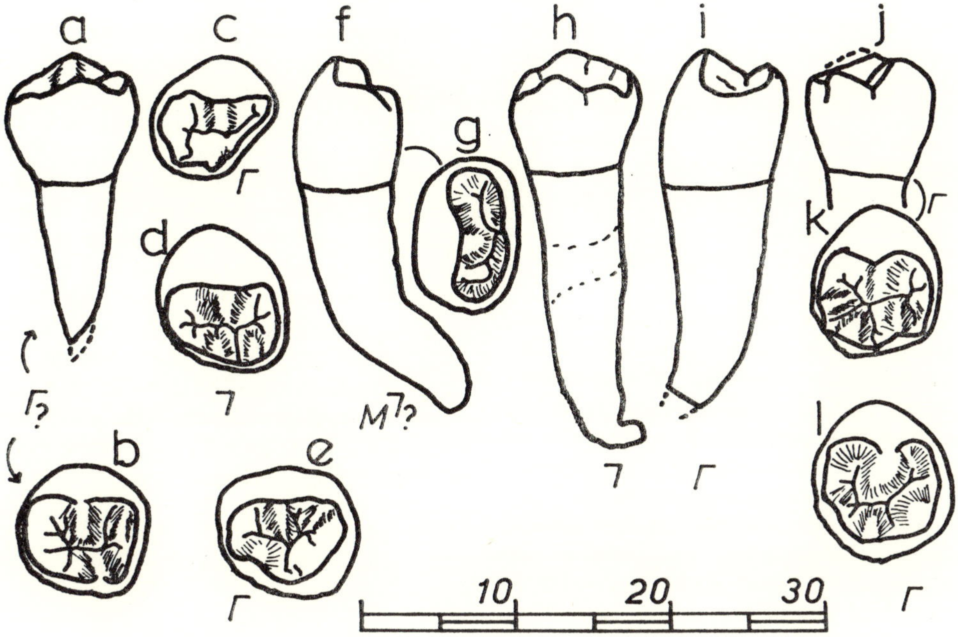

Figure 6-31. Some unusual forms of crown and root in lower second premolars.

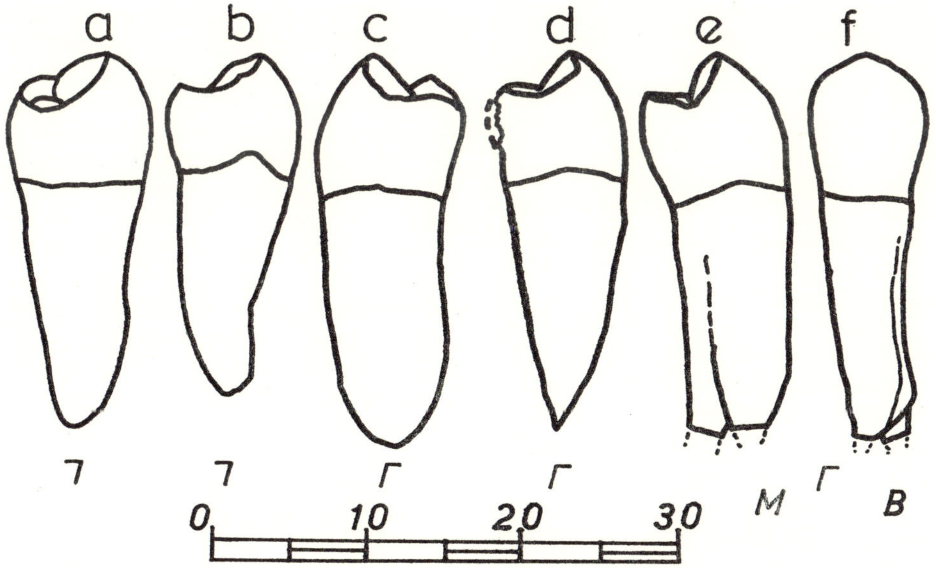

Figure 6-32. Acumination of buccal cusp in proximal view in second premolars. *a,b,* more obtuse examples. Tooth *a* is shown also in Figure 6-33 *a, aa,* and tooth *b* in Figure 6-27 *h*. Teeth *c,d,e* have less obtuse cusps in proximal view. Tooth *e* is shown in buccal view in *f*, and also in end view of the incomplete root in Figure 6-36 *f*.

ly large crown for its small tapering root. There is a prominent lingual cusp and ridge, and like tooth *e* of Figure 6-29 the buccal cusp appears rather small but with prominent shoulders. There is a rather prominent transverse ridge from the buccal cusp, but none from the lingual cusp, so that the occlusal groove is strongly V-shaped. The occlusal surface has a square appearance but in occlusal view the long axis is B-L.

In teeth *c,d* this longer B-L axis is more evident when the occlusal view including buccal surface is checked. The posterior portion of the occlusal surface is much larger than the anterior, but there is no impression of distortion of the crown. Tooth *e* presents an exaggeration of buccal cusp shoulders mentioned for several teeth already described. In tooth *e* the buccal cusp is reduced and the shoulders are more like small cusps. The resulting appearance is molariform with three buccal cusps and two lingual cusps like a lower first molar. If the whole buccal portion is considered as one cusp the tooth would be graded (in the scheme mentioned above) as 4-2-1. If the components of the buccal cusp may be graded for this particular tooth as a special case the formula would be 1-2-1.

The final variation to be examined in this group is found in those teeth where the occlusal form may be described as complicated by additional minor cusps, ridges and grooves. These tend to be in the DL part of the occlusal surface so that there may be two minor D-L cusps (Fig. 6-31 *j,k*), or the additional cusp may merge with the distal marginal ridge which is longer than usual (Fig. 6-31 *l*). In either case the occlusal view outline tends to have six sides rather than five. In tooth *k* each cusp has a well-formed transverse ridge, particularly B and ML cusps, and there are relatively deep and well-marked grooves. In tooth *b* the ridges are more smoothly rounded and only the main grooves are deep.

Acumination of Buccal Cusp

In lower second premolars there appears to be little variation in acumination of the buccal cusp. Whether viewed from proximal, or from buccal or lingual, it is usually a blunt cusp. In proximal view this obtuseness is associated with the buccal convexity of a lower tooth and the degree of prominence of the transverse or triangular ridge (Figs. 6-25 *b,c,* 6-29 *a* and 6-32 *a,b*). In the last two teeth *a* has a small lingual cusp, and *b* has a lingual ridge with no cusp (see Fig. 6-27 *h*). Less obtuse buccal cusps are seen in Figure 6-32 *c,d,e.* Tooth *c* has a well-developed ML cusp and a small DL cusp, and its transverse ridge is moderate. Teeth *d* and *e* are from young people; *e* has a divided root with incomplete apices, and *d* is from a boy aged 14$\frac{4}{12}$ years. It has a completed root with a fine sharp apex.

The degree of prominence of the buccal ridge has been shown to influence one's impression of acumination of the buccal cusp in proximal view. In lingual or buccal view it is the straightness or otherwise of the cusp slopes that is a principal factor. If convex from shoulder to tip of cusp, obtuseness is likely to be the impression one gets, but often slopes differ from one another; one may be less convex than the other, or actually concave. The general relation of one to the other may be that of an obtuse angle, but if there is little convexity they may meet in an arc of such short radius that there is almost a point.

For example, tooth *c* in Figure 6-32 has just been cited as less obtuse in proximal view because the transverse ridge is not prominent. In lingual view however the almost straight cusp slopes form a very obtuse angle with one another, but they nevertheless meet almost at a point (Fig. 6-34 *a*).

In terms of the obtuse relationship the cusp is blunt, but in terms of their junction the cusp tip is sharp. An example of asymmetry in cusp slopes is seen in Figure 6-33 *c*, and a tooth with a marked concavity

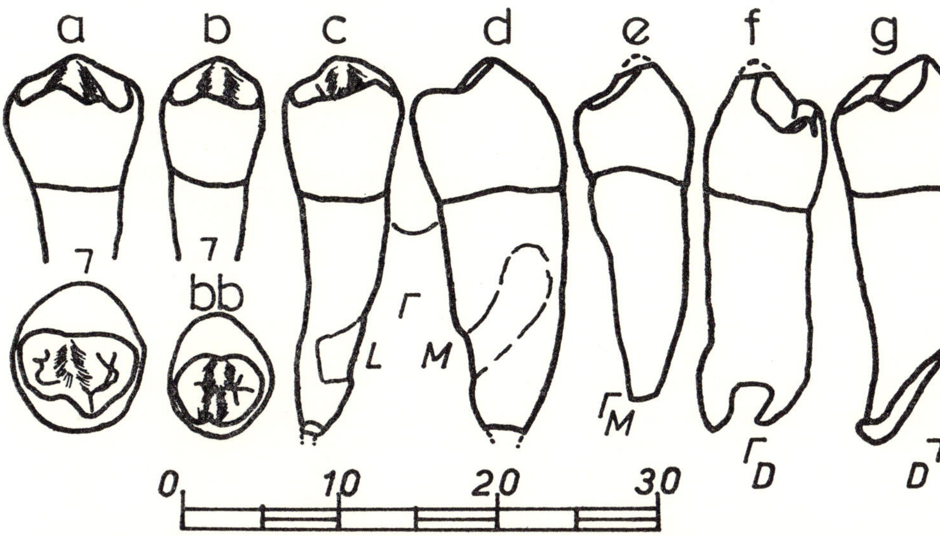

Figure 6-33. Cusp acumination continued, and unusual features in roots. Second premolars.

in each slope is in Figure 6-31 *a*. The shoulders in this tooth are prominent and the buccal cusp could here be described in the contradictory terms of "wide" and "very small."

It is evident that no acceptable criteria for description of cusp acumination have yet been established, but that analysis of variation in this character is complicated, and the objective has been to describe something of the complexity.

With this in mind, comments on acumination of the buccal cusp in lingual or buccal view may be condensed and simplified in summary. Teeth that have been selected as obtuse in cusp outline seen from

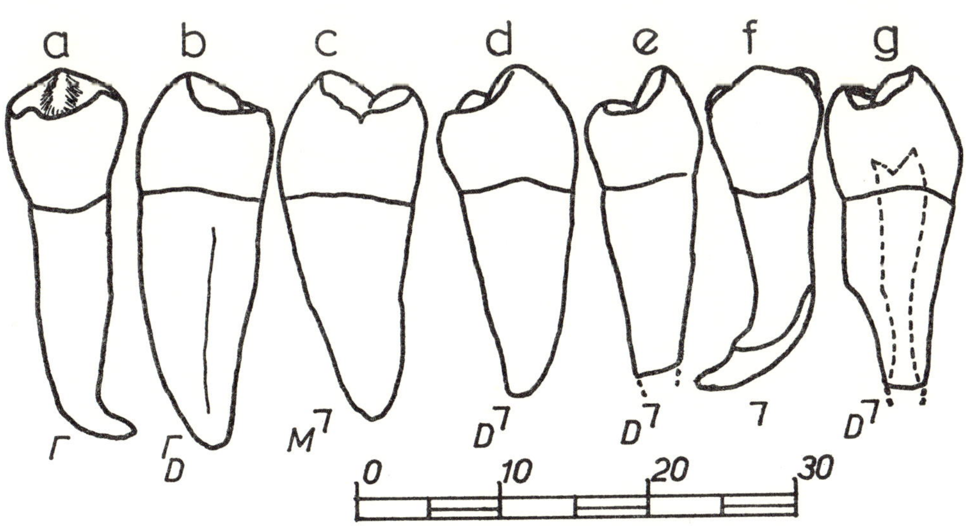

Figure 6-34. Curves and bends in roots in second premolars.

lingual (Figs. 6-25 *d*, 6-26 *d,e*, 6-27 *e* and 6-33 *a*) are also obtuse in proximal view (Figs. 6-25 *c*, 6-34 *b*, 6-34 *c*, 6-34 *d* and 6-32 *d* respectively). One tooth, less obtuse in proximal view, was described in more detail to illustrate difficulties of classification (Figs. 6-32 *c* and 6-34 *a*).

ROOT OF SECOND PREMOLARS

As in other single-rooted teeth, there is much variation in roots of lower second premolars. Teeth already figured have shown long or short, wide or narrow, fine or sturdy, evenly or unevenly tapered, straight or curved roots, and many different forms of apex. These have belonged to teeth selected to illustrate particular features of the crown, but they now serve also in showing many of the characters involved in a study of root variation. The later figures include outlines showing further variation in curves, bends, grooves, folds, and division of roots. Some of the teeth figured present additional details that are relevant to a combination of known anatomy and clinical experience when seeking an explanation of the curves and other characters just mentioned.

Although curves and bends are not always, or precisely, towards mesial or distal, most of these are best seen in buccal or lingual views. Thus, tooth *c* in Figure 6-32 was used to portray cusps in distal view, but its sharp apical bend (Fig. 6-34 *a*) was missed therein. In contrast, teeth *d,e* of Figure 6-26 have fairly straight roots in lingual view, but the outlines are far from symmetrical in Figure 6-34 *b,c* respectively. The next tooth *d* of Figure 6-34, with an apical bend to lingual, bends also to mesial (Fig. 6-27 *e*). The young tooth (Figs. 6-33 *b* and 6-34 *e*) has a slight curve to lingual and distal which evidently arose when the root was about half complete.

The prominent curve in the root of tooth *f* of Figure 6-34 is equally prominent when viewed from proximal. This part of the root has a distinctly twisted appearance. It is quite possible that this right tooth was "crowded" and deflected to rotate anticlockwise and erupt into lingual occlusion. This explanation of the curvature in the root is supported by the location of a carious cavity on the anatomical MB surface, and by the pattern of stain, confirming that caries started on the

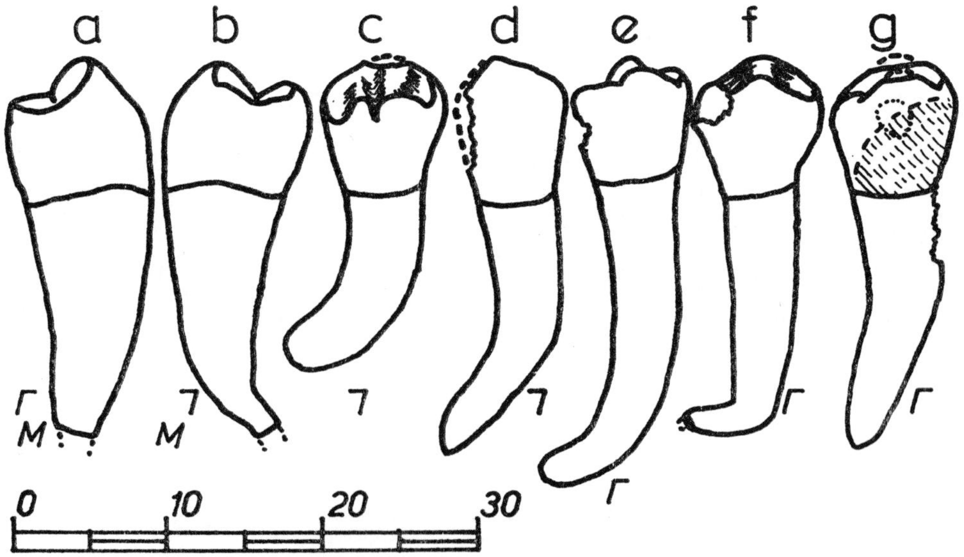

Figure 6-35. Long curves and abrupt bends in second premolars.

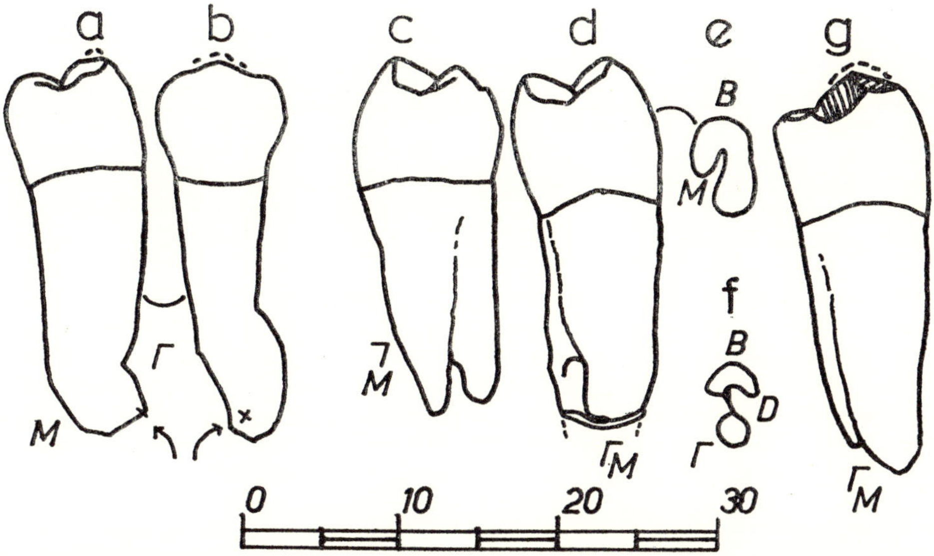

Figure 6-36. Root bends (continued), and root division in second premolars.

functional point of contact. (See also Figure 6-35 *g*, and relevant text.) It is also possible that during development the terminal portion of the root was modified in form by close proximity to the inferior dental canal. Such association has been suggested also for grooves in roots of other teeth (Figs. 6-31 *h* and 6-33 *c-f*).

Tooth *a* of Figure 6-35, although presenting a less obvious curve than that just described, is a similar case and provides further evidence in support of the explanation offered. This left tooth, extracted from a boy aged 15⁹⁄₁₂ years, had erupted in malocclusion, being deflected lingually; and it had rotated a little, also anticlockwise, confirmed by evidence on the tooth in the form of incipient caries and forceps damage. In this case caries was initiated on the anatomical DB surface, and forceps trauma on MB and DL surfaces.

Tooth *b* of Figure 6-35 has a strong lingual curvature of root which accords with its known history. It was removed from a girl aged 15¹⁄₁₂ years; the first premolar and first molar were in contact and the second premolar had erupted lingually. Thus in several cases of root curvature there is a history of malocclusion or other evidence, which appears to allow a satisfactory explanation of their curvature. It seems reasonable to assume that malocclusion may be a causative factor in other cases.

Another tooth which presents developmental and acquired features that seem to invite explanation is shown in Figure 6-35 *g*. Some of these features are like those described for tooth *f* of Figure 6-34, but in this tooth *g* curvature is to buccal and distal. Stain line, and proximal facet on the anatomical lingual surface, show that this left tooth has rotated anticlockwise and erupted buccally. The functional buccal surface (the anatomical mesial surface) has been polished by toothbrushing, but there is a large cervical and subgingival cavity with carious exposure of the pulp cavity.

In a dentition showing first-degree wear in enamel it is likely that cusp interference would cause the principal working stroke of occlusal movement to be lateral rather than protrusive. In such a case one would expect to find fine scratch marks in enamel facets chiefly buccal to lingual, although this is an over-simplification of masticatory movement to make the point. In this tooth *g* the fine scratch marks appear to run anatomically M-D, or parallel with the occlusal groove. This lends support to the conclusion from other evidence that the tooth was rotated on its axis by approximately 90 degrees.

The first premolar shown in Figure 6-20 *a* has an apical bend to mesial. A radiograph taken before the tooth was extracted shows the mental foramen at the level of the apices of the two premolars, lying between them, and with each apex apparently turned or "bent" away from it.

In Figure 6-34 *g* is shown a young second premolar with incomplete apex. In the root there is not a groove but a rather abrupt narrowing. There is no evidence of pathology or trauma visible to the naked eye, and it is thought that if this tooth had been displaced during removal of its deciduous predecessor there would be some such evidence to interrupt the buccal as well as the lingual outline of the root. Attention is drawn to the first premolar in Figure 6-23 *g* where there is a groove, strongly suggestive of proximity to the inferior dental canal or mental foramen and in that tooth also most noticeably on the lingual side. In the second premolar the reduction in width is confined to the lingual part of the root and there is no spiral effect. From a radiograph the outline of the pulp cavity has been traced on to the tooth outline (Fig. 6-34 *g*, broken line), and it is seen that there is a corresponding reduction in width. As this again relates only to the lingual outline, and there is no apparent interruption in outline continuity, it is unlikely that this tooth has suffered injury during development. The form of the root here also appears to be an adaptation to an anatomical structure, and in the absence of any evidence of pathology it is difficult to see what else it could be than the canal with its branch to the mental foramen. This is usually found in the vicinity of the premolars, but root formation in permanent teeth is a relatively late development as compared with that of the canal and its contents.

In making this suggestion one expects to be informed that the canal is too far below the tooth to become involved in this way, although in the third molar region it is relatively common for roots and canal to be closely associated. Variations in the mental foramen and its connection with the inferior dental canal were investigated by Brash (1924) and Warwick (1950). Brash pointed out that the opening of the foramen moves backwards relative to the teeth during the years of growth. Warwick showed that as the surface of the human mandible grows by deposition around the issuing mental nerve, a bony canal is built up that is subject to changes in direction. As a result, this canal which connects the foramen with the inferior dental nerve curves not only laterally but also markedly upwards and backwards. Warwick also recorded the number of foramina, right and left, directed approximately along various axes in a number of adult human skulls. In view of the known variations in this canal, and the many variations in length and curvature of roots which have been demonstrated in the present work, it would seem probable that in some cases premolar roots and canal would be closely associated and involved in growth changes, and we have presented cases which appear to be examples of such association.

The outlines include examples of teeth in which the terminal or apical part of the root has made an abrupt change of direction (Figs. 6-34 *a* and 6-35 *f*). It has been suggested that proximity of the developing root to the inferior dental canal might account for such bends. Teeth are sometimes found which indicate that there has been a more or less abrupt change in direction at an earlier stage of development. In such cases the tooth may also present evidence of trauma or pathology which may be associated with disturbance of the developing premolar by movement of the roots of its deciduous predecessor. This may occur during removal of an abscessed deciduous tooth, and the effect on the developing permanent tooth may amount to dilaceration or "green-stick fracture" of its root.

Tooth *a,b* of Figure 6-36 presents an abrupt change in direction that cannot be explained as such a dilaceration since it has occurred too late in development—the deciduous tooth would have been lost before this stage was reached. Moreover, with so much root completed before the abrupt change in direction, it is unlikely that the tooth would have yielded to a dislocating trauma to produce the result seen. Nor does this tooth bear any resemblance to the abrupt bends where close association of inferior dental canal seems possible as a cause.

The tooth does however present features which collectively may lead to an explanation. The stain pattern indicates that the tooth was in normal alignment and position, and the light faceting of enamel by wear supports this. In proximal view (*a* in Fig. 6-36) it is seen that the earlier formed portion of the root curves slightly but definitely to lingual and then, apparently in response to changed conditions, abruptly changes direction back to buccal. There is no history available regarding this tooth, but it is suggested that firstly it was crowded out of the arch, rotating while erupting lingually. Then, as a result of orthodontic treatment, it seems that the tooth may have been brought into good alignment, to which the normal stain pattern already mentioned bears witness. A further item of interest in this tooth is the position of the apical foramen, namely at the points of the arrow-heads in the two outlines.

Apart from the normal variations of thickness or slenderness of root and sharpness or bluntness of apex described in other groups of teeth, lower premolars also have been shown to present a very considerable variety in changes of direction in root axis. To these must be added the more or less abrupt changes in root contour which have been referred to as transverse or spiral grooves or a twisted appearance, and those other departures from normal morphology which may result from trauma or pathology.

Lower premolars are of special interest in a study of root variation because in some ways they are a unique group. They may be exposed during development to a combination of influences or experiences not suffered by any other group of (usually) single-rooted teeth. Upper teeth, for example, are never far from (and often demonstrably closely associated with) the nasal fossa or maxillary sinus and the many variations found in these and the alveolar ridges or processes. Lower premolars have only one anatomical structure which appears likely sometimes to influence the direction of root formation, and lower anterior teeth have no such structure.

Because of the usual, but not invariable, sequence in which canines, premolars and molars erupt, premolars may meet obstruction during root growth or eruption so that they may be deflected during emergence. This applies to both upper and lower premolars, but conditions are not identical in each jaw even though the causes of a "crowded" type of malocclusion may have much in common. Thus loss of space by interproximal decay in deciduous molars may occur in either, but the considerable differences in morphology and relative sizes of first and second premolars may well contribute to the variety in degree and direction presented in cases of such deflection and the modification that takes place in the root. Crowding of premolars is common when a child subject to early dental caries does not receive prompt or adequate restorative treatment. The fact that caries of deciduous molars may lead to an alveolar abscess (or "gumboil"), and that treatment of decay or abscess is often limited to extraction of the tooth, may well lead to pathological or traumatic injury to the developing premolar or to its total loss. Extraction of the deciduous tooth earlier than it should have been shed naturally may add further to the probabilities of a crowded malocclusion developing.

Abscess of the deciduous molar at an early age may lead to hypoplasia of enamel in the subjacent premolar, or displacement of the premolar during extraction of the deciduous tooth (Fig. 6-38 *c,d*). In some cases the unabsorbed roots of the deciduous molar have so embraced the developing crown that it has unavoidably been removed with the deciduous tooth. Early removal of the deciduous tooth (unless a space retainer is fitted) will, like interproximal decay, lead to loss of space or of normal growth so that crowding is inevitable. Early emergence of a premolar following early extraction of its deciduous molar is common and may introduce another factor in the subsequent development of crowding. Moreover it should be mentioned that incomplete extraction (broken root) is not rare and when the retained fragment is an unresorbed deciduous root it may contribute to deflection of an erupting premolar.

Thus there are many ways in which a developing premolar may be deflected during the course of eruption and it is likely that among them lies the explanation of some of the root curves, etc., in the outlines presented. In most of these the case histories were not known but it might well be expected that in caries-free groups and individuals, or where preventive and conservative treatment has been available, many of these root variations would not be found.

Orthodontic treatment of displaced teeth is relevant in the discussion of changes in root outline. That some teeth which have been subjected to such treatment will later be extracted is certain, but it may be very difficult to obtain adequate records after a more or less lengthy lapse of time. At the age at which orthodontic treatment is carried out it is highly probable that teeth with incomplete roots are involved. It is also likely that premolars are included among these, and that some such teeth brought into "normal" alignment and occlusion have already developed a degree of root curvature as described above. From the time that realignment movement in the tooth commences, it would be expected that further root growth would be reflected by a change in direction of root surfaces. In line with these thoughts it is expected that a root might well acquire some such form as that shown in Figure 6-36 *a,b*. Rosenberg (1972) says that orthodontic treatment can cause dilaceration of a premolar root. Our specimen appears to be from an adult of middle age, and was extracted during the mid-1930s. At the time when this tooth had an incomplete root, orthodontic techniques were different and one can readily believe that the greater forces then sometimes used would also be capable of causing dilaceration.

Also relevant to this discussion, which embraces not only changes in direction of a root axis but also cases of rather abrupt changes in root outline or thickness, are some cases which are considered pathological and some which are not. Of the latter are such teeth as those outlined in Figures 6-23 *g*, 6-33 *c,d,e* and 6-34 *g*. Changes in outline or thickness due to pathology may arise from local or systemic conditions. Examples of local conditions are abscess of adjacent deciduous teeth through advanced decay, or injury to the developing permanent tooth during removal of the deciduous tooth.

Changes in root outline believed to reflect systemic pathology may cause changes such as that in the terminal or apical part of the root shown in Figure 6-3 *b*. This is a tooth from a prehistoric Tongan mandible. This tooth, together with others from the same mandible and similar teeth from a prehistoric burial of a Maori child, was illustrated in a recent paper (Taylor, 1972a). The mandibles concerned are illustrated in an earlier paper (Taylor, 1971b).

Grooving and Division of Roots

In lower first premolars various kinds of grooves and divisions of roots were described and figured. Those found in second premolars are often similar but tend to be less frequently or less obviously present. A quite different kind of groove was also mentioned (Fig. 6-23 *g*), and somewhat similar examples were found in second premolars. It was suggested that these may sometimes indicate close association of the developing tooth root with the inferior dental canal or its branching to form the mental foramen (Fig. 6-33 *c,d,e*). Tooth *f* in Figure 6-33 bears some resemblance to a lower molar root where it has been found to "straddle" the inferior dental canal. It would seem that this might reasonably be called either a grooved or a bifid root.

When describing grooves in lower first premolars attention was drawn to a groove found on the mesial surface of the root. It was shown that when prominent this groove tended to be asymmetrical and to indent the root obliquely. It was referred to as the cleft groove. In some cases the cleft was complete so that the root was branched, but divided unevenly. In these the minor branch was anterior, or mesial and buccal, not unlike the lower premolar roots of some anthropoids.

A good example of a cleft groove is shown in Figure 6-36 *d*. This is a young tooth, and the end view of the incomplete root is seen in *e*, where the cleft groove passing obliquely from mesial towards buccal is well shown. Another young tooth with almost completed root (Fig. 6-32 *e,f*) has two separate canals, but the oblique cleft can still be recognized in the end view (Fig. 6-36 *f*). Further examples of clefts and late branching of the root are shown in Fig. 6-36 *c,g*. In the latter tooth there are also marked buccal and distal grooves for the greater length of the root.

A tooth which presents all three of these grooves, mesial, distal and buccal, all well-marked but with no indication of root division, is shown in Figure 6-37 *e,f*. The crown has three cusps. Two teeth with bifid roots, in one case showing an abrupt bend to lingual in each branch from the point of bifurcation, and the other closely resembling bifidity seen in lower canines, are shown in Figure 6-37 *a,b*. The former has a small lingual cusp and lingual ridge and U-shaped occlusal groove; the latter has a small lingual cusp, transverse ridge and two occlusal pits. It is not unlike a

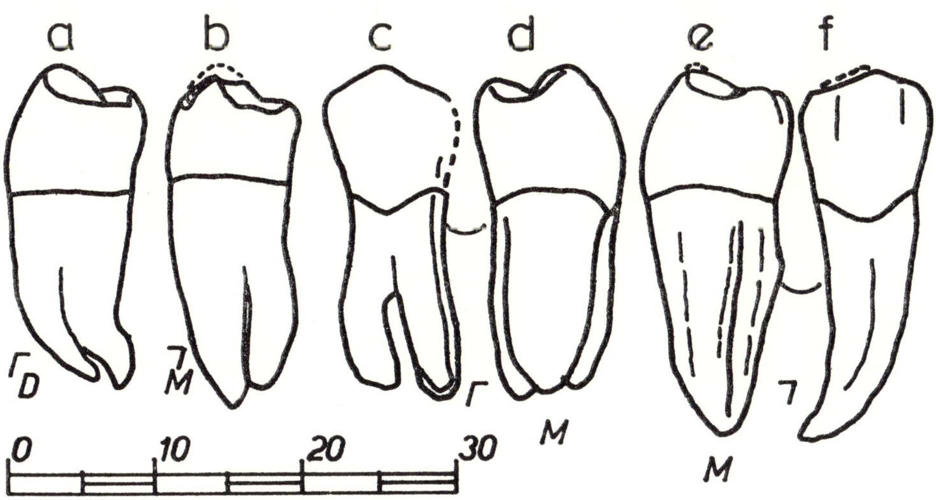

Figure 6-37. Root bends, root branching and root grooves in second premolars.

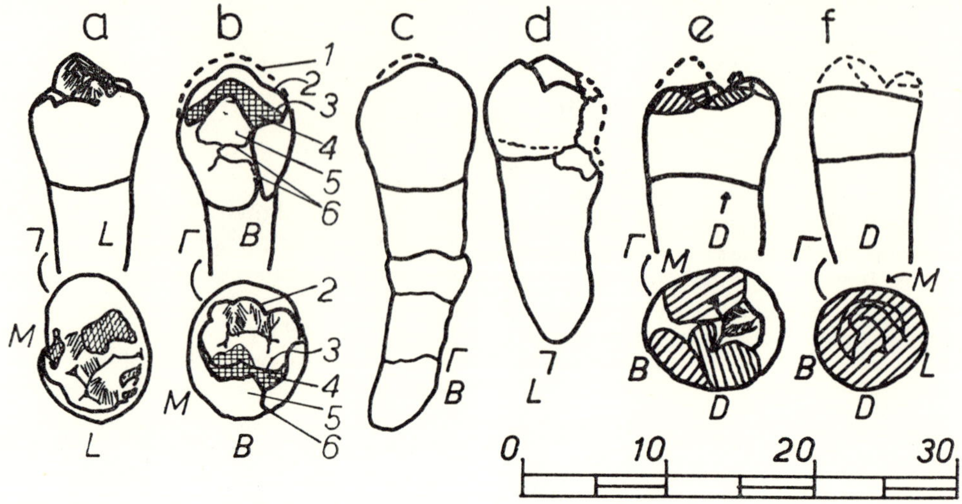

Figure 6-38. Changes in crowns and roots resulting from pathology, wear and trauma. Second premolars.

first premolar, but the stain pattern on mesial is suggestive of contact with a wider tooth than a canine.

Tooth *c,d* of Figure 6-37 is unusual. The crown is clearly that of a second premolar with ML cusp and DL ridge, but the bifid root with M and D branches bears resemblance to that of a lower molar. Unlike a molar, however, the M branch is distinctly minor and the wide D branch has a broad, blunt and bifid apex.

It is clear that in second premolars both crown and root may present considerable variation in morphological detail. No relation has been found between variations in either, so that the form of the crown does not provide the dental surgeon with any clue to complications that may be met in extraction. Some variations in root form may be indicated by X-ray, and it would be advisable to note also the apparent relationship of tooth roots, inferior dental canal and mental foramen as shown in the radiograph.

Occlusal Modification—Wear

The effects of wear in second premolars are similar in most respects to those seen in first premolars. There is some difference in the pattern of exposure of dentine arising from anatomical differences in height of buccal cusp and of lingual portions of occlusal surface. Notching at buccal cervices through faulty toothbrushing is less often seen and less severe, as the more posterior teeth become progressively inaccessible.

An unusual appearance of occlusal surfaces that should not be confused with wear, although it may be involved in wear, is shown in Figure 6-38 *a*. It may be confused with the variation in detail of occlusal grooves and ridges which has already been described, and it is therefore relevant to the present study. It is a pathological manifestation arising from defective formation of enamel in early stages of calcification of the tooth crown. This hypoplasia of enamel may result from an exanthematous illness, or from an abscess of the overlying deciduous molar. In either case, after recovery or removal of the cause, formation of enamel may proceed normally. Subsequently the tooth may be affected by dental caries as has occurred in this tooth in the areas marked with fine shading.

Evidence of occlusal enamel hypoplasia may disappear as a result of wear. The damage to this tooth through enamel hypoplasia is comparable to that shown in the canine tooth in Figure 5-15 *a*. When checked against Schour and Massler's chart of tooth development it is seen that damage to the enamel organ of this second premolar would have occurred between the ages of 2±6/12 years and 3±6/12 years. Unless the child suffered very early and severe caries of the second deciduous molar (the usual precursor of an alveolar abscess), the hypoplasia in this tooth at this early age is most likely to be the result of illness.

A much more severe example of enamel hypoplasia is shown in Figure 6-38 *b*, but in this case the tooth remained caries free. Much of the buccal cusp has no enamel, and in lingual view the broken line (1) shows the presumed outline if the cusp had been normal. The other numbers in the two outlines of this tooth indicate the following: 2, lingual cusp; 3, ridge of dentine forming buccal cusp; 4, exposed dentine indicated by cross-hatching; 5, enamel on buccal side of cusp; 6, further "scarring" of enamel. In this tooth there are several areas on the lingual cusp and buccal surface where enamel formation was defective. Small areas of exposed dentine are seen, and the enamel organ was so badly damaged that one "scar" continues right to the buccal cervix.

Teeth *c* and *d* of Figure 6-38 are examples of dilaceration. In tooth *c* trauma occurred when the root was partly formed. In *d* crown formation had just been completed when it suffered dislocation. Root formation proceeded, but the abnormal relationship of crown and root has been made less obvious by a large carious cavity involving distal surface and cervix.

Tooth *e* in Figure 6-38 is a "tricuspid" second premolar, wider on lingual side. Wear has produced three facets, but removal of hard tissue has in general been fairly even or level. The buccal cusp, and one lingual cusp, have been worn to the top of the occlusal groove. In tooth *f* wear has proceeded further, so that the worn surface is like a transverse section through the crown. Wear of second degree has exposed dentine of the buccal cusp and part of the lingual ridge, and therefore has removed features that assist identification. From the shape of the occlusal outline and of the occlusal groove the tooth appears to belong to left side.

CERVIX OF SECOND PREMOLARS

As mentioned for first premolars, the cervical line does not present features that assist in distinguishing mesial from distal. Reference to the outlines figured shows that, in proximal view, the cervical line may be almost straight, or arched, and the arch is usually low and seldom prominent like that in Figure 6-32 *b*.

A low arch may involve the full length of the cervical line in proximal view (Fig. 6-29 *a,e*), or only part of it as in first premolars (Figs. 6-2 *e,f* and 6-9 *a,b*).

In buccal or lingual view, in both teeth, the cervix is almost straight, or slightly concave rootwards (Figs. 6-8, 6-10, 6-11, 6-12 etc., for first, and 6-28, 6-33, 6-35 for second premolars). Where the root presents a buccal groove the cervix may be somewhat V-shaped towards that groove (Figs. 6-19 *b*, 6-23 *f* and 6-37 *c,f*).

An unusual lingual cervical line is seen in Figure 6-30 *c*. In transverse section at cervix the root of this tooth is almost an equilateral triangle, the lingual angle corresponding with the crest of the cervical arch shown in the figure. The somewhat similar lingual cervical line of Figure 6-38 *b* is a result of damage to the enamel organ which has resulted in severe enamel hypoplasia in this tooth.

LINGUAL PROFILES IN LOWER PREMOLARS

In Figures 6-6 and 6-7 were shown apparent variations in relation of crown axis and root axis in first premolars. Although such axes do not exist, nor can the position of a hypothetical axis be precisely defined, it is often possible to visualize approximately where an axis of crown or root, or of the whole tooth, would lie. This is a useful exercise, for it increases one's awareness of form and contour.

The placing of the root axis is influenced by the lingual and buccal profiles of the root, whether one or both are straight or curved, and by the changes that occur in their length, or by the nature of the tapering that results. In some cases the root axis might reasonably be curved, or might pass through the apex. In others, especially where there is marked asymmetry in the apical region, it will not be so.

The placing of the crown axis is influenced by the dominant buccal cusp and whether or not there is a lingual cusp or ridge. In some second premolars both a mesio-lingual cusp and a disto-lingual ridge, or two lingual cusps, are present. Convexity of profiles and height of crown are other factors to consider, and it has already been shown how in lower teeth the axis tends to be nearer to lingual (and in upper teeth nearer to the labial or buccal side).

As a result of these characters the lower crown may appear to lean lingually, and these are the cases where crown axis and root axis appear to meet at an angle. The nature of this apparent leaning is affected by yet another character that varies considerably, and this is the form of the lingual portion of the crown profile. The character now described may be seen in first and second premolars.

Firstly, there is the lingual profile in a single curve of longer radius, extending from cervix to cusp tip as in Figures 6-3 *b*,

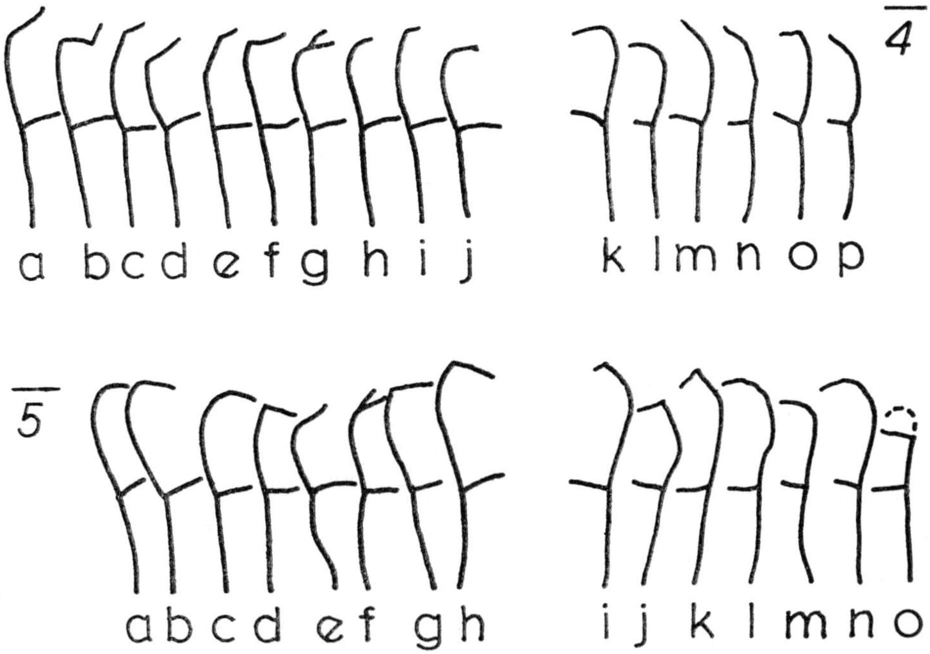

Figure 6-39. Lingual profiles showing variation in cusp form, crown height and curvature, and relation of crown and root outline at cervix. These have been traced from proximal outlines already figured. Top row: first premolars; second premolars below. Some are from mesial and some from distal view, and therefore there is no right and left significance in the arrangement of the outlines.

6-6 *e*, 6-7 *a*, 6-11 *dd* and 6-29 *b,c*. Secondly, there is the curve of shorter radius confined to the cusp region as in Figures 6-3 *c*, 6-11 *bb*, 6-21 *a* and 6-23 *b*. Thirdly, some profiles are more straight than curved, except for the cusp tip portion (Figs. 6-2 *g*, 6-9 *d*, 6-12 *bb*, 6-13 *c*, 6-29 *a*, 6-33 *d*, 6-36 *g* and 6-37 *b*).

As a result the lingual profile of the crown presents a number of variations in its relation to that of the root at the cervix. Some of these are shown in Figure 6-39 as tracings from the relevant portion of outlines of proximal views in earlier figures.

SUMMARY

On page 204 were listed characters that have been attributed to crowns and roots of lower premolars. Evidence has now been presented to show that those characters are not found in all such teeth. However, the following can be said:

(1) *In first premolars*

- (a) There may be two cusps, the lingual being much smaller than the buccal cusp, and they may be joined by a ridge or separated by a groove.
- (b) The lingual outline may appear cusp-like owing to the presence of a groove.
- (c) There may be a small ML cusp and a DL ridge.
- (d) The anterior portion of the occlusal surface may be higher than the posterior part, and may be smaller.
- (e) The anterior portion may present a groove passing towards the mesial surface of the root, nearer the lingual side of the root.
- (f) The root may have a groove in line with that just mentioned. This groove may vary in depth, sometimes forming an oblique cleft.
- (g) The root may have a shallow median groove on M or D surface, or on each of these.
- (h) There may be a groove on the buccal surface as well, so that the root appears to consist of three fused elements.
- (i) The root may actually be bifid in the apical region, and when this is so the MB branch tends to be smaller and the D branch to be larger.
- (j) The root may present a curve or bend, buccally, lingually, mesially or distally, or it may appear to curve in at least two of these directions.
- (k) The root may be flattened, oval or round in transverse section, but it is usually wider on the buccal aspect.
- (l) The apex may be fine or blunt and present much variation.
- (m) In proximal view there is considerable variation in profile of root and crown as regards curvature and convexity.
- (n) The buccal cusp varies in height and acumination in buccal or proximal view.

(2) *In second premolars*

- (a) There may be two cusps, with less difference in size than in first premolars.
- (b) There may be two cusps, the lingual cusp ML and a ridge DL, with much variation in prominence in the lingual cusp and ridge.
- (c) As in first premolars, the anterior part of the occlusal surface tends to be higher, and smaller, than the posterior portion which often is wider B-L. These features assist in identifying M and D of the tooth.
- (d) There may be no lingual cusp, but a somewhat semicircular lingual ridge from ML to DL with

a similar shaped, or crescentic, groove between the ridge and the buccal cusp.

(e) There may be no lingual ridge but two distinct lingual cusps.

(f) The two lingual cusps may be approximately equal in size, but the ML is usually the larger.

(g) The two lingual cusps may together equal, or exceed, the M-D dimension of the buccal cusp, so that in occlusal view the lingual portion is as wide as, or wider than, the buccal portion in this dimension.

(h) Where there are two lingual cusps, the DL may tend to further division into two minor cusps.

(i) The lingual outline of cusps or ridges therefore varies greatly.

(j) The crown in occlusal view may appear compressed, reducing the B-L dimension. Occasionally the M-D dimension appears the greater at the expense of B-L.

(k) In occlusal view the occlusal surface is usually wider on buccal, but the outline of the whole tooth may change the visual impression to that of a large oval, narrow at the buccal cervix. This effect is related to the tendency of the crown axis to be nearer to lingual.

(l) The root shows many of the variations seen in the first premolar, as regards curvature and apex.

(m) Grooves in the root are less common or less marked than in first premolars. This applies particularly to the cleft groove on mesial surface, but it does occur in second premolars.

(n) Branching of the root, more especially in the apical portion, is not common. Neither is it rare, and sometimes there are distinct branches resembling those of a molar tooth.

In brief summary, therefore, it may be said that lower premolars present a considerable number of variable characters. The teeth may be very easy, yet sometimes difficult, to identify. Like other teeth they may also present a number of characters in crown or root that may give information relating to the health, habits, experiences and age of the person concerned, even though no such confirmatory history is available.

Chapter 7

Maxillary Molars

DESCRIPTION of molar teeth with respect to morphological characters is a bigger task than for other teeth, not only because there are six in each jaw, and there is a plurality of cusps and root branches, but also because of the variety that must be considered normal in these teeth. Moreover, uppers and lowers are so different that separate treatment is obviously desirable, but beyond this it is difficult to give adequate description of their morphological anatomy in concise sections.

If each molar, first, second and third, is considered separately, the story is complicated by the fact that some characters may or may not be common to two or all three of these teeth, and the manner of their presence (as regards form, degree of development or other quality) may vary considerably as between these teeth in different individuals. Thus separate treatment demands repetition or alternatively, omission of information, and it is in respect of this information that textbooks have been deficient. The information omitted can be useful in differentiation or identification. Since this study relates to clinical practice, to dental anatomy and to forensic problems, it is necessary to provide that relevant information.

In this case, therefore, discussion is not based primarily on each individual molar, but these teeth are studied collectively as upper molars (and then lower molars in due course). In general the author's analytical procedure is based on the character rather than on the tooth, but comments are related to the particular tooth where necessary.

Because Dahlberg has presented occlusal surfaces so precisely and extensively in his series of plaster plaques, it was intended in the present work to concentrate rather on the roots of molar teeth. It was found, however, that it is not reasonable to examine root styles while ignoring morphological variation in crowns in general and in cusps in particular. Nevertheless the aim has been to confine the study to description of the material, to analysis of its variation and so to recognition of features and characters which may assist identification even though they are involved in these modifications.

At the same time it has been necessary to take into account the way in which additional elements, themselves subject to variation, may be recognized and related to variation of the more "normal" elements. This study is not concerned as to whether variation in normal and additional elements has any particular relation to evolutionary theories, or significance therein. Indeed, it is felt that some physical anthropologists would wander less often in the fields of hypothetical fancies if they were more aware of the biological and behavioural backgrounds of teeth and individuals.

For the present report, illustrations of observations on upper molars have been taken almost entirely from the 1073 teeth selected for mounting on 213 cards in this section of the author's collection, but these comprise only a small fraction of the number of molar teeth which have been studied. The figures in this chapter contain 394 outlines drawn to scale, relating to over 200 teeth.

GENERAL CHARACTERS OF UPPER MOLARS

Starting from the elementary observation that upper molars tend to have four cusps and a root trunk with three branches, one may progress to the disposition of these. The cusps are usually at the angles of a rounded quadrilateral when viewed from occlusal, two being placed buccally, and two palatally. In the same view the tips of the buccal cusps are further from the centre of the quadrilateral than are those of the palatal cusps—in other words the buccal cusps are nearer to the buccal outline than the palatal cusps are to the palatal outline of the figure.

The root branches are located as two on the buccal side and one on the palatal side. They are often approximately equal in length although not in size or shape, and the overall length of root is less than that of the canine tooth in that jaw, and often less than the premolars also from cervix to apex.

The first molar is usually the largest and has the greatest divergence of root branches, while the third molar is smaller and has least divergence. These statements may be negated in some cases, as regards size when there is a large third molar, and as regards divergence where root fusions are involved, or they may be otherwise inapplicable. Thus the second molar may be anomalous in form, the third molar likewise, and the third molar may also be much reduced in size, or it may not have developed at all.

It is well known that the third molar is variable in several respects such as the following: (a) size as above indicated; (b) occurrence, its presence or absence possibly involving one, two, three or all four of the third molars in one person; (c) eruption, or emergence; this may not occur even though the tooth is present; (d) eruption may be early or very late for no obvious reason; (e) eruption may be prevented on account of impaction by bone or against another tooth; (f) complexity of crown or root as distinct from actual size or bulk. These variations are found both in prehistoric and in contemporary skeletal material of varying ethnic relationship.

SIZE OF MOLAR TEETH

Variation in size of molar teeth cannot be dealt with merely by measurement of dimension or bulk or surface area. Description of any tooth as large or small without further information may convey a vague idea, but in the case of molars these terms are seldom satisfactory because of the more complex form and consequent greater number of characters that may vary. It may seem easy to depict small teeth and large teeth (Fig. 7-1 *a-d**). Tooth *a* and *b* are M1, and *b* is longer from apex to occlusal surface, but its P root is less divergent and its maximal root distance P-B is less than that of *a*. Thus it is larger only in some dimensions, and it could be said that for its crown size its root is spread over a smaller area than is the case in *a*. But this relates to M view, and the

* The scale is shown for all outlines in 5 mm intervals up to 30 mm, but the numbers have not usually been entered on the scale. Where it was desired to show features, rather than a projection of true M,D,P or B views, the tooth has been turned or tilted slightly. This accounts for apparently varying dimensions in different views of the same feature. Where it may not be obvious that more than one view is given of one tooth, the outlines are linked by a curved dotted line, or by arrows. Occlusal outlines are always oriented with mesial (M) towards the top of the page. In these, the cusp tips are indicated by X, a small cusp or tubercle by *t*, and a Carabelli cusp by Cc. Accessory cusp or root elements are labelled "Opc" as explained in the text (p. 248). The main occlusal ridges of enamel are shown in broken lines, and occlusal grooves or fissures by continuous lines. Shallow grooves on other crown surfaces and on root branches are shaded as also are near contact or fusion of root elements. A ragged outline, with or without parallel shading, represents dental caries, but shading within a smooth outline usually indicates an amalgam restoration (filling) or an attritional facet; the size and position should identify these. In Figures 7-10 and 7-11 the shadings of attached bone are explained in the legends, as are also the end-view root outlines in Figures 7-12A, 7-21, 7-24, 7-26, 7-32, 7-33 and 7-36. The markings C– or C+ beside outlines from young teeth with incomplete roots, indicate that the amount of root formed at the time of extraction was respectively less than, or greater than, the height of the crown.

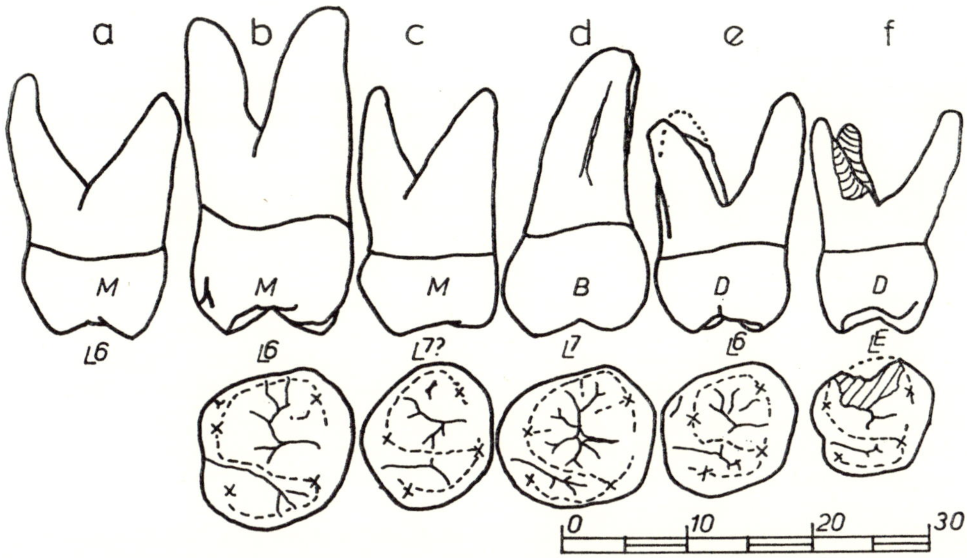

Figure 7-1. Comparisons of size are complicated by such variables as total bulk, or relative bulk of crown to root, number and bulk of root branches, their divergence and curvature, their partial or complete fusion, and the number of main cusps. *f*, a deciduous molar with areas of commencing resorption of roots.

comparison may be different in B view.

Teeth *c* and *d* are M2, *d* in B view. Tooth *c* has the smaller crown although it has four large cusps, while *d* has a scarcely recognizable DP cusp. Tooth *c* has small root branches, but they are all separate and appreciably divergent. In tooth *d* both B roots are fused, its P root furcates at a late stage and is much less divergent than in the case of *c*. In comparing *c* and *d* it is seen that the form of the crowns and roots is quite different. Tooth *d* can present some greater dimensions overall, but its root is reduced by partial fusion and its crown is reduced to almost three cusp style. Surely its designation as a large tooth has some limited significance because of these findings? One must therefore question the value of dimensional measurements for comparative purposes.

The matter of comparison of teeth or dentitions by dimensional measurement and by such terms as large or small will be enlarged upon later, but here it is necessary to say that in comparisons of size in teeth which commonly have branched roots, details of the branching are essential. The same applies to cusps and other characters which are subject to morphological variation, and therefore attempts at a meaningful comparison would involve complications. And this is not all, for it must be remembered that a tooth is part of an individual. It would be unreasonable to assume that tooth dimensions and type do not bear some relation to the stature and physical type of the individual to which they belong. Moreover there is the chance that an individual may be born to parents who differ widely, or perhaps little, in these, and also in other respects such as race. The same is true of other forbears in an individual's ancestry. While certain characters are often recognized in related persons, it is unlikely that a reliable pattern of inheritance of any such character could be elucidated. Surely then it must be fatuous to pretend that dimensional measurements of teeth are of any significance for comparative purposes? For descriptive purposes they are similarly useless, for no particular dimension is more important than another or gives any indication of the morphology of a whole tooth or of parts thereof.

DIFFERENTIATION

As with other teeth, there are characters that enable a molar tooth to be oriented as regards mesial and distal and left and right. Where this may sometimes be more difficult (apart from damage by pathology or fracture), there may be a variety of factors involved. These include reduction in number of cusps, or increase through the presence of an additional element (which may or may not be clearly recognizable as such), and variations in the root. As with the number of cusps in a crown, so also the root may have fewer or more than the usual three branches. The potential for variation in this respect is considerable, for it involves some permutations and combinations not only of fusion patterns and positions of furcation, but also of what may be called identity characters of the three root branches. These identity characters in turn are related to the position of each in relation to crown features of cusps, convexities and grooves. Here also, the whole matter may be complicated by the presence in varying degrees of one or more additional elements which in their turn may or may not be recognizably associated with similar elements in the crown. These additional inclusion elements were classified by Herbst and Apffelstaedt (1930), and this writer has made use of the term Odontopagus parasiticus concretus (Opc) from their work.

Each of the three molars may present a range of variation in characters just mentioned, such as number and size of cusps or root branches, or position of furcation of branches. In a particular individual however there tends to be a relationship between the variations, and this often provides the easiest way to determine which tooth is which. Thus if the DP cusp is diminished in the second molar it will be less so in the first and may be missing in the third. If roots are partly fused in the second, they may not be fused in the first, but tend to be more completely fused in the third molar. From first molar to third, therefore, the relationship could be called a descending order of anatomical complexity, but the "gradient" is by no means a "smooth" one that may be described or defined. In fact either segment may be affected, the first perhaps most often by some degree of development of the Carabelli cusp. In the second portion the gradient of complexity may be reversed by inclusion in the third molar of one or more additional elements (Opc) in crown or root; or it may not exist at all, as when the third molar is suppressed.

The presence of four well-developed cusps, or of a fifth at MP (Carabelli), and three well-differentiated and divergent root branches, makes it highly probable that the tooth is a first molar, but the Carabelli cusp does sometimes occur in second molars. Root branches that are scarcely divergent, especially if the DP cusp is either much reduced or absent, greatly reduce (but do not eliminate) the possibility of a tooth being a first molar. Whether the tooth is a second or third molar may be less easy to determine, but there may be other recognizable features or characters to assist the determination.

Among the most useful of these are acquired characters related to age or function, or to the immediate oral environment. Thus a distal facet at the contact point implies that the tooth is not a third molar (the rare exception of a fourth molar having been present must be allowed for), but the absence of a distal contact point facet will not positively identify a third molar—the tooth could be a second molar where the third molar has been suppressed, or removed early.

Occlusal wear on a third molar requires caution in interpretation and its significance should be judged in relation to other findings. Thus where a first or second molar has long been missing, a third molar may show more wear than in a full mouth, but if the lower tooth is missing the upper may be less subject to wear. In either of these circumstances the tooth may have tipped mesially, and the wear pattern should present evidence of this.

Polish from toothbrushing may reach as far back as the buccal surface of a second molar, but is unlikely to show on a third molar in normal position. By contrast the buccal surface may present evidence of decalcification or stain accumulation, and the area of demarcation by these may in turn indicate whether a more distal tooth had been present.

Further consideration of differentiation between first, second and third molars, and between left and right teeth, involves orientation by features of crown and root and is summarized at the end of this chapter.

THE CROWN

As molars have more cusps and root branches than premolars there is more scope for variation, and this does in fact occur. The tooth may be viewed from B, P, proximal or from occlusal. The cusps may be examined as regards their number and disposition, as may also the sulci, grooves and pits related to them. The shapes of main surfaces are of course dominated by these same features but are themselves subject to variations in convexity, and in orientation as regards the frontal, sagittal and horizontal planes. In the usual views of the crown these variations contribute to the impression of bilateral asymmetry; and so, together with recognition of their morphological relation to occlusion, they often assist orientation.

The Cusps

The disposition of the four cusps is most commonly two each on B and P, so placed that they tend to form the angles of a rounded quadrilateral. Decrease in number of cusps primarily involves the DP cusp but there are many gradations of reduction, and as these are associated with

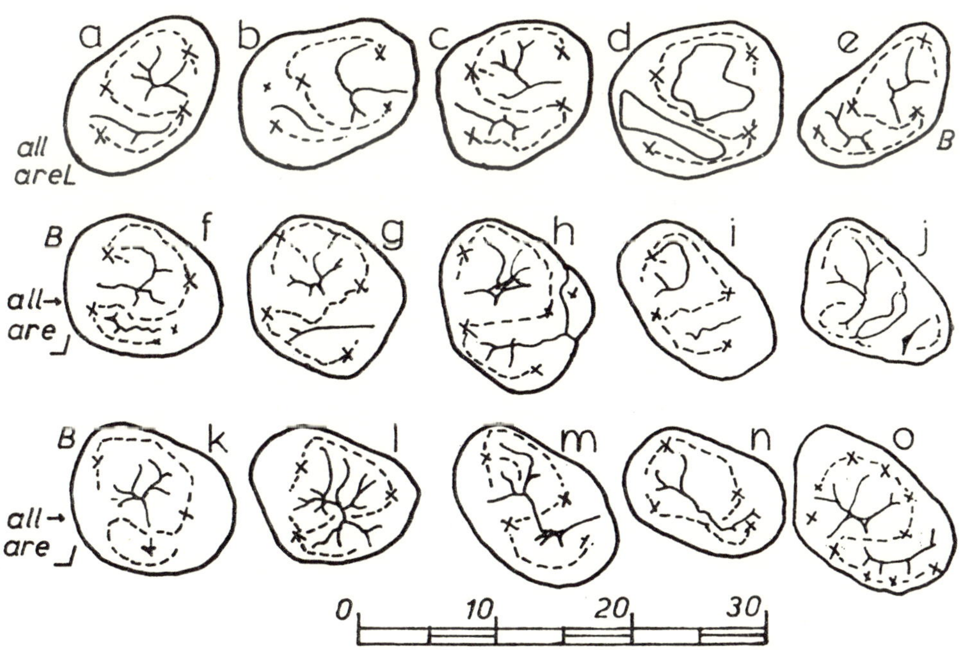

Figure 7-2. Outlines of crowns in occlusal view. The presence or absence of the disto-palatal (DP) cusp is only one of the factors affecting the form of this outline. Note also the variety of occlusal grooves and of pattern formed by main ridges.

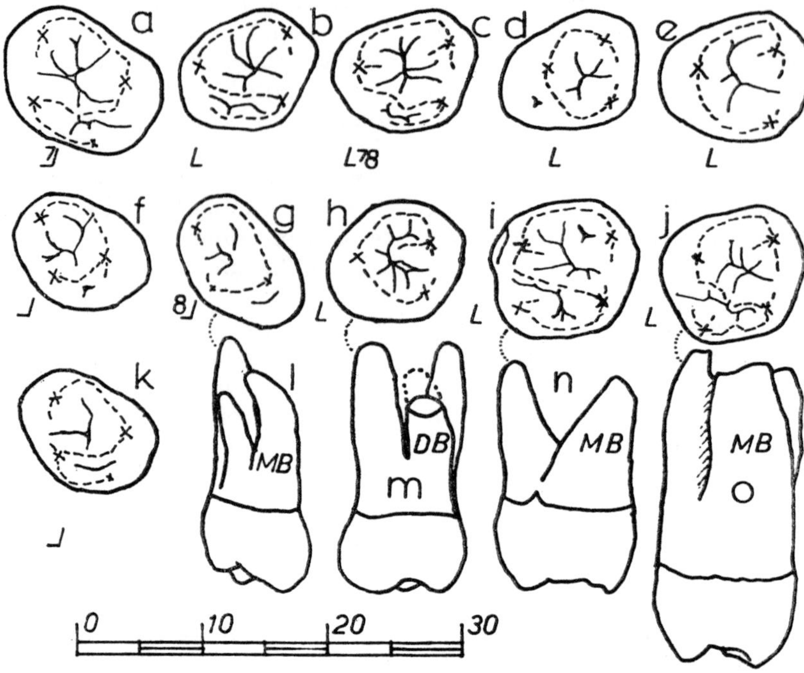

Figure 7-3. More occlusal outlines as in previous figure. Where M and B outlines of whole tooth are also shown, note variation in root styles, crown curvature and cusps. Tooth *f* is shown in buccal view in Figure 7-5 *o*.

variations also in grooves and pits and ridges and tubercles, it is often a matter of subjective judgment to describe what is seen—certainly it is not a variation that can be measured (Fig. 7-2 *a-o*).

In other cases it seems that the MP cusp has been enlarged at the expense of the DP cusp, so that the MP cusp is the largest of all three, and this impression of size is all the more noticeable because of the greater convexity of the palatal surface (Fig. 7-2 *k*). In some cases of reduction of the DP cusp, the occlusal outline may be described as more oval or triangular than quadrilateral (Fig. 7-3 *b-h*).

The DB cusp also is subject to reduction in size, but neither so often nor so much as the DP cusp, for it does not "disappear" (Fig. 7-3 *g,h,k,l,m*). This reduction usually affects the second and third molars rather than the first, as is also the case with reduction or loss of the DP cusp.

The MB cusp, while constantly present and usually prominent, is often occlusally less robust than the MP cusp. If the same character is described another way, by saying that the anterior sulcus may sometimes appear more saucer-shaped at the expense of the MB cusp, perhaps a more satisfactory idea is conveyed regarding variation in this character (Fig. 7-3 *i,n* by contrast with *j,o*).

Increase in the number of cusps may conveniently be considered under two headings—the Carabelli cusp and the non-Carabelli cusp. The Carabelli cusp is thus named when the additional cusp is on the MP aspect of the tooth. In the great majority of cases it occurs in the first molar. It is not uncommon in the second deciduous molar and is also found in the second permanent molar. Its greatest range of variation is found in the first permanent molar. Much attention has been devoted to this feature by many workers, including Korenhof (1960) who gives an extensive list of relevant references. In its minimal degree the feature is a pit rather than a tubercle (Fig. 7-4 *a*). Although the term "Carabelli pit" may not be historically justifiable, it is convenient; but it tends to be rather loosely used to refer either to a true pit or to a small groove in this position.

The term Carabelli cusp also is not a precise term, for although it implies usually a recognizable small additional cusp in a particular position, there is considerable variation in the degree of its development and in the nature of the grooves and other cusps related to it. If, for convenience, the groove between this cusp and the rest of the tooth is also referred to as the Carabelli groove, it will facilitate description of the variations in the relationship of this groove to the posterior occlusal groove which separates the two palatal cusps and often continues on to the palatal surface as a true palatal groove. Thus the Carabelli groove may be separate from both of these grooves (Fig. 7-4 *a,b*), it may join the palatal groove (Fig. 7-4 *c*) or it may join both of them where the Carabelli cusp is prominent (Fig. 7-4 *e,f*). The second of these is a rather extreme example in which the Carabelli cusp is so large that it appears partly to have displaced the MP cusp, or to have "pushed" it into the centre of the tooth. Thus both the anterior sulcus and the DB cusp have been reduced, and instead of having an MP cusp in the usual position, the tooth presents it as an "island" cusp, hemmed in by a wide contact between the DP and Carabelli cusps. Another unusual variant is shown in Figure 7-4 *d*, where the rather small Carabelli cusp presents a shallow longitudinal groove. The impression one gets in this case is of

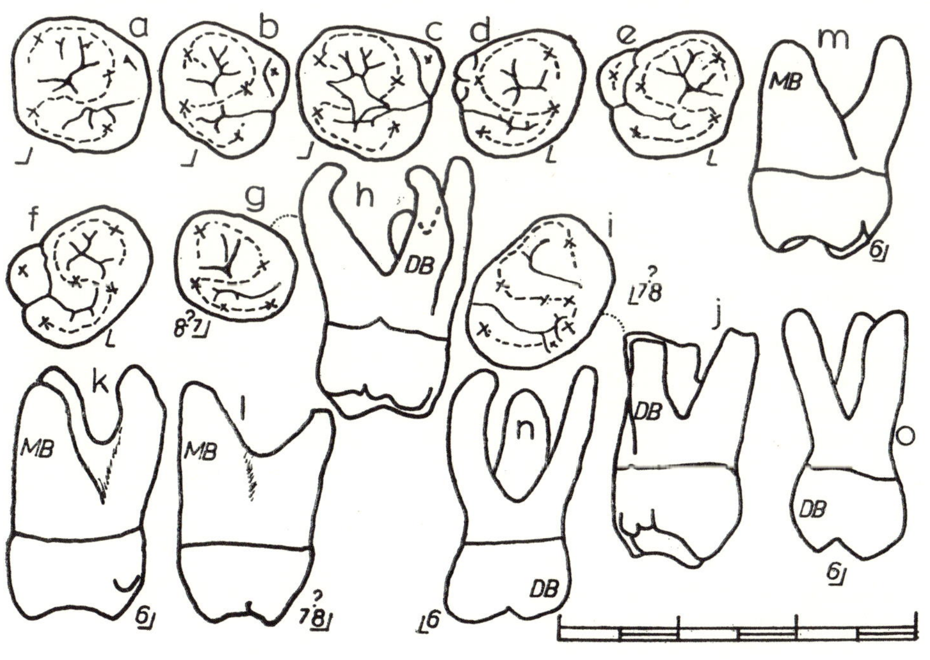

Figure 7-4. *a-j*, the Carabelli feature and other additional tubercles in the molar crown. *k, l*, partial fusion of P root to a B root. In tooth *f* the root does not show any additional element in MB or P roots, but the P root is fused to DB branch. *n,o*, styles of divergence in B roots, and of reduction of DB cusp (see *i,j* also in the latter respect).

a tendency towards bifidity of a "normal" Carabelli cusp, but not of duplication of the cusp.

The additional cusp, which is not a Carabelli cusp, may be present in much more variety. Firstly there are those which are difficult to define by position or description. In some teeth one or more of the four cusps may be reduced in size and replaced by a ridge bearing one or more tubercles, and this may occur as a distal marginal ridge in an almost three-cusped tooth (Fig. 7-4 *g,h*), in the oblique occlusal ridge (Fig. 7-4 *i,j*) or in the mesial marginal ridge (Fig. 7-5 *a*). In some cases these teeth present no appreciable deviation in the root pattern. In others, however, there is a variation in the root, of such a position and nature that it seems reasonable to assume that there is some developmental association with a variation noted in the crown, and Figure 7-5 *a* is one of these. With these cases an approach is made toward the very wide group of variations referred to above as examples of Odontopagus parasiticus concretus (Opc).

The Opc is by no means always a typical cusp, nor is it found only in the crown. It may be found as apparently part of both crown and root, or it may appear to be mostly, or entirely, in one or the other. It is necessary therefore to consider some cases with variation in crown form and deal with others later as involved with root variation. An Opc may resemble in form and size a Carabelli cusp, but because of its different position, such as MB instead of MP, it must be classed as Opc (Fig. 7-5 *b*). Alternatively it may be situated MP, but not on a first molar tooth (Fig. 7-34 *d*).

The question must arise as to whether the honour is justified that was accorded to Carabelli for his observation and description of a feature which does not appear in all teeth, nor in the same degree, but is constant only in its position. In the present study there are so many examples of Opc and its variations that one must object to special distinction for the feature just because it is sometimes found in this particular position. The decision must be influenced by finding whether there is a difference other than locality between the series of Opc on one hand, and Carabelli cusps on the other.

Other differences can be looked for on the basis of structure, form, degree of development, frequency of occurrence and relation to the root of the tooth. Examination of structure is outside the field of the present study. It would require sections and histological examination under magnification, but this survey is limited to only naked-eye studies in morphology. As for classifying the form and degree of development of Carabelli's cusp, it is the variety of Carabelli features such as pits, grooves and tubercles, as well as their prominence, which are used as the basis. The classification is subjective and to be workable it inevitably groups together or ignores obvious variations (their relative importance unknown) such as depth and extent of grooves and fissures, and relation of the Carabelli feature to the form and size of adjacent cusps. But all these variations, including so-called positive and negative features, are involved in the study of Opc in any part of the crown of any other tooth in the dentition.

As for differences between the Carabelli cusp and Opc in their relation to tooth roots, there is no information—no one seems to have thought of looking for it. The well-developed Carabelli cusp was bound to attract attention, and it may well be that such is common in MP position. The more obvious variations in this position would next deserve comment, but the greater diversity of additional features elsewhere in the dentition, and much less frequent in any particular location, would present a much more formidable subject for description. Root involvement or relationship would require much more work even in skeletal material, and it would eliminate the simplicity of reporting by a glance in the living mouth at an easily recognizable feature.

This I see as the setting for the concept and study of Carabelli's cusp, namely as a coronal feature in a particular position on a particular tooth, easily reported in convenient categories for a vast number of observations. Such data are a fertile field for statistics and racial comparison, and with palaeontological data included, the crop of hypotheses has been prolific. No doubt there are now itchy fingers feeding the data to hungry computers.

One might well ask how these concepts have so long escaped rejection as a valid basis for investigation. Rather the writer submits that the difference between Carabelli features and other accessory features is of a contrived nature, and has arisen from a preconception that significance lay in location. It was largely overlooked that an "exposed" location could give undue prominence to the feature; that there were many similar features elsewhere; and that visible presence in the crown did not establish that a coronal feature was exclusively coronal. (See frontispiece.)

With these considerations in mind, the

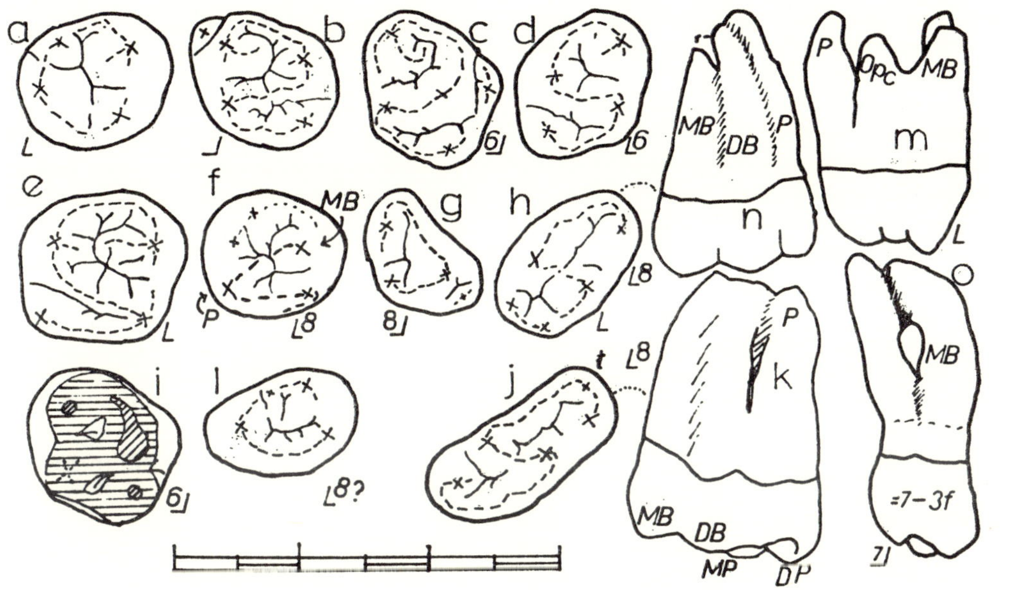

Figure 7-5. Cusps, variation in number. Decrease, by reduction or absence of DP cusp. Increase, by presence of Carabelli and paramolar tubercles, Opc and a variety of small tubercles. *a,* mesial Opc with additional radicle partly fused with MB root. *b,* "paramolar tubercle," (? Opc) on MB aspect (see also Fig. 7-26 *d*). *c,* Carabelli cusp. *d,* four cusps (DP is large) and few grooves with clear S-form of main ridges. *e,* four cusps and many grooves. *f,* two Opc on M, P cusp displaced distally and no DP cusp. Ridge system disrupted and distorted so that only upper loop of S is present. The crown of this tooth is wider on P than on B side, the reverse of the usual. *g,* DP cusp displaced to P and isolated from ridge system so that only upper part of Z is present. *h,* compressed crown and fused flattened root. Four cusps plus Opc on distal with its radicle fused with P root as seen in *n. i,* four cusps evenly worn until dentine is exposed in three of them, and the only remaining unworn occlusal surface is anterior and posterior pits. *j,k,* fused root and compressed crown with four cusps plus Opc tubercle *(t)* on mesial. *l,* three cusps plus mesial tubercle. *m,* three cusps plus a mesial Opc tubercle with associated radicle partly fused to MB root. *o,* same tooth as Figure 7-3 *f,* having three cusps and merely a pit representing posterior groove. The remaining occlusal ridge system is the top portion of the Z-shape. The buccal roots first diverged and later fused in the apical third. In *c* the oblique ridge is prominent with no dip, by contrast with the interrupted ridges in Figure 7-2 *l,m,n.* Teeth *g* and *j,* although apparently very different, both have the DP cusp "pushed" around to the P side. In *g* it is a small cusp and its connecting ridge to DB is lost. In *j* it is a large cusp and retains a long connecting ridge; it also has an additional element *t* on mesial.

hypotheses concerning phylogenetic significance in the Carabelli features lose much of their attraction, and it seems much more likely that they and Opc are ontogenetic variations and do not necessarily have phylogenetic significance.

This concept of the Opc accords most readily with one's observations of the range of variation in their position and degree of development. Thus the aberration may occur, or cease, at any stage of tooth formation with the result that there may be produced anything from an enamel tubercle, or slight enlargement of some part of crown or root, to a recognizable twin formation adherent to the parent tooth, or even separate as a supernumerary or supplemental tooth. It is suggested that in seeking an explanation for these aberrations the major question is not "Why are there so many variations?" but rather "Why are the details of the specific pattern so closely maintained?"

As for examples, space will permit illustration of only a few of the great number in the collection. It might at first seem that they could conveniently be considered in three groups separately, namely those confined to the crown, to the root, and those involving both regions. The demarcation of these groups however is not precise, for classification of some specimens is arbitrary or subjective, and so illustrations will be deferred until root variation has been considered.

The Ridges and Grooves in the Crown

These features are no less characteristic in upper molars than are the cusps, and they also vary widely. As in other teeth, some molars may have little more than the main ridges and grooves while others may present a number of subsidiary grooves and pits. These may extend on to the ridges and thereby complicate description of the details of their irregularities (Fig. 7-5 *d,e*).

As with premolars, upper molars also tend to have M and D marginal ridges but the form of the latter varies much more because of the many degrees of reduction that may occur in the DP cusp. Cusp ridges of both buccal cusps tend to be almost continuous except for a wide buccal groove, while those of both palatal cusps are nearly always separated by a groove which, although often a deep fissure, may also vary considerably in length and depth. Often this groove is confined to the occlusal surface, especially where there is some reduction of the DP cusp. In the three-cusp molar this posterior occlusal groove may be reduced to a short groove, or to a pit, or there may be no visible trace of it (Figs. 7-3 *d,e* and 7-5 *f,g,l*). But where there is a well-formed DP cusp, this groove is usually prominent, and continues on to the palatal surface as the palatal groove, a very common variety (Fig. 7-5 *d*).

Further contributions to the variations in grooves are made by the range of development of the Carabelli cusp and by additional elements (Opc). It has been mentioned earlier that the former may contribute a pit, a small groove, a larger one continuous with the palatal groove, or an extensive modification of the occlusal groove pattern in extreme examples (Figs. 7-4 *f* and 7-31 *a,b,c*), but variations arising from the Opc cannot be encompassed so descriptively as a series. This is because they are not confined like the so-called Carabelli feature to a particular region of the crown, and they may involve also the tooth root. Some of these grooves may be seen in outlines of Opc below.

Although the cusp ridges of MB and DB cusps are almost continuous by contrast with those of the palatal cusps, there is nevertheless often a concavity of the buccal surface in this position. This is not a prominent character, but by contrast with the more angular concavity of the palatal groove it can be helpful in identifying these surfaces when the more usual distinguishing characters are missing. It is illustrated by a tooth where occlusal features have been worn flat, leaving a trace of the two occlusal grooves and exposing dentine of the mesial cusps (Fig. 7-5 *i*).

For ready identification and orientation of the crown of an upper molar tooth, probably the most consistently present and helpful character is the oblique ridge joining MP and DB cusps. The ridge, though prominent, is seldom of the same height as the cusps and is not straight in direction between the cusps; it bends distally, thereby making the anterior occlusal fossa larger and more saucer-shaped than the posterior one. This same feature contributes on the one hand to the oblique direction which may be so noticeable in the distal groove, and on the other to the saucering referred to, for the anterior surface of this oblique ridge tends also to be more oblique to the tooth axis than its distal surface.

The near continuity of cusp ridges on the buccal side and their abrupt interruption on the palatal side, together with the continuity between both mesial cusps and between both distal cusps through mesial and distal marginal ridges respectively, is specially noteworthy. This continuity through the oblique ridge produces a pattern which permits orientation for mesial and distal, and for left or right, to be rapidly determined in the great majority of upper molars when other features are missing.

These ridges collectively form either an S or a Z shape, always S for left and Z for right teeth. The middle bar of the letter, i.e. the oblique ridge, always points forward to the midline, so that it is easy to place the tooth in an imaginary palatal view of a dental arch, and check its identification. To stress the infallibility of this test it may be pointed out that neither an S nor a Z can lose identity by inversion, and that if either is placed in the wrong side of the imaginary dental arch the "oblique ridge" points backwards to the midline. In most teeth there should be no difficulty in distinguishing mesial from distal, or buccal from palatal.

This is not to say that all teeth may be readily identified by this method. There are some which at first sight do not present the series of ridges just described, and some of the reasons for this are: (a) the DP cusp may be reduced or missing; (b) the occlusal pattern is complicated by a Carabelli cusp, or an Opc; (c) the oblique ridge is not prominent, or appears to be interrupted; (d) the crown has been damaged or modified by pathology, fracture or wear; (e) the crown form has been modified in outline by distortion (the "compressed" outline), and perhaps further complicated by any of the conditions mentioned in (a) to (d) above, with the probable exception of the "conventional" Carabelli cusp, for this is unlikely to be associated with a "compressed" type of tooth.

These possible complications will be dealt with briefly: (a) if the DP cusp is reduced to or beyond the degree where the posterior occlusal groove is represented by an elongated pit it may still be possible to trace a modified S or Z, or at least to recognize the upper section of the letter (Figs. 7-2 and 7-3 give examples). Root elements may reinforce one's judgment; (b) in these cases it is often possible to distinguish between the additional element and the "basic" features, but there are some which severely tax one's ability to recognize these; (c) this group also may present problem cases (Fig. 7-2 *l,n*); (d) in these cases one must make the most of any remaining clues, such as stained or polished areas and facets, which may indicate position in the mouth; (e) the "compressed" tooth is considered in the next section on occlusal outlines.

Occlusal Outlines of Crowns

It was shown in Chapter 1 that some tooth outlines resemble a geometrical figure (Figs. 1-2, 1-14, 1-17, 1-25, 1-33), and this applies also to the occlusal view of upper molars. Variations of the kind noted for incisor teeth, which were related to types such as square or tapering, convex or more straight-sided, or other characters which are "personal" in a dentition, may not be so easily recognized in occlusal views. The most obvious factor related to variation is the number and arrangement of cusps. It has been seen that while, as a group, all upper molars share in the range of this variation, yet there are differences in the nature of such variations in the individual teeth, whether they are first, second or third molar. Thus, as the first molar usually has four well-developed cusps, its outline is more nearly rhomboid, whereas the outline of the second molar, by reduction of the DP cusp, tends to change the quadrilateral outline towards a trapezoid or triangular form (Figs. 7-2 and 7-3).

A large DP cusp or a large Carabelli cusp may give a trapezoid outline to a first molar, so that the noticeably longest side is on palatal or mesial (Fig. 7-4 *c,e*). An unusual reversal of relative dimensions is seen in Figure 7-5 *f* where two Opc elements lie between MB and P cusps, and are associated with a separate fourth root branch.

The rhomboid character of equality of opposite angles allows for variation in angles, and this is readily observable in occlusal views of upper molars, especially if the angle between M and B surfaces is studied. In normal teeth this is an acute angle, more so than its opposite angle, and its recognition assists in orientation of the tooth. The comment that the DP angle is less acute recognizes that true rhomboid characters are not present, and leads to an examination of the embrasure between molars.

It will be observed that the M side of the rhombus tends itself to be angled nearer to the B side, while the D side of the rhombus is more arc-like. This has the effect of bringing the contact points of these teeth nearer to buccal so that the palatal embrasure is longer and wider, and acts as a spillway towards the tongue during mastication. As the angle just mentioned is also nearer the occlusal region of the M surface, the contact point also is nearer occlusal. This in turn makes for greater efficiency in mastication and contributes to protection of the interdental gingival tissues. Severe occlusal wear may well extend beyond the contact point, but such wear is usually accompanied by interproximal wear also. In the absence of complicating conditions such as tooth loss, pathology or malocclusion, the loss of the contact is compensated for. The interproximal wear changes the contact from a point to an area, and the usual tendency for teeth to drift forward maintains contact in this area. The result of failure in this or of excess fibre in the diet may be the impaction of food between teeth, with the usual sequelae, namely inflammation, pain and resorption of interproximal tissues.

There are two groups of upper molars where the variation in occlusal outline appears not to be primarily influenced by increase or decrease in number and development of the usual four cusps. These are the teeth with an Opc, and the teeth we may describe as compressed, for want of a better term. As a group, these teeth vary considerably, but always the B-P dimension is greater than the M-D. Mostly the teeth are third molars, but some are second, and they give the impression that during development the tooth bud was restricted distally and forced to assume an apparently compressed or distorted form (Fig. 7-5 *j*). These teeth include those where the usual degrees of reduction of DP cusp are easily recognizable (Fig. 7-5 *l*), and also some where there are four cusps, and the DP cusp appears to have been "pushed around" to lie palatally of the MP cusp (Figs. 7-2 *e*, 7-5 *g,j* and 7-6 *b,f*).

The author does not know what evidence there is to account for the apparently compressed morphology of these teeth, and there is no indication that inheritance has been considered as a factor. In the first instance the most logical field of study would appear to be anatomical relationships during development and growth of the face and jaws. As the alveolar process lengthens to accommodate the increasing number of teeth in the permanent dentition, its immediate relations include the nasal fossa medially, the maxillary sinus above and the palate and sphenoid bones with the pterygoid process and fossa posteriorly. Most directly posterior to the alveolar region is the external pterygoid plate, the lateral and medial surfaces of which give partial attachment to the external and internal pterygoid muscles respectively. These are the structures therefore that are most closely related to the developing last molar, but it should be noted that this relationship changes during growth, and no doubt variations in the time and extent of these changes occur among individuals.

Thus, in the child, the width between pterygoid processes "lags behind" the increasing width between the growing alveolar regions. The difference seen in density of palatal bones and these alveolar regions bears testimony to the greater vascularity and growth in the maxillary bones at this stage. Attention was drawn to these differences in the author's earlier work (Taylor, 1963a, Plate 1 in that paper), and also to variations in length of tuberosity, and in its relation to the maxillary sinus (same paper, Plate 9, Fig. 49). In that paper, and in a preceding one also (Taylor, 1962b), there are many illustrations which show variations in the relation of the tuberosity to the pterygoid process in the adult skull. In some the juvenile relationship has persisted to a certain degree. In others the pterygoid fossa and external pterygoid plate are more directly behind the alveolar ridge, and the post-dental alveolar process is short. Two such cases associated with a "compressed" type of third molar are well shown in the photographs (Taylor, 1962b, Plate 2, Fig. 20; and Plate 8, Fig. 72). In the first mentioned case the third molars have four cusps, but the DP cusp has been displaced to lie palatally to the MP cusp. In the second, the remaining 8| has three cusps, and the other third molar that was present (|8), is represented by a very "compressed" socket from which the tooth was lost post-mortem.

In earlier papers (Taylor, 1962a, 1962b, and 1963a), graphs and photographs of well-formed palates show variation in the size or length of the post-dental alveolar process, and in its relation to the maxillary sinus. In some of them the molar teeth appear to have insufficient space, and some third molars have "compressed" crowns. But it is important to note that a short alveolus has no relationship to crown morphology, for crown form is fixed and calcified before formation of the alveolar bone which will finally support the tooth.

Crowns of these teeth are formed in crypts high up in what later becomes the posterior wall of the maxillary sinus. Initially the occlusal surface faces almost posteriorly, and as it descends it rotates to face eventually its antagonizing lower molar. If the shape of these so-called "compressed" teeth is the result of crowding of the tooth bud before calcification, certain questions arise. Among these are, firstly, what structures could be involved; secondly, what are their relationships; and thirdly, what stresses might be present?

The structures would surely have to be the tooth germs, and later perhaps the dental crypts with their contained developing crowns of second and third molars. The relations, in brief, are that the third is superior and deep to the second, and uncalcified when calcification in the second is appreciably advanced. The question of stresses is more difficult. It is complicated by variations in growth rhythm and development of other nearby parts, including at least the sinus and maxillary tuberosity, nasal and pterygoid fossae, the dentition in general and functions related to mastication and respiration.

The writer is unwilling to speculate as to how these complicated factors work together and with other factors produce such varied results. Suffice it to observe that delay in descent of the second molar crypt, or acceleration in the third, could conceivably distort the softer (less calcified) germ and crypt of the latter. It is relevant to point out that the major axis of the compressed outline would become relatively greater in an MB to DP direction (as is found in Fig. 7-2 *n*); also that the flattened, or even concave, region of "compression" would become the medial surface of the crown (as also is found in these cases, Fig. 7-6 *c-g*).

The process of movement of the tooth crypt through the bone is concomitant with its movement with the bone of the growing face. The manner of growth-changes in these bones was demonstrated by Brash (1924), while Brodie (1934) reviewed studies of tooth movement and "eruption." The latter were made mostly with lower teeth, and even with uppers it seems that second and third molars have received little attention.

Thus it seems reasonable to regard the "compressed" appearance of some of these teeth as an imposed character in the absence of evidence that it is of genetic origin, but it is advisable to repeat that compression of the crown has no relation to restricted space in the alveolar ridge. Such restriction however (sometimes in association with sinus variation) might well account for the compressed appearance of roots of some of these molar teeth (Fig. 7-6 *h,i,j*). Sometimes a compressed crown is associated with a root that has three

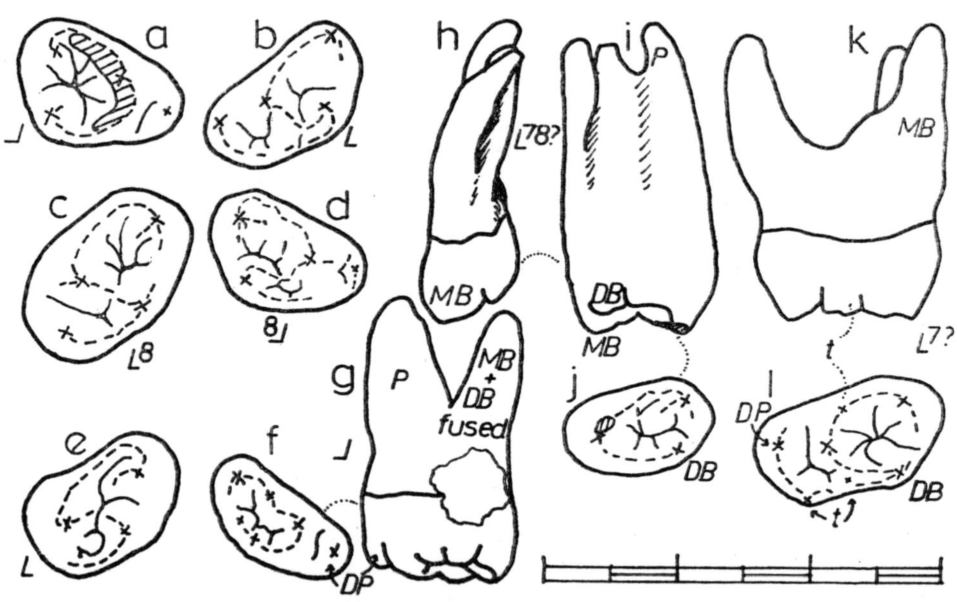

Figure 7-6. Teeth with compressed crowns or roots, or both. *a,* tooth with facet of occlusal wear. The DP cusp appears to be "pushed" in a MP direction so increasing the BP dimension at the expense of M-D. *b,* a similar distortion but to a greater degree (or with a larger DP cusp), so that the occlusal outline appears compressed against its adjacent tooth giving a concave M surface. *c,d,e,* more examples of compressed crowns with four cusps. The S or Z pattern of main ridges can be recognized, although in *e* the oblique ridge is interrupted. *f,g,* two views of a tooth having a compressed crown, and fusion of both B roots. The ridge pattern is confused by extra tubercles, one on M and two in place of DB cusp. The DP cusp is displaced so that the distal limb of Z is missing. *h,i,j,* three views of a tooth with a small DB cusp and no DP cusp, so that the root as well as the crown appear compressed. In the root this is probably an imposed character related to the posterior wall of the maxillary sinus. *k,l,* two views of a tooth with three well-spaced roots. There are three additional tubercles *(t,t).* Two of these appear to have displaced the DP cusp more palatally, and a third on mesial appears associated with an additional element on MB root. This is not a typical compressed crown, although its B-P dimension has been increased.

well-developed branches (Fig. 7-6 *k,l*). In such case the root will appear to have been compressed near the cervix, because it is of course essential for root and crown to conform in this region.

Although the use of the term "compressed" may tentatively have been justified by showing that it could be an imposed character in some teeth, this certainly does not cover all cases. It follows from this discussion that in some it is the crown and in some it is the root that has been compressed, and that a differing combination of factors may have been involved at the development stage of either. The term "compressed tooth" would be better replaced by "tooth with compressed crown, or root, or both." And this is not all, for there are so many teeth where the changed outline of the crown may arise in some degree from the presence of additional elements, or Opc.

Teeth with an Opc were mentioned above as a group where variations in the usual four cusps were not the main cause of variation in the occlusal outline. In these it is rather the Opc itself, its position and degree of development, or its style, that changes the outline. But these additional elements may also occur in the presence of cusp-related and compression variations (Figs. 7-30 *b,c,* 7-31 *a,b,c* and 7-24 *d*). This adds considerably to the variety of shape that may be seen in the occlusal view of the crowns of upper molars.

THE ROOT

When summing up the observations of variation in an earlier chapter, it was remarked that except that crown and root must identify at the cervix, they appear to vary independently. The same can be said for upper molar teeth. There are certain characters that may be found most often in the first, second or third molar, characters in the crown or root that relate to the form of the outline of a transverse section at the cervix. The root itself tends to have three branches, each with its own basic or type characters, but subject to fusion in almost any degree with one or both of the others. Additional elements in the form of Opc, sometimes present in crown and/or root, must also be included in this study. The scope of variation in regard to personal characters, thickness, slenderness, breadth, length, type of apex and curvature was very considerable even for single-rooted teeth.

Since in upper molars each of the three root branches has its own characters, and their divergence or otherwise tends to be recognizably different in the three molars, the range of variation is potentially much greater in these teeth. The inclusion of additional elements further extends it. But this is not all, for there are yet other factors which, although apparently external to the teeth, seem likely to exert considerable influence in some cases on the final form of the root. These are mainly concerned with the maxillary sinus and the alveolar ridge.

The first has been cited in relation to curves or bends in upper premolar roots, but its own varied morphology frequently results in an intimate relationship to the roots of molar teeth. The length or backward extension of the alveolar ridge, closely associated as it is with the form of the maxillary sinus (Taylor, 1962b, c; 1963a), must in some degree determine the bone space available for root formation; so also must the height of the ridge (or depth of palate). For these many reasons the study of variation in upper molar roots is complex and therefore restrictions on description and illustrations are unavoidable.

Characters of Molar Root Branches

Some general comments on molar roots and the manner of variation were given earlier under the heading "Size of Molar Teeth." These must now be extended, and illustrations presented.

Apart from personal or family characters which have been shown to apply to the roots of any or all of the teeth of a denti-

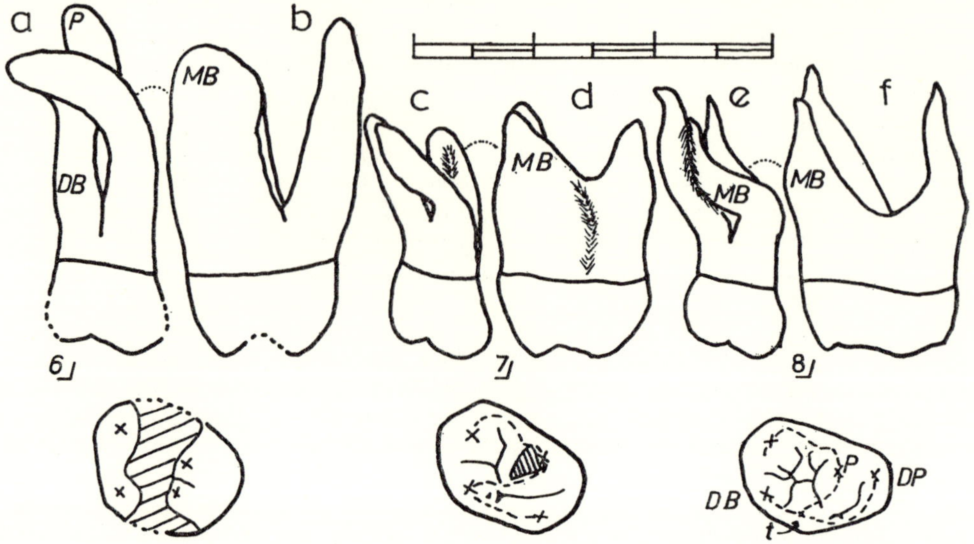

Figure 7-7. Three teeth, with three views of each. Excessive root curvature, especially of MB root, appears to be an imposed character associated with maxillary sinus. In the first and second molars, association with the zygomatic or lateral wall of the sinus is the most likely relationship, and in the third molar the posterior wall appears to have involved the P root also.

tion, upper molars have more type characters because of their complex form. And since these teeth are close to other variable anatomical structures it would seem reasonable to refer also to imposed characters. It is not intended to imply that these can be described or defined in the same way as one can define personal and type characters. They are visualized rather as the morphological result when certain variations of these anatomical structures are present in association with certain personal characters.

Thus the personal character of long and

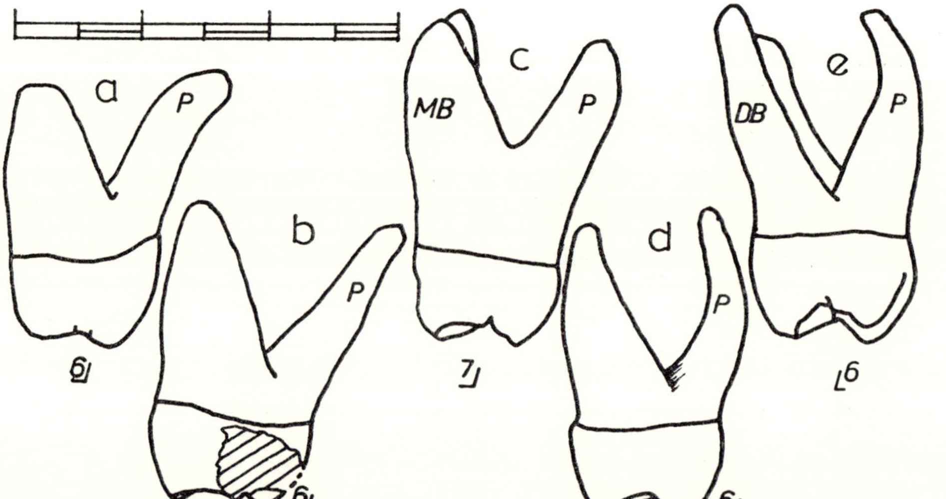

Figure 7-8. Teeth with three roots which present much variation in the degree of divergence and the style of curvature of the P root.

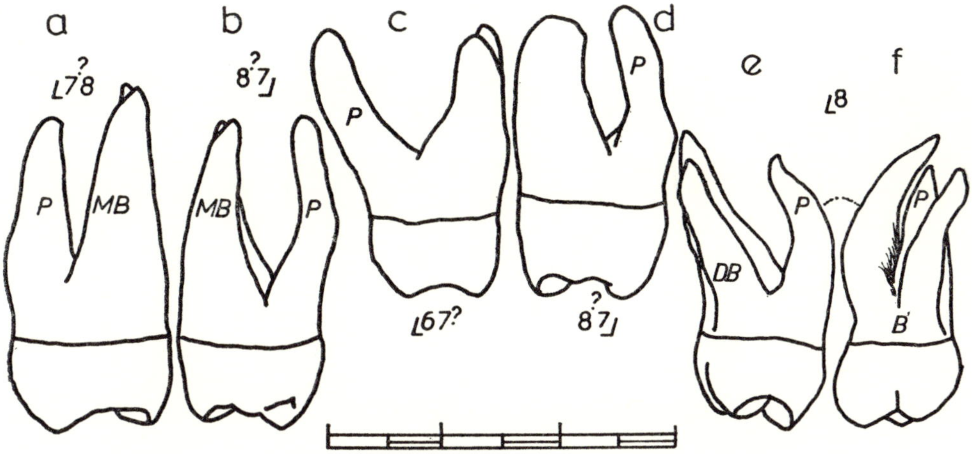

Figure 7-9. Five more examples of variety in P root. Note also variation in size of crowns, sturdiness of roots, and crown-root proportions. See also Figure 7-10 *c-f* in these characters.

relatively thin roots in association with a large maxillary sinus extending towards the zygomatic process may well account for the root form seen in Figure 7-7 *a,b*. A different effect, such as that in Figure 7-7 *c,d* and *e,f*, may result when the tendency for root fusion in a second or third molar is associated with the posterior wall of the sinus.

It seems unlikely that there is a close genetic relationship between personal dental characters and variations in these other structures. On the contrary, it would appear reasonable to regard the relationship as a propinquity of structures which have a partial independence as regards variation, whereby the earlier establishment of form in one may sometimes affect the morphological detail of another during its growth. For example, long thin roots may be found to diverge more or less to B and P; they may curve, or be almost straight (Figs. 7-8 and 7-9), so that whether, or to what degree, these characters have been imposed or influenced by adjacent anatomy may only be surmised. But there may be direct evidence, in the form of attached sinus wall, as in Figure 7-10 *a,b*, that the sinus has dipped deeply between roots. In such a case a radiograph with the tooth *in situ* may appear as though roots entered the sinus, but the teeth in Figure 7-7 would convey to the dental surgeon contemplating extractions their own warning of imposed characters. Radiographs prior to extractions in this region should always be planned to record the relation of sinus to tooth roots, but unfortunately the small size of standard films would usually require additional exposures to produce satisfactory results. For third molars, especially where the second is already missing, a radiograph indicating close relationship of root and sinus may enable special precautions to be taken, thus avoiding a possible fracture of the tuberosity. Such fractures are by no means rare; and they may not only complicate healing, but also the construction of an efficient artificial denture. Examination of extracted upper molars, particularly second and third molars, frequently shows evidence of their close relation to the sinus in the form of smooth areas of sinus wall attached to their roots (Figs. 7-10 *a,b* and 7-11 *a-d*).

When an extracted molar is to be identified it is likely that personal and imposed characters will be first to attract attention, but it is by awareness of type characters that identity is established. In the root this involves recognition of form and arrangement of the three root elements regardless of whether there is complete fusion, or

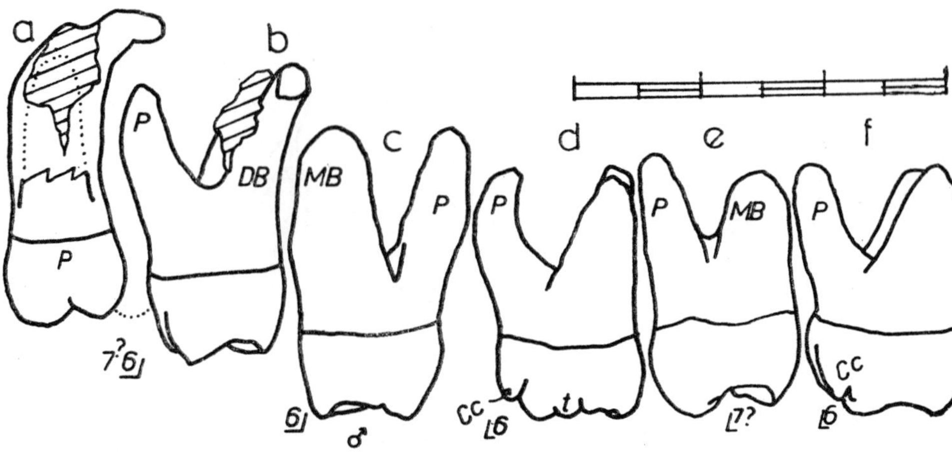

Figure 7-10. *a,b,* a tooth with a portion of wall of maxillary sinus adherent to B roots; it had fractured at time of extraction and shows how the sinus wall or floor may dip down between molar roots. In *a* the P root has been largely omitted from the drawing. (See also Fig. 7-11). *c-f,* more examples of variation in actual size, and proportionate size of crown and root; *c* has a small crown and large sturdy root; *d* has a large crown and a short sturdy root with a recurved P root; *e* has straight roots, P being longest and partly fused to B; *d* and *f* are both first molars of similar length and crown-root proportion, both have a Carabelli tubercle but proximal outlines of crowns are quite different.

partial or total separation of one or two, or of all three root branches.

Although there is a size relationship that is fairly consistent, it is the disposition and shape of each root element that provide the more reliable information to their several identities, and so also to orientation and identification of the tooth. Three different methods have been used to illustrate these characters of size, disposition and shape. In the first (Fig. 7-12A *a*), three-rooted first and second molars have been sectioned close to the root trunk. In the second (Fig. 7-12A *b*), the open, incomplete roots of young teeth (mostly third molars) have been drawn. In the third

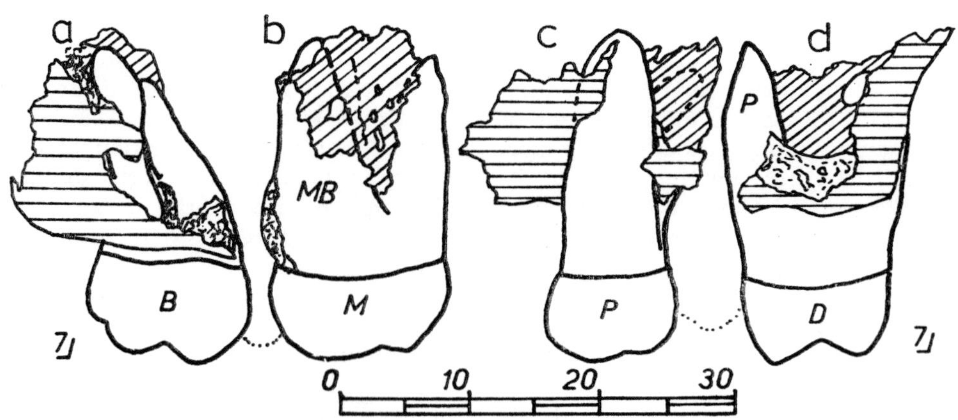

Figure 7-11. Two more examples of extracted teeth with adherent bone. External alveolar bone surface is shaded horizontally; sinus wall or floor is shaded obliquely and cancellous bone is clearly indicated. Both are second molars, and in *a* the indicated portion of tuberosity contains the crypt of the developing third molar. The small unshaded areas in *b* and *d* are root surface. The conformity of roots to sinus wall suggests that root curvature in these cases was an imposed character.

method (Fig. 7-12A *c*) a soft copper wire loop has been moulded around the root, cut and opened, if necessary, for removal; contact of cut ends is restored and held on wax; then copied with the camera lucida. This last method is most suitable for fused and grooved roots.

The MB and P root branches are large. Because they are so different in form there is no need to know which one is larger. In the transverse section the MB root is approximately oval, often more flattened on the mesial aspect, and the long axis lies in a general B-P direction; this axis may sometimes incline distally as it passes from B to P (various examples in Fig. 7-12A). In these latter cases the transverse section of the root trunk often presents a rounded

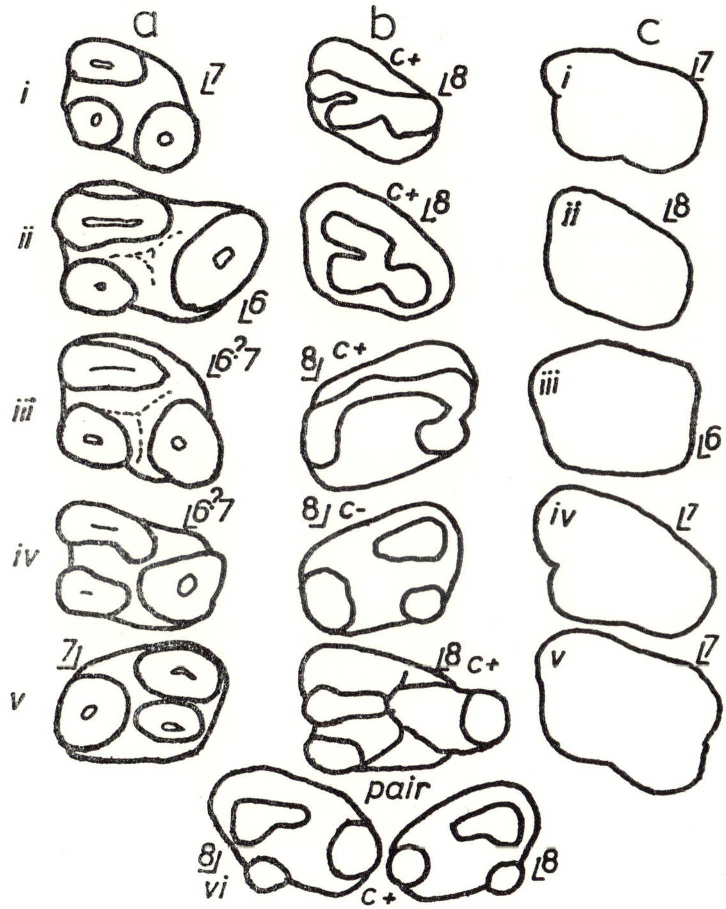

Figure 7-12A. Shapes in transverse section of the three root branches and their relation to root fusion and cervical outlines. Column *a* outlines are from mature three-rooted teeth in which the roots were cut off close to the furcation, and pulp canals are indicated. Note tendency for MB to be more flattened and larger than DB, and for P to be "thickest" but variable. Column *b* outlines are from "apical" views of young teeth with wide open, incomplete roots. All except *b,iv,* are C+ i.e. the formed portion of root was longer than crown height. *b,v,* had a very divergent palatal root. All in this column are third molars and *vi* shows a pair from one person in which some bilateral asymmetry is already apparent. Column *c* shows cervical outlines, from apical aspect, of mature teeth with all roots fused. In *iii* the tooth had a Carabelli cusp, and in *v* the P root element is grooved. This tooth *v* has a large DP cusp as in Figure 7-12B *g*.

acute angle at the mesial cervix, especially in teeth with compressed or rhomboid crowns (Fig. 7-6). Where the MB root branch joins the trunk it usually extends beyond the half-way point of the mesial cervical dimension. This character is very useful for identification and orientation, for it tends to hold also for most cases of fusion, so long as limits of root elements can be recognized. The presence of additional elements (Opc), however, may disturb the usual relativity of size and shape.

The DB root is smaller than the other two. It is often elliptical in section with the long axis of the ellipse approximately parallel to that of the MB root, except when that root is strongly inclined as mentioned earlier. This elliptical outline is most common in first molars, but a smaller and more circular outline is often found in the other two (Fig. 7-12A *a,b*). The P section tends most often to be circular, but may also present a broad ellipse, especially in first molars. In these cases the long axis runs M-D and not B-P (Fig. 7-12A *a,b*).

If the size of root branches for each tooth is considered as a group, their length, thickness, style of apex etc., might seem best described as personal characters, but here also there are type characters involved. These concern relative height and length, which here are different characters, since height may be affected by changes in orientation. If the tooth is viewed from proximal, and levels are visualized almost parallel with the cervix, the root branches may seem almost equal in height as judged by apices. But if the P root is strongly divergent or curved, it may well exceed the other branches in actual length (Figs. 7-7, 7-8, 7-9 and 7-10). In the same view, or from B, the DB root could be judged smallest, but it may stand higher or lower than MB (Figs. 7-7 and 7-8). The lower level of the MB apex may be associated

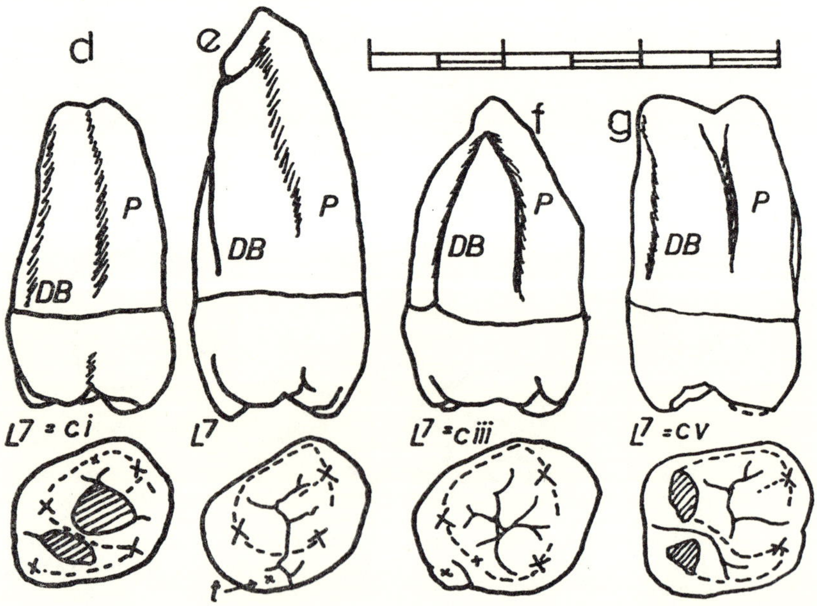

Figure 7-12B. Identification and orientation. In these four second molars all three roots are fused. In each case the root grooves clearly differentiate the three root elements and their type characters. In the crowns, *d* and *g* have four well-defined cusps and the full S-ridge pattern. Tooth *d* has two small amalgam fillings, and *g* has facets of wear on two cusps. Teeth *e,f* have three main cusps and DP tubercles, so that the distal limb of the S-ridge is missing.

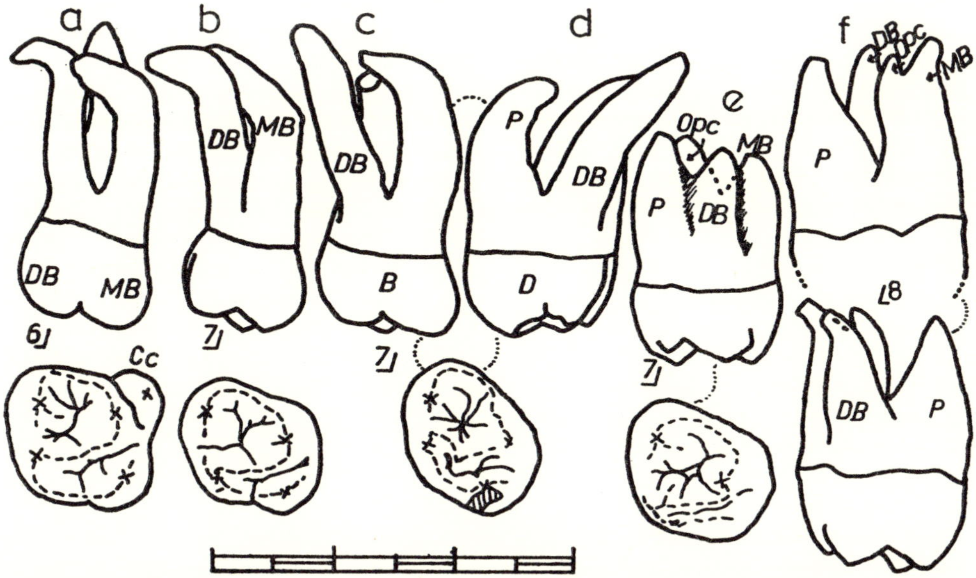

Figure 7-13. Imposed characters, and additional elements. *a,b,c,* buccal roots initially divergent may later tend to make contact, as bends or curves in the lengthening roots are imposed by proximity to sinus wall. The recurved P root in *d* (same tooth as *c*) is uncommon. See other such teeth in Figures 7-9 *d,e* and 7-10 *d*). Tooth *a* has large DB and DP cusps, an MP and a prominent Carabelli cusp. Teeth *e,f* have additional root elements partly fused to MB root on its palatal aspect so providing a fourth apex. Neither tooth has an additional crown element or tubercle to correspond. The occlusal of tooth *f* is shown in Figure 7-6 *c*. Additional outlines of tooth *a* are shown in the frontispiece.

with the distal curve so common in this root (Figs. 7-7 *e,f* and 7-13 *a-d*). When identifying the several root elements it is not their bulk but recognition of their peculiar morphological characters that is of most importance. Even where fusion has largely replaced the "separateness" of root branches, there are often grooves or differences in surface convexity which indicate the various root elements (Figs. 7-12A *c* and 7-12B). It goes without saying that characters of crown and of root are read in conjunction wherever possible.

There are of course variations in the relative bulk of root branches, or in the root elements of fused roots. Many of these no doubt reflect normal variation and would have no special significance. However, awareness of appreciable departure from relative size or from normal morphology in these parts should alert the observer to consider whether this may result from fusion with an additional tooth element. For example, the palatal root, instead of being between the other two branches, may extend beyond one of them, or the MB root may have a second apex (Fig. 7-13 *e,f* and 7-14 *a,b*).

Fusion of Root Branches

Some degree of close approximation or actual "fusion" of root branches is common. It may involve one or more of the usual three branches, as well as additional elements. With the former, the tooth may be described as having three apices, but fewer than three roots (Fig. 7-14 *d,e*), or it may be impossible fairly to describe the root form and there are many such cases. But where additional elements are involved, the morphology of one or more branches may be changed considerably. This may result from combining reduction of normal branches by any degree of fusion between them, with one or more additional elements in root or crown, or both, which are themselves fused to any degree with the main elements (Fig. 7-15). Within these two broadly-defined groups there is scope for great variation, and this is what does occur. These variations may profoundly affect the apparent disposition and recognition of normal elements, and so confound one's efforts to identify and orient a particular isolated tooth.

This is not the best place to pursue the study of variation involving additional elements, since the crown is involved probably as often as the root, and it is preferable to discuss both together. For the present the concern is with fusion involving the three primary root elements.

In such fusion the first molar is least, and the third molar most involved, and this applies both to frequency and to degree. Neither of these adverbial terms may here be precisely defined, but both are useful in describing a tooth's likely relationship to a particular group. Thus in one mouth roots may be widely divergent in the first molar, and less so in the second, while the third molar may have separate but almost contiguous roots. These second and third molars show a tendency towards fusion in root elements but in different degrees, and could reasonably be included in a survey of the incidence or frequency of fusion. The same third molar might well have shown two roots completely joined, and the second molar two contiguous roots, or two or three of its branches partly joined. Thus fusion may be described in a particular tooth, but it can be so complex in variety and degree that it would be futile to attempt a useful classification.

One might further confound the issue by demonstrating the unscientific use of the word "fusion" applied to the character in question. The root elements cannot fuse if they were never separated. Alternatively, should the term be applied only to the subsequent or pathological joining of contiguous roots by cementosis? In the sense in which the term has been used, the great-

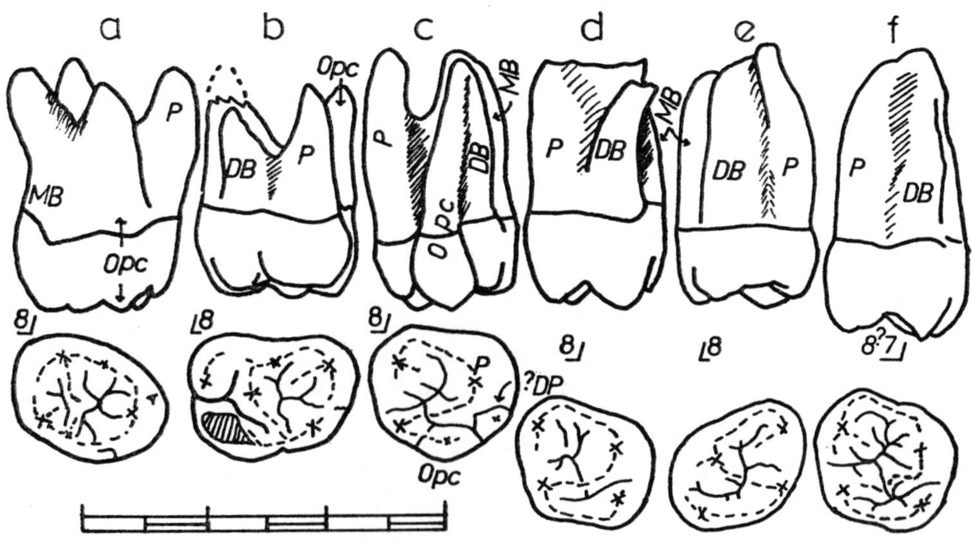

Figure 7-14. *a,b,c,* teeth with additional elements, Opc, in both crown and root. In *a* and *b* the additional root element is partly fused to MB root (as in Figure 7-13 *e,f*). In *c* the prominent Opc is distal and fused to DB root, while MB root is partly fused to P root. The DP cusp is reduced and displaced palatally. *d,e,f,* teeth with four cusps and with varieties of root fusion, but root elements easily identified. In *d,e* the occlusal Z- and S-ridge patterns are easily seen, but in *e,f* the oblique ridge is interrupted.

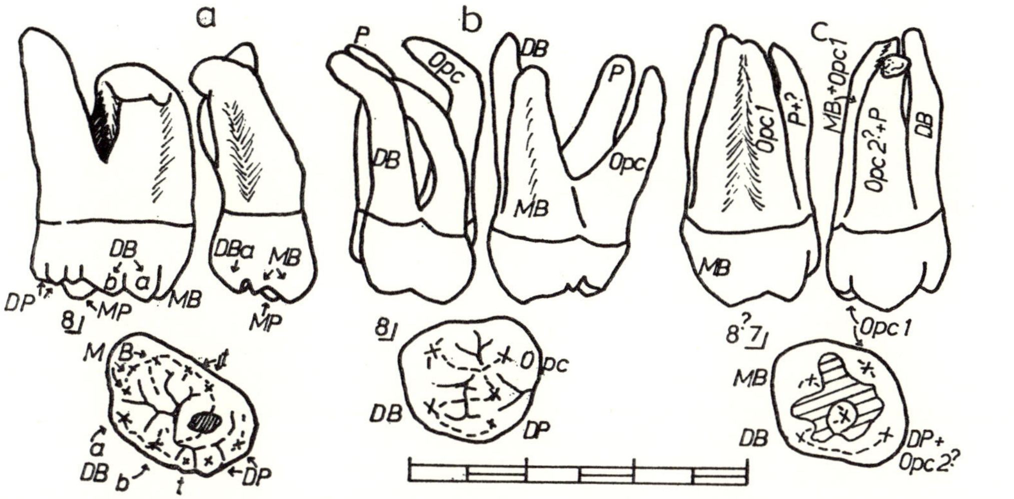

Figure 7-15. Additional elements in crown or root or both, and with variation in type characters which collectively complicate identification. Three teeth and three views of each. *a*, B roots fused, but DB element itself is grooved. Crown has many tubercles, two or three of which may together represent one of the type cusps. Thus MB cusp has three tubercles, and DB and DP two tubercles each, with another between them. The large P cusp with a facet from wear is almost surrounded by tubercles, two of which share the ridge from P to MB. Tooth *b* has four separate root branches, one of which is associated with a prominent crown element between MP and MB. This Opc is joined by a ridge to the top bar of the Z-pattern, while the oblique ridge is interrupted. Tooth *c* has an amalgam filling surrounding the centrally placed main P cusp. There are evidently two Opc each with crown and root elements. Opc 1 is fused to MB root and Opc 2 shares the P root and DP cusp.

est degree of fusion is envisaged as a developing together of tooth elements of enamel organ or dentinal papilla. These elements may alternatively differentiate to varying degrees to produce recognizable different morphological features. Partial separation of contiguous root elements, complete separation, or divergence of part or of the whole of the root elements, are conveniently visualized as degrees of the same character. The term "fusion" is reasonably descriptive of one extreme degree in which this character is found, and I therefore regard it as a permissible and convenient term to use for this purpose. It also conveniently embraces the concept of the inclusion of additional elements during tooth development, which has already been referred to by the abbreviation "Opc."

In regard to frequency and degree of fusion in the three basic root elements of upper molars, it has been seen that there is difficulty in presenting precise information because the character is too complex for treatment either qualitatively or quantitatively. Nevertheless some progress can be made in analysis of the character, and the results are relevant to fields of special interest, namely forensics, physical anthropology and dentistry.

If all root branches were essentially straight, the study of their divergence from one another, or from the tooth axis, would be easier. But like the single roots of other teeth, each molar root branch has both type characters and personal characters, so that there is much variety in the details of length, breadth, taper, and in style of apex. To these may be added curves and bends related to normal bone morphology and perhaps accentuated by variation in adjacent anatomical structures. These latter variations have been called "imposed characters." Thus a root branch which initially, i.e. in the proximal or first-formed portion after the furcation, diverged at a particular angle may change direction (Figs. 7-7, 7-13 and 7-16). The change may be abrupt or otherwise, and the result is that divergence is reduced or increased. These changes may affect two, or all three, root branches in varying degrees. In some cases root branches which were initially divergent from one another may make contact in their distal portions (Figs. 7-7 *c,e*, 7-13 *a,b* and 7-16 *a*). These changes in direction sometimes appear to be imposed characters, such as may be associated with the extension of the sinus into the malar process of the maxilla (Figs. 7-7 *c,e* and 7-16 *d,e*).

In imagination one may visualize the formation of teeth speeded up, and represented as a motion picture on a screen, by a series of radiographs or drawings. A study of the development and growth of the maxillary sinus and of the sequential development of the three molar crowns would show the stage and anatomical relations when crowding (if any) must occur to produce the so-called "compression" of second and third molar crowns. What conditions there are that might produce that effect are not known. But it is known that they would have to operate before the crown was rendered rigid by calcification, and that this happens long before the formation of roots or of alveolar bone which will support the roots.

In this imaginary animated film there might well be depicted the later conformation of roots to the expanding sinus, and to limitations imposed by availability of alveolar bone. The film could thus show the production of imposed root characters

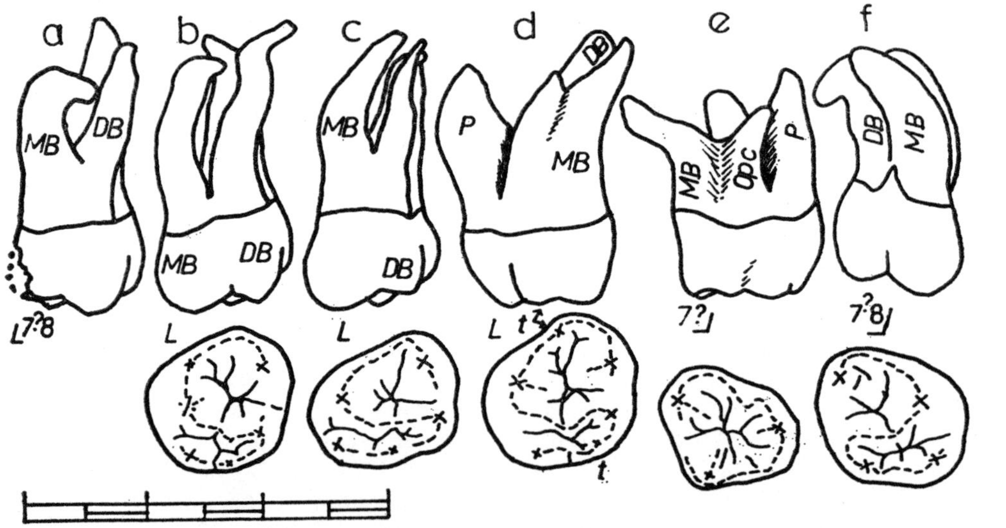

Figure 7-16. Variation in many features of crown and root. In roots, length, sturdiness, abrupt and gradual curves in various directions. In root furcation at an earlier or later stage of root formation contrast *b* (early, giving short root trunk and long branches) with *c* (late, giving long trunk and short branches). In crowns, compare form and size outline, number of cusps and tubercles, ridge and groove patterns. (Crown of *a* had large carious cavity, and details of features had been lost). *b* has an additional tubercle at M and D; they participate in ridge pattern but there is no visible root element. *c* has a distal tubercle but no root element. *d* has tubercles distal and mesial, the latter associated with a root element partly fused with MB root. *e* has only three cusps and no tubercle, but there is a distinct Opc root element partly fused with MB but having its own apex. The occlusal groove pattern is complex. *f* has four distinct cusps with no occlusal complication of grooves or ridges, but the root has imposed characters of curvature and evidently of fusion also.

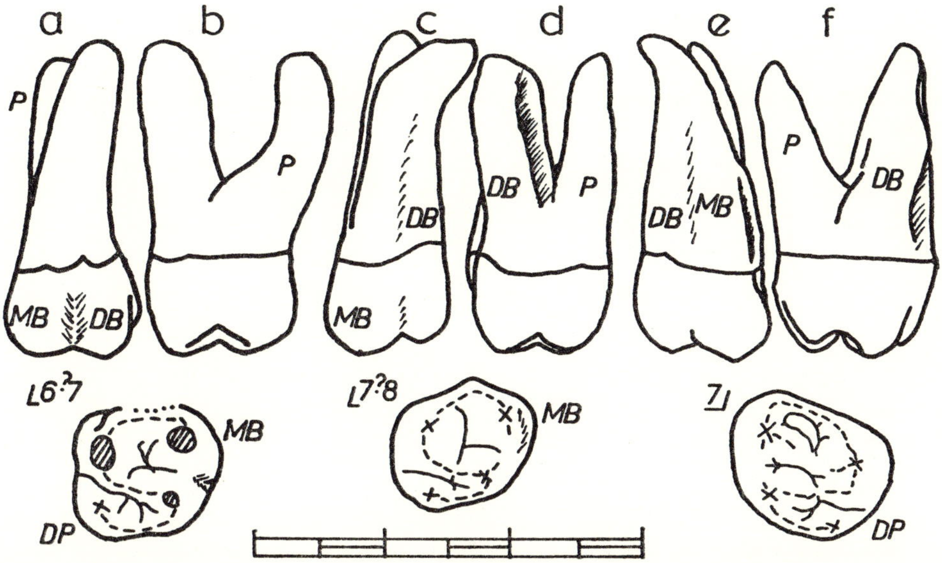

Figure 7-17. Styles of root fusion. *ab,* a tooth with complete fusion of B roots, so that there is a resemblance to the root of an upper premolar. *cd,* fusion of B roots, but the combined root is sturdy and grooved so that its constituent elements are easily recognized. *ef,* another example of fusion of both B roots, and here also the constituent elements are evident. Note the different styles of divergence of P root in these teeth, and that there is no apparent reduction of the four cusps in any of them.

of curvature and of varieties of root fusion. It might also be designed to show incorporation of additional crown and root elements, establishment of occlusion, and so on.

As there are three root elements it is easy to see that the basic patterns of fusion of two branches would be a fusion of both buccal roots, or the fusion of either of them with the palatal root. The other possibility is fusion of all three. All these do occur, but the scope for diversification is widened, not only by combinations of these with other variations to which the "normal" tooth is subject, but also by involvement with additional elements.

As for the basic patterns just postulated, complete fusion of two roots is unlikely to occur in first molars unless the roots are short. While buccal roots, even if long, may not be widely separated, actual contact is more likely to be an imposed character in this tooth which tends to have more divergent roots than the other two. In the second and third molars fusion of roots is common, and may occur in any style. Even complete fusion of buccal roots is found, so that the tooth has a bifid root like an upper premolar (Figs. 7-17 *a,b*).

Fusion of the palatal root with one other arises more often with the DB (Fig. 7-18 *a,b*) than with the MB (Fig. 7-18 *c, d,e*). Awareness of this tendency is important when root fracture occurs during extraction. This note of caution is relevant also when a deciduous maxillary molar is extracted. Because of greater divergence of roots, or of partial resorption from the axial surface of the MB root, it very easily breaks, and it may be found to lie further to mesial than might be expected. Moreover, resorption tends to be less advanced in this root than in the DB root.

Because of the difference in size between the buccal roots, there is likely to be a marked difference in appearance between teeth with this style of fusion, according to the roots involved. If the MB branch

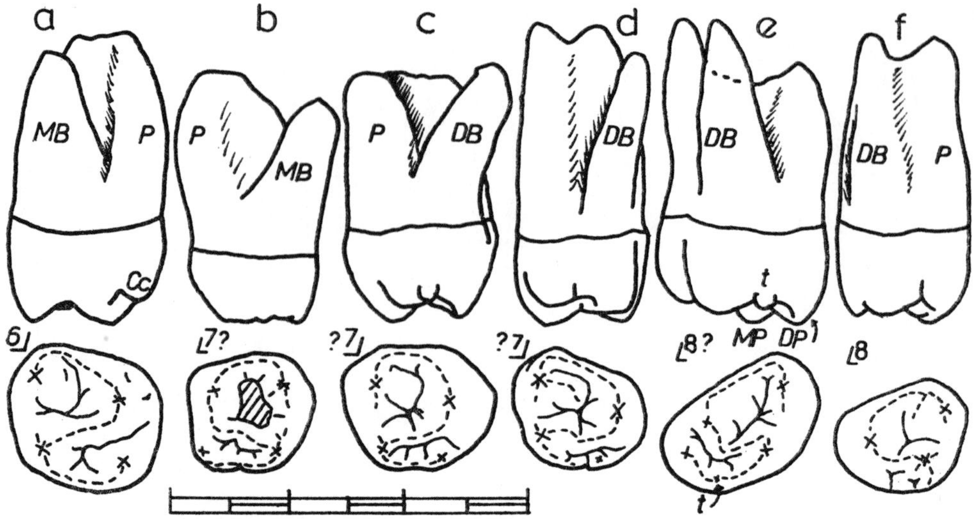

Figure 7-18. Styles of root fusion. *a-e,* fusion of P root with a B root. *a,b,* the most common style, fusion of P and DB roots, with a separate sturdy MB root. *c,d,e,* a less common style, in which the smaller DB root appears relatively slender. See also Figure 7-33 *d. f,* almost complete fusion of all three roots. In this case there are only three cusps; the DP cusp is absent and the posterior groove is represented by a mere trace and a pit.

is joined to P, the separate DB branch may appear very small (Figs. 7-14 *d,* 7-18 *d* and 7-33 *d*). If the DB is joined to P, the separate MB branch appears relatively quite prominent (Fig. 7-18 *a,b*).

To say that fusion may be "partial" in any degree of length is an oversimplification. Essentially it means that furcation may occur anywhere from near the cervix to the apex. Whether apical notches as in

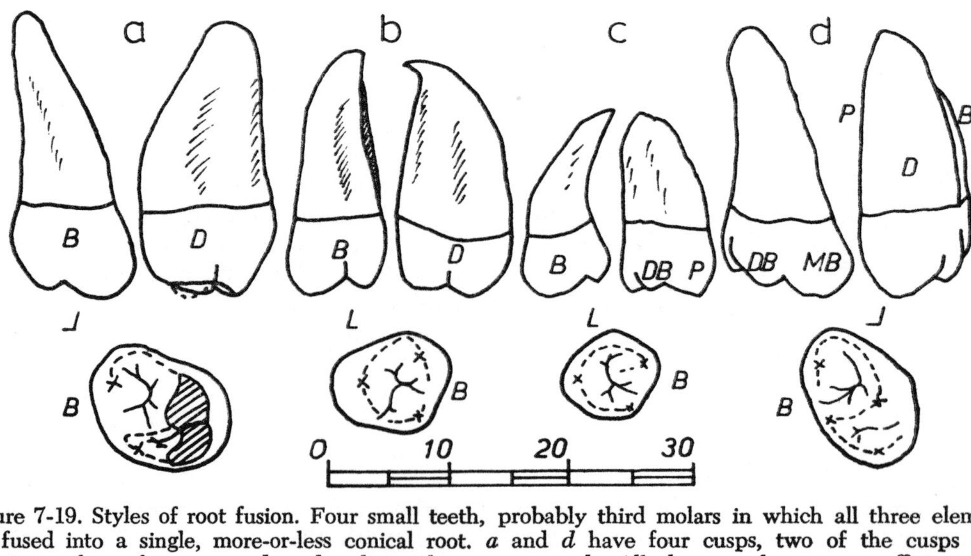

Figure 7-19. Styles of root fusion. Four small teeth, probably third molars in which all three elements are fused into a single, more-or-less conical root. *a* and *d* have four cusps, two of the cusps in *a* showing a facet from wear. *b* and *c* have three cusps each. All these teeth present sufficient type characters in crown and root to permit identification and orientation.

Figure 7-18 *d,e* and *f* should be regarded as furcations or incomplete fusings is one difficulty. Another is seen in the condition presented in Figure 7-14 *f*, a tooth where the palatal root canal obviously branches off at an early stage, but the palatal root remains attached by a band of tissue to the buccal elements right to the apex. For this morphological study it is classed as fusion of all three branches, and there were many such cases. The deep groove was so consistently on the distal surface that it can assist identification of a tooth. Sometimes there is a deep groove between buccal root branches but this was found as well as, rather than instead of, the distal groove (Fig. 7-21 *a*). This particular tooth has been drawn from B, D and O, and the outline of the apical region, in apical view, has been added (Fig. 7-21 *aa*).

It is probably true to say that when a definite furcation has occurred between two root elements the latter do not normally fuse later. Separation and later contact may occur as an imposed character (Fig. 7-13 *a,b*) or by subsequent deposition of cementum, but in either case the histological relationship of the rejoined branches is different from normal (in the sense in which that word has been used here).

To return to "partial" fusion, namely those cases where furcation occurs during approximately the second half of root length (from cervix to apex), clearly it is not feasible to attempt description or classification; variation is too great, especially in third molars. The scope for variation is widened, not only as regards imposed characters, but also by the greater tendency for variation in size, in reduction of cusps, or for inclusion of additional elements in crown and root. The apparent coexistence of reduction of normal elements and inclusion of additional ones is a further complication, but it may provide an interesting challenge in identification of the various parts (Fig. 7-25 *c* and frontispiece, lower tooth).

In like manner Figure 7-21 *b* shows a tooth which at first sight presents a small root branch partly fused to a larger root with a blunt apex. The crown has two good-sized cusps and three smaller ones, and the root has several shallow grooves which indicate its constituent elements. When these are considered together with the cusps, it is not difficult to identify M, B and P, and to recognize the small oblique root branch as an Opc with its crown element as a small M cusp between the large MB and P cusps. Of the remaining two small cusps, one is clearly DB and the other is an Opc with a root element fused throughout with the main root and indicated by two shallow grooves on the D surface. It fills the position of the more common deep distal groove mentioned above in relation to Figure 7-21 *a*.

In Figure 7-21 *c*, there are outlines of another third molar with two Opc, each with a crown and root element. In the crown there are six well-defined cusps of varying size, but although the apex of this young tooth has not been completed, there is no indication that any of the normal or Opc root elements would have formed a separate apex. The usual O, B, D outlines are shown, and with *cc* is given the outline at mid-root, oriented similarly to the occlusal view. This shows the shallow grooves which assist identification and orientation of crown and root elements and of the tooth itself.

Thus even among the many cases of complete fusion of root elements, with or without the inclusion of additional elements, there may be recognizable characters of this kind. Careful examination of an isolated tooth may therefore be rewarding.

Personal characters in these teeth seem responsible for further variation, particularly as regards the kind of apex. In general the fusion of all root elements may thus produce an irregular dome or pyramid shape (Figs. 7-19 and 7-20), but some degree of flattening is very common. In these latter cases change of viewpoint completely alters the effect. A common variation arises when one or more elements

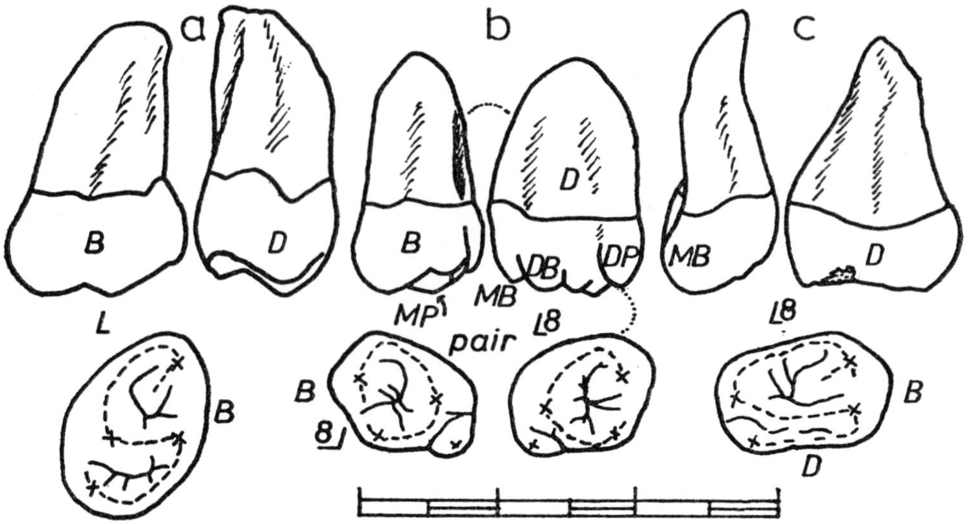

Figure 7-20. Four more small teeth with root fusion to a single root with recognizable type elements in crown and root. *b* gives three views of |8, and the occlusal view of its pairing tooth from right side. Tooth *c* has a "compressed" crown with marked concavity at mesial cervix.

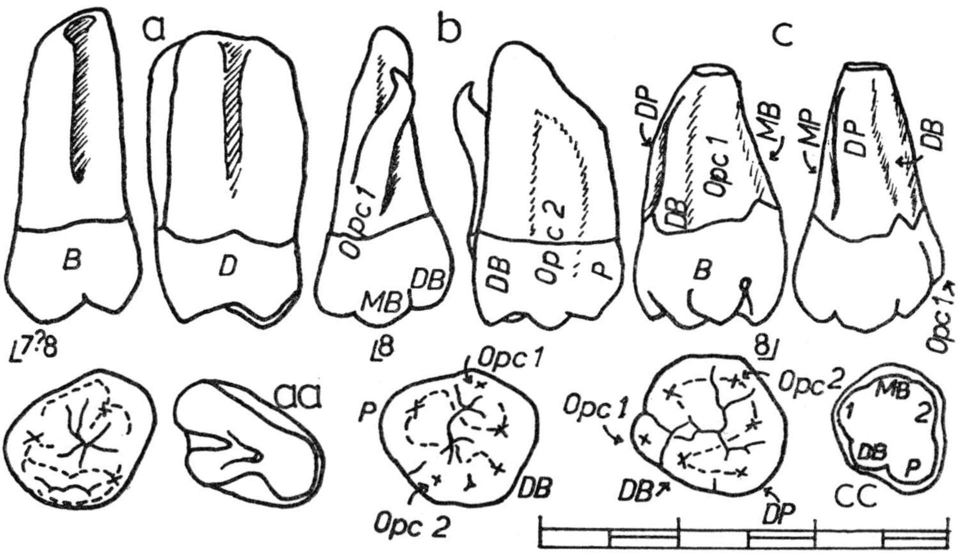

Figure 7-21. Three teeth showing further styles of root fusion. *a*, three roots fused, but deep grooving between elements. The DP cusp is absent, but there are a posterior groove and a ridge completing the S-pattern. *aa*, the outlines at the cervix, and at mid-root showing the deep grooving on B and D. *b*, a tooth with three main cusps and two Opc, the second of which may replace the DP cusp. But this Opc clearly has a root element fused with the three main elements. Opc 1 on mesial has a prominent cusp and its radicle separates from the root trunk at an early stage. The occlusal ridge pattern is disrupted. *c*, a tooth with four main cusps plus two Opc, mesial and distal. Their root elements are recognizable but both are fused with the main elements, all five fused into one. This is a young tooth with incomplete apex. *cc*, outlines at cervix and mid-root as in *aa*, but root opening is omitted.

form small terminal branches with a separate apex (Figs. 7-6 *i*, 7-14 *e* and 7-18 *d,e, f*).

It has already been shown that variations in the maxillary sinus and alveolar ridge appear responsible for characters or variations imposed on roots of some upper teeth (p. 48) and that this applies also to upper molar roots. It has further been noted that extracted teeth sometimes present portions of sinus wall attached to the root. Elaboration of these observations is relevant to this study. In the first place the presence of the attached pieces of very thin bone not only confirms the very close relationship of some molar roots to the sinus, but also provides much information concerning morphology and variation of the inferior and posterior walls of the sinus.

The implications of close relationship of roots and apices to the sinus are well known in dentistry. Conditions involving the dental pulp and the periodontium are sometimes associated with sinus involvement, and evidence of chronic infection may be seen in skeletal material. Conversely, maxillary sinusitis may sometimes cause considerable discomfort in the upper teeth.

There is another aspect of the association of sinus and tooth roots. This is the probability that characters of root divergence or otherwise, and root curves, may be largely imposed by the relation of these structures during growth. Consideration of this involves the further variable of bone bulk or the potential for production of basal and alveolar bone.

Evidence of the considerable variation that may occur in palate depth was shown for groups of well-developed Polynesian adult skulls (Taylor, 1962a, Plate 18). Those contours were in a coronal plane through the second molar tooth sockets, and width at the palatal alveolar margin is greater than width of the floor of the nasal fossae. The result is that from above downwards the palatal alveolar wall slopes outwards. The molar palatal root conforms to this, and the medial sinus wall is virtually that of the nasal fossa.

The width of the sinus is not limited to that of the alveolar ridge, for while it may extend downwards into the ridge it may also extend laterally, well into the malar or zygomatic process (Fig. 7-22). If the basal and alveolar bone is thus reduced there is limited space for development of molar roots, especially if they carry a "personal" potential for long roots. Completion of roots of the first molar takes place entirely below the sinus so that there may be conditions that impose on buccal roots a curve to distal (Fig. 7-10 *a,b*).

With second and third molars conditions may be somewhat different, when their roots grow in relation to the posterior wall rather than below the sinus. Their root morphology, particularly the distal curve

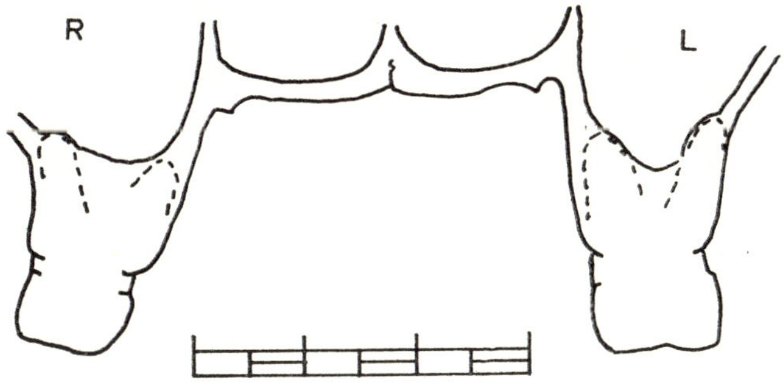

Figure 7-22. Drawing, approximately to scale indicated, of section through skull fragment at second molars, showing relation of tooth roots to sinus wall. In this case the sinus floors are both well below the nasal fossae and dip between the roots. The roots are of medium length but the palate is deep, and bilateral asymmetry is evident.

of palatal root sometimes seen, would thus appear to be largely imposed by variation in the extent of the sinus and in the amount of alveolar bone available to accommodate their roots (Figs. 7-7 and 7-16). Some of these teeth certainly appear to have developed in "cramped" conditions, and this may be a factor in their tendency towards root fusion (Figs. 7-15 *a*, 7-17 *e,f*, 7-19 and 7-20).

Examination of a young skull shows that in the early stage of crown formation of second and third molars their crypts may be high on the posterior wall of the sinus. As each tooth descends, and the occlusal surface turns through nearly ninety degrees, it does not project beyond the maxillary tuberosity. The bony crypt, containing firstly the partly formed crown, and later the root trunk as well, is accommodated within the sinus. Well before emergence of cusps through the "gum," the eruptive process reduces this projection in the floor of the sinus in spite of the increasing length of developing roots. It would be convenient to visualize this as an expansion of the sinus which forces the teeth downwards. However, Sicher (1960) states that it is a confusion of cause and effect to claim that bones enlarge because the contained air sinus expanded, but that expansion of the sinus is secondary to bone growth, and that skull sinuses enlarge again when normal growth has ceased. On this basis the appearance of root apices thrusting into the adult sinus floor could be explained rather as the result of expansion or lowering of the sinus floor around or between completed roots. Furthermore—recalling that these roots are formed after the sinus—there appears to be no clash with the author's view. This regards root curvature, divergence, compression and near fusion as largely reflecting an interplay of basic characters and other such variables as personal characters, potential for basal and alveolar bone, shape of sinus and other local anatomy with which the growing root must conform. In other words, there is good reason to accept that many variations in root (and crown) morphology as described are imposed characters.

ADDITIONAL DENTAL ELEMENTS AND THIRD MOLARS

The additional elements considered here are those which form part of one of the three upper molars.

Much consideration has been given, and evidence presented, to show the potential for variation in upper molar roots. Similarly, molar crowns have previously been studied. Some physical anthropologists whose dental studies are confined mostly to skeletal material acquire a certain familiarity with tooth crowns, but their difficulty in identification of isolated teeth or in replacing such teeth correctly in fragmented material speaks for itself. They may have little familiarity with common root morphology, much less with its variations, and the same is true also of some workers who have dental qualifications. In this study the importance of both crown and root characters in identification of teeth has been repeatedly shown.

Anyone who has studied a great number of teeth would agree that this report has covered many aspects of morphological variation in crowns and roots of upper molars, but that so far it has said little about a large group of them. These are the teeth, mostly third molars, but not only uppers (and by no means only molar teeth), which are sometimes dismissed under some such collective term as malformations, anomalies or abnormalities. The most "dramatic" specimens may be called "gross anomalies," but there is a tendency to avoid further description even of the less aberrant forms. This is understandable, because the very wide range of variation both in nature and degree, and the unavoidability of subjective judgments, combine to frustrate attempts at classification.

Among the attempts to resolve this difficult situation is the classification by Herbst and Apffelstaedt (1930) which the author has found helpful in the effort to sort these variations morphologically by naked-eye examination. In their classification Herbst and Apffelstaedt gave the name Odontopagus parasiticus concretus (Opc in the author's abbreviation) to a wide variety of these aberrant forms.

The majority of "dramatic" specimens of variation featured in dental museums or case reports may have been from known third molar positions, but attempts at meaningful description or identification of their elements are conspicuously absent. It was explained earlier that it is not the intention here to include gross anomalies in the study of variation. The fact that it is difficult to "draw the line" testifies to the variety of anomalies met with. The recognition among them of so many characters found in "more normal" teeth shows that in some sense there is a gradation between normal variation and anomaly, and this has called for some extension to the intended scope of the study. That has been done, subject to obvious limitations, with encouraging results. Increased awareness of the interplay of biological and physical factors has seemed to give a reasonable explanation of morphological results, so that many more of these so-called anomalies can be "analyzed," their parts recognized and the tooth identified. Thus some of their morphological features can now be associated with variation in adjacent anatomical structures during development.

This has also facilitated the recognition of additional elements in crown and root, but whether these have evolutionary significance is quite another matter and forms no part of the present work. Indeed, as the study of more and more such teeth has brought an increasing awareness of the great variety and degree of development in which these additional elements occur, evidence for any such significance seems to have faded. Anyone might select a few examples to support an hypothesis, but these will not establish it by them-

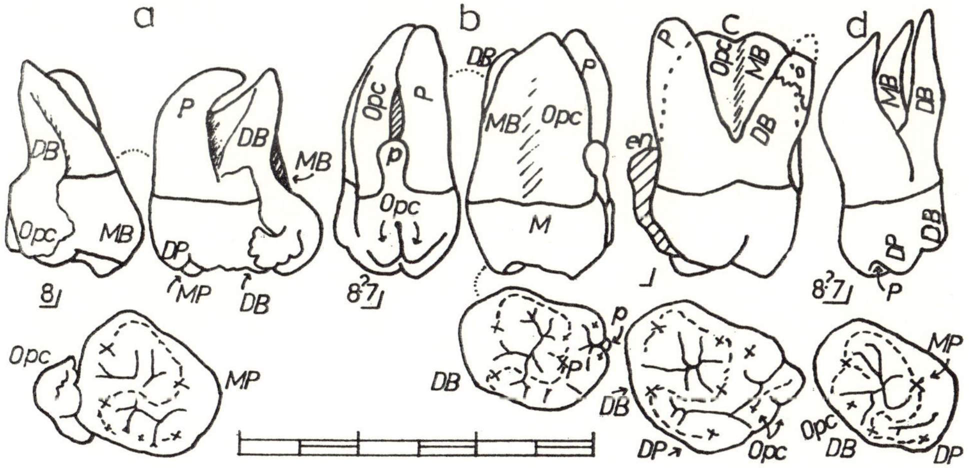

Figure 7-23. Unusual or non-typical additional elements. *a,* both enamel and dentine seem to be present in the portion adjacent to, but separated from, the crown of the autosite. The root portion merges with the DB root. *b,* there are apparently three Opc crown elements on the P aspect of the tooth. Two of these are continuous with a prominent enamel pearl-like structure, *p,* but associated root elements are not evident. *c,* description of additional elements is somewhat similar to that for tooth *b,* but while *b* has no DP cusp, tooth *c* has four main cusps, a Z-pattern of main ridges, and a distinct Opc root element fused with MB root. *d,* this tooth has an Opc crown element between the buccal cusps, and two prominent P cusps. The root is viewed from DP aspect to show the three sharp apices.

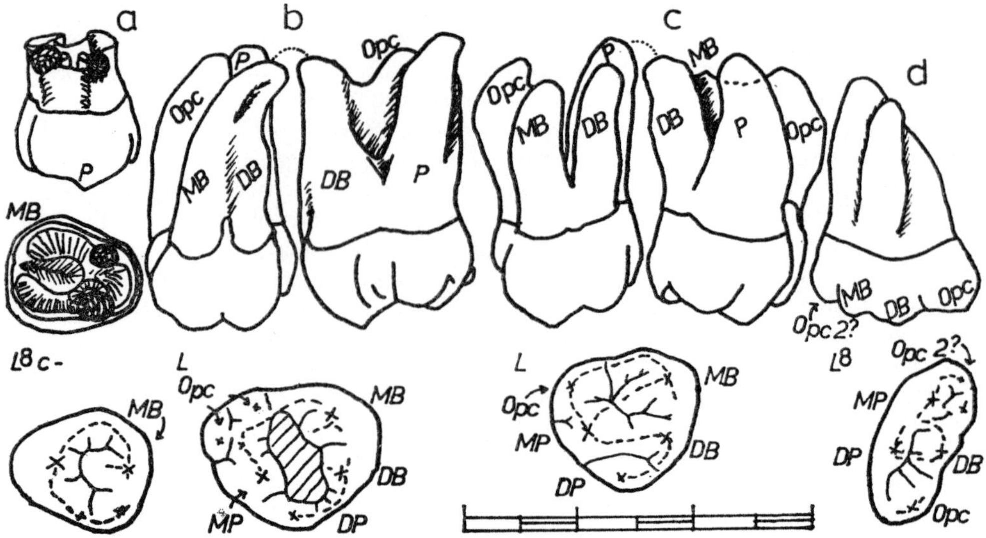

Figure 7-24. Further varieties of additional elements, and enamel pearls. *a*, three views of a young third molar. In the crown there are three cusps and a tubercle. On the root two enamel pearls have formed M and D in root grooves, but they are not connected to the cervix by enamel tangs. *b*, a large tooth with occlusal amalgam filling. Several Opc crown elements on mesial appear to have displaced the main cusps. There is a prominent Opc root element fused to buccal roots, and these are fused to one another. In the groove between the B root elements there is a prominent enamel tang, but no pearl. *c*, three views of another tooth having a prominent Opc crown element on mesial, with its prominent root element fused partly to MB root. In this case the B roots are separated, so that there are four apices. *d*, a much compressed tooth with two Opc at opposite ends of the crown. All root elements are fused to form a flattened conical root.

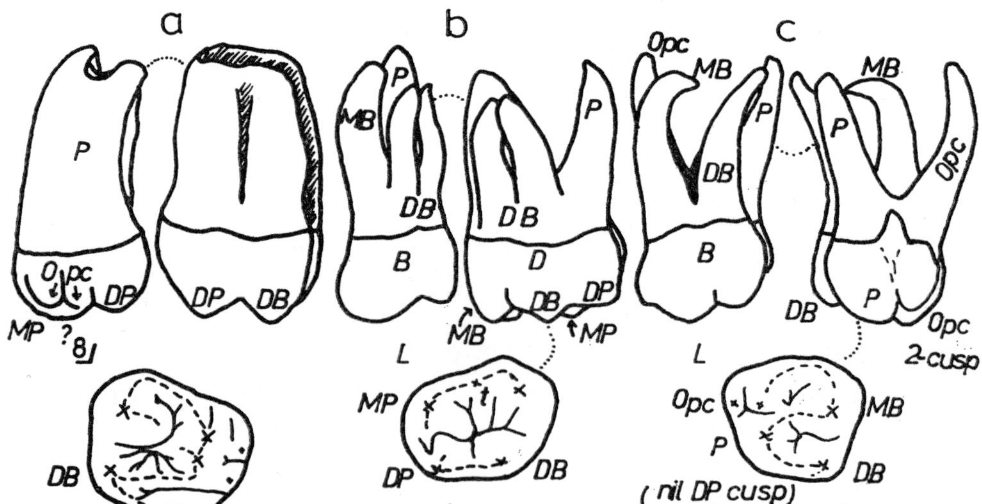

Figure 7-25. More variations in Opc, three views each, of three teeth. *a*, three Opc grouped around MP cusp, but no root elements to correspond. In the main roots, each B root is fused to P, and the B roots are separated by a prominent groove. The root is not conical, so that there is a broad complex apex and all root elements are recognizable. *b*, an unusual root in which the DB branch is represented by small twin roots of approximately equal size, so that there are four distinct roots. The crown has four cusps, plus a mesial tubercle. *c*, a tooth with four separate and divergent root branches, one of which is clearly associated with a two-cusp Opc on MP aspect. The main MP cusp has been displaced and there is no DP cusp. This tooth *c* is also shown in the frontispiece.

selves, especially when the evidence can be interpreted differently (Tomes, 1887).

Although at the moment illustrations of Opc will be confined to upper molars, it should be understood that some comments apply also to other teeth of the dentition. Illustrations of Opc in lower molars will be presented later. There has already been reference to the pit, groove, tubercle or cusp (in its various degrees) that has been associated with the name of Carabelli. The Opc now to receive attention may vary much more in form, in position and in degree of development. Unlike the Carabelli cusp, they may involve either crown or root, or both, and are not confined to the MP region of the molar tooth.

Just as there is great variation in the normal or type characters of crown or root of a tooth, so also do the additional elements of crown or root show wide variation in Opc. But there is a basic difference in the scope for variation. The Opc is not limited by type characters, although type characters may sometimes appear. Thus the kind of Opc which has been called a geminated incisor will present incisor characters, and in the molar region an Opc may present some molar characters. In such cases also there may be some recognizable personal characters such as a tendency for enamel to present grooves or to lack them. Imposed characters may be recognized, such as the sharing in root curvature imposed on the "host" root (Figs. 7-24 *b,c* and 7-27 *b*).

If one were to seek a general observation concerning the Opc it might well be that it does not necessarily conform to any particular morphological concept, other

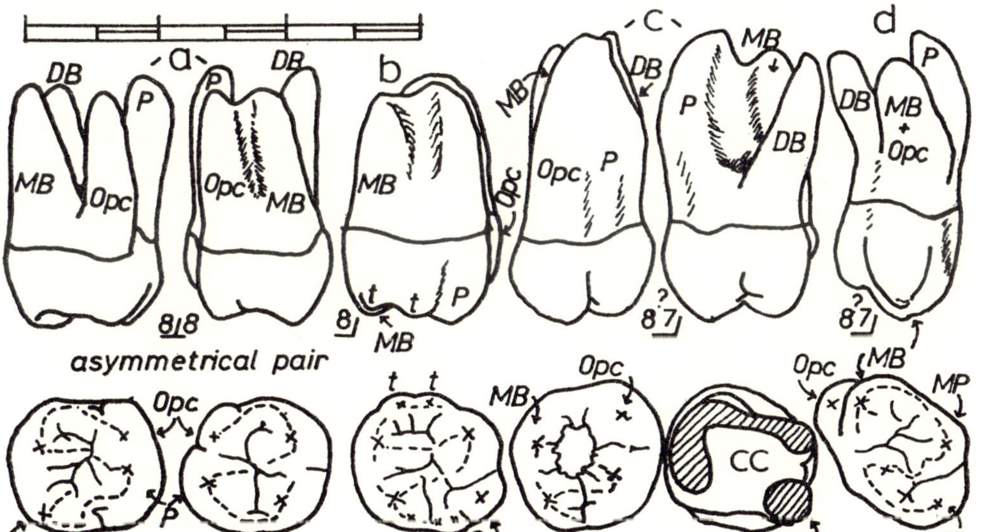

Figure 7-26. Further varieties of root fusion and Opc. *a*, an asymmetrical pair of third molars, each having a prominent Opc at MP in both crown and root. In one the root element is fused with the MB root, but in the other it forms a separate branch. *b*, this tooth has a prominent Opc cusp and radicle, and three tubercles all at DP but no DP cusp. There are mesial tubercles also, and the occlusal does not present the typical ridge pattern. In the root, MB is fused to P, and DB fused to Opc. *c*, four views of one tooth, where *cc* is a diagram of the root pattern seen in apical view. There is occlusal caries, a prominent Opc cusp and radicle at MP, and no DP cusp. The Opc radicle joins both P and MB branches. *d*, a four-cusp tooth with prominent Opc cusp lateral to the MB cusp. If this Opc radicle is ignored, the additional cusp in this position would be designated as "tuberculum paramolare," according to Korenhof (1960). (See also Fig. 7-5 *b*.)

than to form part of a tooth. Histologically no more need be said here than that apparently normal enamel and dentine are found where they would be expected, and in normal relation to one another. Thus dentine is not externally found coronally of the cervix of the host tooth, nor enamel on the radicular side. This statement should perhaps be qualified, to allow for specimens like Figures 7-23 *a* and 7-35 *a* and enamel pearls. The latter occur in great variety of form and position, and although the views of several workers are discussed by Herbst and Apffelstaedt it is not difficult to find cases that obviously have the characters of Opc (Figs. 7-23 *b,c* and 7-28 *a*).

In some teeth the Opc elements can be recognized only in the crown (Figs. 7-15 *a*, and 7-26 *d*), or in the root (Fig. 7-28 *b*). Figures 7-28 *c* and 7-29 *a* present borderline cases which show the difficulty of classification. In each there is a small enamel tubercle below the additional root element, and in the second case (Fig. 7-29 *a*) there is another tubercle on D, but there is no trace of a root element above it.

If cases are examined where both the root and crown elements are obvious, there is also variation in their relation to the root and crown of the autosite or host tooth. Thus in Figures 7-14 *c* and 7-27 *a* the crown and root of the Opc are both clearly recognized but merged with the autosite. In Figure 7-29 *b* there are two Opc, one as just mentioned, but the other has a crown that is completely separate from the autosite. Its root then joins that of the

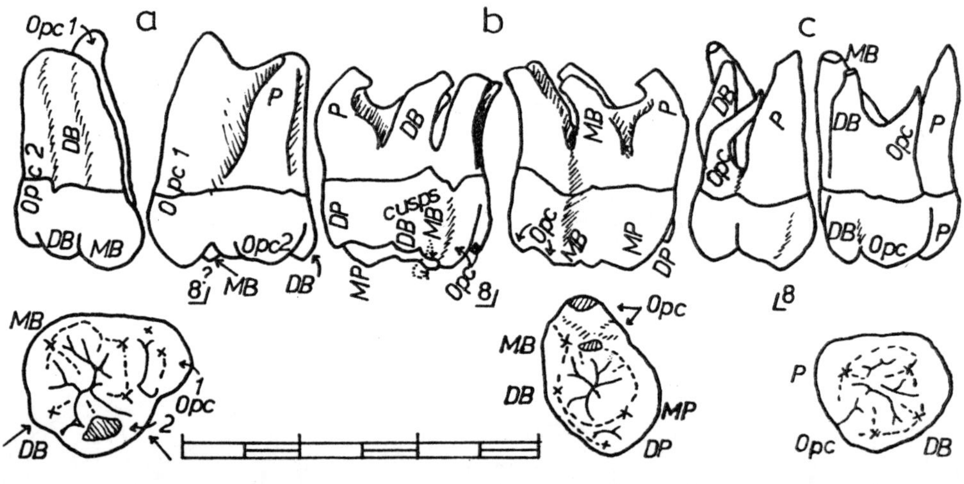

Figure 7-27. Three teeth with multiple Opc having crown and root elements. *a,* Opc 1 has two cusps with one long root fused on the palatal aspect of a fused root which includes the three basic root elements plus the radicle of Opc 2 which is placed distally. The crown element of Opc 2 has a facet from wear (shaded). Of the four main cusps of the tooth, MP and DP are joined by a continuous ridge instead of being separated by a palatal groove. The two external straight arrows with the occlusal outline show the directions from which the tooth is viewed in the upper outlines. *b,* a young tooth with the four basic cusps and three root elements easily recognized though partly fused. On the mesial aspect is a complex Opc with a major and minor cusp; the former is merged at its tip, into the MB cusp. These two cusps of the Opc are associated with a separate root which is deeply grooved but has one continuous pulp cavity. This tooth may seem to resemble the tooth in Fig. 7-31 *b,* but they are not a pair, and the Opc are placed differently. *c,* a tooth with three distinct basic cusps, and an Opc on distal with its radicle partly fused to the DB root. Whether the DP cusp is partly represented in the P cusp or the Opc is obscure. Both are prominent, but the ridge pattern is irregular and no oblique ridge can be recognized.

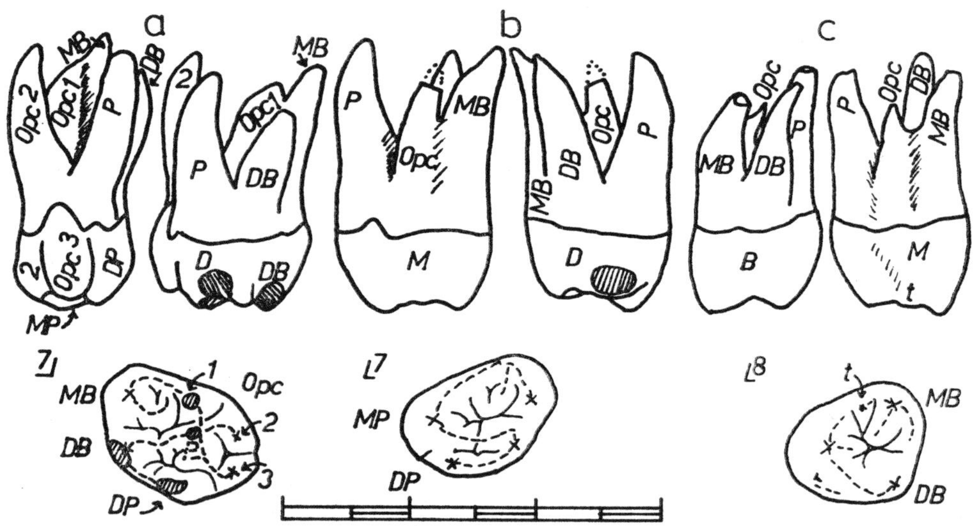

Figure 7-28. Three teeth with further variety in Opc in crown or root. *a*, a tooth with four basic cusps, but the MP cusp is displaced by a complicated Opc mass extending from mesial to DP. This Opc appears to have three components in the crown and two in the root. Part 1 is in the usual position of an MP cusp but its radicle is fused almost to its apex with the MB root. Part 2 has a prominent crown component and a separate prominent root. Extending above this root and the separate P root towards the furcation between them is Opc 3. Its enamel is prominent and the cervical portion bears some resemblance to a large enamel pearl in spite of its smooth continuity with its coronal part. There is no evidence of its association with a root element. The tooth has several facets of wear, including one on D surface which identifies it as a second molar. The tooth has five distinct apices. *b*, this tooth also has a distal facet, but by contrast with *a* it has a simplified crown. The DP cusp is small, but the S of the ridge pattern is clear. On mesial there is no occlusal tubercle. There is however a prominence of occlusal ridge at MB, an irregularity of mesial cervical line, and at mid-root a quite prominent Opc radicle separates from MB. This tooth therefore is close to having Opc in root but not in crown. *c*, this tooth has three main cusps and a mere trace of DP pit and ridge. It does however present a mesial tubercle (*t*) which is clearly associated with a radicle like that in *b*. See also Figure 7-29 *a*, both tubercles.

autosite, as in the lower molar described in an earlier paper (Taylor, 1968a). Examples of Opc with crown element fused to autosite, but with a separate root like that in Figure 7-25 *c*, may truly be called four-rooted molars. But there are many intermediate forms which still have four apices. The most obvious are those where two of the usual three roots are partly fused and the Opc stands alone (Fig. 7-27 *b*), or where bifidity divorces the Opc root from one of the basic three (Fig. 7-27 *c*). The less obvious cases of separate Opc roots may not have a fourth branch or apex if two, or all three, basic roots are involved in fusion, although the Opc root may be partly, or completely, separate (Figs. 7-27 *a*, 7-29 *c*, and 7-21 *b*, 7-30 *a* respectively).

The morphology may become more complex where there is more than one Opc. Thus in the crown these may be of different sizes (Fig. 7-27 *a*) or more similar (Fig. 7-29 *b*); they may be small or relatively large; they may be in the same vicinity (Fig. 7-29 *b*) or in more or less opposite parts of the crown (Figs. 7-21 *b,c* and 7-26 *b*). A somewhat similar diversity is found in root elements. As with a single Opc these multiple cases do not necessarily

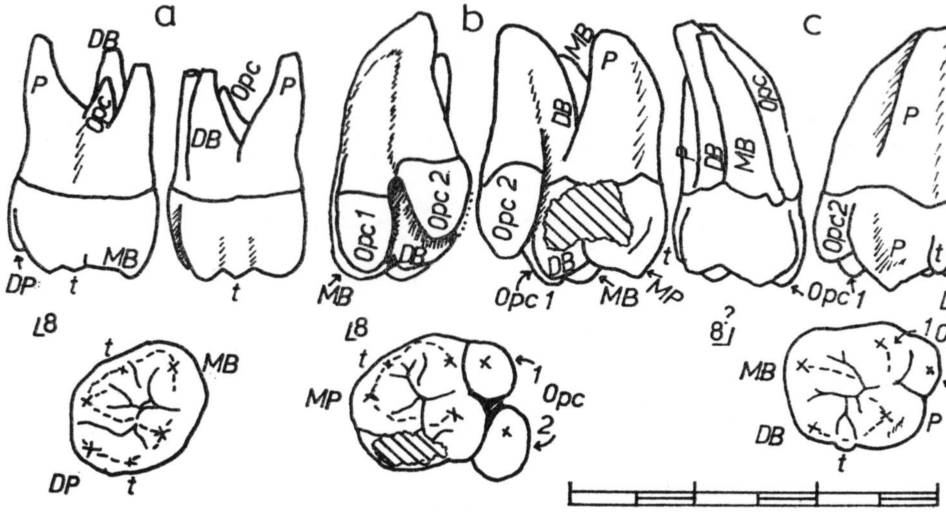

Figure 7-29. Three teeth showing further variation in style and prominence of Opc. *a,* a tooth with four main cusps and normal S-ridge pattern. There are two tubercles, one each in M and D marginal ridges. The M tubercle is associated with a radicle but there is no trace of one for the D tubercle. *b,* this tooth (with a carious cavity, shaded), has two extremely prominent single-cusped Opc on the buccal side. Each has a root portion, but both are fused in with the tooth's MB and DB roots which themselves are fused. There is a separate P root, which is large and lightly grooved but one cannot confidently associate this character with the small mesial tubercle in the crown. *c,* this has no normal DP cusp, but the groove in the large P cusp may represent the posterior occlusal groove. This cusp has been displaced by Opc with two prominent cusps. These appear to share one prominent root element which, together with the normal three, are all fused to form one grooved but more or less conical root. The Opc represented by a small but distinct distal tubercle *(t)* cannot be traced beyond this feature.

show similar prominence or "matching" characters in both crown and root, so that decisions and descriptions concerning them may be biassed subjectively.

An extensive study, as in the present case, tends to overwhelm the worker as he finds the infinity of variety and gradation that occurs. The variety serves to emphasize that a classification which embraces all cases must either be so complicated as to be unworkable, or it must accept a common cause for considerable diversity in morphology. This appears to be the basis of the classification by Herbst and Apffelstaedt (1930), and while it does little to reduce the task of descriptive analysis, it offers a reasonable explanation of the diversity. It is easier to see the results as an aberrant extension of the accepted normal genetic potential for variation, than as a partial awakening of a dormant genetic pattern. The diversity of the variations found should effectively dispose of an atavistic explanation for their origin.

This report has shown the advantages of descriptive analysis of variation in normal teeth, or of normal variation in teeth, and it has also accepted that normal and abnormal are not to be distinguished one from the other by a precise definition. Since there is no clear distinction as to whether some teeth present a rather "extreme" degree of normal variation, or a minimal Opc element, there are many such borderline cases. Add those of obviously aberrant form and one finds ample scope to test ability in identification of upper molars by recognition of basic or type characters, personal and imposed characters and additional elements.

As has been seen, some additional elements are easily recognized, not only because of their size or form but also because of their position. They may be so placed as to lie outside of what is a familiar or common form of crown or root outline (Fig. 7-26 *d*). An Opc may still be easily recognizable as additional even though the usual morphology has been reduced, as in a crown lacking a DP cusp (Figs. 7-25 *c* and 7-30 *b*), or a root with branch fusion (Fig. 7-29 *c*).

Less easily recognized is the Opc in the form of an additional tubercle within the crown outline (Fig. 7-31 *a*), especially where one of the usual cusps is reduced, giving the appearance of that cusp having been replaced by one or more tubercles (Figs. 7-2 *o*, 7-21 *c* and 7-29 *a*). In some the whole occlusal surface may be so nontypical that it is difficult positively to identify the various elements (Figs. 7-26 *a,c* and 7-27 *c*). Again, there may be difficulty in recognizing what corresponds to the oblique ridge; it may be interrupted by a groove (Figs. 7-2 *l,n*, 7-12B *e*, 7-14 *e* and 7-30 *c*), or further complicated by compression, or by reduction or loss of the DP cusp, so that the S or Z pattern of ridges is obscure (Figs. 7-5 *j,l*, 7-30 *a* and 7-31 *b,c*). Some crowns present a number of rather poorly defined tubercles and accessory grooves and ridges (Figs. 7-5 *e* and 7-32 *a*). Reduction of size of main cusps in some of these gives an impression of exaggerated shoulders to the cusps. It is questionable whether Opc are involved here, or whether some cusps are rather extreme examples of normal variation in enamel. (These are not to be confused with the pits and irregularities seen in hypoplastic enamel.) By contrast with this

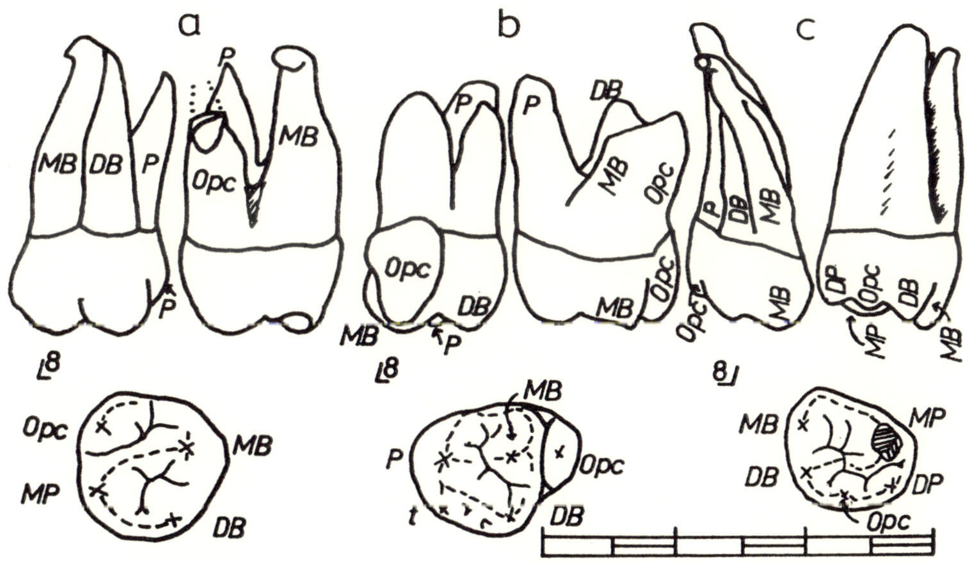

Figure 7-30. *a*, at first sight this appears to be a tooth with four cusps and three roots. On this basis the apparently simple ridge pattern is abnormal. But examination shows that the two buccal root elements are fused throughout, and the other two roots are P and Opc. The Opc cusp has partly "pushed" the MP cusp distally, and there is no trace of DP cusp or of the posterior groove. *b*, this tooth has no DP cusp, but there is a small tubercle in that position. There is a prominent Opc at MB and its radicle clearly is fused with the MB root branch. This tooth, like that in Figure 7-29 *b*, should effectively dispose of hypotheses concerning "paramolar" cusps reviewed by Korenhof (1960). *c*, in the crown this tooth has the usual four cusps, a prominent Opc tubercle between the distal cusps, and a recognizable Z-ridge pattern although the oblique ridge is interrupted. The fusing and grooving of root elements leaves some doubt as to whether there is a root element associated with the Opc.

undulating or ridged enamel there are teeth with smoothly rounded cusps, the main ridges and grooves well-developed, perhaps having an Opc which is clearly defined, but where other minor or accessory irregularities are virtually absent (Figs. 7-2 *m*, 7-5 *d*, 7-6 *c*, and 7-30 *a*).

Evidence of Opc in a root may vary considerably. One of the three normal root branches may be disproportionately large (Figs. 7-15 *c*, 7-32 *b*, *c*) or nontypical in transverse section, or it may fuse with another and yet maintain its own direction in the presence of a personal character of divergence of root branches (Fig. 7-23 *c*). Another variant is a wide root with a wide apex which is out of harmony with the personal character of root and apex in the other branches (Fig. 7-23 *b*). Yet another, although closely allied to the last, is the wide root with bifid apex, a variation which must attract notice in a tooth that normally has a maximum of three root branches, each with a single apex (Fig. 7-24 *c*). The Opc fused to a root branch, and presenting a bifid apex therewith, may occur in the presence of some degree of fusion of the three primary branches (Figs. 7-24 *b* and 7-30 *a*). In some cases root branches which are widely divergent are yet joined by a broad band of tissue. It is questionable whether this band represents an Opc (Fig. 7-32 *c*). The author is inclined to regard it as a normal variation in fusion of primary root elements, and has observed it to be common in deciduous upper molars, where it joins P and DB roots leaving the MB branch separate.

The Opc fused to a root branch, and presenting a bifid apex, is intermediate between the Opc completely fused with one of the root branches, and the Opc which

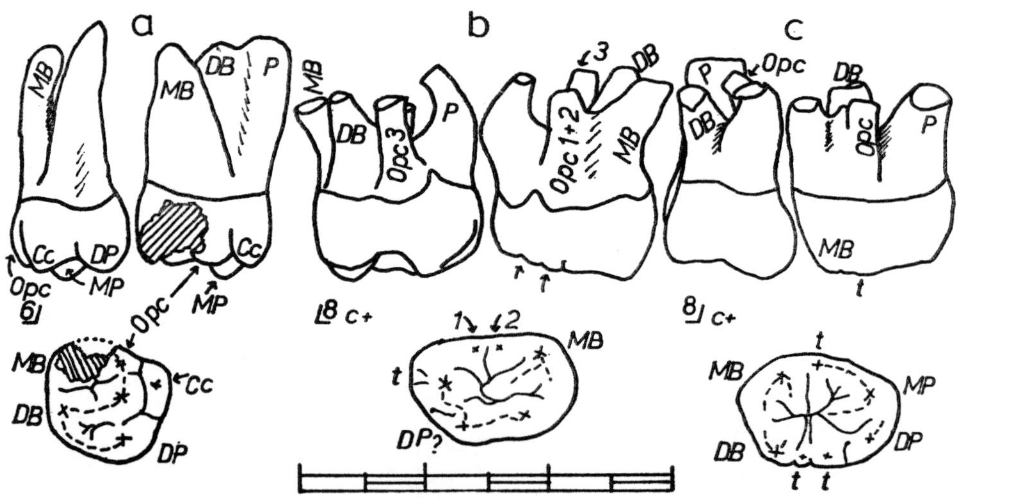

Figure 7-31. Three teeth having enamel tubercles which lack, or do not have, associated root elements. *a*, a first molar with a prominent Carabelli cusp (Cc) and a mesial Opc tubercle. Only the usual three root elements are present, the DB and P being fused almost to their apices. There is a carious cavity (shaded). *b*, a four-cusped tooth with two mesial tubercles which are associated with one Opc root element almost completely fused to MB root. There is another separate root element (Opc 3) which is in the position of DP cusp which never (?) has a separate root. Is this an Opc root without a crown element? There is some additional enamel material (*t*). Is this an Opc crown element without a radicle? This is a young tooth with incomplete roots. (See also legend to Fig. 7-27 *b*.) *c*, this tooth has four basic cusps and three tubercles, one mesial and the others distal. The first has a rather complex radicle partly fused with a reduced MB root. The other two have no identifiable radicle. The occlusal ridge pattern is interrupted by grooves related to the additional tubercles. This is a young tooth.

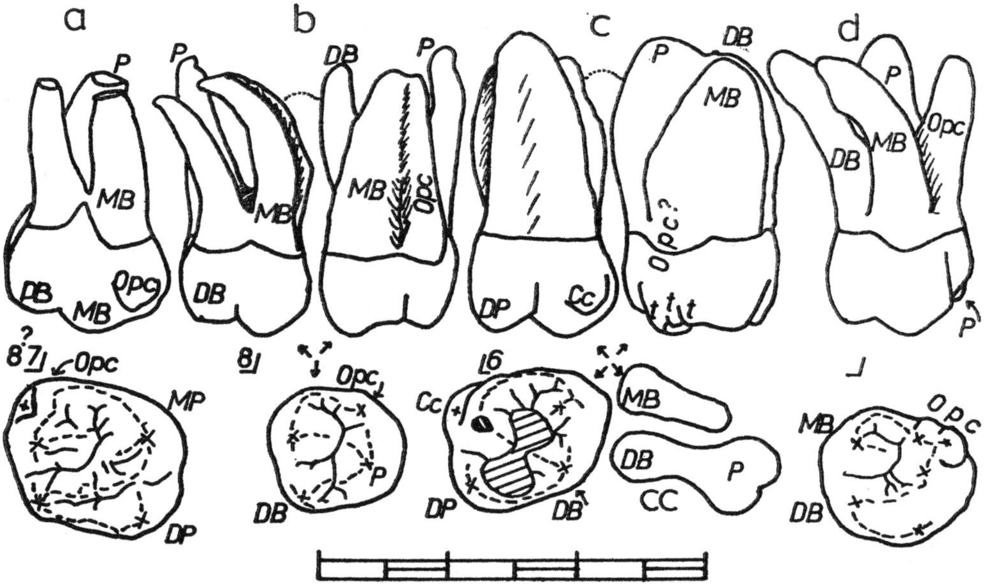

Figure 7-32. Four teeth presenting further variation in Opc with crown elements lacking, or having, root elements which may be separate or fused with a main root branch. *a*, a large crown with four main cusps, a Z-ridge pattern and many minor grooves. There is an Opc cusp on MB, but no radicle. There is a prominent enamel "tang" into buccal root furcation but no "pearl." (See also legend to Fig. 7-30 *b*.) A young tooth. *b*, a small crown lacking a DP cusp, and with grooves interrupting the remaining sections of the Z ridges. There is a prominent Opc at MP and an associated root element fused with the full length of the MB root. The resulting root is relatively very wide and there is a prominent groove for the full length of its mesial surface. *c*, a first molar with four main cusps (MP with small facet from wear), a clear S pattern of main ridges and an amalgam filling. There is also a Carabelli cusp (Cc) and several small indefinite tubercles at mesial. Above these there is a widening of MB root for part of its length suggesting that the tubercles and root enlargement are Opc elements. The P root is wide and grooved on P aspect, and a band of tissue connects P and DB roots. In *cc* is shown an approximate transverse outline at mid-root. *d*, a tooth with four prominent, separate, root branches and three main cusps, the DP cusp being represented by a ridge only. The Opc root is associated with a crown element with virtually two small cusps on MP.

is a completely separate root. Where the other roots also are separate the result is the four-rooted molar. There is no simple corresponding term to describe an Opc addition to the tooth crown. Where the root element of an Opc is so prominent as to present a separate root, it is likely to have also a recognizable crown element associated with it (Figs. 7-25 *c*, 7-28 *a* and 7-32 *d*).

It has been seen that the tendencies towards reduction of the DP cusp, reduction of divergence between root branches, or fusion of branches, are greater in the second molar than in the first, and greater still in the third molar. But there is no constant style in these tendencies; the root branches may be fused although the crown has four well-developed cusps (Fig. 7-33 *a*), or a three-cusped molar may have three separate root branches (Figs. 7-28 *c* and 7-33 *b*).

Teeth with moderate additions in the form of Opc, and those with more complex additions in crown or root or both (often referred to as anomalies) are much more commonly found as third molars, or in that position, although the less dramatic examples of Opc are by no means absent from first and second molars. The anomalous forms are well known to result in complicated root morphology, and this report shows that some such features of curvature or fusion are reasonably accounted for as imposed characters. These anomalous forms often find their way into a collection; so that there are many available for study.

Identification of these teeth as upper or lower, or left or right, may sometimes be very difficult. Neither crown nor root may resemble a normal tooth, but it is seldom that close study does not result in recognition of some character which may serve as a starting point. This may be a root groove that suggests the position or form of one of the root branches. From this, a trial orientation as upper or lower may be supported by some slight resemblance of part of the crown or occlusal surface to that of a normal tooth. At the same time mesial or distal regions may be distinguished by a wider and less convex (mesial) surface, opposite to a smaller and more convex (distal) surface, and the probability is that root curvature is to distal (or partly to buccal in a lower).

Another clue, sometimes useful in determination of buccal and lingual, may be found by turning the tooth on its long axis and comparing opposite profiles. The differences looked for will be discussed later when showing the profiles of both upper and lower molars in relation to occlusion (p. 329).

Reduction in Size, and Duplication

It is well known that third molars may vary much more in size than other teeth. This has been briefly considered and will later be relevant when considering diminutive teeth (p. 322, and Fig. 8-23 *g,h,i,*). The teeth of unusual form just described, especially those including additional ele-

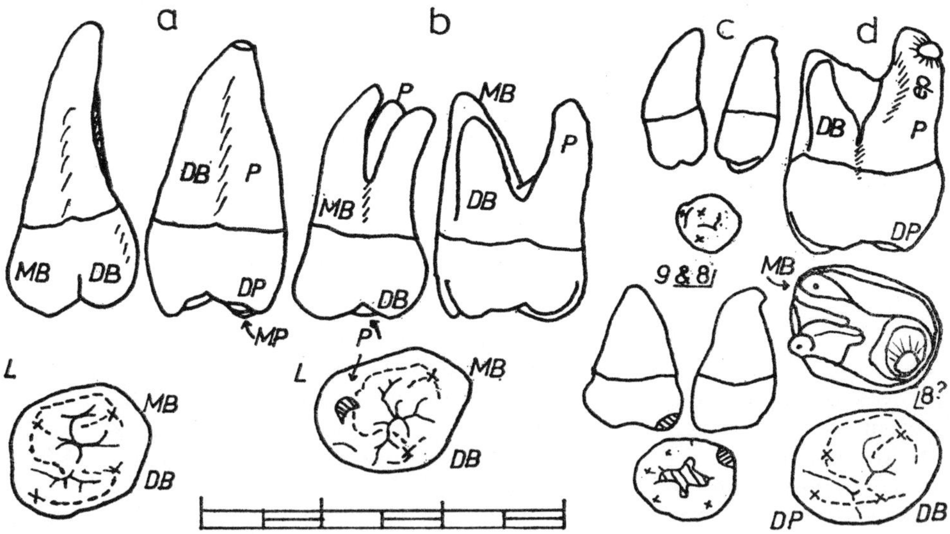

Figure 7-33. *a,* a tooth with four well-developed cusps and a clear S pattern of ridges. All the root elements are fused to form a single, more or less conical root. *b,* by contrast with *a,* this tooth has only three cusps, but it has three separate and divergent root branches. *c,* "twin" third molars, upper right, extracted from a middle-aged white woman. Three views of each tooth. *d,* an upper molar with a prominent enamel pearl *(ep),* set in a concavity on the palatal side of the palatal root, near the apex. There is no enamel tang between it and the cervix. The MB root is partly fused with the P root, and the middle outline is an apical view of the tooth. The lower outline shows a normal four-cusp tooth with clear ridge pattern and main grooves only.

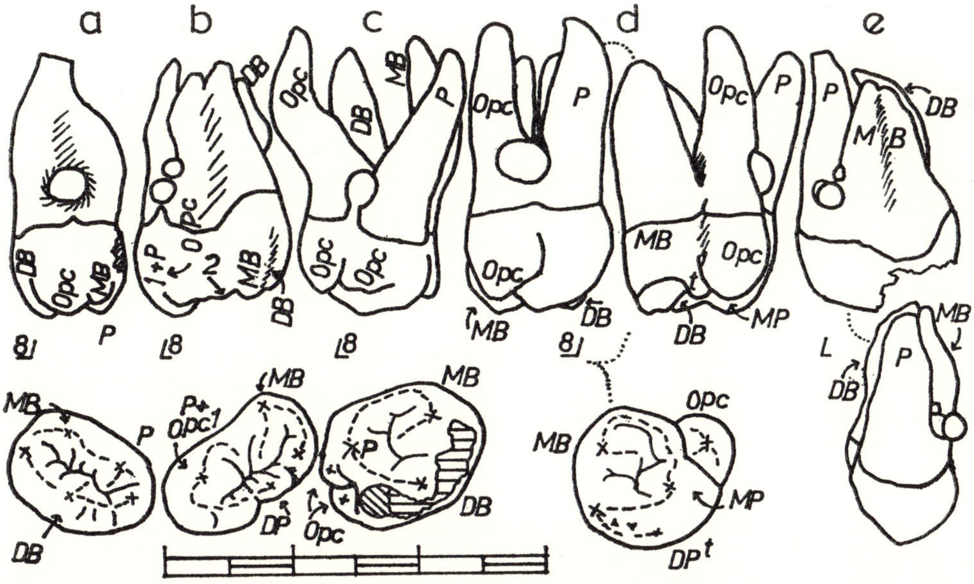

Figure 7-34. Five teeth showing variety in enamel pearls. Teeth *a,c,e* have carious cavities (irregular outlines), and *c* also has a small facet from occlusal wear. *a*, a tooth with five cusps, one being a prominent Opc, and all root elements are fused into one. The pearl is on the side of the root, but not connected to the small point of cervical enamel directed towards it. *b*, a tooth with two pearls in line with, but not connected to the more prominent enamel tang, or to one another. They are in a groove apparently between two Opc radicles, one of which is fused to P, and the other to the MB root. The first of these has a crown element evidently fused with and contributing to the large MP cusp, but the second is represented by a mesial ridge or tubercle beside the MB cusp. *c*, this tooth has four diverging root branches, one of which is an Opc continuous with a large Opc cusp. Beside this is a second Opc cusp with no discernible radicle. Between these Opc there is an enamel extension continuous with a prominent pearl in the adjacent root furcation. The horizontal shading represents decay. The oblique shading is an area of fractured enamel presumably weakened by decalcification and dislodged during extraction of the tooth. Evidently a DP cusp had been present. *d*, three views of a tooth with three main cusps (the DP is represented by a tubercle only) and a large Opc. There are four root branches, one being Opc between MB and P, and there is a large pearl partly embedded at the furcation of Opc and P roots. It is on a dentine base which is partly covered with enamel, and although there is no connecting enamel tang, the cervical line points slightly at each side of the Opc. There is a very prominent cusp in the position of a Carabelli cusp, but it is obviously associated with the Opc root. Is this an exception to the rule that a Carabelli cusp has no radicle? Alternatively, is the traditional morphogenetical concept of Carabelli's cusp so sacred that this tooth *d* and similar variations must be explained by yet another hypothesis? *e*, this tooth has three distinct root elements, but MB is grooved suggesting that an Opc is involved. So much of the crown has been destroyed that little more can be said regarding this. There are two enamel pearls at a root furcation, but no irregularity of cervical line or enamel tang in this region of the tooth. A further point of special interest is that the larger pearl has a distinct dentine "stalk" connecting it to the tooth root. Is this truly an enamel pearl? It appears closely related to the formation shown in Figure 7-35 *a*.

ments (Opc), are mostly relatively large teeth. But it is by no means rare to find, in the third molar position, teeth that are relatively small; some may include Opc elements and some are of almost "normal" form. It must be a subjective decision as to whether these are at the lower extremity of normal variation in size, for the term "diminutive" cannot be clearly defined and is merely convenient for embracing a large number of small teeth of varying morphology.

It is very uncommon, but by no means unknown, to find two teeth distal to a second molar. The writer noted several Tasmanian skulls with such teeth in the Queen Victoria Museum in Launceston in 1946. Some of these teeth were relatively large, in good alignment and worthy of being regarded as fourth molars. But both the third molar and the additional tooth may be reduced in size like the two shown in Figure 7-33 *c*. These two teeth in right upper third molar position were extracted from the mouth of an adult white female by the writer's father in 1917.

Thus one has on the one hand the observations that third molars may be reduced in size overall, or the crown or root may have fewer cusps or root branches, or show fusion of branches, or the tooth may not even be present. These observations have sometimes been interpreted in support of the notion that there is an evolutionary trend towards reduction of the dental formula of man.

On the other hand, third molars are commonly found larger than normal, with more complex crowns or roots or Opc, or there may be an additional tooth in this region of the mouth. These findings, by the same token, should indicate a tendency towards increase in the dental formula. The author prefers to regard these various

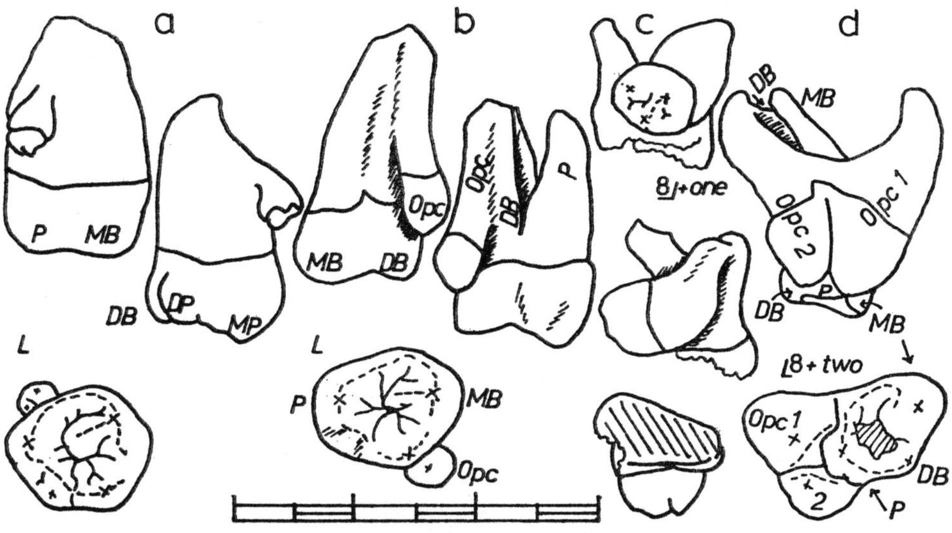

Figure 7-35. *a*, a tooth with an additional element which, although attached at mid-root, has its own separate crown or enamel portion. Although larger and less like a "pearl" than the structure in Figure 7-34 *e*, it is clear that the manner of formation is similar. It should be noted that the "parasite" grows into rather than from the autosite, which in this case presents complete fusion of all three root elements. Whether this tooth has a reduced DP cusp or another Opc in that position cannot be determined, but like a normal DP cusp it has no associated radicle. The radicle of the parasite soon loses its identity by merging with the autosite and apparently does not continue to its apex. *b*, by contrast with the preceding case the Opc in this tooth has a radicle which can clearly be traced right to the apex of the autosite. *c*, a small third molar (crown destroyed by caries) with a relatively large Opc so that both are approximately equal in size. Both crowns are separate but fusion has then taken place in the roots. It might be noted that with crowns initially placed at such different angles development would cause the roots to grow towards one another. Might not this account for the different result in Figure 7-33 *c*, where separation was mentioned in twin teeth developing side by side? *d*, a tooth with two large and very similar Opc partly fused together and to the P side of the autosite. Each has its own widely divergent radicle, one being connected by a fusion band to the B roots.

observations merely as evidence (as mentioned above) that in addition to normal variation there is potential for aberration beyond the "normal" range.

If this is so it would seem reasonable to include among these aberrations the so-called enamel pearl.

Enamel Pearls

Variation in characters of enamel pearls is illustrated in Figures 7-34 and 7-33 *d*. These small structures, usually covered with enamel, are attached to the tooth on the root side of the cervical line. They are often spherical and are mostly found at the furcation of a root trunk; but this is by no means the only place where they are found. They may be found when root elements are fused and there is no furcation (Fig. 7-34 *a*), and in a depression in a root end (Fig. 7-33 *d*).

There may be more than one pearl, on opposite sides of a tooth (Fig. 7-24 *a*), or in axial line on one surface (Fig. 7-34 *b*). The cervical line may, or may not, rise to a point below the pearl *(a,b)*, and this point of enamel may, or may not, continue as a fine tang or ridge of enamel to connect with the pearl (Figs. 7-23 *b* and 7-34 *b,c*). Sometimes the enamel tang may be relatively wide at its commencement, so that there is an appreciable irregularity in the level of attachment of periodontal tissue at the cervix, and this may present a threat to the integrity of gingival health and so also to the tooth itself. An Opc element (Figs. 7-25 *c* and 7-28 *a*) may have a similar effect. (See also Figs. 7-16 *f*, 7-31 *b* and 7-32 *a*.) The writer recalls extracting a lower first molar for a healthy boy aged about fourteen years. The mouth was well cared for and clean, except for an acute paradental abscess involving the root bifurcation. Into this region extended a rather wide enamel tang, but there was no associated pearl. It appeared that infection had arisen in plaque debris associated with the defective gingival attachment in this region.

Herbst and Apffelstaedt (1930) review some of the studies of enamel pearls. As regards their formation, histological sections have shown that in some pearls there is continuity of dentinal tubules from the autosite into the pearl, so that in these cases formation of both root and pearl dentine take place together. Presumably formation of pearl enamel is closely associated with this in time. As pearls vary so much in size and position it is possible that they vary also in the time and manner of formation. It is not known whether pearls may be formed without the inclusion of dentine, or without even being attached to the tooth. The last supposition envisages the possibility of an enamel pearl becoming "detached" and lost at the time of extraction of the tooth, or through decay of soft tissues in skeletal material. This possibility comes to mind when observing the varied form of enamel tangs that may or may not be found associated with enamel pearls. In other words, why are there large pointed tangs with no pearl, small or narrow tangs with pearls continuous or discontinuous with them, and pearls with no tang in view? May the pearl-forming ameloblasts "come apart" from the tooth root and rejoin it, and be capable of forming a pearl while separated from or after rejoining the root-forming tissues?

A spherical pearl, only partly covered with enamel, is seen in Figure 7-34 *d*. This pearl, and a large Opc cusp on MP (but not to be called a Carabelli cusp?), with a prominent separate root element, are associated with a third molar which otherwise has three cusps and three root branches (the DP cusp is represented by a tubercle). Apparently different is the larger of the two pearls in Figure 7-34 *e* where the enamel is like a cap to a small dentine "stalk." A further development of the kind is seen in Figure 7-35 *a* where the stalk is prominent, and the cap has depressions like an "occlusal" surface. In Figure 7-35 *b* the additional element is readily acknowledged as an Opc, with both crown and root elements, but still distinguishable from the larger autosite which resembles a normal tooth.

In this same tooth *b* attention is drawn to the enamel tang extending from the buccal cervix on to the root, but with no trace of pearl formation. In another case, not figured, the tang is quite different. It arises just above the distal contact point and proceeds as an increasingly distinct ridge, crossing the cervix and continuing for a distance approximately equal to the height of the crown of the tooth. It terminates as two small pearls in a deep groove between the fused DB and P root branches.

In the next case (Fig. 7-35 *c*) apparently the autosite was reduced in size (it had been carious and the crown is broken off), and the Opc is relatively larger than in the

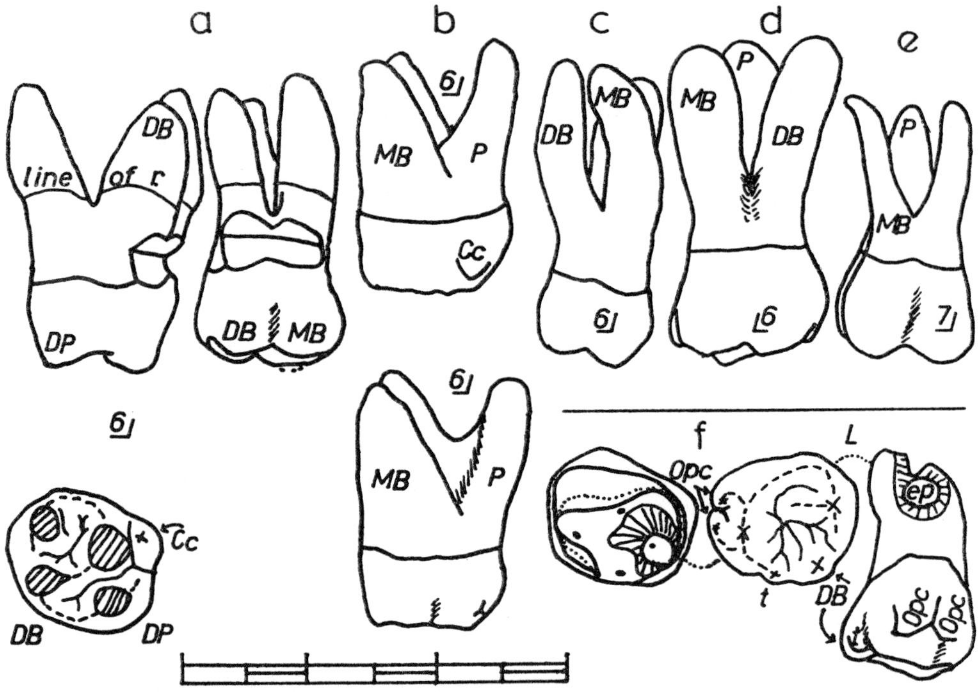

Figure 7-36. *a,* three views of a tooth with a prominent Carabelli cusp (Cc) and a facet of wear on each of the four main cusps. The tooth bears witness to trauma to soft and hard tissues caused by faulty technique during zealous prophylactic performances. There is a line of demarcation above the root furcation indicating the level of recession of the gingival attachment. From this line down, the entire B surface is highly polished, and there is a deep V-shaped notch in the less hard dentine above the cervix, with sharply defined horizontal apex to the V. The damage has been caused by friction from bristles and dentifrice. Such abrasion is rare on second or third molars (Taylor, 1971a, 1973b). *b,* two left first molars which bear close resemblance in many respects. As regards differences, one has a Carabelli cusp and three quite separate root branches. The lower tooth has a Carabelli pit, and a fusion band between P and DB branches. *c,* a first molar with very small crown and three long separate root branches. *d,* a large first molar with three separate, divergent, very thick roots. *e,* a second molar with moderately large crown, but three separate very short and slender root branches. *f,* three views of a tooth with fused root branches and an enamel pearl *(ep)* embedded in a concavity near the apices. The crown has three main cusps, and a tubercle at distal. There are two adjacent Opc crown elements on P, but no evidence of additional elements in the root. In the apical view the outlines are (from outside) crown, cervix, contour at mid-root (dotted) and at apical vicinity, and concavity with enamel pearl embedded. The positions of the three apical foramina are shown.

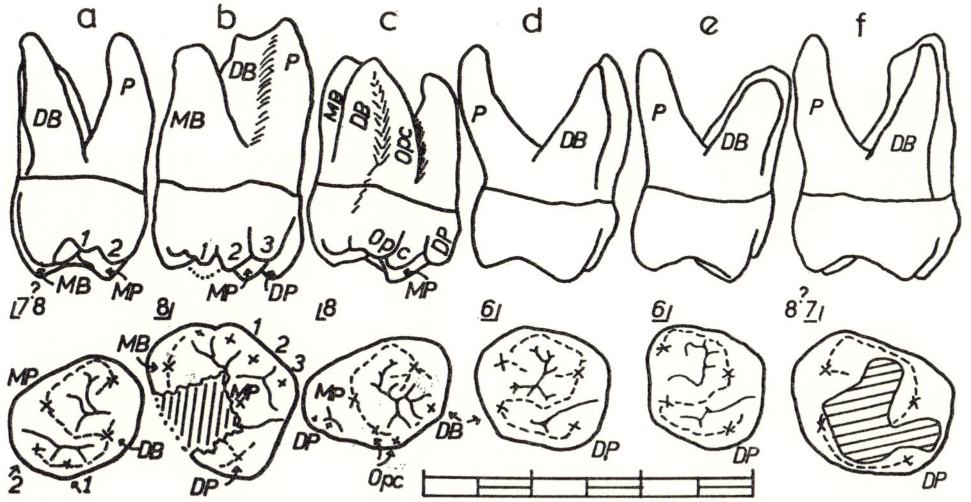

Figure 7-37. *a,* a tooth with three root branches and no Opc root elements. The DP cusp is duplicated. Is this to be regarded as DP cusp plus a tubercle, or as two Opc which replace the DP cusp but participate in the S of the main ridge pattern? *b,* a tooth with part of the crown including the DB cusp destroyed by caries. There are three (or 4?) Opc occlusal tubercles in line from M to P but little evidence of additional root elements other than a wide-based MB root. *c,* a tooth with two pairs of tubercles at DP and D. (Whether one pair represents the DP cusp displaced (see Fig. 7-6 *a,b*), or whether both are Opc features is not clear, but details of crown and root are in strong contrast with tooth *a.*) In *c,* the crown outline is elongated in its B-P dimension, the ridge pattern lacks the posterior limb of the S, and the occlusal grooves are very different. In this also it is clear that additional elements are present in the root, fused to the DB branch. *d,e,f,* distal and occlusal views of three right molars. Teeth *d* and *e* are approximately similar in size; *d* has widely divergent root branches like a deciduous second molar (but it is definitely M1), and *e* has three thick stumpy roots, the B branches separate but touching. Tooth *f* has a very large crown in occlusal view (and an amalgam filling). In proximal view the crown is not high, nor the root branches heavy or long. (See also Fig. 7-36 *c,d,e.*)

previous case (*h*), so that the two parts are not much different from one another in size. The autosite is recognizable also in Figure 7-35 *d,* although it appears to be less in bulk than the two additional elements, each with crown and root, which make up the whole. Whether this is more correctly described as gemination, twin formation or Opc is not the main concern. Rather it is desired to establish the fact that in a study of many specimens it has been possible to find a series of gradations from the smallest enamel pearl to the complexities of crown and root illustrated or described herein. These testify to the potential of dental formative tissues for variety in division and combination. An alternative assumption, that they are genetic attempts to demonstrate past, present or future evolutionary experiments and trends, leans for support on selected cases. It ignores the great majority of irregular cases and also the finding established by the present study that there are innumerable examples intermediate between them. Add to this the extensive evidence of normal variation which never oversteps the generic type, and surely that "alternative assumption" becomes incredible. (See also Fig. 8-16 *j* and pp. 310, 336.)

Figure 7-36 gives further examples of the Carabelli cusp, of Opc and of the enamel pearl. There are also features which will be referred to later (p. 334). In Figure

7-37 the first three teeth present aspects of variation and of Opc which involve the identification and designation of cusps and tubercles. In their crown morphology some of the usual features are lacking but there are unusual characters present. The question arises as to whether the latter represent the missing features. Alternatively, may the unusual features be regarded as additional elements (Opc) in a tooth which has lost "normal" elements? Thus in *a* there is a familiar form of crown, a clear S-pattern of ridges and uncomplicated occlusal grooves, but instead of the usual DP cusp there are two small non-typical cusps. They could be reasonably accepted as replacing the DP cusp. There is no unusual feature in root style. Tooth *b* evidently had a reduced DB cusp; there is a displaced DP cusp, and an MP cusp which is almost surrounded by additional tubercles. These last may be related to the widely based MB root. In *c* there is certainly an Opc root element. The crown has a large anterior sulcus with complicated grooves; there is no distal limb to the S, and instead of a displaced DP cusp there are a number of tubercles.

These three teeth support the view that variation may involve at the same time both the loss of "normal" features and also the presence of additional features which may replace the former, or be situated in other regions of the crown. In view of the many other variations on this theme that are presented in this study, one must question the generic significance evidently implied by some workers in their naming of coronal tubercles. Such systems not only ignore the possible relationship, or lack of it, between root elements and crown elements demonstrated in our figures, but also have perforce confined their designations to teeth which conform to the system. Can credibility condone exclusion of so many other teeth? The present study contributes to the understanding of variation in these other teeth.

Identification of Upper Molars

This recapitulation may assist the identification of maxillary molars by naked-eye examination.

There are relatively few complete molar teeth that cannot confidently be identified as upper or lower, but their placing as left or right, or as first, second or third molar can be difficult. Where the tooth is incomplete, or damaged by fracture or pathology; or where crown or root elements are reduced in number or fused, positive identification may be impossible. In the great majority of cases however there should be no difficulty in recognizing an upper molar and assigning it to left or right side. This is because a maxillary molar tooth has potentially so many characters in crown and root, and because in spite of wide variation in characters, or absence of some of them, there are usually a sufficient number present to allow the tooth to be identified as such. The first determination therefore is that the tooth is an upper.

There are only two other determinations involved in the present summary, namely laterality or sidedness and serial position (whether the tooth is a first, second or third molar). Although sex cannot be ascertained from tooth morphology, it has already been shown that much other information can be obtained from evidence of wear and pathology, and from stains, calculus deposits, etc. Some of these, or incomplete roots, may give indications of the age of the person at death, or at the time the tooth was extracted, and may even indicate something of the habits or physical character of that person. In a sense some of this information bears upon identification; but having determined that the tooth is an upper molar, the concern here is only with characters that assist its correct placement in the dental arch.

Left or Right

Determination of laterality has two steps. First it is necessary to recognize buccal, palatal, mesial and distal, and then by placing the tooth in an imaginary dental arch as described earlier (or against a skull, one's own face or in any other preferred way), it is simply a matter of trial and error until correct orientation is achieved. A number of characters of root and crown may be used in the first step.

If there are three root branches, they may be distinguished by their most common type characters: MB, wide and flat where it joins the root trunk; DB, sometimes flattened similarly on its M and D surfaces, but certainly the smallest root; P, the thickest, occasionally flattened on its palatal surface, and often diverging noticeably to P. If buccal roots are curved it is most likely to distal.

If the crown has four well-developed cusps, MB and MP cusps are large, the former often somewhat flattened where it forms part of the anterior occlusal sulcus. The DB cusp is smaller, and DP cusp smallest. These are the teeth where the occlusal oblique ridge is usually most easily recognized. Viewed with the crown uppermost the ridge dips and bends to D as it passes from DB cusp to MP cusp; its posterior surface slopes steeply to the posterior groove and its anterior surface slopes gently to the anterior sulcus. The two P cusps may be sharply separated by the posterior groove continuing on to the P surface, but the groove separating B cusps is more shallow and less fissure-like.

The oblique ridge may be virtually interrupted at its "dip and bend" by small secondary grooves from the anterior sulcus and from the posterior groove. In spite of this it may still be clearly recognizable; if so, it is of much help and almost provides a short-cut to orientation of the tooth. It has been shown (a) that by passing from DB to MP this ridge is directed medially and anteriorly, never posteriorly; (b) that together with anterior and posterior marginal ridges the oblique ridge forms an S-shape in a left tooth and a Z-shape in a right tooth; and (c) that these letter shapes cannot be interchanged by reversal. Thus, in a trial orientation, if the oblique ridge appears directed backwards, or if the ridges make a Z on left side or S on right side, the tooth has been wrongly placed.

If the crown does not have four well-developed cusps, but they are reduced to "three and one-half" or three cusps, it will be in the DP position that the change has taken place. The "half" cusp may be a small cusp, one or more tubercles, or merely a ridge-like area posterior to a short groove which represents the posterior occlusal groove. In these cases the one P cusp is often large. In these cases also it may be possible to recognize the upper two sections of Z or S, and so enlist this as an aid in orientation. The short groove referred to may be reduced to a pit or there may be no trace of it at all (Fig. 7-3).

In many teeth of unusual crown morphology, such as the "compressed" form where the DP cusp may appear "pushed" to palatal of MP cusp, it may still be possible to recognize that Z or S pattern of ridges, but in a distorted style (Figs. 7-5 *j*, 7-6 *b* and 7-18 *e*).

Root branches that are partly or completely fused to other branches may still retain some feature of type characters which can be recognized and so assist in orientation. Recognition of these usually follows examination of grooves, which may for example mark out the wide and flat character of MB root, or the distal groove that often indicates P and DB root elements. If these can be related satisfactorily to cusp positions, progress towards identification has been made. Another groove of this kind is that usually found on the buccal surface of fused MB and DB root elements.

The presence of additional elements may greatly complicate the procedure of identification. It is seldom that great difficulty is experienced when the additional element is the pit, groove or tubercle associated with the name of Carabelli. This feature varies in degree over a considerable range, but there are some respects in which it has almost had consistency thrust upon it so that failure to conform in these respects deprives the feature of the Carabelli appellation. Consistency in the Carabelli feature lies chiefly in its location on the MP surface of the crown.

An additional cusp may at first sight look like a Carabelli cusp, but it may be on a different surface, such as MB. Such a cusp therefore should be of secondary importance in orientation; a surface is not assumed to be palatal because it presents such a cusp, but rather the surfaces are identified by other characters. We thus determine whether the additional feature is, or is not, a Carabelli cusp.

If characters of root and occlusal surface have not established orientation, the tooth may be rotated on its long axis while profiles are examined. Buccal cusps are further from the axis than palatal cusps, and their tips are sometimes ridge-like, sometimes more domed. Convexity of crown profile is asymmetrical in these cases. It may be described as greater on P, forming a long arc from cervix to cusp tip, but on B tending to form an angle near the tip. These differences may also be described for "root plus crown" profiles, noting that the root portion tends on P to diverge more markedly from the tooth axis. Thus the B profile may be almost a straight line from root across the cervix to the cusp angle just mentioned, but P profile forms an angle at the cervix (see Fig. 7-36 *b*).

Comparison of crown profiles M and D in buccal view may also reveal differences. In this case the M contour tends to be longer and straighter and the D contour shorter and more convex. It may have been noted at the same time that in this view the MB cusp tends to be wider and its tip further from cervix.

If these contrasts in opposite profiles can be recognized, and are found compatible with tentative assignments of M, D, B, P regions to the tooth under examination, they tend to confirm one's judgment. But there are further possible sources of data which may assist in the decision. These are imposed characters and acquired characters, and there is a clear distinction between them.

The term "imposed" has been used for characters arising during formation of the tooth. Omitting those of pathological origin, the interest is with morphological effects such as the "compressed" crown, or certain divergencies, curves or bends in roots. It has been seen that a compressed crown has its long axis B-P and not M-D. As for the root branches, it was shown why buccal roots tend to curve distally, or why the reverse may occur in a third molar with fused roots.

Acquired characters are those that arise after the tooth has emerged to a functional position, and they are seen mostly in the crown. They comprise decay, stains, deposits and evidence of wear. Bearing in mind that molar teeth are less often in malposition than are premolars and anterior teeth, particularly in respect to rotation or torsiversion, a maxillary molar tooth often acquires characters that assist not only the identification of its surfaces, but also its position as first, second or third molar. The immediate matter at hand is with surface identification.

Decay is more common on proximal (M and D) and occlusal surfaces. In a caries-susceptible person buccal cavities are common and are often distinctive in appearance. They vary according to the tooth and to efforts at dental prophylaxis (Taylor, 1971a). The persistence of stain or calculus deposits also varies in these respects. Interproximal wear may show in the form of a small facet on M or D, and although a facet may be found on P surface, this should easily be distinguishable from the interproximal facet. A buccal surface, especially in a first molar, may bear evidence of toothbrushing abrasion in the cervical region, like that seen in more anterior teeth (Fig. 7-36 *a*). Stain, and sometimes calculus deposits, may be limited cervically by a curvature of outline that bears witness or otherwise to the form of the alveolar margin, or interdental septum, so that proximal or other surfaces may be indicated.

It should be evident from the above that type characters, imposed characters and acquired characters may collectively provide much data that can be used to identify surfaces and so determine the laterality of a maxillary molar even when it is of unusual morphology, or incomplete.

First, Second or Third Molar

The serial position occupied by an isolated upper molar cannot always be determined, but in doubtful cases one can usually say there is a strong probability that it was first or second, or that it was second or third. This is because, although in some characters there is an overlapping in the range of variation, there is a tendency for some characters to be more noticeable, or to occur more often in one than in another. Thus there may be found in one individual a decreasing complexity of crown or root form, or a decreasing divergence of root branches (or increasing tendency towards root fusion), from the first to the third molar.

But this "gradient" of complexity is not necessarily similar for crown and root in one person, nor is it always lowest in third molars. Thus complete fusion of roots may be found in a third molar which has four well-developed cusps, or second and third molars may show reduction to three cusps, but may present three root branches that show no fusion and sometimes marked divergence.

Complexity in root or crown may alternatively be greater in second than in their first molars, but it is third molars that usually present the greatest contrasts from the most common four-cusp and three-root style. These so-called aberrant forms have been discussed previously. Some appear to present imposed characters, but most were assumed to include additional elements which arose from the potential for division and a range of variation inherent in tooth-forming tissues. It follows therefore that most such teeth are tentatively classed as third molars, and this impression may be supported by acquired characters mentioned above.

Teeth with three root branches (especially if these are divergent) and a well-developed DP cusp are most likely to be first molars, and doubts are reduced where there is also a Carabelli cusp or pit. Some uncertainty regarding the last feature must remain when it is recalled that these have been found in first and second molars, both teeth *in situ*. First molars may have roots with little separation (especially buccal roots). They may have some root fusion, especially buccal roots, sometimes DB with P, occasionally MB with P. A tooth with a much reduced DP cusp is unlikely to be a first molar.

A second molar often has a reduced DP cusp, or that cusp may be absent, leaving three cusps, of which the P cusp may be the widest or largest. The DP cusp may be represented by a ridge. The posterior groove may not extend to P surface, and it may be reduced to a mere pit, or completely absent as in the full reduction to a three-cusp style. Reduced divergence of root branches or fusion in the styles just detailed for first molars is common. Complete fusion is not rare, so that the tooth may present a single, more or less conical, root. Such a root usually presents grooves indicating its constituent root elements.

Third molars may vary in crown and root in any of the styles just described for second molars, but as in seconds, so also in thirds, there may be three distinct root branches or four well-developed cusps as in first molars.

It has been shown how acquired characters may assist in identification of sidedness of a molar. These also may assist determination of its serial position, but there are pitfalls. Perhaps the most useful such character is the facet of interproximal wear on adjacent teeth. First and second molars may present two such facets, M and D, and third molars on M only.

And now for some pitfalls. It is possible, but extremely rare, for a third molar to have a distal facet where there is a fourth molar in functional occlusion, as in the Tasmanian skulls mentioned earlier. It is not uncommon for a second molar to present only one such facet which may be on M or on D. It is missing from D where a third molar has not erupted, or has been extracted early. It is missing from M where the first molar has been denied contact through dental caries or operative procedures (which include early extraction for orthodontic reasons). Other acquired characters may indicate that the second molar had tipped mesially as a result of these. Alternatively a second molar may have been extracted early and its place subsequently occupied by the third molar, with resulting complication of identification.

Dental decay and other forms of pathology, operative treatment and personal habits, and their possible effects on teeth in a contemporary society, may certainly complicate identification of teeth, but they also add greatly to the data available. Interpretation of such data from a background of the science and practice of dentistry can give much information of forensic value in identification of human remains.

Chapter 8

Mandibular Molars

FROM THE AUTHOR'S collection of lower molars approximately 410 teeth have been mounted. From these the figures for illustration of this chapter, comprising some 348 outlines, represent 174 lower molar teeth. Diminutive teeth are not included in this count.

Description of lower molars follows the same broad plan as for upper molars. In general the lower has at least four cusps and usually two root branches. Also, first, second and third lowers have many features in common, but there are some features that are more likely to be found in a particular one of the three teeth. Thus there are type characters concerning number, disposition and form of cusps, root branches and grooves. There are personal characters related to length, divergence, and sturdiness of roots, and the usual differences in prominence and acumination of cusps, and in convexity of surfaces.

As with upper molars, there is wide scope for variation in all of these characters, and to them may be added divergence, fusion and curvature of roots. These additional features may in part reflect type and personal characters, while curvature in some cases merits recognition as an imposed character.

Imposed characters were defined as those likely to arise at a very early stage of crown development, but more often during root formation, through the necessity to conform to the morphology of adjacent anatomical structures and supporting bone. It was shown that amongst such structures those mostly concerned were the maxillary sinus, nasal fossa and canals or foramina carrying blood vessels and nerves. While the variations in these structures as regards their form and relation to tooth roots have not been examined in detail in this study, they have been accepted as expressions of normal variation which may be associated with tooth variation. In the case of lower molars there are no sinuses involved. The chief features concerned are the inferior dental canal and bone morphology, and their influence on root form is most likely to be seen in the third molar. Many writers have reported on aspects of this relationship, and some of the effects on root morphology are well illustrated by Miles and West (1954).

In the lower jaw, variations in the amount of basal and alveolar bone may create conditions for the developing molar (especially the third molar) quite different from those encountered in the upper jaw. These must be considered as a likely factor sometimes involved in root curvature, and it seems reasonable to regard their results also as imposed characters. Morphological details of the completed root may therefore bear witness not only to the range of normal variation in regard to type characters, but also to the influence of suspected personal characters and of conditions external to the tooth. These external conditions are themselves subject to change during the growth period, but their effects on the growing tooth are permanent and irreversible, and these are the imposed characters. But this is not all.

As with upper molars, there is an extensive range of variations in tooth form arising from the presence of additional elements in crown or root. These were examined in considerable detail in Chapter 7 and referred to as Opc. For that reason the subject will receive less attention here. Nevertheless it will be considered, and not only to demonstrate differences in the Opc of lower molars. By so doing it will also be shown that by their range of degree and variety they give emphasis to the contention that they are ontogenetic rather than phylogenetic in origin.

THE CROWN

The textbook description of lower molar crowns refers to the normal first molar's five cusps, the second molar's four cusps, and the third molar's tendency to be like one or the other. Reference may also be made briefly to variation in the first two molars, and it may be hinted that the third molar is so variable in many respects that it is beyond description. This, then, is the task, namely, an attempt at analysis of variation in all three molars.

Inevitably reference will be made here to some features mentioned by others, or covered by such meticulous records as Dahlberg's plaques already referred to, but the method here is different, as is the purpose. Examination of as many morphological characters as possible, and of the manner of their variation, in both crown and root and their interrelationships, must facilitate a comprehensive and more accurate awareness of the nature of variation. With the additional familiarity that may come from clinical experience and study of skeletal material, it is found that isolated teeth or parts of teeth may enable one to contribute usefully in forensic work. At the same time one may gather data that are relevant in the hypothetical fields of dental anthropology, dental surgery, or oral hygiene and nutrition (Taylor, 1975, 1976).

Whatever may be the order of priorities, it is essential to study the whole tooth, crown and root. Failure to recognize this has unfortunately devalued much otherwise careful work. Partly for convenience this study is reported under separate headings for crown and root, and some characters (such as occlusal grooves and root curvature) clearly merit separate treatment. Other characters, such as size, cannot satisfactorily be given separate treatment.

Size of Crowns

It has been shown earlier that the term "size" in reference to a tooth requires qualification. It may refer to teeth that are easily described as large or small when one looks at the whole tooth (Figs. 8-1 *a,d,* 8-2 *b,c,** 8-3 *a,e,* 8-9 *b* and 8-12 *f*). In some cases there is a quality of sturdiness or slenderness of root, or of length, that prompts one to use a particular adjective (Figs. 8-1 *e,f,* 8-6 and 8-11 *e*). In others (and examples were illustrated for single-rooted teeth), rotation of a tooth between proximal and buccal or lingual views may merit a change of adjective if the root is flattened. Thus there is the character of proportion, not only of dimensions of crown and root, but also of, say, length and breadth of crowns or of roots themselves. A further consideration in assessment of size in a multi-rooted tooth arises from the character of divergence or fusion of root branches.

The large-crowned tooth in Figure 8-2 *a* may be said to be small because of root fusion, while that in Figure 8-2 *b,* which

---

* Although this Chapter deals mostly with mandibular molars, it includes a little material involving both upper and lower molars. In the figures, occlusal outlines (unless otherwise indicated) are always oriented with M (mesial) towards the top of the figure. The positions of cusp tips are marked by X, but the size of the X does not indicate the prominence of the cusp. A small cusp or tubercle may be marked with a *t*. Grooves and ridges are indicated by continuous and broken lines respectively on occlusal outlines, and by lines or light shading on others. Carious cavities and fractures of crown or root are shown with irregular outlines, amalgam fillings by regular or curved lines, and facets of wear are shaded obliquely. Recognition of these should present no difficulty. As in the figures of upper molars, additional elements in crown or root are marked *Opc*. Orientation and identification of parts of teeth in any outline may be assisted by the further labelling of mesial, distal etc., in the usual way. The scale is in 5mm intervals.

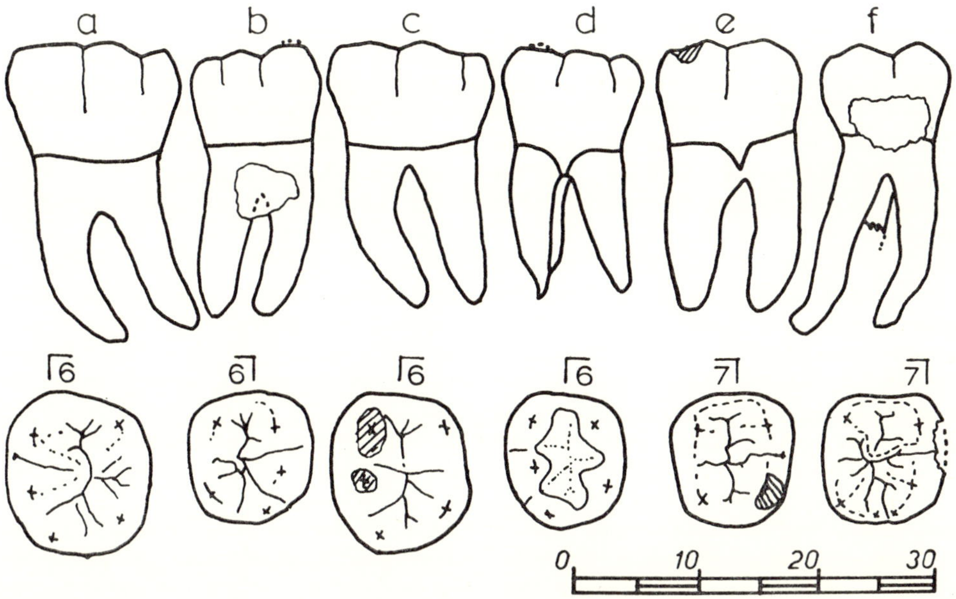

Figure 8-1. Buccal and occlusal views of six lower molars varying in features concerned in description of size. (Tooth *f* has a third root which fractured during extraction. See Fig. 8-15 *d*.) Note in occlusal views the variety in main and secondary grooves.

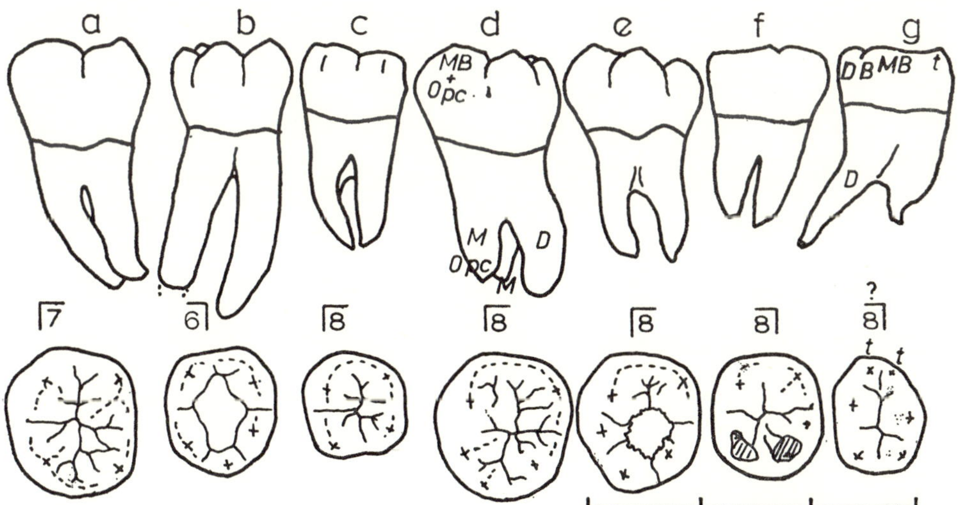

Figure 8-2. Further examples as in Figure 8-1. In tooth *g* note that the crown has two additional tubercles, paired at mesial, and that the M root is much shorter than D. All these are unusual characters. In tooth *b* the D root apex had been lost by fracture.

has a smaller crown but a longer divided or divergent root, might be described as a large tooth. Therefore, when describing the size of a tooth, it is essential to elaborate and to specify whether it is the overall dimension, the proportion of crown or root, or the dimension of either, and the viewpoint or anatomical character that is referred to.

The teeth of Figures 8-1 and 8-2 *a,b* (all first or second molars) well illustrate the differences that are found in proportions of crown size to root size. When third molars are studied, not only is the variation in proportions much greater but so also is the variation in actual size of crown and root. There is however a noteworthy observation regarding disproportionate teeth. Variation in actual size of third molars of approximately "average" proportions of crown to root ranges from a small tooth (excluding diminutives, Fig. 8-2 *c* is a fair example) to a large tooth (Fig. 8-2 *d*). With disproportionate teeth the range tends only in one direction, namely to a decrease of root size and increase of the crown (Figs. 8-2 *e,f* and 8-3 *a,b*). The author has not found the opposite extreme where there is a small crown and a very large root, and indeed it is difficult to see how crown and root formation could proceed to such end.

It should be noted that the more likely finding, a relatively large crown, is usually characterized by some additional features rather than as presenting an "oversize" version of the common four or five cusps. It may not be easy to identify such additional elements, because, as with upper molars, they may be in the form of ill-defined tubercles, ridges and grooves or pits which complicate the "normal" pattern (Fig. 8-3 *a,b,c*). Others can fairly be described as additional cusps (Opc?), or as obvious Opc with additional elements in crown or root or both. These will be referred to presently. When the Opc is more prominent in the root one may be reminded of the missing extreme mentioned above. One would feel that such a structure when found might

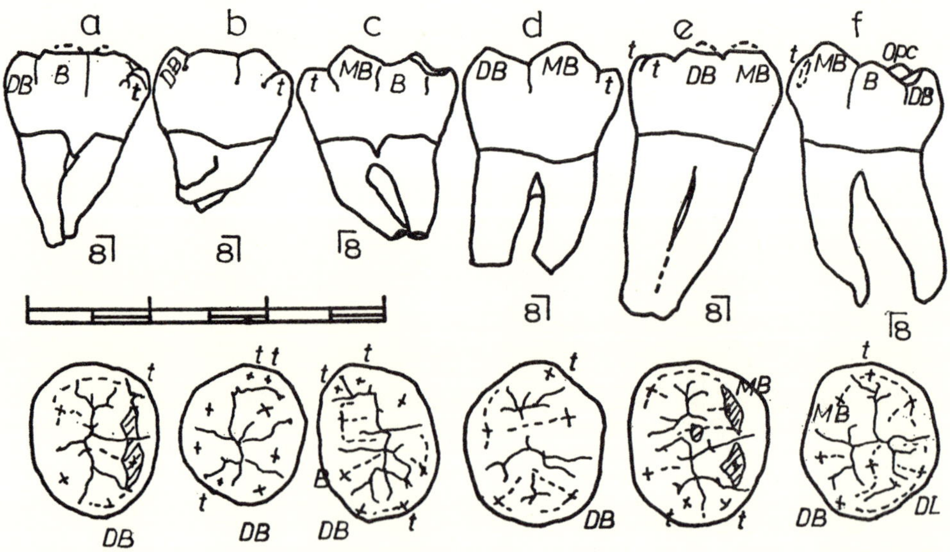

Figure 8-3. Buccal and occlusal views of six third molars illustrating characters involved when describing the size of a tooth. Is it large or small overall, either as regards crown or root, or as regards relation of crown to root, and does fusion or divergence of roots influence the choice of adjective used? The occlusal views extend the awareness of variation in disposition of cusps, tubercles, ridges and grooves, and of actual and relative dimensions of length and breadth of crown.

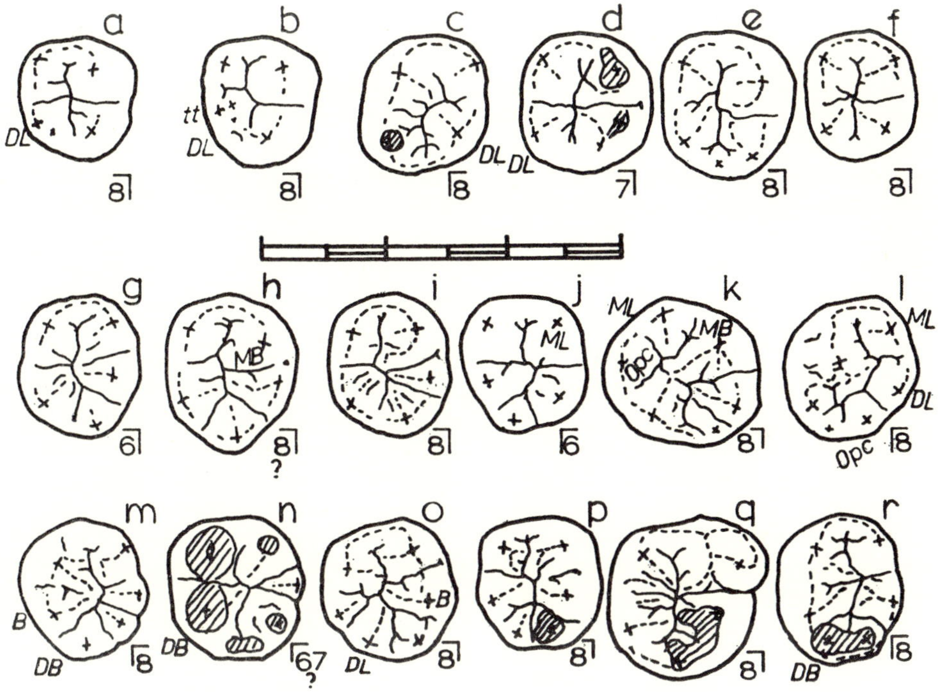

Figure 8-4. Occlusal views of eighteen lower molars. Apart from emphasizing differences in size and shape of outline, the camera lucida has facilitated accurate plotting of cusp tips, ridges and grooves. The great diversity in these is obvious. (Other views of tooth *q* are shown in Fig. 8-8 *b*.)

more properly be classed as an odontome, and not a variation within the scope of the present work.

In spite of what has just been said it must be noted that there is no consistency of pattern in the relative size of cusps. In lower molars it is most common to find the MB cusp largest. Similarly the smallest cusp, where there are four cusps, is usually DL; in a tooth with five cusps it is the DB cusp mostly, but sometimes it is the DL which is smallest.

In Figure 8-4, tooth *a* has a mere tubercle at DL while tooth *b* has two such and a small ML, but two relatively large B cusps. Tooth *c* has a large DL cusp, but the DB is larger still, so that the B-L dimension of this crown is widest at D, the reverse of the usual. But this tooth also has a bifid D root indicating the presence of an Opc element. It would be convenient to describe the large DB, or DL, cusp as having together absorbed or annexed the crown element of the Opc. (The suggestion that this may occur is considered again when discussing tooth *a* in Fig. 8-21.) Tooth *i* in Figure 8-4 is another style of "disproportion" in cusp size, this time involving B and DB cusps.

In Figure 8-7 *a* the second molar has virtually five and a half (5½) cusps, namely a DB cusp plus tubercle beside it. The young tooth *g* in Figure 8-16 has four cusps. The DL cusp is very large and the D root formation had already divided showing that an Opc was involved. The notion of a crown element being absorbed or annexed is convenient for description, but will be considered later (p. 314, and Fig. 8-21 *a*). On the same basis one might say that a cusp may annex or take over part of the material of an adjacent cusp.

Thus in Figure 8-4 *i* the B cusp is reduced and the DB is much larger.

Variation in crown size therefore is seen to involve a number of factors. Some characters obviously must be of genetic origin. Other features might well be so, and this probability is sometimes strengthened when teeth of related individuals are examined. But this is of limited practicability since the complexity in detail of variation inevitably frustrates efforts to pursue such comparative studies. Thus, apart from those personal characters evidently related to body type and stature of the individual, and sometimes perhaps inherited more from one parent than from the other, there are the characters that may collectively be described as complexities. These have been indicated by the examples just given. They are seen to involve variation in relative size of "normal" features and variation in the number and nature of additional features. The latter, such as ridges, tubercles and additional cusps, may sometimes be obviously associated with additional root elements, or apparently be confined to crown or root only. The more obvious cases are conveniently designated as Opc, but there are also a very great number and range of such variations that cannot clearly be described, and are certainly not classifiable in any meaningful way. The writer prefers to regard them as expressions of normal potential for variation inherent in dental and other tissues.

Occlusal Features

Some of these complexities will now be examined. In Figure 8-4 the eighteen occlusal views illustrate diversity in number, relative size and position of cusps. Teeth *m* and *n* each have an extra lingual cusp. In *m* its equality in size with the DL cusp suggests the description "twin DL cusps," but in *n* the designation of Opc appears preferable. In neither tooth is an additional root element apparent. In *l* the D root is bifid. While primary grooves and ridges are all different, secondaries are much more so, not only in position and style but also in number. Thus teeth *d,e,f,g,j* have few secondaries, but *k,l,o,p,q* are complex. (Many more such variations are shown in other figures.) In the bottom row, all teeth except *q* have virtually a sixth cusp but no matching additional root element.

In Figure 8-5 there are four corresponding outlines of each of seven teeth. While the occlusal views add to examples of variation in features noted in the previous figure, the B, L and M outlines illustrate variation in other characters. With regard to crowns, there are differences in height, width and acumination of cusps, and in convexities of corresponding profiles. In B and L views, while there is no marked difference in convexity of M and D profiles, there is a difference in B and L profiles seen in M view. In the B and L views the crown appears to be higher at M than at D. Another way of describing this is to say that the M marginal ridge and contact point are further from cervix at M than at D.

In proximal view however there is a more consistent and noticeable difference between B and L outlines. A similar but opposite difference is found in upper teeth, and in Chapter 9 these characters are discussed in relation to occlusion and to identification of teeth. Perhaps the most obvious result of this particular character in occlusal views of lower molars is that B cusps are located further from the outline than are the L cusps. This is because the occlusal view sees beyond the cusp to the true buccal surface, but does not usually include more than the cuspal portion of the L surface. The effect is very clearly presented in the six lower molars from one person where cusps have been virtually worn away (Fig. 8-6).

The upper outlines in Figure 8-6 are drawn from teeth *in situ* in a prehistoric mandible from Tonga which was figured in another paper (Taylor, 1971b). As the mandible was broken in the anterior re-

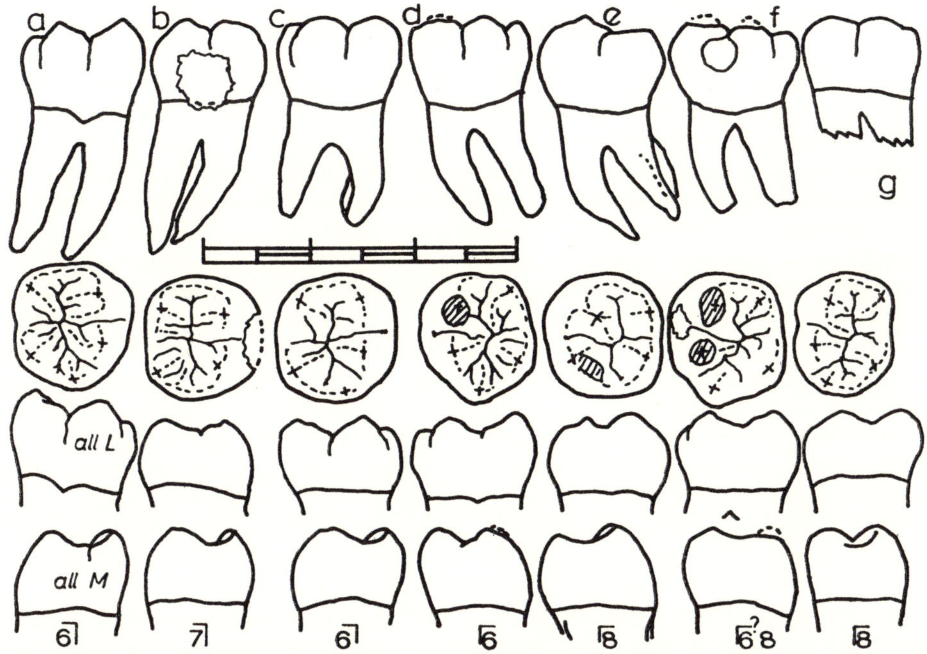

Figure 8-5. Four outlines of each of seven teeth. Top row B, third row L, bottom row M. Note differences in height, width and acumination of cusps, in occlusal ridges and grooves, both primary and secondary. In proximal views (bottom row) there is a consistent difference in B and L outlines. In tooth *e* there is a third root branch on L, but no trace of corresponding additional crown element, and in tooth *g* both root branches had evidently fractured at time of extraction.

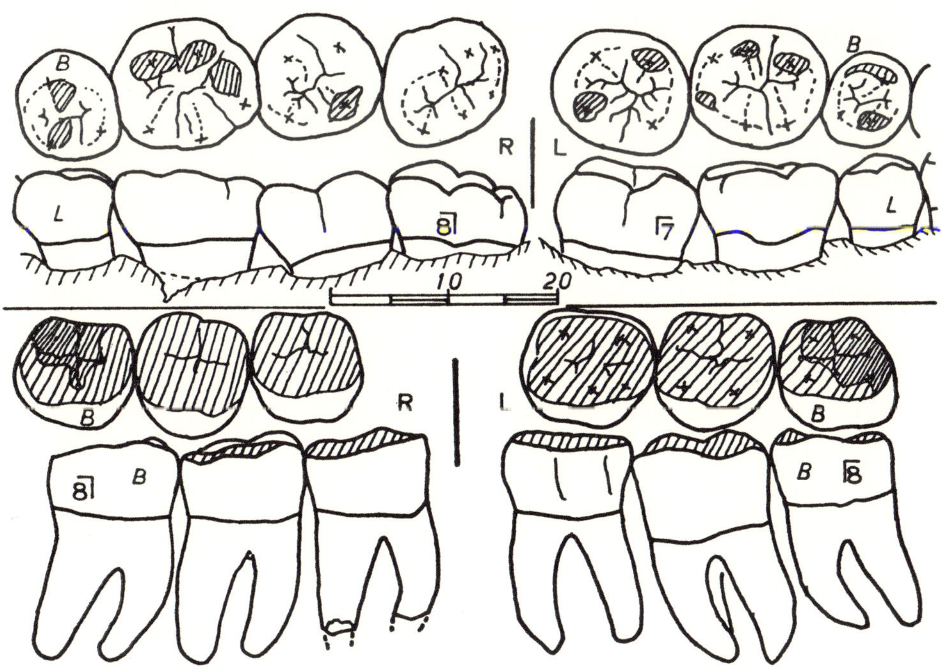

Figure 8-6. Comparison of first, second and third molars in the same individual—two cases. In the top example are occlusal and lingual, and in the lower, occlusal and buccal. Direct comparison between the dentitions is not intended because of different orientation in presentation. (Note that in this figure occlusal outlines are not orientated with M towards top of page.)

gion, each portion was placed "B-side down" for drawing with the camera lucida. The lateral views therefore are of lingual surfaces, and because of the difficulties of procedure, the scale for these particular drawings is approximate. There is no third molar on the left side, and that on right side was out of alignment and tipped distally, an uncommon irregularity.

One of the objectives in this figure was a comparison of size and form in first, second and third lower molars in left and right teeth of two persons. In the Tongan, left and right teeth are not mirror images, particularly in regard to occlusal grooves and ridges. In the other dentition which has heavy occlusal wear, outlines show closer resemblances in corresponding teeth (and this applies for roots also). Although wear was severe throughout this dentition, it is seen to be more advanced on right side. A similar difference in wear was reported in Maori and Chatham Island skulls (Taylor, 1962b, 1963a). In each third molar, part of the worn area had become darkly stained, and this suggests that occlusion had recently changed.

The writer was given twenty-seven teeth removed from this person, but upper third molars are not amongst them. However, examination of upper second molars shows that each has a well-worn distal contact facet, but both are covered with stain whereas mesial facets are clean. Thus the surmise is proved correct, for it is apparent that the functional occlusal area had been reduced by recent removal of upper third molars.

This comparison is continued in Figure 8-7, using specimens of known race (Maori), some from skeletal material of

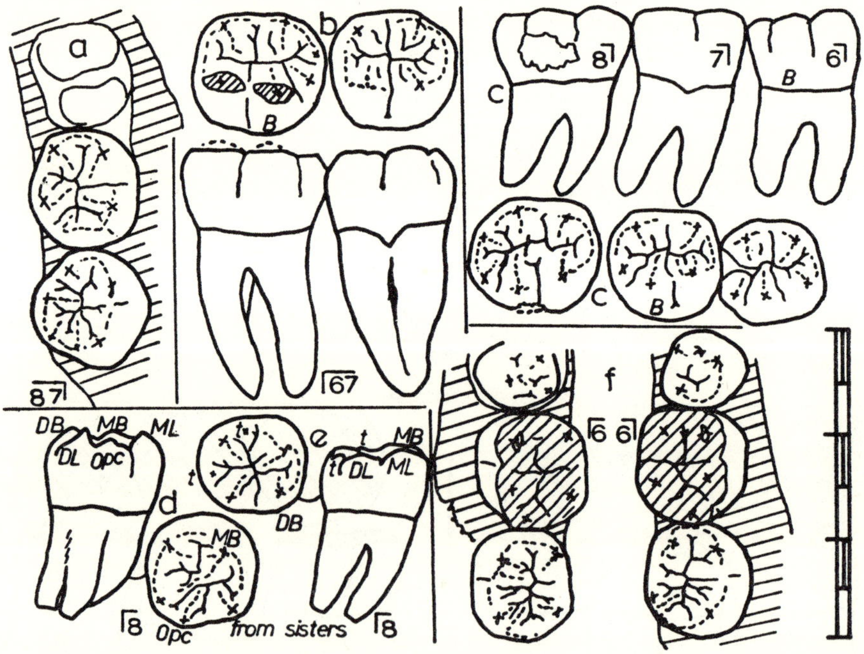

Figure 8-7. Comparison of first, second and third molars, continued. *a* and *f* from pre-European Maori skeletal material. *b-e*, teeth extracted by a dental surgeon from Maori persons. *a*, mandibular fragment with second and third molars *in situ*. *b* and *c*, from adult males. *d* and *e*, from sisters 18 and 16 years respectively. *f*, pre-European mandibular fragment of Maori child aged approximately ten years. (Note that in this figure occlusal outlines are orientated with M towards top of figure only in *a,f* but not in *b-e*.)

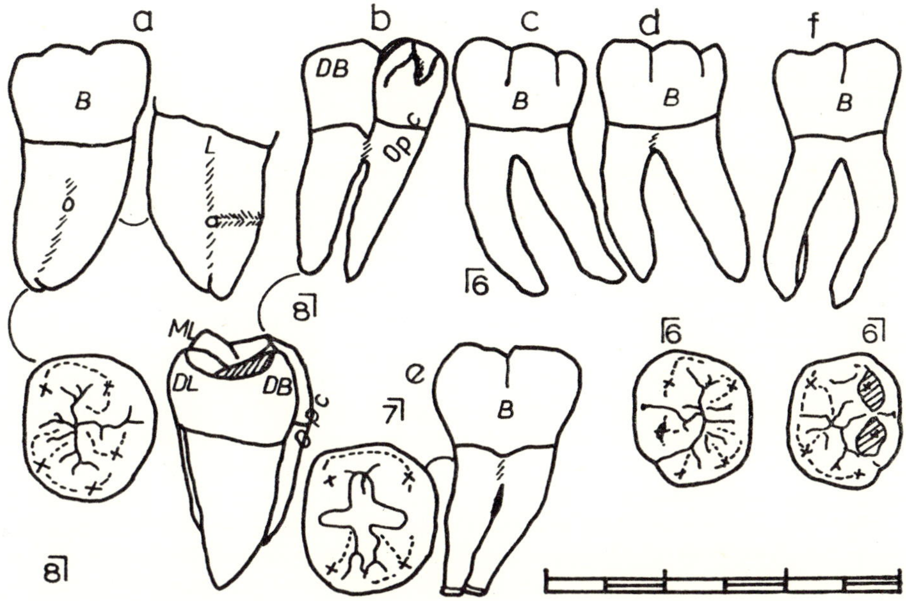

Figure 8-8. Further examples of root variation. Tooth *a* has fused root elements which are perforated at mid-root by a canal which is continuous with a lingual groove crossing the D portion of the root. Tooth *b* has an easily recognizable Opc fused with MB cusp and continuous with M root. The abrupt step in the cervical line is noteworthy. The tooth was tilted for the D view, and the occlusal of this tooth is shown in Figure 8-4 *q*. Teeth *c,d,f* are first molars with varying curves and divergence of root branches. Tooth *e* has a curved and fused root but M and D elements are easily identifiable. It is a young tooth with incomplete roots and is from the same person as tooth *a* in Figure 8-2.

unknown sex and some of known sex and age, these being extracted teeth given by a dental surgeon. Teeth *d* and *e*, both left third molars from sisters aged eighteen and sixteen years, are quite different in crown and root. When compared, wear on first molars is found to be negligible in the two adult males on modern diet, but already considerable at ten years of age in the child from pre-European times (Taylor, 1963a, 1975, 1976). At the time of death of this child the left second premolar was emerging from its crypt, and the right third molar crown could be seen through the gubernacular canal. In this case corresponding left and right teeth were closely similar in crown morphology.

THE ROOT

In most of the previous figures teeth have been drawn in B or L view, so that some of the diversity of style of bifidity and of fusion of M and D roots has already been shown. Without this it was not possible to demonstrate that it is ambiguous and inadequate as a description to say that a tooth is large or small or average. It was shown that length, divergence or fusion of root branches may prompt such descriptions, although size of crown and proportionate size of crown and root are essential considerations in any such assessment. A description therefore should include at least a qualifying phrase showing the character to which the adjective applies.

Few of the teeth in these earlier figures have shown a third root branch, so that variations concern the length, thickness, divergence, fusion and curvature of more or less "normal" roots. The distance from cervix to root furcation bears no special relationship to root length or to root divergence. The style of furcation as seen from B or L may be variously described as an arch or an angle and varies considerably from wide and rounded (Figs. 8-2 *e*, 8-5 *c*), to a very acute angle (Figs. 8-2 *f* and 8-5 *b*), with many modifications related to divergence of branches and curvatures in the same. Divergence itself is a vague term and therefore unsatisfactory since it varies not only in different teeth but also frequently in a particular tooth; this is mainly because of curvature in the root axis, but also through twists in the axis and through the qualities of thickness, taper and type of apex. The description also is subject to change with the viewpoint.

Divergence may be considerable and continuous (Figs. 8-8 *d* and 8-10 *b*); it may appear to be so as a result of an abrupt curve or bend, or because a root is long (Figs. 8-10 *c* and 8-11 *d*). Divergence may be minimal and yet the branches remain separate (Figs. 8-9 *c* and 8-10 *a*), or it may not be continuous where one or both branches change direction and restore contact between them (Figs. 8-2 *a*, 8-3 *e*, 8-10 *e,f*, 8-11 *c* and 8-12 *c,d,e*).

Fusion also occurs in great variety. To do justice to this it would be necessary to include outlines of pulp cavities obtained with the aid of radiographs and sections of teeth, but this is outside the present report although it comprised an extensive part of the study on which the report is based. Excluding what might be called pathological fusion arising from deposition of additional cementum, there still remains a considerable variety for consideration, both as regards the internal anatomy of the pulp cavity and the external morphology of the root.

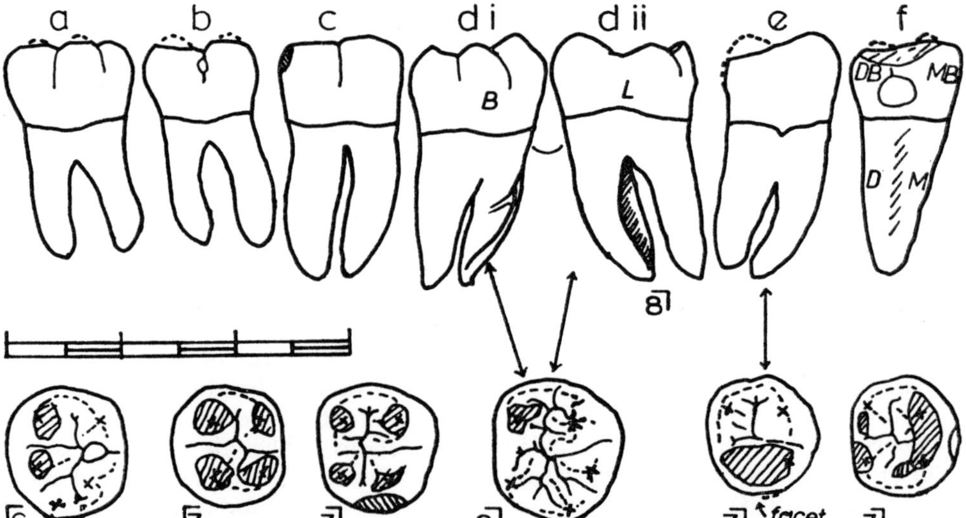

Figure 8-9. Teeth presenting a variety of characters, which are unusual or which can be of use in identification. *a,b,* teeth with well-marked primary grooves on occlusal surface, but lacking secondary grooves (as also does tooth *f*). *c,* although the root branches are separate throughout their length they do not diverge. Wear on all four cusps is light but even, suggesting good occlusion, but the D facet is unusual in position and degree of wear. It shows that the tooth could not be a third molar. Removal of lower third molar and over eruption of the upper could have produced this D facet. *d,* the M root is very wide, giving appearance of a twisted root and different divergences when viewed from B and L. *e,* there is no wear on M cusps but D cusps are severely worn, and there is also a D facet. This tooth must have been a second molar that tipped mesially after the first molar was extracted. *f,* an unusual case of root fusion, similar to that in Figure 8-11*f*.

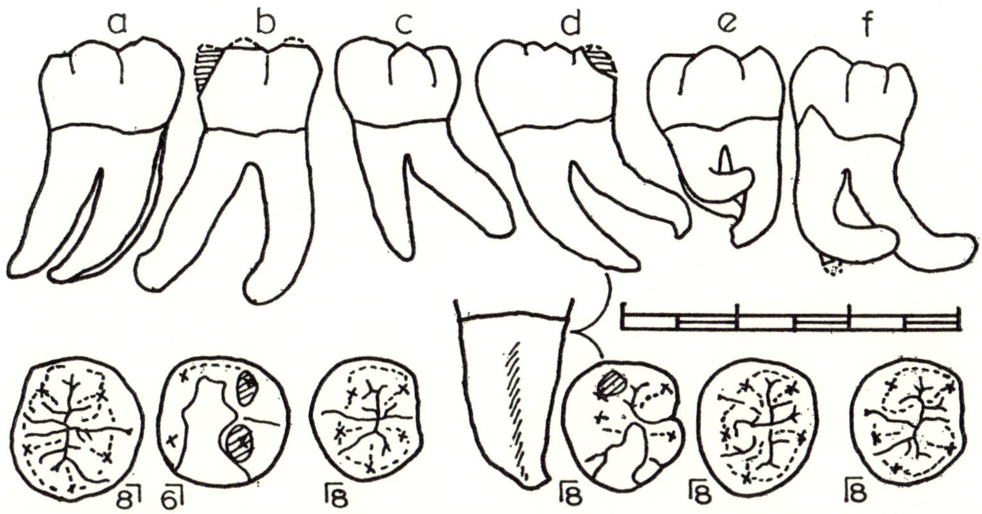

Figure 8-10. Root curves, imposed characters and crown features. *a,* both roots have a long sweeping curve, the M root has a prominent groove on M surface, and the occlusal surface has many secondary grooves. *b,c,* excess root divergence which would complicate tooth extraction. In *b,* M root curves markedly while D root diverges. In *c,* M root is straight while D root bends abruptly from its furcation. *d,* both roots curve as in *a* but are more divergent, and M root has a marked M groove. *e,f,* M roots are bifid and curve abruptly through 90 degrees. In *f* the lingual apex of M root is fractured.

Comparing first and second molars, it is common to find less divergence in the second, and even full length fusion as in Figures 8-7 *b* and 8-8 *e.* In each of these teeth the pulp chamber and canals will surely be those of a two-rooted second molar, just as those in Figure 8-8 *c,d,f* will be those of a normal first molar. But when the furcation is much further from the cervix, and more widely arched as in Figure 8-2 *d,e,g,* examination of the pulp cavity sometimes discloses a deep pulp chamber reminiscent of that described as taurodont. Such teeth are reported from time to time (Lunt, 1954 and Miles, 1954). Examples of complete fusion, with so little indication of separate M and D root elements that B views look like proximal views of a normal tooth, are shown in Figures 8-9 *f* and 8-11 *f.* Pulp cavities were not examined in these.

In lower molars not having additional root elements one can therefore find as great a variety of division or fusion of root elements, of divergence and curvature and of thickness and slenderness of branches and bluntness or sharpness of apex, as was described for the roots of upper first premolars. All these and many more are found when teeth having additional root elements are examined.

As with upper molars, it is proposed that teeth with additional elements should not be considered separately for crown and root. Again as with upper molars, some such elements are easily recognized in crown or root, or in both, but also there are many "border-line" cases where the degree of development of these elements is such that their recognition or identification must be subjective.

ADDITIONAL TOOTH ELEMENTS

It is appropriate here to draw attention again to the case of left third molars which differ so much in two sisters (Fig. 8-7 *d,e*). Tooth *e* has four main cusps and two additional tubercles on D and B but the root has the usual two branches with no evidence of an additional root element. Tooth *d* has a crown with four main cusps, and an oblique ridge dividing the primary groove and joining MB and DL cusps, and this is continuous with an Opc root element which is partly fused with the D root.

Tooth *d* in Figure 8-9 has a very wide M root which appears to include an extra element on B side, and this gives the root a twisted appearance. The occlusal pattern is complex and may well incorporate an additional crown element corresponding with that in the root. Two "borderline" teeth are seen in Figure 8-10 *a* and *d*. Each has a large, grooved M root. In *a* the crown is not unusual except as to style of secondary grooves and ridges. The crown of *d* however may well have additional elements, although details are somewhat obscured by an amalgam restoration. With teeth *e,f* there is no doubt of the presence of root Opc. Each M root is bifid and bends abruptly to D from about mid-root. As both are third molars these bends are probably imposed by proximity to the inferior dental canal, but why the D root of *e* should curve to M is difficult to explain.

Figures 8-11 and 8-12 present a further thirteen teeth, each with some feature of special interest as regards root divergence, convergence or fusion, or of crown shape, grooves and ridges. Attention is drawn to these in the legends to the figures. Carter (1914), when discussing root curvature in lower third molars, showed that in certain conditions of eruption and emergence the changing direction imposed on the crown must produce a particular style of curvature of the root. His hypothesis, however, does not explain many cases presented here, a good example being the tooth in Figure 8-11 *a*. Figure 8-13 gives more variations. Teeth *a* and *b*, each in lingual view, present roots that are joined right to the apices on B side and yet show separation at an early stage on L side. In these two teeth also it is of interest to note the contrast in proportion of root size to crown

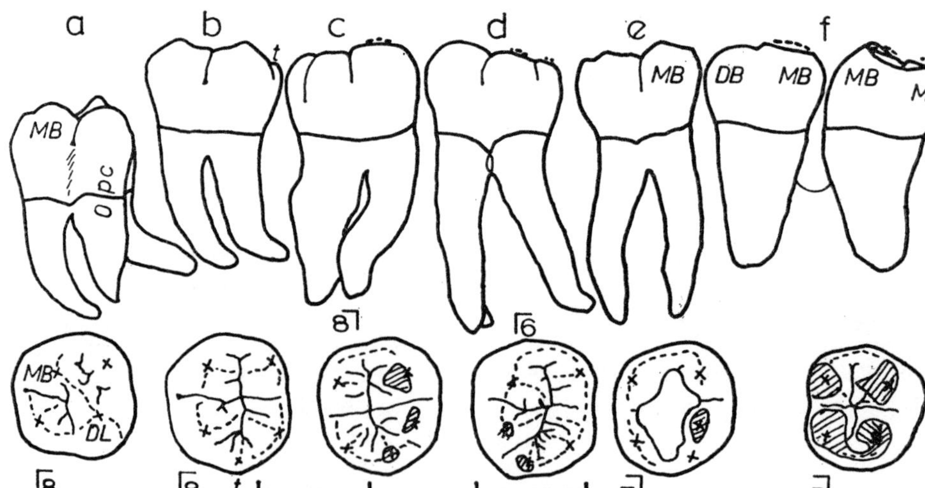

Figure 8-11. Further examples of curves and fusion in roots, and variation in crown features. *a*, a third molar with an "assortment" of root curves. *b*, abrupt curve in apical region. *c*, double or reversed curves in both roots. *d,e*, in each the M root is almost straight, but the D root while at first similarly divergent continues so in *d*, while in *e* it bends at half way to be parallel with M root. *f*, three views of an unusual style of fusion. (See Fig. 8-9 *f*.) The great variety in occlusal ridges and primary and secondary grooves is further demonstrated in *b,c,d,f*.

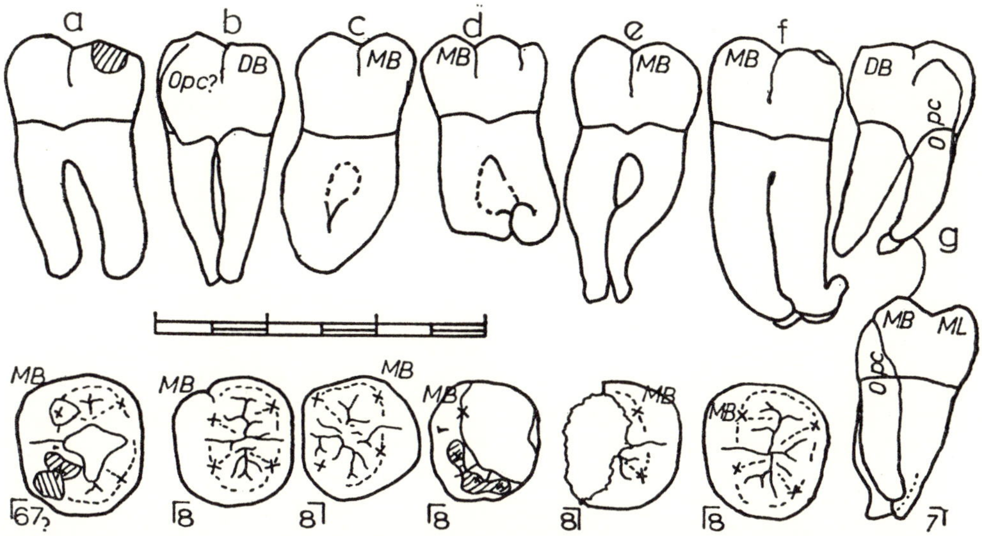

Figure 8-12. Variation in root curves and fusion, continued. The apical curves and grooves in *f* are imposed characters related to the inferior dental canal. Tooth *b* has a trace of Opc at MB of crown and an irregular cervix, but the root is normal. In g, the Opc is again at MB and easily discernible in crown and root and it leaves that root by furcation and termination before the apex is reached.

size, and in sturdiness or slenderness in the root elements. All teeth in Figure 8-13 are third molars.

Teeth *c* and *d* have imposed root curves which suggest adjustment to the inferior dental canal, but tooth *d* must surely have erupted to malocclusion. Tooth *c* obviously had additional crown elements, but full evaluation is frustrated by the destruction caused by caries. In tooth *e* the abrupt curve of the fused root is to B rather than the common curve to D. Facets of wear show that the tooth was fully functional in occlusion. The pointed conical fused root of tooth *f* appears to have root elements of different length. The crown has six cusps, but the style of grooves has been partly obliterated by an amalgam restoration.

Figure 8-14 presents further examples of curves and grooves imposed on third molars, some being associated also with additional root elements. In tooth *a* there are four apices, two being on additional elements. These branch abruptly from the fused main root elements in their apical half, and their form suggests that they may have "straddled" the inferior dental canal. Tooth *c* suggests that its relatively long roots passed beside the canal rather than the more common style of curving, to lie more or less above and straddling it as in *d,e* and *f*. Tooth *g* appears to have resembled *c* in its relation to the canal.

Figure 8-15 presents seven lower molars with a variety of Opc elements in crown, or root, or both. Tooth *a* has a prominent Opc at MB of its crown, but there is no trace of any such in the root. Tooth *b* has a very similar Opc in the crown, and although the tooth has a fused root the Opc is continuous with a well-defined Opc element in the root as well. Tooth *c* has a small Opc root branch which arises on the buccal side of the root furcation. Tooth *d* has a much larger strongly divergent Opc root element on the lingual side. This branch, half of which was lost by fracture at time of extraction, appears to have been formed partly at the expense of the D

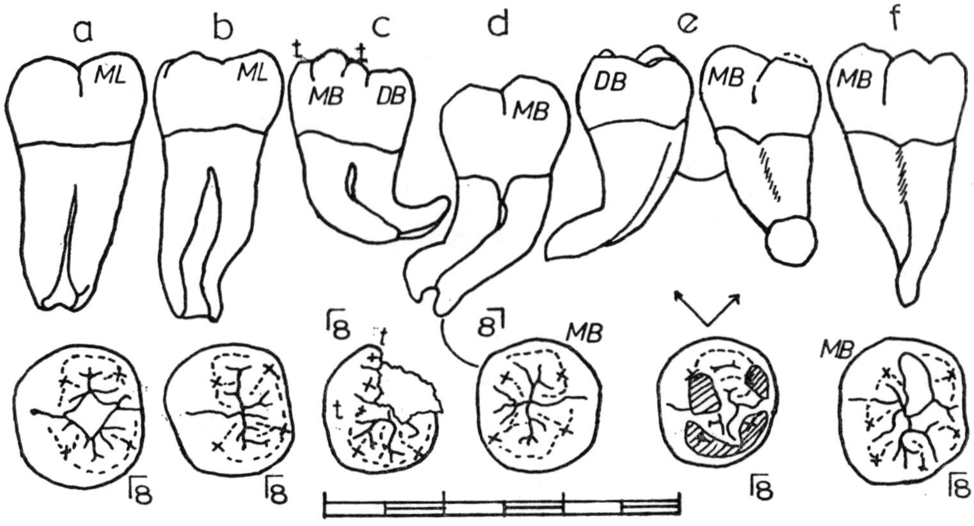

Figure 8-13. Third molars presenting various unusual features.

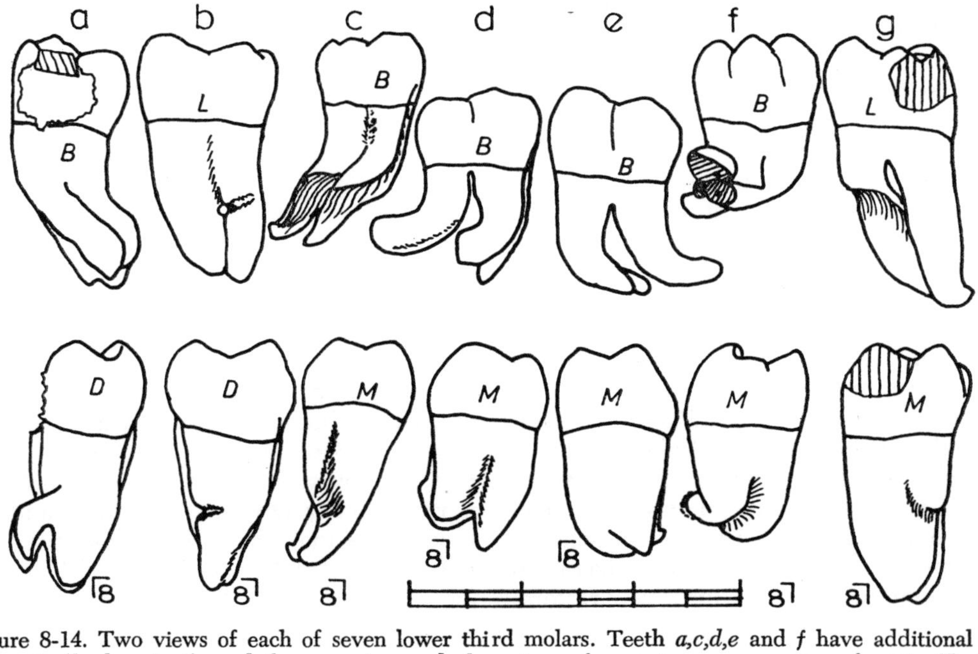

Figure 8-14. Two views of each of seven lower third molars. Teeth *a,c,d,e* and *f* have additional root elements (broken in *f*), and there are imposed characters of curvature or grooving of roots. Tooth *b* also appears in Figure 8-8 *a*.

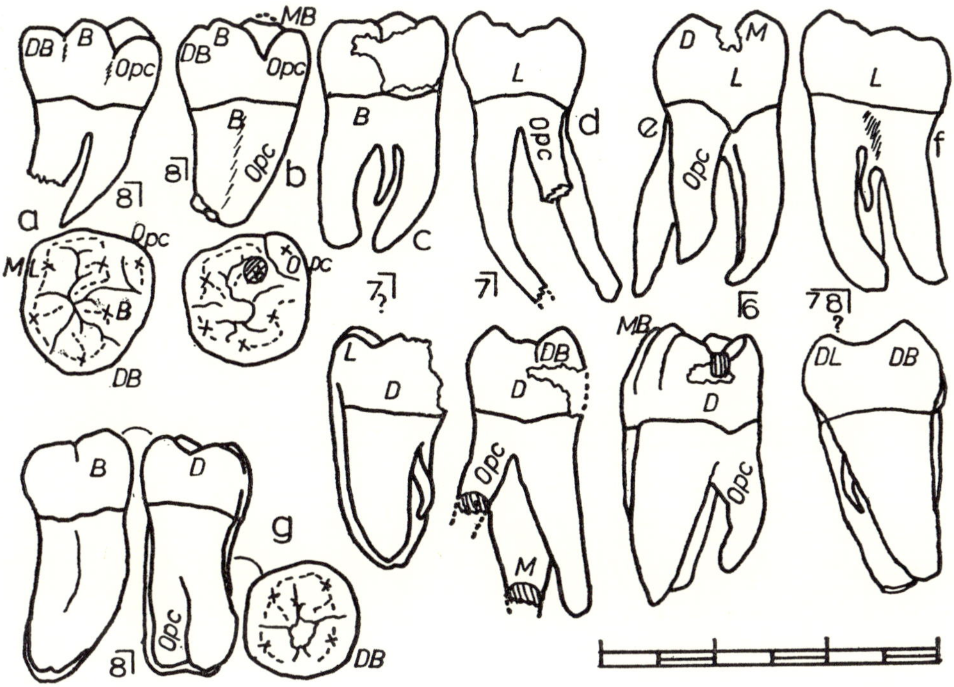

Figure 8-15. Seven lower molars presenting a variety of Opc elements in crown or root, or both.

root which is disproportionately slender.

Tooth *e,* a sturdy first molar, has a sturdy Opc root element diverging from the DL of the autosite, while tooth *f* has a short and slender Opc root arising from the DL aspect of the furcation. All these teeth, *c-f,* have no evidence of Opc in the crown, and yet the Opc root element branches from the autosite at an early stage of root formation. Tooth *g* also has no trace of Opc in its crown, but the root Opc is different from the preceding examples. It arises later, but is clearly defined, in spite of remaining fused to the already fused root of the autosite.

The teeth in Figure 8-15 collectively demonstrate variety in style, size, position (B, L, etc.), and extent (crown or root or both), but they also underline a question that has not yet been discussed, and certainly has no simple answer. Why in some teeth is there differentiation, branching and divergence even of "normal" roots, while in others this does not occur but there is fusion or even an early branching and a later convergence and fusion (Fig. 8-12)? From this question will be omitted the changes in direction that appear to be imposed characters, but can some of the variations in crown form and "complexities" that have been described be omitted as well? For example, is the failure to form the usual number of cusps, or the reduction of secondary grooves and ridges, to be seen as failure of differentiation in crown elements?

If the present use of the word complexity is extended so that it connotes not only crown features but also root furcation of normal elements and of Opc, there is another problem. The degree of complexity "laid down" in the crown does not determine that to be followed in the root. Thus in Figures 8-3 and 8-19 *d,f* there are a num-

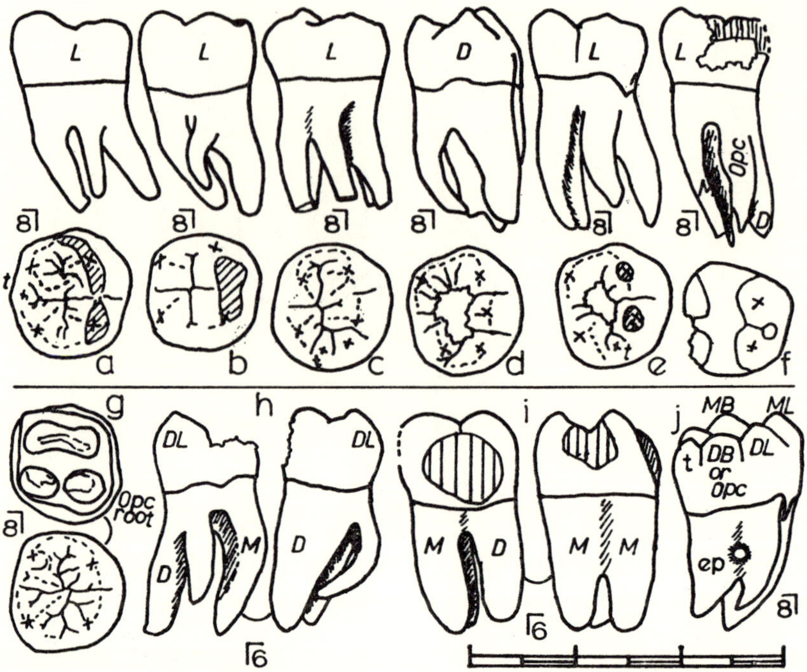

Figure 8-16. Ten lower molars with further examples of Opc. *a* to *f*, third molars from right side, having an Opc branch on L. Except for *c*, the Opc branches from D root rather than from M or the furcation. In *c*, it is associated more with M root; but it is uncertain whether the crown Opc has displaced the DL cusp or is represented by a DL tubercle. In tooth *d* there may be an Opc crown element merged with the large DL cusp. In the young third molar *g*, the D root divided at a very early stage and evidently a DL Opc is associated with the large DL cusp. In tooth *i* there is no crown Opc, but the M root is evenly bifurcated in its apical half. Tooth *j* has a prominent tubercle at DB. The D root has an enamel pearl *(ep)* at mid D surface and bifurcates soon afterwards. There is a long and prominent enamel tang entering both the B and L furcations.

ber of complex crowns without complex roots. In Figure 8-16 *f* and some later figures (as well as in upper molars shown in Chapter 7), there are a number of examples of complexity of root but not of crown.

To suggest that the Opc in Figure 8-15 *g* conforms to a fusion trait (as distinct from a noncomplexity trait) would be absurd. The absurdity would be emphasized through the nonconformity of the Opc which diverges abruptly in the later stages of formation of a fused root (Fig. 8-14 *a*).

To sum up, a great variety of style and degree of fusion and of branching of normal root elements, and of Opc elements, so complicates the question of why these differences occur that it is unreasonable to attribute a phylogenetic origin to them.

While this conclusion receives further support in outlines in subsequent figures, the value of the latter lies also in the provision of a graphic record of many actual examples.

Figure 8-17 presents seven more varieties of Opc, by even division of one root *b*, of both roots *c*, "twin" Opc roots at DL in *d*, starting in crown and becoming prominent in root *e*, and Opc in both crown and root but in different regions, in both *f* and *g*. Figure 8-18 presents six teeth, five certainly

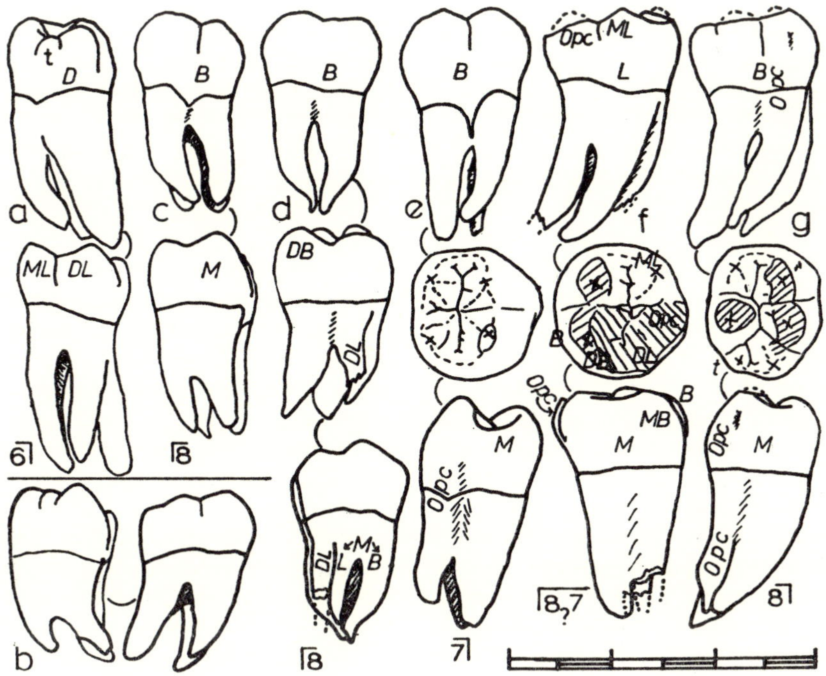

Figure 8-17. Seven lower molars with various styles of Opc, mostly in roots. *a,* on L, by division of D root. *b,* on L, by division of M root. *c,* two Opc on L, by late division of each root. *d,* three views of tooth with two Opc roots at DL. In these four teeth, *a-d,* there is no Opc in crowns. *e,* the Opc starts in the crown at MB and becomes prominent by division of MB root. *f,* three views of tooth with prominent Opc cusp on L, and ML root element fused with M root until slight separation in apical region. In the upper outline the tooth is rotated to show the grooved and divided M root, and that the Opc root and Opc cusp do not correspond in position. *g,* three views of tooth with prominent Opc on B of M root, and corresponding slight Opc at MB of crown. There is also a prominent DL tubercle in the crown but no corresponding root element.

being third molars, in which Opc elements may clearly be identified in both crown and root. In *a* and *b* the Opc has some characters of a separate but adherent tooth with its own cervix, but in neither case is there a separate apex. The Opc in *d* has prominent occlusal ridges, quite different from the cusp-like form of that in *e.* This tooth has a prominent D cusp and an M tubercle, unrelated to the Opc and with no root element. Tooth *f* has a very complex crown and four root branches; it might well be regarded as a fusion of twin teeth, or alternatively as incomplete separation. Such conception receives some support from two unequal occlusal groove systems which are separated by major ridges. In total there appear to be five cusps and four tubercles, one being almost central and surrounded by grooves. A similar view might well be taken of tooth *f* in Figure 8-19 where a prominent ridge virtually divides the occlusal into two areas of cusps and grooves.

The recording of variations in Opc is continued in Figure 8-19. Teeth *a,b* are a pair from one person, but they are certainly not mirror images, for they are dissimilar in both crown and root. The pattern of grooves and ridges is different, and although each has a large Opc at MB, these also are different. In the left tooth the Opc crown is clearly defined and tends to present a cusp and tubercle, but its root element is merged or fused in the M root. By contrast the right Opc has a single cusp, but its prominent root element begins to separate from the M root at an early stage, is divergent and sturdy, and is as long as the main root branches.

Tooth *c* of Figure 8-19 is very complex in crown and root, but full evaluation is impossible owing to partial destruction by caries. Even so there appear to be two Opc crown elements on B side, but root elements are not easy to identify separately. Tooth *d*, one of a pair, has an Opc element at M and another at D, with the ML and DL cusps between them. The root elements are much less complex. They are fused together, but there are grooves at M and D indicating four elements in all. Tooth *e* has no clear Opc in the crown, although it is unusual in outline, which is prominent at MB and DB. From B the bifid root does not attract attention except that the branches are of unequal length. But from the lingual side it is seen that a slender Opc branch leaves the D root at about the level of the main root furcation. It is shorter than the D root and approximately parallel with it.

Tooth *f* is a right third molar, as is *c*, and both have complex crowns, but they have little else in common. The disposition of main cusps and Opc elements, the form and size of these, and the occlusal outline, are quite different. As for their roots, where that of *c* has a number of twisted and partly separated or fused elements, tooth *f* has only two elements, separated but close together so that they almost form a cone.

In two other third molars (not figured) there are three distinct root elements, almost equal in size and placed in line. In one, where the crown is almost destroyed by decay, the three branches are separate.

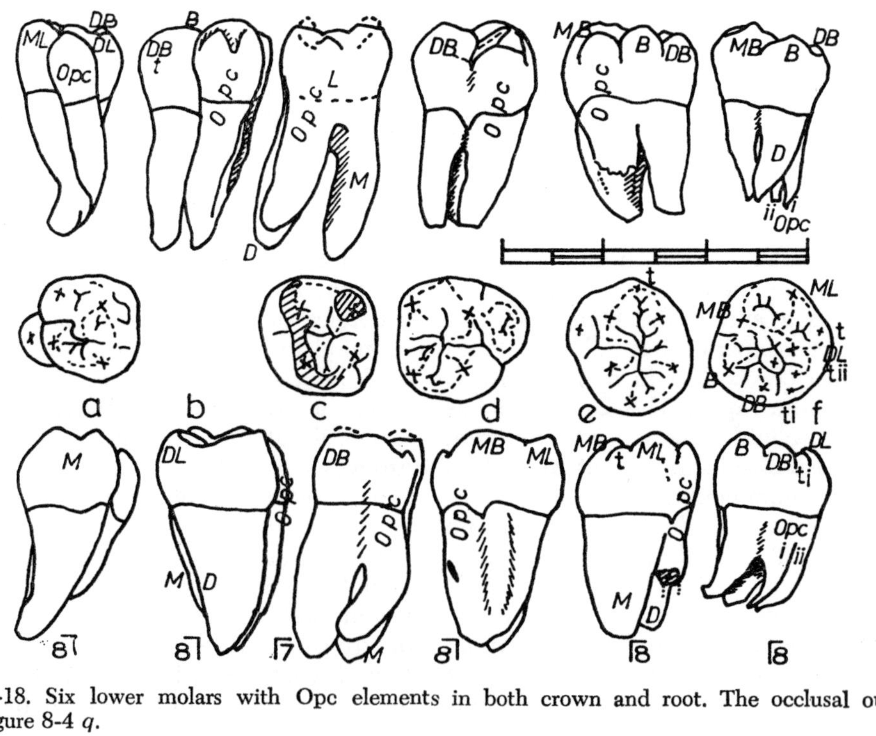

Figure 8-18. Six lower molars with Opc elements in both crown and root. The occlusal outline of *b* is in Figure 8-4 *q*.

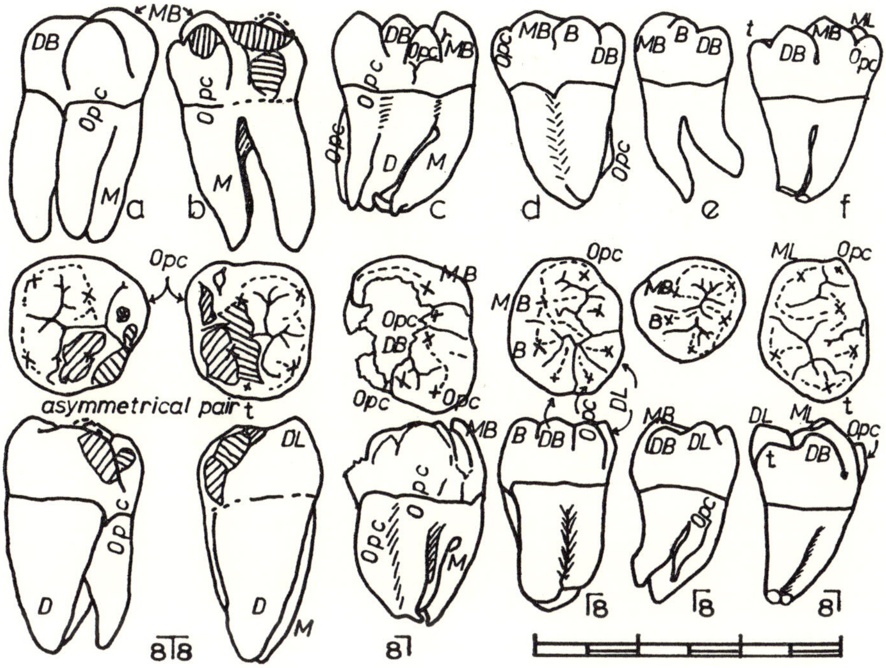

Figure 8-19. Six lower molars with Opc of varying complexity in crown and/or root.

In the other the mesial branch is separate, and the others are fused but deeply grooved on B and L. Most of the crown is intact and both it and the root have the appearance of two teeth that have merged their contiguous cusps and root elements. These two teeth might be described better as incomplete twin formations than as having large Opc crown and root elements placed distally.

(Figure 8-20 is discussed later on p. 319.) Figure 8-21 *d* shows a tooth that combines characters found in such dissimilar teeth as in Figure 8-19 *e* and *f*, and yet is not like either of them. Thus it has an occlusal surface uncomplicated by additional cusps or tubercles (Fig. 8-19 *e*), and a root that in one view consists of M and D elements almost fused to conical form (Fig. 8-19 *f*). But unlike the latter it does have an additional root element (Opc) which separates at almost mid-root and is shorter than the autosite root, as in Figure 8-19 *e*. But that Opc was on L of D root whereas the present example has the Opc on B of M root. Again, whereas the former Opc had no trace of a crown element, there is such an element in Figure 8-21 *d*, although it did not arise until the occlusal part of the crown was complete, and it has not the prominence of a cusp or tubercle.

These three teeth comprise an interesting group. They demonstrate that a crown may be virtually uncomplicated and yet have the usual bifid root complicated by an Opc branch (Fig. 8-19 *e*), or even have a fused conical root plus Opc branch (Fig. 8-21 *d*). Alternatively the crown may be very complicated, while the root is fused to a simple cone (Fig. 8-19 *f*). If Figure 8-19 *c* with its very complex crown and root, and the great number of more common variations presented earlier are included, there must have been presented an appreciable number of permutations and combinations. At least it has been shown that

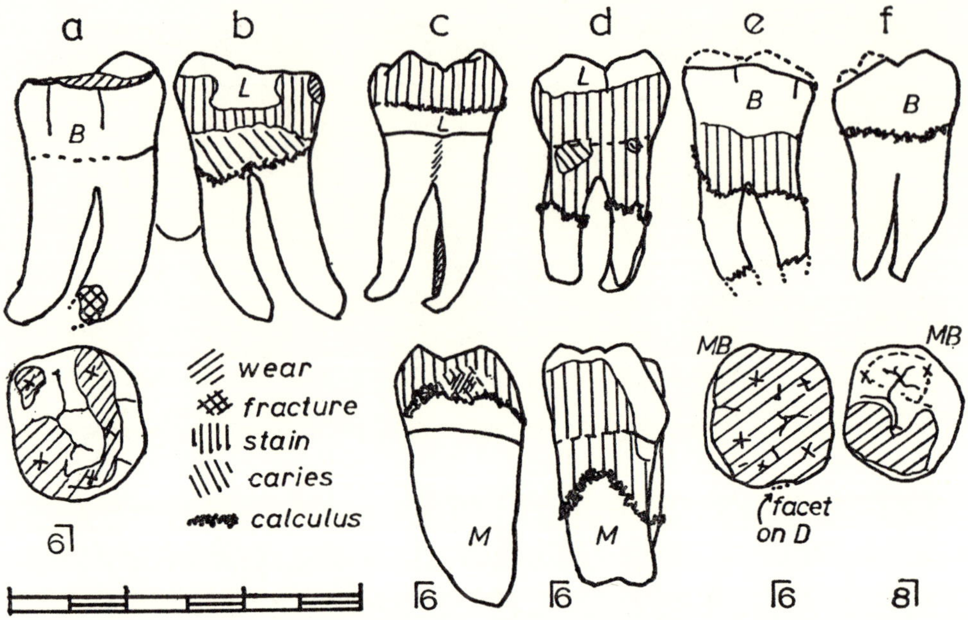

Figure 8-20. Teeth presenting evidence of wear, stains or other acquired characters which have relevance to identification and forensics. (These are discussed on p. 319).

variations and combinations in crown and root are largely independent, but with the requirement (as stated early in this study) that the two must conform at the cervix. In other words, there is no pattern of consistency whereby the presence (or absence) of a character or any quality or degree of its development in the crown of a tooth will be followed by the same in the root. Not even in a pair of teeth from one person, where there are comparable Opc in each crown, does it follow that additional elements will be present, or comparable, in each root (Fig. 8-19 *a*). The dissimilarity found in left third molars of sisters (Fig. 8-7 *d,e*) is also relevant to the finding of inconsistency in variation. The significance of this finding will be referred to later.

Returning to the illustrations, Figure 8-21 *a* presents a style which has not yet been described. There is a prominent Opc cusp plus root, at DL, but only one other recognizable cusp on L, and two on B. However, there are two distinct tubercles, one each at M and D. The first arises in the M marginal ridge, but the latter is isolated by grooves. Does it represent the normal DL cusp, but with most of its substance annexed by the Opc? Alternatively, should the distal tubercle be regarded as the Opc? If so, it is separated from its root element which is an obviously robust Opc and itself continuous with a cusp already oversize, and so it is ineligible for designation as the normal DL cusp.

Acceptance of the former view, namely that the Opc has annexed a part of the substance that might otherwise have become the normal cusp, seems by far the more reasonable conclusion. If this is correct it is important, since such explanation greatly facilitates identification and understanding of many hitherto puzzling details of dental morphological variation. And not only so, but the designation of the additional element as *Odontopagus parasiticus concretus* is appropriate for the implied procedure in tooth development whereby the incomplete differentiation of an additional element may involve the annexation of part of a "normal" element.

Many examples have been given to show that an Opc root element may leave the root trunk on B or L side at its furcation into main branches, and continue to develop independently and form its own apex. Or it may initially be fused to B or L aspect of M or D root branch, and either remain so fused, or at some stage diverge from it. In the crown the Opc may apparently occupy any position relative to the normal cusps of the autosite, and where two Opc elements are close to a normal cusp they may in effect surround it. An example apparently of all these relationships may be seen in three views of one tooth in Figure 8-21 *b*. Two adjacent Opc crown elements at DL cause the DL cusp to be surrounded by grooves. The broken roots show that the root element of Opc 1 diverged from the L furcation, but for Opc 2 the root element was fused (at least initially) with the D root. The lost fragment could have shown whether it remained fused or whether it left the D root at some later stage.

In Figure 8-22 *a* the only trace of an Opc crown element is a groove and pit on MB cusp. M and D roots remain fused on B side for half their length and then form parallel branches separated by a wide arch. At about the same stage a groove appears on the M surface of M root, and this root later divides into B and L branches. At a much earlier stage a separate Opc root arises on L side from the usual position of root furcation.

In Figure 8-22, teeth *b,c* are young left third molars with roots at the C− and C+ stages respectively (see p. 93). In tooth *b* the crown presents five cusps in the usual positions, plus a well-marked tubercle at M. The root, even at this early stage, had differentiated into M, D and an Opc branch on B. Tooth *c* has unusually large B and DB cusps. There are the usual M

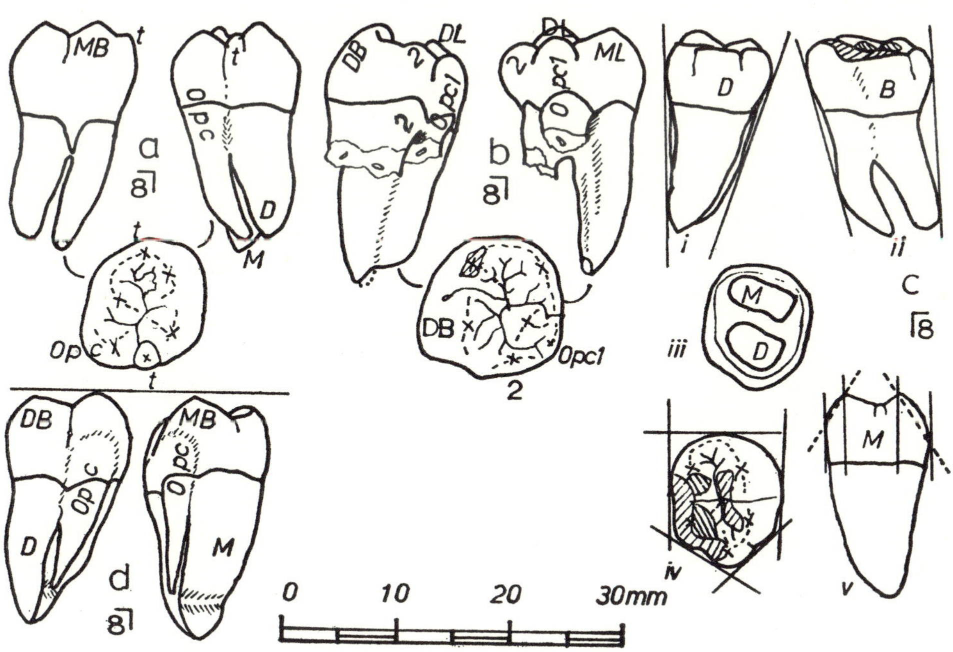

Figure 8-21. *a,b,d,* further styles of Opc in crown and root. Teeth in this figure are discussed also in regard to identification. See page 320, and Figure 9-5 regarding tooth *c*.

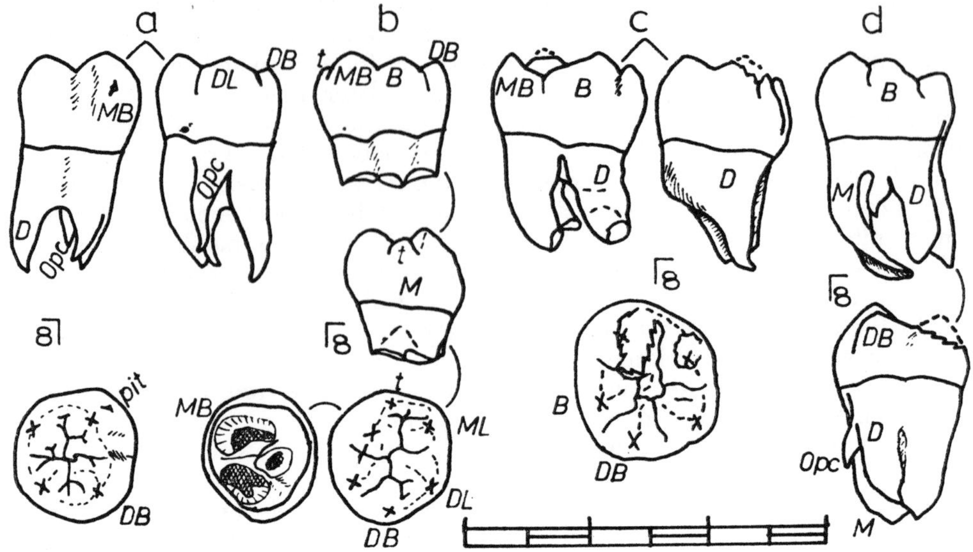

Figure 8-22. Identification of lower molars including young teeth with Opc.

and D root branches initially, but while the M root later divides into B and L branches the lingual branch is abruptly deflected between the other two, so that the three uncompleted apices in this young tooth lie almost in a straight line.

Tooth *d* in Figure 8-22 has a wide and deeply grooved M root and the D root divides into B and L portions approximately equal in size. From the B arch of the main furcation arises another small but divergent root element. The crown is partly destroyed by caries but it would appear that the DB cusp is an Opc with its own DB root element in D root, and that the small branch is a second Opc without a corresponding crown element. (Figs. 8-21 and 8-22 are used again later to illustrate problems in identification, see p. 320.)

Cervical Line

It was shown that in some teeth, particularly upper canines, there is usually a difference between the mesial and distal arcs of the cervical line. The difference can be recognized so often that it is a character that is useful in tooth identification, especially when wear, pathology or fracture may have removed the more commonly used characters. No such consistent feature of the cervical line has been noted in lower molar teeth, but irregularities do occur and should be given at least brief attention here.

Because molar teeth are wider B-L than anterior teeth, the alveolar ridge also is wider and the crests of the interdental septa are much less arched. To say that the proximal cervical lines conform to these may be convenient for describing the almost straight or slightly arched cervix, but it must be remembered that the cervix is established before tooth emergence. It is the alveolar bone that adapts to the cervix, whether the tooth attains a normal position or is in malocclusion.

Cervical lines on B and L of lower molars are nearly straight or level in most cases, except for necessary conformity with the convexity of tooth surfaces. However, it is not uncommon for this smooth curve to be interrupted opposite the root bifurcation, particularly on the B side. The form of this irregularity varies considerably in accord with its degree of development and of its adaptation to the local tooth anatomy. As with upper molars, these irregularities are often associated with enamel pearls but by no means mostly so, and it is those cases without pearls that are here considered.

In its minimal development the irregularity is no more than a slight dip or point in the cervical line. This may be towards the furcation arch between roots (Figs. 8-1 *e*, 8-2 *a,b,e*, 8-3 *a,c*, 8-5 *a*, 8-7 *c*, 8-11 *a* and 8-12 *a,d,e*), or into the groove between fused roots (Figs. 8-3 *b*, 8-7 *b*, 8-8 *e*, 8-9 *e*, 8-13 *e,f*, 8-19 *d*, and 8-22 *a,b*).

As a more prominent enamel tang extending into the furcation, examples are seen in Figures 8-1 *d*, 8-11 *d*, 8-13 *d*, 8-16 *j*, 8-17 *c* and 8-18 *d*. It is noted that in Figure 8-11 *d* there is an interruption in the deposition of enamel.

Irregularities in the cervical line where it is associated with Opc are common but by no means always present. In Figure 8-21 *a* there is a prominent B tang but the Opc is on DL where there is no interruption of cervical line. In Figure 8-21 *d* the cervix dips slightly at each side of the Opc, and in tooth *b* of that figure, with two Opc, the cervix dips strongly each side of Opc 1 in the root furcation at L. In Figure 8-15 *e* the dip is prominent on L at one side of the Opc, but it is slight on the other or D side. In a somewhat similar style of Opc (Fig. 8-16 *h*), the cervical line is scarcely affected.

In Figure 8-18 *d* where the prominent Opc is completely fused in crown and root, the cervix dips markedly to a long point on each side of it. This is in contrast to tooth *e* beside it where the cervix is only slightly involved with another prominent Opc which has a diverging root element. Inconsistency in this feature is again illustrated in Figure 8-19 *a* where a similarly divergent Opc is bounded on one side by a slight dip and on the other by a long point.

Another case of prominent but completely fused Opc (Fig. 8-12 *g*) shows straight continuity with cervical line on M, but a wide deep tang entering the furcation on B. Another style of interruption of the cervical line in association with Opc, which may be described as complex, is seen in Figures 8-12 *b* and 8-8 *b*. In these the cervical line of the Opc is at a different level, at least on one side.

A quite different irregularity is seen in Figure 8-10 *f*. In this case the cervical line turns abruptly crownwards instead of rootwards, as in all other cases illustrated. In this specimen the irregularity is below the MB cusp. There is no evidence of Opc in the crown, but the M root divides in its apical half and the lingual apex has been lost by fracture.

Comparable examples of these variations were found in upper molars and presented in Chapter 7. Collectively they illustrate and add emphasis to the finding mentioned above, namely that variation has a very wide range in style and degree, and that there is no consistency in the association of style or degree of the variations.

IDENTIFICATION, WEAR, AND FORENSICS

The identification of a tooth as a lower molar or as first, second, or third molar may either be easy or very difficult. Anatomical morphology may clearly indicate the identity as regards a maxillary or mandibular tooth, and this may be the main aid to recognition of the tooth as first, second or third, and also as a left or right tooth. But the wide range of morphological variation that has been described shows that a number of characters may, in a broad sense, be common to any tooth as regards the categories, upper and lower, left and right, or first, second and third molar. For example, although an upper molar usually has three root branches and a lower molar two branches, teeth with a simple fused root, or with two, three or more branches, do occur amongst first, second and third molars in both jaws. Similarly with regard to the number of cusps.

However, it is known that variation is

not only "dispersed" in this way, but also that it is more likely to present a degree or particular style in some of these teeth than in others. Thus there is an element of probability that can be of assistance. Further help comes through a heightened awareness of type characters—the more common disposition or placing of features such as root branches or cusps, as well as their relationship to one another. The recognition of divergence of root branches, of the presence of fusion or of additional elements (which may or may not reduce or increase the complexity of the tooth), and the recognition of personal, imposed and acquired characters may all contribute to data used in identification. Acquired characters (as distinct from imposed characters) include effects of pathology and of its treatment, effects of function such as occlusal wear, and facets on proximal contacts or elsewhere, stained or polished areas and wear and abrasion from prophylaxis, habits, ethnic customs, etc.

It is clear that familiarity with the varied anatomy of tooth roots is essential, so that a person who lacks this knowledge is poorly equipped for identification of teeth.

Positive identification of teeth is useful for work in various other fields bearing on basic dental sciences. Not only may this be assisted, but also much additional data, which could be important in forensic work, can be obtained by a worker's training in biological sciences and experience in clinical practice. Thus the microhistology and pathology of sectioned teeth provide a rich field of data, but so also does naked-eye examination of unsectioned teeth to which the present report relates.

These comments apply to molar teeth as well as to all other types or classes, not only as individual teeth, but also collectively as parts of the human dentition. The reference just made concerning acquired characters might well be elaborated to show how teeth may become modified in appearance during life. Their morphology may be changed by the addition or loss of substance by pathology and by loss of substance through functional wear or through abrasion, fracture or solution. Addition of substance may accrue to the root by deposition of cementum, or to crown or root by deposition of calculus or of various stains. These changes may occur singly or in a variety of combinations. They may affect similar or different regions of teeth (although some tend to be confined to particular regions). There may be merging, or clearly defined, areas of demarcation between the regions so involved. It is even possible for the effect in one case apparently to be the reverse of that found in another. This is well illustrated in teeth *c* and *d* of Figure 8-20.

Some of these changes may reflect fluctuations in nutrition, organic or functional disease during tooth development or later, or they may concern the oral environment of the tooth resulting (perhaps at different periods) in tooth decay, gingival recession, and calculous deposits. Stains may testify to neglect of oral hygiene or to habits such as smoking or chewing, e.g. betel nut. Wear or abrasion, according to its nature and position and extent, may result from one or more factors—type of food, masticatory stresses and patterns, holding of objects or materials between teeth, ethnic customs, artificial prophylaxis (materials and techniques involved), dental restorations, missing teeth, malocclusion, stable and unstable prosthetic appliances, sudden trauma, etc. The writer has presented examples in the present work and in published papers (Taylor, 1948b; 1955; 1962b, c; 1963a; 1970a, c; 1971a, b, c; 1972a, b; 1975 and 1976).

Recognition and interpretation of the kind of changes mentioned may provide much data concerning the person whose tooth is studied. If the tooth is one amongst others in a skull, bone as well as teeth contribute data concerning the person at time of death. An isolated tooth may relate also to time of death, but may alternatively indicate certain conditions existing at the time of extraction of the tooth, and may often present instrument abrasion as proof of that operation.

Facets of wear and the nature and position of stains on teeth are sometimes of great assistance in identification and orientation of teeth, particularly in molar teeth where variations in characters of type, etc., may lead to uncertainty. For example, a tooth tentatively identified as either first or third lower molar, if found to present a distal contact stain or facet, could not be a third molar. Absence of such evidence however does not positively establish it as a third molar—it could be a first molar where the second molar has been lost. Therefore the possibility of a missing tooth being extracted or congenitally absent, or possibly unerupted, must always be kept in mind. If this absence applies to a third molar where a second molar presents some characters of a third molar, absence of a distal contact facet might wrongly be construed as evidence for identification of the second as a third molar. And further, it is known that removal of a second molar "at the right time" may enable the third molar to take its place, and in some circumstances be mistaken for it.

Some of the pitfalls or difficulties of identification have been indicated. Some are peculiar to or absent from ancient, recent or contemporary material, and vary according to whether the sample is accompanied by other skeletal material, or is an isolated and complete or incomplete tooth. The part played in this exercise by the presence of dental restorations or other evidence of surgical intervention also is very relevant but cannot be considered here. As a subject it merits separate treatment, but its potential and importance, especially in forensics, is obvious. So also should be the value of training in basic biological sciences, as well as sound clinical experience, for recognition and interpretation of relevant evidence.

Application of these in the examination of a prehistoric fragment of mandibular bone with anterior teeth was reported by the writer (Taylor, 1971c). As regards lower molar teeth, a few examples are given here to illustrate recognition of clues that may assist identification of individual teeth.

The tooth in Figure 8-20 *a* is easily identified as lower right first molar, and confirmed by the distal contact facet. It is a sturdy tooth with moderate occlusal wear on all cusps, yet having more sharply defined facets along the buccal cusps. There is some calculus indicating gingival recession, incipient lingual cervical caries and some heavy dark stain at proximals. It is assumed to be from a middle-aged man who was a pipe smoker and careless regarding oral hygiene. He had formerly enjoyed masticatory efficiency (wear on occlusal and contact points), but this had changed (stain over contacts); and since acquiring an upper artificial denture (buccal occlusal facets) mastication had changed to less efficient "mashing" (buccal surface cleanest). A lower partial denture (a small lingual area cleaned by friction but not faceted, *b*) had been unsatisfactory, and in view of the unhealthy periodontal condition (calculus level) the remaining lower teeth had been removed and a full denture made. All this is surmise, but it is what does happen, and the tooth bears evidence in support of each assumption.

A left first molar with clean contact facets has been worn almost flat (Fig. 8-20 *e*), exposing dentine in cusp positions, and leaving only partial traces of the main central grooves. Occlusal, buccal and lingual surfaces are polished, but on B and L surfaces there is cervical caries and a line of calculus showing that gingival recession and associated pathology had involved the root furcation. Both roots had fractured during extraction which had evidently proved difficult on account of dense bone. This person had always had efficient and vigorous masticatory function with unimpeded lateral movements. Artificial prophylaxis was practised habitually if not efficiently. The periodontal condition had been neglected until replacement of otherwise good healthy teeth by artificial dentures in middle age had been accepted.

The clearly defined, mirror-smooth facets formerly produced by contact with porcelain artificial teeth have been largely superseded by contact facets arising from use of acrylic (or "plastic") artificial teeth. But any facets, from whatever cause, give much information concerning masticatory movements, whether they are normal or impeded by malocclusion, and they may indicate that a particular tooth itself was malpositioned. The lower right third molar in Figure 8-20 *f* has stain on lingual, mesial and occlusal surfaces (anterior grooves only), with a mesial contact facet that is decalcified. This tooth at first in normal occlusion had gradually tipped forwards after the second molar had been lost, and wear had occurred while it was in this position.

The contrast noted above in the teeth in Figure 8-20 *c* and *d* is interpreted as follows: Tooth *c* probably was extracted from a young adult, for the gingival line was supra-cervical and the white area is enamel that was subgingival and protected from mouth conditions. The remainder of the crown surface, evenly stained a light brown, testifies to lack of friction from either mastication or artificial prophylaxis. Tooth *d* had been removed from a middle-aged man whose pipe smoking had stained black the sheltered areas of lingual surface. Periodontal involvement and alveolar resorption had exposed the root furcation, which had become chronically septic. The tooth however had remained functional, and habitual prophylaxis "cleaned only where it touched" and that included polished cementum at the buccal cervix. The white (clean) areas are those which were subjected to friction during mastication and toothbrushing.

Figures 8-21 and 8-22 show more examples of teeth that have some "irregular" features of crown or root that make them more difficult to identify, and it will be shown how aids to solving the problems can be recognized and applied.

Tooth *a* Figure 8-21 has four cusps and two tubercles at M and D, and two of the cusps are virtually joined by an oblique ridge, as with upper molars. Moreover, there are also three root branches, one flattened and widest like the MB root of such. But the third root branch is quite unlike a palatal root and more like that of an Opc. It is associated with the largest cusp which (if the tooth were an upper molar) would be DP; but DP or DL is the position for the smallest in four-cusped upper and lower molars, and is likely to be represented by the small distal tubercle on this tooth. So far then, interpretation of characters favours identification as a lower molar with bifid distal root, the minor branch being the root element of an Opc cusp. This diagnosis receives strong support from the proximal profile which is typically lower molar, and the reverse of an upper molar profile (see section on tooth profiles below). This tooth was discussed for another purpose on p. 314.

The tooth in Figure 8-21 *b* has four main cusps, the smallest of which is axially placed and bordered by two minor cusps, so that the occlusal pattern is unlike any particular molar tooth. There were three root branches, the two which fractured during extraction having two and one pulp canals respectively. The latter and smallest root branch is evidently the root element of an Opc, namely one of the minor cusps. The other minor cusp, placed almost distally, evidently had a root element with pulp canal fused with the distal root (at least to beyond the fracture line). The largest root branch, typically wide, flat and mesial, bears the usual curve and proximal profile that enable M, B, L to be positively identified from the surviving intact root alone. The M proximal profile of the crown is in accord with this.

Tooth *c* in Figure 8-21 is much less complex, but is a good illustration of the value of profiles in identification. It has five cusps, all worn to first degree (no dentine exposed), but the fifth cusp is placed precisely to distal of central groove. Viewed from occlusal it is not obvious (as is more usual) as to which are B and L sides. Viewed from proximal however, the profiles of crown and root dispel any such doubts (*ci, cv*).

Figure 8-22 shows more examples of irregularities for identification and description. Tooth *a* has a cruciform groove and four cusps, the MB of which has an Opc pit on its B surface. The bifurcation of main roots is late on the B side, but an Opc root appears at the earlier L furcation. Tooth *b* is a young tooth at the C— stage, i.e. root formation shorter than crown height. There are five cusps and a mesial tubercle, but the root formation which has just reached the furcation shows that an Opc branch between the main roots is forming on the B side. This position is much less common than L location. A young tooth at the C+ stage, tooth *c*, has an irregular crown with five cusps, and an Opc root on ML. The profile contours establish identity and orientation without difficulty.

Tooth *d* presents several unusual features and orientation is complicated through loss by fracture of much of the crown. Enough remains for B and M to be identified by profiles. There is a distal Opc cusp which establishes its root element by division of the D root. But there is also a small Opc root arising from furcation of M and D roots, and here again this is in the uncommon B position. If this tooth were described as presenting "three and one-half roots," one could hardly object.

This last tooth lends emphasis to our contention that statistics concerning the occurrence of additional root branches cannot be compiled to have any accuracy in regard to frequency, location or size. For example if it were proposed to determine the relative frequency of "an extra root" occurring on B or L, by taking only well-defined cases, this would not accord with reality and so the resultant figure would be useless. If an attempt were made to include all cases, variations must either be ignored or noted. The first ob-

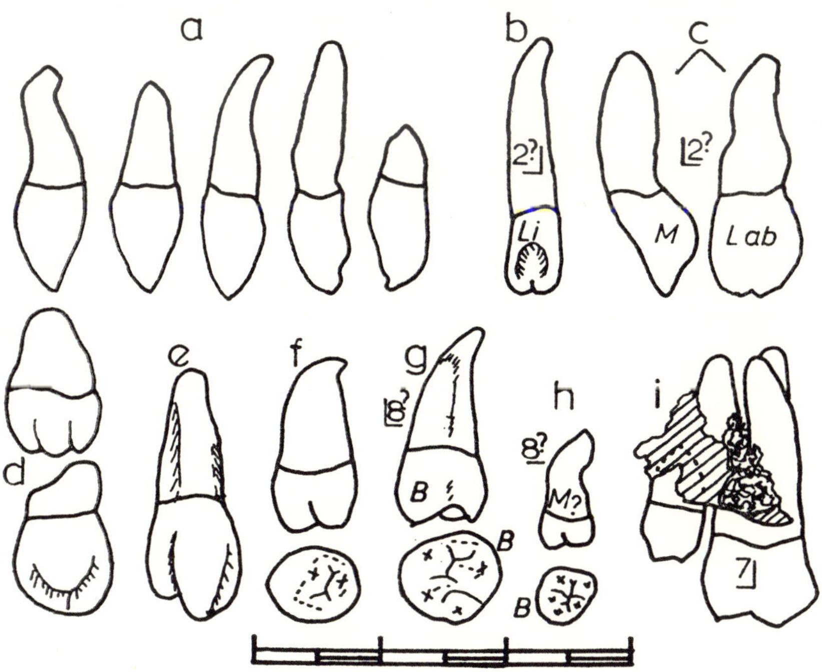

Figure 8-23. Diminutive teeth in maxilla and mandible.

viously is not feasible. The second would founder in the attempt to define categories and subjectively sort the specimens. It has been seen that they occur in all degrees of fusion or separateness, with or without identifiable crown elements, in size from minute to large, as part of any normal root branch or at the furcation of any such, separately in the presence of fused or branched normal roots or joined thereto, and this last completes the circuit to the first style mentioned. Additional elements cannot be precisely defined, or measured or counted.

DIMINUTIVES

The present collection included 221 mounted diminutive teeth.

Diminutive teeth appear to fall into two main groups, namely peg teeth and those that apparently form part of the dentition. Peg teeth (of the general style of Fig. 8-23 *a*), also "humped and cornet" teeth, are stated to be "tooth-like structures or odontoids" (Herbst and Apffelstaedt, 1930). They are found in the embryonic clefts of the body, which in the mouth limits them to the anterior part of the maxilla.

Diminutive teeth which are part of the dentition always have a flattened root when they occur in the incisor region (Fig. 8-23 *b-e*). They may in other places resemble a premolar *(f)* or bear distinct resemblance to a molar. Tooth *g*, for example, has a crown with two cusps and a tubercle separated by grooves, and also clearly recognizable three root elements (though fused) of an upper molar. Such distinctive molars may be very small (*h* and *i*), the second specimen having been retained *in situ* with a second molar during extraction with an attached fragment of alveolar bone.

Teeth of this miniature form are usually third molars. Three cases in Chatham Island skulls were illustrated by the writer (Taylor, 1962c. Plates 6 and 8, Figures 51, 70 and 71 in that work). In the first of those skulls the empty socket leaves some doubt as to whether the small tooth was separate from the third molar, or attached to it as an Opc. In the present study there was no evidence of an Opc attached in this distal position of M3.

It is evident that diminutive teeth as part of the dentition are themselves subject to much variation in occurrence and form, and therefore cannot be excluded from the present study. But since so many of them are atypical it is important to know the position in which these teeth occur. As this information is lacking for the majority of such teeth in the present collection, it is not intended to illustrate or discuss them further.

It is uncertain also whether any of these specimens occurred in the mandible. It has been suggested that a diminutive third molar is a "part-way stage" to a congenitally missing third molar. Data concerning the presence or absence of third molars in the Chatham Island material studied were presented in earlier papers (Taylor, 1962a, b, c).

Chapter 9

Occlusion, Dental Profiles and Arches

OCCLUSION

DENTAL SCIENCE has given much attention to the study of occlusion of human teeth since it has relevance to art and practice in most dental fields. Ideal or normal occlusion has been defined in varying detail, and often illustrated by a photograph of a person or skull in which the dentition closely approaches the description of the chosen ideal. Much less attention, however, has been given to the manner in which many dentitions fail to conform and yet suffer little disability because of their nonconformity. Obviously there are many variable factors concerned.

The orthodontist has enlarged his field of study beyond the noting of nonconformity, and he considers the prospects of realigning crowns of teeth to conform with his desires. Biological studies of growth of bone, basal and alveolar, and of tooth roots and their response to the application of pressures arising from mechanical appliances and muscular action have contributed to the planning of treatment. The dental surgeon and periodontist are concerned with anatomical restorations to restore function. They may further modify the existing conditions so that changing positions or wearing surfaces of teeth do not cause interference during masticatory movements or injury to periodontal tissues, and in this way they work to prevent the establishment of a "traumatic" occlusion.

The dental prosthetists at first regarded a knowledge of occlusion and of masticatory movements as the basis of their work, but later studies have shown that the nature of biological responses of soft and hard tissues to functional stresses is more important. Some artificial dentures "set up" with the aid of much measurement, "anatomical" articulators and other sophisticated paraphernalia proved useless, while others, prepared with a combination of a simple hinge articulator and "experience," served the patient well. This is not a condemnation of the former procedure nor an acceptance of the latter, but it is mentioned as evidence of the involvement of more variable factors than had been provided for. Among these are the anatomy of bone, of the temporomandibular joint, and also the nature of muscle function, as well as the habits and psychological urge of the patient to adapt and succeed or otherwise.

Amongst anatomical factors that vary are the arrangement of the natural teeth, the manner and vigour of their function, and their collective efficiency as a masticatory mechanism. That human dentitions can vary considerably in their "set up," and yet function efficiently under considerable stresses has been amply shown in the many illustrations in earlier papers (Taylor, 1962b, c, 1963a). Amongst these there is convincing evidence that overlapping and interdigitation of cusps is not necessary for vigorous and efficient function. The significance of this was further demonstrated more recently (Taylor, 1975, 1976).

In the present study attention has been frequently drawn to the form of cusps as part of tooth morphology and to variations in this character. This is part of the reason why a study of occlusion is important in the overall study of variation in tooth morphology. It provides the setting for showing the significance of tooth profiles, so often referred to in earlier chapters. It also facilitates recognition of the consistency of certain characters in buccal and lingual profiles, and awareness of how and why they are different in upper and lower teeth.

These observations provide the basis for a useful aid in identification and orientation of isolated teeth, and this will often apply when part of the crown or root is missing and when variation or the presence of additional elements renders a tooth atypical, thus complicating its identification. In the present work, therefore, the study of occlusion is not directed towards a detailed description of an ideal dentition which may have only hypothetical existence. Reality is of greater interest. Although in almost every character there is a wide range of variation, yet for each tooth we have recognized type characters, sometimes the imposed characters, and often its personal characters. The last have been shown to relate to the whole dentition rather than being confined to the tooth type, whether incisor, canine, premolar or molar.

We now look at characters which again relate to the whole dentition, but which, instead of differing as among individuals, are not personal, but differentiate upper teeth from lowers. These characters are in a sense complementary as between upper and lower teeth, and between facial (buccal or labial) and lingual profiles as seen from proximal. Like other characters they vary considerably, but it is the consistency of their presence in some degree that provides assistance in identification and orientation.

Recognition of these profile characters in a crown may sometimes be assisted by association with more easily recognized characters in a root, but the reverse may sometimes hold, *mutatis mutandis,* so that an atypical or incomplete root may be orientated by recognition of profile characters in the crown. In this sense also the profiles of crown and root have a complementary relationship. These profiles and their axes, as well as the whole tooth axis, may often be described as characteristic as regards convexity or position. However, it is in the crown rather than in the root that differences in lingual and facial profiles are more often or more easily discernible.

Although the presence and nature of profile characters was indicated when each tooth was described, attention is now directed to their place in the anatomical relationship of upper and lower dental arches.

TOOTH PROFILES AND DENTAL ARCHES

Profile characters of upper and lower canines (Fig. 9-3 *b*), enabled the writer in 1937 positively to identify the controversial canine fragment, and to show that the dentition portrayed in the generally accepted restoration of the Piltdown skull could never have existed (Appendix 6). Many years later, proof of the fraudulent association of the Piltdown fragments testified to the soundness of the writer's studies in tooth morphology which form the basis of the present report.

Traditional teaching that human maxillary incisors and buccal cusps occlude outside those of the mandible "because upper teeth are arranged in a wider arch" is not acceptable. It is always untrue in some respects, and often misleading in others. Teeth are irregular bodies enclosed within exceedingly irregular curved surfaces. There is no point within the tooth body or on any surface that is "the tooth." There are no corresponding points on individual teeth of a dentition which could be joined to truly represent a curve or arch in which the teeth are arranged.

One may attempt a compromise and imagine a line to touch each apex, each corresponding cusp, or each cervix, and there would then be an irregular curve or arch at each region. But which apex in multi-rooted teeth is selected or which cusp where there are more than one on a tooth would have to be specified. And why should any particular root-tip or cusp-tip rather than another be more representative of a tooth? Neither the tip of a cusp nor the tip of a root is a point of precise location, and the cusps and apices themselves have been seen as subject to considerable variation, especially with wear in the former, and curves and fusions in the latter.

Arches determined by tangents to unworn incisal edges and tips of buccal cusps would be wider for upper than lower. This difference would decrease if tangential arches were determined by facial margins of facets as wear increased, and in the anterior region the arches may be almost identical when the "edge-to-edge" bite becomes established. It should be noted that the "edge-to-edge" bite is acquired, not by tooth movement but by wear that progressively removes those parts which, in the unworn state, mostly contribute to the differences between upper and lower crown profiles. In cases of extreme wear where anterior teeth have lost their crowns completely (Taylor, 1963a, Plate 6), the relationships between wear, edge-to-edge bite, occlusal plane and tooth axes are well seen.

For comparison of dental arches, an alternative compromise might be attempted by adopting a curve tangential to buccal (or lingual) cervices of teeth *in situ*. In a large proportion of dentitions this comparison would result in curves approximately similar and equal in size for upper and lower. In many more, the lower curve would be wider than the upper in the molar region, and yet the upper buccal cusps would still overlap the lowers.

Returning to the concept of arches or curves determined by positions of apices and cusps, for convenience apical and cervical arches and cuspal arches will be referred to and also (again for convenience) lingual roots and other than buccal cusps will be ignored. Apical arches might well be found very different as between upper and lower and very often wider in lowers. With cuspal arches as just mentioned, uppers would mostly be wider in the anterior portion and less so, or even similar, in the molar area. In the cervical arches the change to a wider lower takes place approximately at the first molar.

The differences in comparison of arch size or width in these three regions result partly from the difficulties indicated above as arising from the irregular and varying morphology of teeth themselves. In great part also the differences may arise from variations in the arrangement of teeth as between individuals. In this question the essential aspect of morphology is the tooth profile and it is the interplay of variation in this, with variation in arrangement, that gives rise to the normal range of variation in the "set up" of dentitions. The result is that much difference in some respects, and similarity in others, presents a wider concept of normal occlusion. At the same time it must be emphasized that the appellation "normal" is justified by abundant evidence that efficient function and dental health have been maintained for a long period in spite of considerable wear in tooth substance and concomitant physiological adjustments.

The term "axis" was applied to teeth in Chapter 1, and it was shown that there are both a crown axis and a root axis which separately may not coincide with the tooth axis. A tooth axis may not be straight, nor may the crown or root axes, as a result of curves or bends in either. This sometimes happens in an incisor crown, but more often in the root, and this may apply to any single-rooted tooth (Figs. 1-5, 1-6, 1-19).

There is no reality in any of these axes, but they are visualized when examining a tooth. The concept however is useful. It makes one more aware of the morphology of a particular tooth, and how this may be useful has been mentioned often. It is variation in axes as regards their form, and in their position relative to tooth profiles, that contributes to identification of upper and lower teeth. Also it is variation in direction of corresponding upper and lower tooth axes that bear on the different

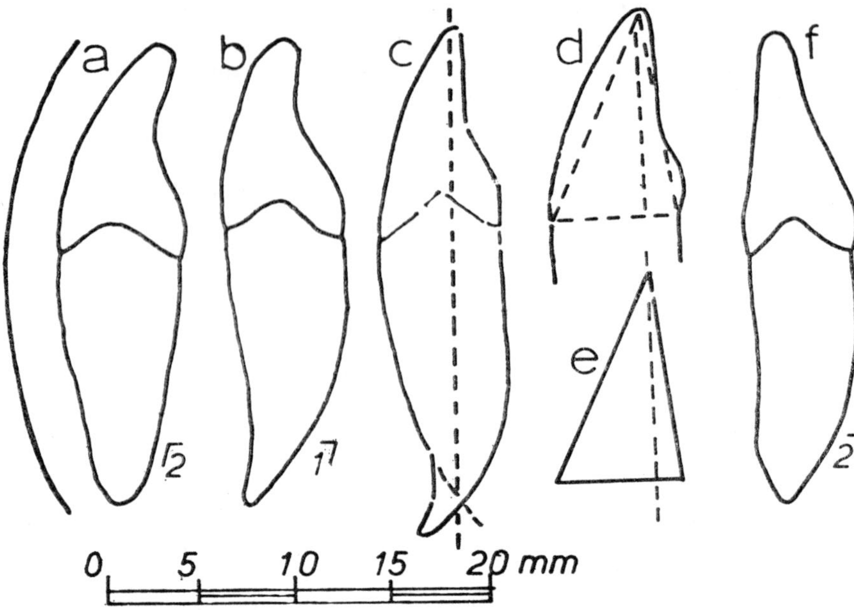

Figure 9-1. Lower incisor outlines and diagrams relating to occlusion style. *a,* a lower incisor showing the arc-like labial profile which is very common in the crown and often includes the root as well. *b,* in this lower incisor the labial profile, root-portion, is less arc-like because of a root bend. The root bend is usually to the labial so that in this case the arc is labially in the crown and lingually in the root. *c,* diagram showing how the tooth axis may be visualized as excluding the small bend at root tip. *d,* the crown profile is visualized as a triangle with its base extending from labial cervix to lingual cervix. The crown axis or height is the perpendicular to this base from the incisal edge as apex of the triangle. *e.* the crown profile triangle showing the perpendicular intersecting the base nearer to the lingual. This is the most common pattern for lower incisors. *f,* profile of an unusual lower incisor in which the perpendicular and the tooth axis are nearer the labial side. This is a character found in most upper anterior teeth. Profiles *a,b,f* are made from extracted teeth to the scale shown.

widths of upper and lower dental arches. Although bone size of maxilla and mandible are also concerned here, it is the tooth profile, and axis inclination of upper and lower teeth (in part no doubt a result of bone size), which will be concentrated on here.

PROFILES OF ANTERIOR TEETH

In its clearest form the labial curvature of a lower incisor produces an arc from incisal to apex (Fig. 9-1 *a*), and the chord of such arc, as the tooth axis, cuts the cervix nearer lingual than labial. Two main variations, one in the root and one in the crown, may reduce the length and curvature of the arc, and both are seen in one tooth in Figure 9-1 *b*. The first is a curve to labial in the apical part of the root, which sometimes, as in the case illustrated, gives an arc-like profile to the root on the lingual side; but if the curve is shorter one may imagine the root without it, as in the apical part of the diagram, Figure 9-1 *c*. The tooth axis then visualized as in this figure is again nearer to lingual.

Description of the second main variation, in the crown, is facilitated by visualizing a crown axis as in Figure 9-1 *d*. This is a perpendicular from the incisal tip to a base line from labial cervix to lingual cervix, or a scalene triangle drawn through those points (Fig. 9-1 *e*). In these the crown axis is the perpendicular shown, and in lower anterior teeth it tends to lie nearer to lingual, as shown for the whole tooth axis. Occasionally an exception to this general rule is found, and an extreme example is shown in Figure 9-1 *f*, a mesial view of the lower right lateral incisor. Lower teeth presenting this character will have other features of crown shape and root flatness that mark them unmistakably as lower incisors, and so it is unlikely to lead to confusion in identification.

A third but minor variation in curvature which tends to interrupt the continuity of the labial arc from incisal through the root is a fullness in the cervical region of the crown. This is more common in deciduous teeth and resembles the cingulum seen in the brachydont teeth of some mammals. Mummery (1924) uses the term cingulum whether the ridge partially or completely surrounds the tooth.

The position of tooth axis or crown axis, just described as unusual in lower anterior teeth, is found to be usual for upper anteriors. In other words their axes tend to be nearer the labial. Because of these differences, the blade of the unworn upper incisor is able to overlap the lower, while the labial cervices of both are in near-vertical relationship in normal occlusion. This relationship is more easily recognized as wear progresses and the so-called edge-to-edge bite is established (Fig. 9-3 *a* and *b*).

To suggest that maintenance of the vertical relationship is assisted in normal occlusion by normal balance of lips and tongue is not to imply that arch form is the result of muscle activity. Indeed, McNulty et al. (1968) presents evidence that it is not. Manson (1968), while recognizing that the effect of abnormal physical

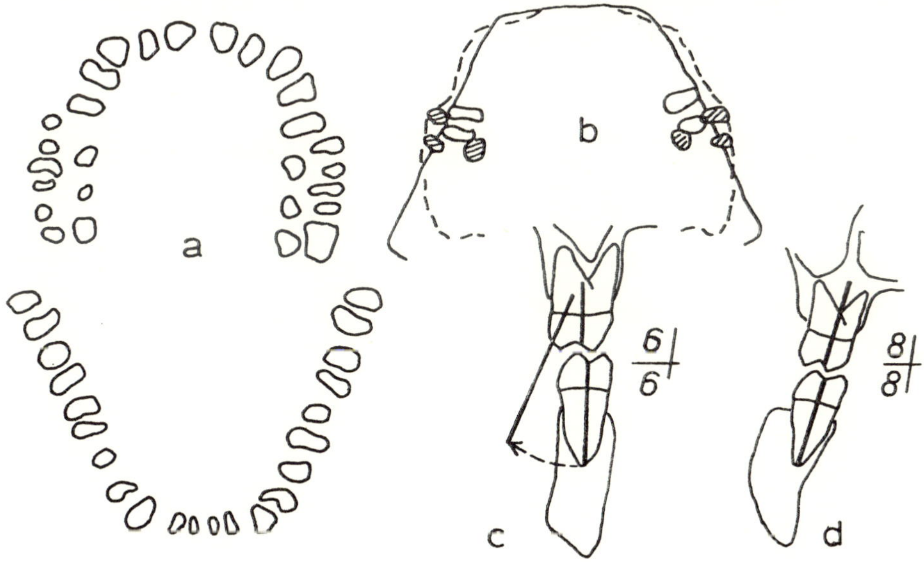

Figure 9-2. Outlines and diagrams relating to occlusion of upper and lower teeth, and of the dental arch in each jaw. *a*, outlines of tooth roots in horizontal sections of the jaws of a cadaver. The sections are made just beyond the free margin of alveolar bone. These were traced from Cryer (1901). *b*, arch forms obtained by drawing lines tangential to the root outlines of *a*. The first molar roots are included. Upper jaw, broken line and shaded roots. Lower jaw, continuous line. *c*, relation of teeth commonly found in first molar region. The tooth axes are nearly parallel to the sagittal plane when viewed from mesial. The indicated swing away from this position shows the different position of the axes commonly found in second and third molars as in *d*. The angle is greater in third than in second molars. In such cases the lower arch width between buccal cervices must be greater than the upper, in the posterior region. When arch width is compared at a position rootward of the cervices, as in *a* and *b*, the difference tends to be even greater.

stresses on growing and already developed bones has been amply demonstrated, concludes that "the pattern of activity is quite clearly dictated by the drive to achieve the morphology of maturity," and that "the motive power is inherent in the tissue which, given a normal environment, will develop according to a genetic template." Sissons (1956) considers genetic factors significant as determining the specific growth and development of the skeleton, and later adds emphasis by saying that "under normal circumstances intrinsic factors are of overwhelming importance in determining the form of bones."

The vertical relationship of crowns of anterior teeth is not upset by some variation in curvature of their roots or inclination of tooth axes. These variations may be associated with dental prognathism in

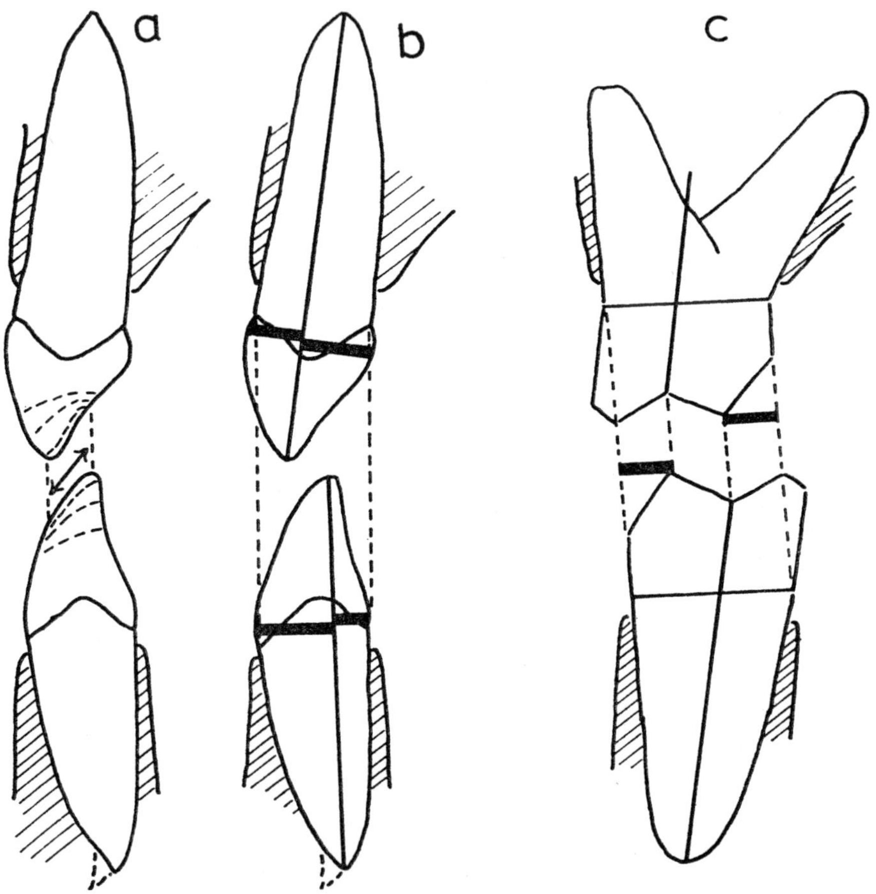

Figure 9-3. Diagrams relating morphology of upper and lower teeth to occlusion, and to vertical relationship of dental arches. *a*, distal view diagrams of left upper and lower canines to illustrate the initiation and development of attritional faceting in cases of normal slight over-bite leading to an edge-to-edge bite. *b*, the relation of upper and lower canines to one another (apart from mesio-distal interdigitation) and the relation of the axial lines to the labial and lingual outlines of these teeth. *c*, the vertical relationship of right upper and lower molars (apart from mesio-distal interdigitation). This diagram shows how, in the presence of vertical relationship of the cervices, there is bucco-lingual interdigitation of the cusp lines. This relationship is made possible by the fact that the lower buccal cusps and the upper lingual cusps are "set in," as shown by the short thick lines. The curved outlines of the crowns have been represented by straight lines.

some ethnic groups or with the range of normal anatomical variation in any group. It should be stressed that such variation is normal and in no way incongruous with the notion of a genetic template, and so the importance sometimes assigned to the quantitative investigation of variation and its statistical expression as a means of comparison is to be deprecated.

Williams (1967) draws attention to the infinitude of variation in normal individuals and states that "marked variations in normal anatomy are found wherever we look for them." Studies of variation in jaws, arches and teeth have shown that the extent of variation is too great to permit presentation of specifications of tooth or arch as typical of its group (Taylor, 1962a, b, c; 1963a). The present study, while closely related to the theme of variation, examines characters that tend to be common to certain teeth, and shows their relation to the anatomy of occlusion and their usefulness in identification of teeth.

Long before the development of techniques which could be applied to the actual fragments enabled the Piltdown fraud to be confirmed (Weiner et al., 1953; Weiner and Oakley, 1954), the present writer had demonstrated that the "Piltdown Canine" had been wrongly placed as a lower right, and that it was an upper left tooth. This identification was determined partly from a study of the convexities and axis position of the tooth profile (Taylor, 1937b). Figure 9-3 and its legend are reprinted from that Piltdown paper. Parts *a* and *b* represent canine teeth and were used in demonstrating how the "Piltdown Canine" could be positively identified as an upper tooth although it had been regarded by the maker of the "restoration" as a lower. In the present discussion, parts *a* and *b* serve to demonstrate the vertical relationship of crowns of anterior teeth where initially there is normal over-bite, and this relation is maintained in spite of the changing position of the facet of wear as the edge-to-edge bite is acquired. In *b* the short heavy lines show that the over-bite results from the different positions of axes in upper and lower teeth—nearer to labial in uppers, and nearer to lingual in lowers, as described above.

PROFILES OF POSTERIOR TEETH

These differences in convexity and tooth axis position between upper and lower anterior teeth are found also in posterior teeth, but in modified form on account of anatomical differences. Thus, in teeth with buccal and lingual cusps, the crown axis does not pass through cusps; similarly the tooth axis in the branched roots of upper molars and first premolars is not related to a particular branch. In the crowns the greater convexity on buccal of lowers and on palatal of uppers is easily recognized. Because of this, posterior teeth occlude in a manner corresponding to anterior teeth, namely with the upper buccal cusps overlapping, or outside of, lower buccal cusps, and with buccal and lingual cervices (upper and lower) in almost vertical relationship (Fig. 9-5). For many cases this is a fairly correct statement as regards premolars and first molars, and we may regard the crown axes of these teeth (as visualized from proximal) as almost in line or parallel. The widths of upper and lower arches taken at cervical level from these teeth are often approximately equal, at least for premolars and first molars.

For second and third molars there is usually a variation, not in the relation of upper and lower crowns judged by those axes, but in the orientation of axes. If it can be visualized that the upper and lower molars fixed to one another in occlusion, and the rigid axis now of both together rotated on a point superior to their occlusal surfaces, the apices of lower roots will swing outwards (Fig. 9-2 *c* and *d*), and the swing is greater in the third molar region than in the second. This variation of tooth orientation is often found. It is clear that as the molar axis diverges more from the vertical, so the width of arches at cervical level will become greater in the lower, and the difference in widths will be greater the further back it is measured (Fig. 9-2). The change in orientation from premolars to third molars is seen in illustrations to a paper by Dempster et al. (1963, their Figures 1d and 10) but it should be noted that their direction lines relate to root-branch sockets individually and not to tooth axes.

DENTAL ARCHES

To prevent any possible confusion, it is preferred that here the term "dental arch" should mean the shape of the curved row of tooth crowns as viewed in norma superioris (lower teeth), and norma inferioris (upper teeth); that is, when the outline in each case is projected on to a horizontal plane. But the term is used less precisely to refer to the curves obtained from various sets of landmarks. Thus, in a particular individual, there may be several different curves for each jaw. Also the corresponding curves from both jaws will reflect differences related to the particular set of landmarks chosen. This means that the resulting curves or arches representing upper and lower teeth for that individual may be almost similar or quite different. It has already been shown that among the chief factors concerned are the direction of teeth axes, and the convexities of tooth profiles associated with morphological differences in the various kinds of teeth. Arch form has been presented in considerable variety by many workers without giving sufficient heed to these factors. Comparisons of form and size have often been made between ethnic groups and between individuals in particular groups. In the results are found pronouncements on racial characters and affinities and suggested forms for the normal or ideal arch, but there are so many variables that even those measurements with statistical indications of variation may be misleading. It has been shown that form and size have a considerable normal range in any group, that measurements and indices do not adequately express these variations, and that they ignore asymmetry (Taylor, 1962a). It is very difficult to define anatomical landmarks related to teeth in such a way that measurements on different individuals may be so standardized as to be fairly comparable within a group, or between different observers. Outlines of arch form may be little more than "tangents" to anatomical features, and there is always the difficulty of representing three-dimensional form in a two-dimensional medium.

Representation of arch form by a line tangential to buccal margins of tooth sockets would seem to minimize the effect of variations in direction of tooth axes, but it is sometimes desirable to use landmarks readily accessible on the living person or on models made from dental impressions. For this the regions of labial and buccal cervices are the most satisfactory and convenient, and even in young persons their positions may be determined fairly precisely.

In skeletal material upper arches were examined both with calipers and with a craniostat giving a high degree of precision for the plotted projections. Results were presented both graphically and statistically (Taylor, 1962a). For a comparison of upper and lower arches a trial sample from these skulls was taken where the mandible was present and the dentition good. In six skulls the upper and lower arches tangential buccally to upper and lower teeth at cervices (4), socket margins (1) and worn occlusal surfaces (1), were plotted and the results superimposed. In three the lower arch was wider in the third molar region. Apart from this the superimposition in each case was so nearly coincident that it was impracticable to illustrate the small differences with separate lines.

For the present study observations are expressed in qualitative terms. Thus arches related to the labial and buccal cervical region tend to be similar in form and size, and in near-vertical relationships to one another, from the incisors to the first molar. Posterior to the first molar the lower arch tends to become increasingly wider than the upper. It has been already observed that in spite of these similarities and differences in arch width the upper teeth overlap the lower teeth throughout the dentition. Moreover, as viewed from proximal, the relation of axes of upper and lower premolar and molar teeth are approximately in line or parallel. Thus the upper teeth are not arranged in a larger or wider arch than the lowers, and the traditional view therefore does not explain the overlap.

Mechanism of Overlap

Overlap of upper teeth in man results from such anatomical differences between uppers and lowers as are seen in the profiles in Figure 9-3. Viewed from proximal the cusps of posterior teeth appear to interdigitate when occluding (Fig. 9-3 *c*), but this is not strictly true owing to the more mesial placement of the lower tooth in relation to its corresponding upper. It would be preferable to describe the relationship as interdigitation of rows of cusps in a bucco-lingual direction when visualized from proximal. The manner of this interdigitation in the presence of nearly vertical cervices may be represented diagrammatically.

Figure 9-4 presents an analysis of the characters of profile curvature, and *a* gives the plan for the other diagrams *b,c,d.* There is a rectangle, ABCD, divided by vertical lines into four equal parts. On the upper and lower portions of the rectangle are represented proximal views of hypothetical teeth with equal-sized cusps placed evenly between buccal and lingual. In this case the diagram shows mesial views of teeth from the right side of the mouth. The lines AB and CD represent cervical lines in vertical relationship to one another; buccal (DA) and lingual (CB) surfaces are vertical to the cervical lines.

The remaining drawings *(b,c,d)* use this diagram to show how the actual teeth differ from the hypothetical teeth and how they are able to present interdigitating rows of cusps while maintaining a near-vertical relationship of crowns. In diagram *b* the upper cusps are about to be displaced buccally and the lower cusps lin-

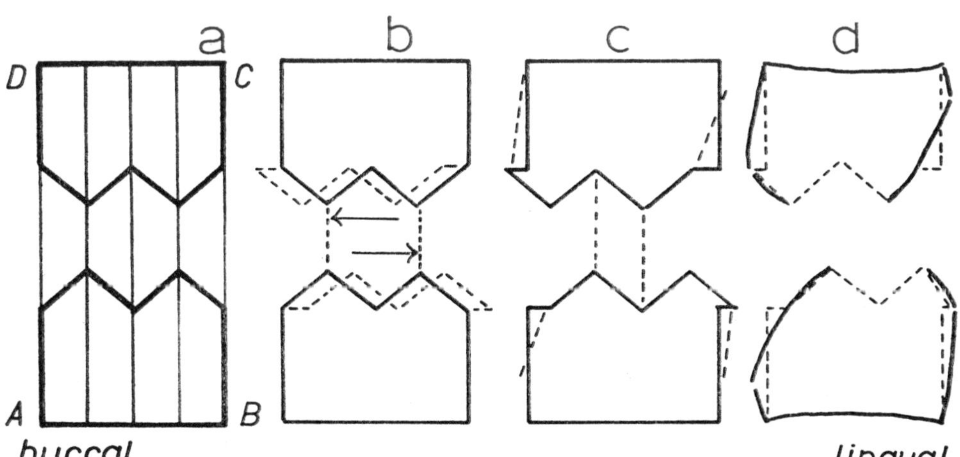

Figure 9-4. A diagrammatic analysis of buccal and lingual curvature of molars seen in proximal profile. This elaborates the theme of near vertical relationship of upper and lower crowns as presented in Figure 9-3. The diagrams show how the rows of buccal and lingual cusps are offset to allow overlap while the dental arches as a whole are similar in size. The upper arch is not wider than the lower.

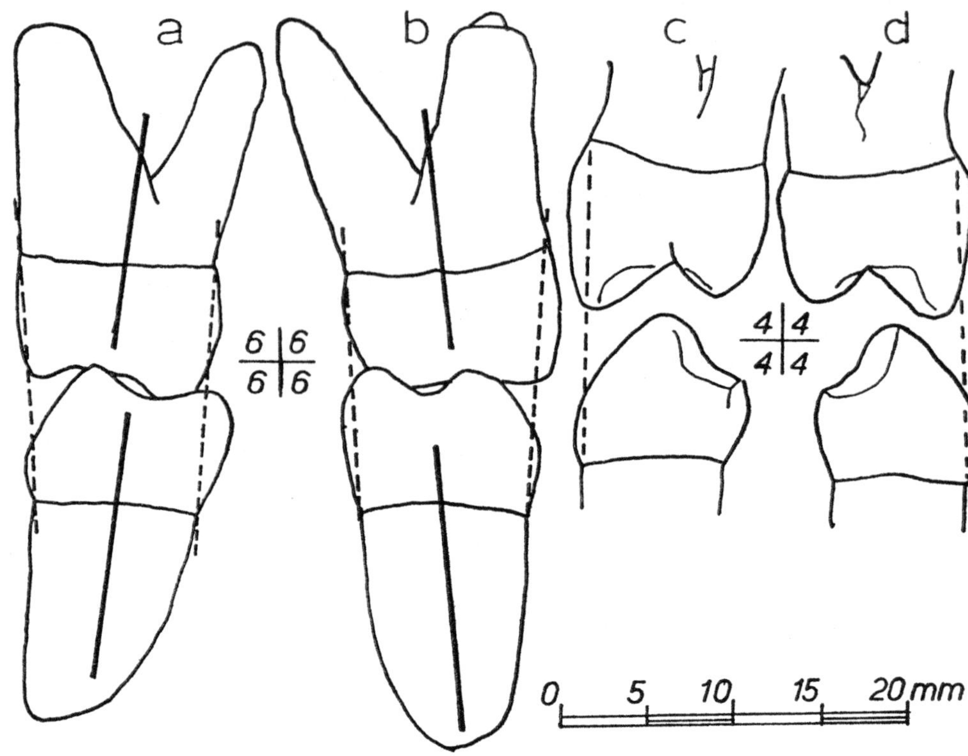

Figure 9-5. *a* and *b*, four first molars extracted from an adolescent. The teeth have been cemented together in exact anatomical occlusion and drawn from mesial aspect. The relations of curvatures and crowns demonstrated in Figures 9-3 and 9-4 are apparent. The broken lines draw attention to the nearly vertical relation of crowns and cervices of the tooth row from this viewpoint. The heavy lines show that the axes of upper and lower teeth on the same side are nearly parallel in proximal view. (They are not parallel in buccal view.) *c* and *d*, four first premolars from a boy aged eleven years. Apart from the fact that the lowers are narrower than their uppers (because of the small lingual cusp in the lower tooth), there is a relationship between curvatures, crowns and buccal cervices similar to that seen in *a* and *b*. See also Figure 8-21*c*.

gually, as indicated by the arrows and the broken lines. This changes the vertical relationship of cusp tips to an interdigitating one, indicated by vertical broken lines in diagram *c*. In this diagram *c* the shoulders resulting from cusp displacement are shown in continuous lines; the oblique broken lines indicate how the shoulders may be eliminated by slight remodelling of the buccal and lingual outlines. In diagram *d* this remodelling has been done (continuous lines), and gives the form and relative positions found in actual teeth. The broken lines in *d* repeat the continuous outline of diagram *c*. The close relationship between the diagrammatic or basic analysis and the form presented by actual teeth is obvious.

With regard to the bucco-lingual relationship of cusps, and near-vertical relationship of crowns and cervices just illustrated, it should be emphasized that this has been represented in proximal view ignoring perspective. It represents bucco-lingual interdigitation of cusps of upper and lower teeth as arising from a displacement, not of teeth themselves, but of upper cusps, a "quarter cusp width" towards buccal, and of lowers, a "quarter cusp width" towards lingual. In these diagrams a cusp represents a row of cusps, as for example all the buccal cusps of upper teeth mesial and distal to the tooth shown. The corresponding cusps of the lower teeth, although apparently fitting into the groove between the upper cusps, are actually "out of phase" in that they are in different frontal planes from their opponents. Thus when occluded teeth are viewed from the buccal aspect there is the appearance that cusps interdigitate similarly in a mesio-distal relationship.

Occlusion, Buccal View

From this aspect, interdigitation is achieved differently. The upper cusp is not "pushed back" nor the lower cusp "pushed forward" (each by a distance of one quarter cusp width), with the crowns retaining a near-vertical relationship in the antero-posterior direction. Instead of this the whole lower tooth is "pushed forward" so that it is half a cusp width to the mesial of its corresponding upper tooth. Compensation for the resulting forward placing of the lower arch is provided largely by the difference in mesio-distal widths of lower and upper incisors. There is no near-vertical relationship of proximal cervices in posterior teeth, except at distal of both third molars, and this arises from the greater mesio-distal dimension of the lower crown. In making this statement one is aware of the many exceptions or modifications that arise from variation in size and form of molar teeth, from the presence of diminutive third molars or from the absence of one or more of these teeth.

Effect of Tooth Wear

After cusps are worn away, the posterior teeth acquire the equivalent of what is called edge-to-edge occlusion in anterior teeth, and they maintain this relation. Where no unusual or pathological conditions are present to cause local malocclusion in individual teeth or groups of teeth, this near-vertical relationship of crowns may persist in the presence of advanced wear of teeth. This is amply illustrated in earlier reports on Moriori and Maori skulls (Taylor, 1962b, c, and 1963a, Plates 2, 5, 6 and 10).

In some cases where the long axes of molar teeth are inclined at a greater angle, i.e. less acute, to the mid-sagittal plane, the cervical width is of course appreciably greater at the lower than at the upper cervices; in spite of this the "edge-to-edge" bite of the second and third molars may be retained and their long axes remain nearly in line and almost parallel in proximal view. A good illustration of this in a Maori skull has been shown (Taylor, 1963a, Plate 6, Figure 34).

It has been taught that cusps assist the holding and crushing of food, but it is a fallacy to regard this as their only, or main function. An alternative conclusion receives overwhelming support from evidence associated with tooth wear.

Ethnic groups presenting much tooth wear have mostly been those that used their teeth vigorously, although wear has sometimes been increased through contamination of food by abrasive matter. The writer's reports of wear in skeletal material have shown many cases of severe dental wear accompanied by clear evidence of vigorous and efficient mastication. At the same time, evidence of good bone structure and generally healthy mouths shows that neither mastication nor nutrition suffered impairment, although cusps had long since been worn away.

It is clear therefore that the primary function of cusps had been fulfilled at a much earlier stage, and yet (if cusps were necessary to hold, crush or grind food), these people were most in need of such aid. It seems obvious that the function of cusps is to guide erupting teeth into normal occlusal relations with those in the opposite jaw. When such relationship becomes established muscle function assists in maintaining it, and cusps are no longer required. Clinical dentistry, whether conservative or prosthetic, while noting the implication must reconcile its application with the effects of existing malocclusion, lack of wear or other evidence of impaired function elsewhere in the mouth (Taylor, 1975, 1976).

ENAMEL PEARLS, AND CARABELLI'S CUSP

Enamel pearls showed so much variation that it is not feasible to present them as separate entities, and the associated features should be included when studying them. From naked-eye observation alone, and this embraces criteria of variation for the present study, it is clear that enamel pearls present no consistency in size, form, structure or location. Although examples have been described in the literature together with photomicrographs, and the origin of the formative cells suggested, there does not seem to be a satisfactory explanation of why they are formed. Certainly there is no explanation that is acceptable in view of the variation that has been noted here.

Just as one worker is able to select examples to support a particular hypothesis, another may, like the present writer, view some differences as degrees of a particular character. It is easy also to select and arrange a number of specimens that seem to form a series in support of the latter view, but because of the number involved it is not so easy to present them.

Thus, while it may seem reasonable to deny that there is a connection between the enamel pearl and the Opc, even a short series will suggest that there may very well be such a connection.

In Figure 7-34, teeth *c,b,a* in that order show actual connection, probably relation, and possible independence of enamel pearl and cervical enamel. Tooth *e* in that figure presents an actual connection of pearl to root, not by enamel but by a dentine stalk or bridge or tang. In Figure 7-35 *a* is seen a structure with distinct resemblance to the preceding one, but in this case there is no evidence that the enamel ever was formed from an epithelial remnant of the main enamel organ of the autosite tooth. It might readily be granted that the enamel was formed from a small bud of the original tooth germ, and that it in turn was associated with a dentine papilla, which in due course merged with the developing root of the autosite (Taylor, 1968a). What is this but an Opc? This case seems closely allied to those in Figures 7-35 *b*, 7-29 *b*, 7-27 *b*, the Opc in 7-34 *d* and so to the whole range of variety in Opc that has been shown.

If one can accept such a series, and the multitude of available intermediate specimens that smooth out the steps of the series so that the metaphor becomes more appropriately a chain, the connection between them must be acknowledged. Inevitably Carabelli's Cusp must be looked at again even if then the almost sacred concepts concerning it, and even the soundness of the data upon which they are founded, will have to be questioned.

The sources and so-called statistics of the data are varied and profuse. Great numbers of dentitions, deciduous and permanent, in men of all races, and in other primates both living and fossil, have been viewed, recorded and pronounced upon. It is known that the cusp in various "degrees of development" from pit, groove, tubercle, through to a prominent cusp on the MP aspect of the crowns of upper molars was widespread, and is common. It is known that additional elements in similar degrees of development are found in other positions, and on other teeth, both maxillary and mandibular, and not only on molar teeth. In upper molar teeth, such elements may most often be found in the MP position, and most often in first permanent (and second deciduous) molars, but it is not known why. And it is not even known whether this is a fact. Why? Because there are so many occurrences in so many degrees in so many teeth, and their grading and recording at best is highly subjective, exclusive and therefore unacceptable.

We do know when we have found a "true" Carabelli cusp, because there is a concept concerning it, but is it certain that it has significance in phylogeny or ontogeny? No. Is there an alternative conclusion regarding its significance? Yes, surely, and this must be considered. Instead of fitting a hypothesis to a particular morphological concept, the concept is re-examined in relation to what actually happens. The variety of occurrences has been referred to in the preceding paragraph.

In Figures 7-32 *b* and *c,* and 7-34 *d,* are three teeth with additional elements at MP. It appears less important that they are not all first molars than that all have recognizable additional root elements also, as have many other Opc found elsewhere than at MP. This study therefore confirms that additional cusps at MP may, or may not, have root elements also. Many teeth in the present study have been shown to have more cusps than root branches, or the reverse, and in a great many more the details of groove, tubercle, ridge and cusp in crown, and of fusion, groove, furcation and apices in root, make it quite impossible to recognize any consistent relation between crown and root. The locations of Opc in crown or root or in both are further complications in recognition and analysis of morphological elements. This is part of the wide range of characters and their association analyzed in this study and recognized as normal variation.

Part of the concept of the Carabelli cusp is that its morphogenetical significance in evolution of the number or pattern of cusps lies in its location at MP. It has been shown that the Opc with a root element is common in almost any position, and that it is often obvious that crown and root elements were related in development of the tooth. If an Opc at MP is without a root element, is it therefore to be assigned more significance in the evolution of cusp patterns than one in the same position that has a root element? Who could know how many Carabelli cusps have root elements when no one has tried to find out? The data concerning Carabelli cusps have come from dentitions *in vivo,* and *in situ* in skeletal material, with virtually no information concerning the root elements of the teeth examined. The fact that degree of development of crown elements has been shown incapable of analysis is difficulty enough; the difficulty is twice confounded by their relationship to variation in root elements. To ignore this and to take a relatively select few Opc in a special position, knowing nothing of their root associations and yet imputing to them some special significance, is unscientific (see frontispiece).

Korenhof (1960) has reviewed the very extensive bibliography concerning the Carabelli features. Many opinions have been proved untenable; many more remain unproved; and it seems that there is no common agreement in any respect. This is not surprising; for the question is analogous to an argument about the meaning of a phrase in a sentence when the context is ignored. In this case the context has two parts, the rest of the sentence and the associated sentences. The rest of the sentence is the rest of the tooth as regards crown and root elements. The associated sentences are the relation of Carabelli features to all the other accessory features that occur.

The Carabelli cusp in the present work is seen as a small part, unjustifiably isolated and inadequately explored, within the much larger field embracing accessory elements in crown or root or both, anywhere in the dentition. The cusp's wide range of variation in form, location and degree of development and of fusion with, or separation from, the basic or type elements of the various kinds of teeth, is seen as a further expression of the potential for variation inherent in developing dental tissues.

It seems to follow that to encompass normal variation a wider net must be cast than hitherto, but who is to define the net's perimeter or say what is abnormal? It has been shown that as a study becomes more widely based almost any specimen loses its individual dramatic impact, and is seen in obvious relationship to others. This writer believes that only limitations of material have prevented the recognition of corresponding variation in other biological groups. In dental variation the presence of square, tapering and ovoid as basic and mixed types of incisor tooth form were convincingly demonstrated long ago in man and anthropoid by Williams (1914).

Less obvious perhaps in some respects, but much wider in scope, have been the variations in all human teeth presented in the present study. There is no reason not to believe that corresponding variations could be found and did occur in other groups. In earlier work with skeletal material, including teeth, it was shown that one seeks in vain for a specimen that may be regarded as typical of its group (Taylor, 1962a, b, c; 1963a). The scientist therefore may not assume that fossil fragments are any more likely to be representative than is contemporary material. Much of the meticulous examination of isolated fossils therefore, while certainly a valuable exercise in technique and observation, has been followed by assumptions and pronouncements that are not soundly based, and the specific significance of such is still unproved.

So also must be the significance attributed to Carabelli's cusp. It has been shown that so-called statistics concerning its occurrence are worthless; firstly because they cannot eliminate subjective assessment of its degrees; and secondly because observations have overlooked information concerning tooth roots (Dietz, 1944).

Certainly let us honour the name of Carabelli. In his day and age he was observant beyond his fellows. But with the infinitely greater material and data now available, what does occur should at least be recognized and accepted, although neither reasons for, nor even the nature of the intriguing cause, is known.

In the author's experience various accessory elements in upper molars tend to be more common in the MP position than elsewhere. Where there is a recognizable Opc radicle in this position, it tends more often to fuse with MB root than with P root. A DP cusp is seldom associated with an apparently unusual P root branch. But the P root varies considerably in transverse section and sometimes it is fused to DB. Not infrequently it presents a longitudinal groove, usually on its P aspect. Such a groove is sometimes present when there is a prominent Carabelli cusp. Who is to say that this is not an Opc crown element with a radicle fused with P root? (Frontispiece.) Again, who can deny a possible association between the commonly found irregularity on palatal edge of an MB root, and a tubercle or ridge irregularity on the M or MB aspect of occlusal surface (Figs. 7-28 *c*, 7-29 *a*, 7-31 *c*, 7-32 *c*)?

These are variations in form and degree of Opc, perhaps more common in this position, but nevertheless consistent with variations in what the writer recognizes as, or suspects to be, Opc elements in other positions.

It was earlier explained that in honour of the work of Herbst and Apffelstaedt (1930), their term Odontopagus parasiticus concretus has been adopted in the abbreviation Opc in the present study. If the term has been applied more widely than they intended, may its use be taken as a tribute to their contribution in a field of study that has long confounded workers in dental anatomy, pathology and physical anthropology. Hitherto there has been offered an illustration of a "malformation," or a few selected specimens have been presented to support an hypothesis concerning significance in dental evolution. But the present survey of what is actually found in a very large number of extracted teeth (in roots as well as crowns) offers a much more acceptable understanding of variation. In effect it is suggested that freedom of ontogenetic diversification expressed in the great range of obviously interrelated variations is preferable, as an explanation of what is actually found, to the conventional subservience to an hypothetical phylogenetic dominance. To cling to the latter requires the acceptance of a few carefully selected specimens as evidence of a struggle to reproduce a lost pattern, the odd hit amongst innumerable misses. This also would endow a minor part of a tooth with the status of a vestigial structure, which the variety of reality shows that it is not. A vestigial structure that is reproduced consistently and similarly, in foetus, embryo, juvenile or adult, one can readily accept as evidence of a genetic pattern that has been modified in the evolution of a species, and as evidence of relationships now partly obscured by changes in other groups also.

The generically limited expression of the potential for variation must inevitably result in the reproduction of details in many combinations of pattern and degree. That it does so has been demonstrated, and the demonstration has been evaluated as just that.

The expression of normal variation in other related groups must inevitably sometimes produce details that are similar. But surely such parallels when found have been given a degree of significance which is unjustified in view of differences in the scarcity or abundance of material available? The taurodont molars of a Neanderthaler are still well within the generic type of *homo,* but if a selenodont or secodont molar in a human jaw is found the Piltdown story will be remembered (Fig. 3-12 *a,b,c,* and Lunt, 1954).

Search for a suitable term for the accessory dental element confirmed the acceptability of Odontopagus parasiticus concretus (Opc). With the connotation of consolidation in the Greek verb *pagio* the notion of a parasitic concretion consolidated with hard tissues of a tooth is presented. Metaphorically this is an acceptable description of many Opc (such as those in Fig. 7-29). In view of the many intermediate examples that have been designated here as Opc, it is reasonable to apply the term also to irregularities in morphology of crown or root which are recognized as tubercles, or to an apparently additional bulk in part of a crown or root. Equally acceptable are the further terms "autosite" and "parasite" for the normal and additional tooth elements respectively. There should be no risk of confusion with their more usual meanings, and in the present usage they are explicit and they simplify description.

Chapter 10

Concepts of Variation

THE FACT OF VARIATION has always been quite obvious; its nature and limitations less so; and its significance an attractive source of speculation. Even a brief study of variation is enough to discourage documentation, while analysis and interpretation have presented a challenge so formidable that only dauntless dedication has prevailed against it. The challenge has always proved provocative, but attempts to meet it have evidently underestimated the complexity both of the subject and of requirements for dealing with it. The present study has made contributions in these respects.

The meticulous recording of occlusal features by Dahlberg has already been acknowledged. Although inevitably some similar features are covered by both studies, the differences in presentation are in part related to objectives. Dahlberg's plaques present a variety of three-dimensional records in the form of casts, the intensive study of which could enable one to liken a particular crown or feature to an indexed specimen in a plaque. This report also is essentially morphological in presentation, but the graphic method adopted has enabled much more data to be presented in a convenient form accompanied by detailed description. The result is a comprehensive analysis and report embracing many of the hitherto neglected areas containing "intermediates" or degrees of variation, as well as those cases often conveniently dismissed as anomalous or abnormal.

To use a pictorial metaphor, the present study is factual, like a photograph. Whether in colour or monochrome, and limited only by the sensitivity of the medium, it records details which are not all contrasty but may merge in pastel tints or shades of grey. But the picture presented by the "-ologist" has so often been that of the artist whose cursory glance provides a notion and an urge to impress it. It has become a story, and he chooses bold outlines or bright colours to tell it. He omits some details that he never saw, and others because he did not comprehend their relevance. Other features he perhaps accentuates, for his purpose is to tell a story that will command attention.

The photograph may at first sight have less impact, or from sheer weight of detail discourage careful study. But how often is it that the detail establishes perspective, and affects the relationship of the features first noted? In other words, the photograph presents things as they are, and another photograph taken from a second viewpoint contributes to the perspective or relativity of detail in the first. The photographic record of reality may therefore convey a different message from that of the artist's picture.

The scientist, like the artist, has free choice. He may select his subject and choose his data to present it. He may further choose to support his interpretation, by skilled placing of detail data. Resemblance implies relationship—this is his message. Resemblance is a very vague adjective when not further defined as to its nature—chemical composition, morphology, dimensions, hardness, specific gravity, function and so on. The dental anatomist selects a feature, perhaps a cusp, like Carabelli's, or the fifth cusp in a lower molar, and grades it by one subjective feature, not more, for relative size would complicate the tally. He seeks no data of the tooth root in relation to this cusp, or additional cusp, or additional cusp elsewhere. He counts his cusps and seeks the statistician's aid. Impeccable statistics confirmed by electronic computer establish that his sample is acceptable, while significance of the result is, or is not, statistically established.

But going back along the line of procedure, at every step compromise is found, even at the first assumption, that resemblance implies relationship. Is this the only interpretation? Far from it. Have not similar cusps been found in ancient fossils and in later ethnic groups? Of course they have, and so have indefinite or unclassifiable cuspal or other details (*if* the examination embraced a large enough sample of teeth that were positively identified, unworn, etc.).

The nature of variation, the evidence of so many characters and so many degrees of permutation and combination, must surely dispose of the concept that variation recalls some details of phylogenetic evolution. Such a notion ignores much of the data, or detail, as does the artist's picture.

As for the statistics, even a computer cannot give sound results from unsound data (Taylor, 1970c), as will be explained under the heading "the incomparable tooth." Use has been made of qualitative records of the occurrence and grading of certain features (Taylor, 1962b, c) and they have been found to be at least convenient. Metrical and nonmetrical studies of dental and other skeletal material have led to a modification in the writer's view of variation. Early realization that variation does not take place around an average (such average is a hypothetical conception) that does not exist, led to the abandonment of any further effort to define it. Nevertheless, the author recognizes that the conception presented both advantages (as a working convenience) and pitfalls for the worker. Having accepted the normality of variation, this endeavour has been to learn something of its nature and limits, and to seek applications of such knowledge. Quantitative and qualitative studies have played their part, but these have decreased in significance as realization has deepened that they were merely tools that aided awareness, and that they have often been wrongly used to produce false images. All images so produced should be critically re-examined, and most of them discarded.

When presenting a paper at a Science Congress on the Piltdown "Restoration" (Taylor, 1937b) the author noted that the canine fragment had been questioned, and quoted: "Judgments . . . as to the characters of the canine tooth seem likely to remain subject to individual opinion and experience . . . after these opinions have been expressed, little more can profitably be said" (Appendix 6). The author did not accept that view, and working only from casts, presented proof of the identity of the canine, of its wrong placing in the accepted restoration, and of the impossibility that any such dentition as in the restoration could have existed. That this was soundly reasoned was confirmed many years later when tests by others on the actual fragments proved their fraudulent association as already mentioned. That report is now history.

The principles on which this author was able to discredit the Piltdown restoration long before exposure of the hoax have been applied here. Not only has this focussed attention on the nature and detail of variation, but also it has offered a wider concept and appreciation of morphological anatomy of teeth, individually and collectively, in the dentition.

Having studied what does occur in presenting to us such a variety in tooth morphology, one is tempted on to the thin ice of speculation as to how or why such variation occurs. One may rephrase the question, "Why do teeth vary so much?" and ask, "Why is there so much resemblance between them?" The ramifications of difference are no more provocative of thought than those of resemblance. For example, how does an upper tooth produce the morphology so well adapted to that of the lower? Or, how is the bilateral symmetry or mirror image of left and right determined throughout the body? Again one might ask why genetic patterns have been unchanged for such ages in some cases, such as the tree shrew, and yet have varied in others to the delight or discomfort of those who seek to unravel the story of evolution?

The scientist must modify his conclusions when he is able to appreciate significance in new data in his own or allied fields. Is he entitled to define his "own" field? Nature is not like that. The sorting of data into fields should be no more than a temporary expedient for convenience, a stage in one's development. The "field" is everything within, and beyond, man's ability to comprehend. A metaphor to illustrate the scope of anthropology is that of the view from a high airport control tower. Around the 360 degrees, through windows one may call physical and social anthropology, ethnology, archaeology, psychology, philology, and even palaeontology, geology and all the other "ologies,"' there may often be seen the same feature but in different relations to other features. To properly comprehend the nature of one, it is essential to consider its relation to others.

This metaphor merely illustrates the nature of the problem of interpretation. A hypothesis is no more than a convenience, a step along the way. The hypothesis may in due course appear established, and yet later be discarded. A "by-product" of the present study is the writer's conviction that the time has come to discard the hypothesis attributing phylogenetic significance to some variations in tooth morphology. Interpretation of certain similar or apparently similar features in different individuals or groups, as significant indicators of a common genetic ancestry, recent or ancient, appears unjustified. Firstly that hypothesis does not adequately cover the facts, and secondly there is at least one alternative explanation of variation.

Some of the relevant facts are as follows:

(a) So-called normal features may be missing, or so much altered or reduced that their identity is uncertain.

(b) Additional features may be found in great variety of position and form, and of degree of development.

(c) They may apparently involve the crown only, or the root only, or be recognizable in both crown and root.

(d) There is evidence that similar variations occur in other races of man, in hominids and in other primates; the lack of comparative statistics must be evaluated in terms of the scarcity of material and of the unsuitability of the features for qualitative and quantitative assessment.

(e) Evidence submitted in support of atavistic significance in these features has been largely confined to carefully selected cases which obviously are not random samples, or in any sense typical for the species.

(f) This so-called evidence ignores the much greater incidence of "nontypical" examples of the feature concerned.

(g) It does not discriminate between examples confined to crowns and those involving tooth roots because of lack of awareness as to whether there is such an association; the evidence is gathered often by observation only of part of the crown of a tooth *in situ*.

(h) The atavistic hypothesis leaves the great majority of obvious and less obvious variations unaccounted for.

(i) It implies the existence of a kind of genetic memory which sometimes endeavours to resurrect a particular feature.

(j) It does not explain why this implied memory so often fails completely to resurrect anything, or what happens to make it forget or remember some character.

(k) It does not explain why the great majority of "resurrections" apparently lack any consistency as to resemblance to a particular feature in form or position; to change the metaphor, the target is missed far more often than hit, and many of the misses suggest lack of awareness of any target.

In summary this list lends support to evidence that the tooth-forming tissues have an inherent potential for variation. Obviously, expression of this potential cannot exceed taxonomic bounds—a hypsodont, or secodont carnassial, tooth cannot appear in a human jaw. Within these reasonable limits and type of tooth (in the sense in which the word has just been used) this potential for variation has relatively wide expression. This is the "alternative" explanation which is offered here, for it fits the facts known at present. It does not answer all questions that could be asked, but this is true of any field that attracts the mind of man. Conclusions must not ignore known facts that are in opposition. Until all facts are known a conclusion cannot be final but only tentative, and it is essential that alternative conclusions be sought and given due consideration. An investigation that does not meet these requirements is not scientific.

In the light of these statements, and of this analysis of morphological variation in teeth, mensuration will be evaluated as a tool in dental studies.

THE INCOMPARABLE TOOTH

From time to time in this study, certain characters have prompted the suggestion that teeth are unsuitable for measurement. All teeth in the permanent dentition have now been examined as regards their morphological variation, and their modification by wear. Attention has also been given to variation in the orientation of teeth individually, and to their arrangement collectively as upper and lower dental arches, as well as to the interrelationship of morphology, orientation and occlusion. It is clear that considerable variation in all these respects can be recognized as compatible with evidence that the individual persons concerned had lived normal lives as regards the anatomy, physiology and function of these parts.

Therefore the conclusion cannot be avoided that wide variation is normal in the respects noted, as it has long been known to be in other respects such as stature, body weight and physical type. The intensive analysis of dental variation now presented is quite different from the many metrical analyses that have been made, but it is factually descriptive rather than statistically so. It is important that it be considered whether the statistical analysis is necessarily factually true, and whether it can be partly so. If this is the case it is essential to know in what respects it may be open to question, and whether these are related to inferences or conclusions that have been made from statistical studies.

The value of statistical studies depends basically on two criteria. Firstly there is the suitability of the material to be counted or measured in a particular way, and secondly there is the statistical analysis of the data. The first must be decided by a thorough knowledge of the material, which includes awareness of the significance of certain variables, and this cannot necessarily be determined by the statistics (although this is sometimes assumed to be the case). The correctness of the statistics themselves is a mathematical question and involves requirements that must be met. Assuming that these are fulfilled, it does not necessarily follow that the requirement of suitability of material has also been met. This is the crux of the present thesis. We will therefore proceed to show why teeth are unsuitable for measurement, and to establish that comparisons and conclusions made from dental measurements are not necessarily true, quite regardless of the mathematical soundness of the statistics on which they are based. The interpretation of statistics based on measurements of teeth in the past, present or future must therefore be suspect.

Analysis of morphological variation in teeth has disclosed many characters that cannot be described in conventional ways. This may be why the subject of variation has been largely avoided and why so few data are available. The reason that efforts at expressing variation in metrical or quantitative terms are of little value is found in the nature of variation. For example, size for a tooth must involve so many dimensions that no particular selection from these could provide a valid basis for comparison. Again, although a certain point on a single tooth may be defined or fixed, variation is such that the establishment of a corresponding precise point for all teeth of that kind is not feasible. Such terms as "most prominent point," or "root apex" or "cusp tip," for example, do not define landmarks from which can be made measurements whose accuracy or significance justifies their use for comparison. Large or small size overall must bear some relation to the normal range of variation within a group, but obviously such relation itself is not constant for all characters. It is equally obvious that sex has some bearing on variation, and that this effect also is variable. There must be a normal range of variation within each sex and within ethnic groups, but so many variables are involved that one must not readily accept any claim to definition of the limits of such ranges. This is said not only because of the obvious complexity of interplay of variable factors, but also because some analyses of skeletal material by conventional methods of dimensional comparison may merit strong objection. This certainly applies in dental studies.

What are these methods and why are they unsuitable? In essence, the methods are comparisons of measurements of so-called length, breadth, width, height and depth, or of indices formed from two or more such dimensions. The confusion arising from different connotations of length and width, for example, when measuring molar crowns or complete anterior teeth, would be difficult to justify; nor could one justify comparisons on a basis of weights or volumes, for neither measure may remain constant in any particular tooth on account of depositions of secondary dentine or cementum or changes in mineralization, or as a result of wear or deposits of calculus.

The unsuitability arises essentially from the allocation of metrical figures concerned with one or more of the conceptual three dimensions of a solid body, and their manipulation as if they constitute a significant basis of comparison. This objection arises from the nature of the solid bodies compared, because teeth are very irregular and variable. Although they obviously vary in what is understood by the terms length, breadth, etc., it has been shown that there are no satisfactory landmarks in teeth for linear measurements, which therefore lose significance. In such short dimensions even tenths of a millimeter should be important, but in these circumstances they become irrelevant, regardless of the degree of accuracy of which the measuring instrument is capable; but this is not all. Teeth vary appreciably also in orientation so that landmarks cannot be defined in relation to the three primary planes as can be done with landmarks on the skull (Taylor, 1962a).

Already we have a somewhat formidable array of objections to descriptions or comparison of teeth by measurement, but there are others which emphasize the difficulty of obtaining an acceptable result. The objective of description of the material with a view to comparison with similar samples is reasonable enough, but the error lies in attempting to do this without sufficient study or awareness of its morphological complexity. Teeth vary in themselves in many characters which, while not directly related to length, breadth, etc., do

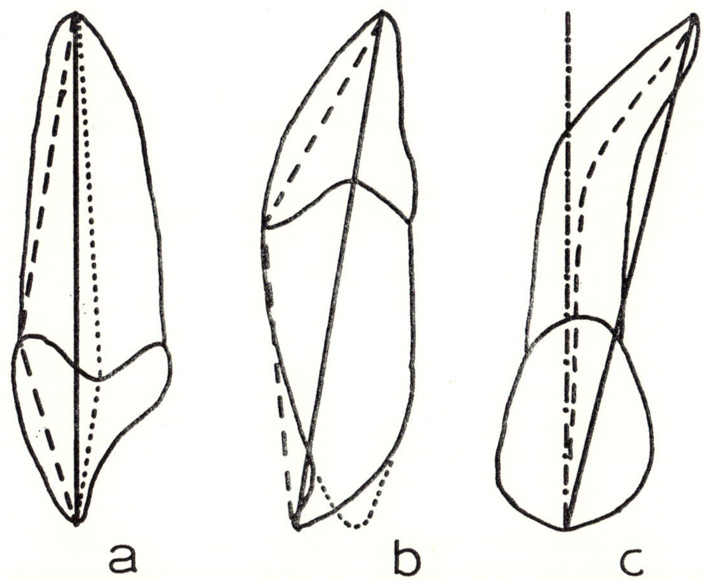

Figure 10-1. Diagrams illustrating some problems in the measurement of tooth length. *a*, length of crown plus length of root, measured with calipers either labially (broken line) or proximally (dotted line) give different proportions, and in each case give a different total length of tooth from that measured directly between apex and incisal edge, or cusp tip (continuous line). *b*, similar difficulties illustrated as for a lower anterior tooth, but with the additional complication of a curved apical region. Should the position of the apex be estimated as indicated? If so, how is the measurement made, correct to one tenth of a millimeter? *c*, three choices for tooth length which may be presented by a tooth with a curved root. These are, length between cusp and apex, length along curvature of tooth axis, and the projection length as indicated. Few roots are straight, and many are curved in more than one direction. Such roots are not abnormal, but how may they be measured accurately?

in fact complicate or frustrate one's efforts to find a convenient quantitative basis for comparison. For example consider the following:

(a) Length of single-rooted teeth. The total length of an incisor or canine should equal length of the crown plus length of the root. But these parts "interdigitate" so irregularly at the cervix that the dimensions vary also according to which of the surfaces (labial, lingual and proximal) is being measured.

(b) Is the total or maximum length of the tooth the straight line distance between incisal edge or cusp tip and apex, or is it a curvilinear dimension along some surface (and there are a number to choose from) between these termini? The former would seem preferable, but if the root is curved to mesial or distal or otherwise (a normal variation), the straight line measurement will be incorrect. A tooth with a curved root may not be fairly excluded merely because it is curved (Figure 10-1 *a,b,c*).

Root length and crown length are most conveniently measured between caliper points applied between cervix and apex, and between cervix and incisal edge or cusp tip, respectively, but these together will differ from total tooth length, both in the straight-line and surface methods of measurement.

(c) Does the labial cervix provide a satisfactory terminus to enable crown length to be compared with root length? Measurement to proximal cervix would give a quite different ratio, but would it be less valid (Fig. 10-1 *a*)? The relative height of the cervical curve obviously varies as between teeth of different persons, but it has also been shown that the curve may differ on mesial and distal of the same tooth, at least in upper canines (Taylor, 1969b and Fig. 1-29). But measuring crown height to the cervical line on proximal surfaces would present further difficulties, and be impossible for a canine tooth. A measurement cannot be imagined that could be acceptable as a record of crown length or height for anterior teeth. Measurement of root length would present almost as great a problem. One has only to mention the considerable variation in apices, sharpness or bluntness, and such root characters as flatness, thickness, grooves, curves or bends and sometimes root division, to become aware of the complications, and of the absurdity of ascribing to any particular dimension a significance that might justify its use as a basis of comparison.

(d) The term "cusp tip" is used here, but definition of a particular anatomical point as such is virtually impossible. Some teeth may almost present such a point, but within a collection of teeth there are relatively few such cases. Moreover, even in cases of slight modification through wear, an estimation cannot approach the degree of accuracy required for such small measurements. All in all therefore, measurements defined as from "tip of the cusp" are unacceptable as measurements for comparison.

(e) Length of multi-rooted teeth. In upper premolars the variety of division pattern in roots has been demonstrated, but in the case of molar roots the problem of defining root length (and also tooth length) is greatly complicated by differences in length and curvature of the root branches. These variations are so numerous that a few teeth which may at first be considered measurable could not possibly be regarded as representative of a group.

(f) Teeth are subject to wear in different parts and to varying degrees. Wear is most often occlusal or incisal, but may also be interproximal. The first variety will obviously invalidate measurements of crown height or crown-to-root proportions. This kind of wear, and more particularly interproximal wear, is commonly found in skeletal material of many ethnic groups. Measurements purporting to give the length of the dental arch, or of certain sections of it, must be invalid in the presence of interproximal wear since it is impracticable to determine the degree of its effect.

In any series proposed for measurement only those having complete permanent dentition could be considered. Limitation to individuals without tooth wear would presumably imply young adults, and these are a minority in most collections of skeletal material. Admission of all adults to ensure a larger group would generally embrace those with wear of immeasurable amount, and attempts to make allowance for loss by wear must further vitiate any so-called "findings."

(g) Teeth of the same kind vary considerably in curvature of corresponding parts. With anterior teeth this can mean that maximum width of an incisor crown between parallels may appear simple and obvious in some teeth but not in others. The types described by Leon Williams (1914) do occur in almost pure type of square, tapering and ovoid, and so also do variations

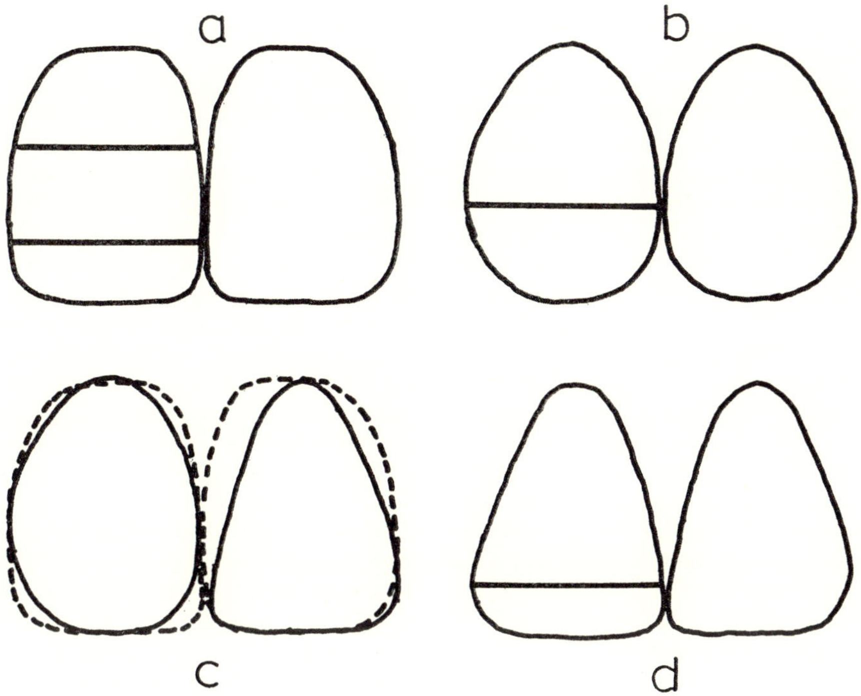

Figure 10-2. Measurements of tooth widths or mesio-distal diameters. Diagrams of pairs of upper central incisors of the three basic types, square, tapering and ovoid, to illustrate some of the problems presented by measurement. The maximum diameter is in a different position varying with the type, and wear may similarly affect this measurement differently. Measurements of crown width or crown length, or height, give no indication of the great differences in morphology presented by the basic types and by combinations or modifications of them. In *c* the outlines of *a* (square) have been compared in turn with one from *b* (ovoid) and one from *d* (tapering).

within the types, as well as combinations of these (Chapter 1). As a result, the position of maximum width (and of contacts with adjacent teeth) may be found in different regions in different teeth (Fig. 10-2). As a further consequence, the effect of interproximal wear varies as between dentitions of different types, for contacts are opened at an earlier stage in some, in spite of the general tendency of most teeth to drift mesially and to maintain contacts. These differences therefore add to variable factors that complicate efforts at consistency in method, and therefore invalidate comparisons of widths of teeth of a kind, or of portions of the dental arch.

The diagrams in Figure 10-2 *a,b* and *d* show the three basic types of tooth form. The horizontal lines suggest the position of maximum crown width, and it is clear that the position may vary with the type of tooth. In the tapering type *d*, a moderate amount of wear will soon have removed the greatest width, and the width measurement will continue to decrease. However, in a square type the apparent width may remain almost unchanged even when excessive wear has taken place. Figure 2 *c* takes the outlines of *a* and compares them with one outline each from *b* and *d*. These differences add emphasis to our statement that it is impossible to make allowance for losses of dimension through wear.

When teeth are compared by measured differences, in spite of the objections indicated above, no recognition is given to differences other than those "measured," mainly length or width. But it has been seen (Chapter 1) that there is infinite morphological variation through a great number of characteristics. If two teeth, one with a fine light root and sharp-pointed apex, and the other with a heavy root and thick-rounded apex, happen to have a similar length overall, and similar breadth at cervix, or maximum width, they must (by conventional mensuration) be regarded as similar. The absurdity of such conclusion is obvious. Similarly two teeth of the same general morphology, but differing in length and width, may be presented as supporting a claimed difference between ethnic groups regardless of the lack of data concerning sex or stature, and so on. Other examples, with their corollaries, come to mind to support objections to such comparisons. Conclusions that are reached by such methods must be rejected, and one must not be impressed by the accompanying statistical formulae concerning variation, or by indicators as to whether the results are "statistically significant" or otherwise. If the methods are unsound, or unsuitable for the material being studied, the results amount to mere statistical irrelevance, whether obtained by computers or otherwise. This surely applies to measurement of teeth.

Goose (1963) lists some inherent difficulties in dental measurements and in surveying attempts to deal with them shows the chaotic situation that has been reached. He stresses that "no amount of statistical refinement will be of any use, unless the basic data are sound." The present survey has shown why teeth are unsuitable for measurement. It follows that compromise at any stage cannot produce sound basic data.

There are other methods of mensuration besides linear measurements and the indices derived from them. It would not be difficult for example to obtain data of weight or volume, or of areas projected on to a plane, but it would be easy also to show that any of these are by no means free from objections. All in all, therefore, the study of size or form of teeth presents many problems, and the methods that have mostly been used—mensuration to gather data and statistical treatment of the data—have been shown to be unscientific. It is essential to recognize the nature of the material and to devise methods of study accordingly, but workers have been trying to make the material conform to the method.

Analysis of variation is clearly a rich field for study, particularly the morphological variation of teeth. Certainly there must be dental characters arising from their evolutionary or ethnic history. Although these may be recognized and sometimes their occurrence may be subjectively graded or counted, it is unlikely that they can ever be measured mathematically and there seems to be no good reason for attempting to do this. But this does not make them unworthy of study, and some are quite acceptable as nonmetrical characters.

Much has already been learned in other rewarding fields of study, such as the manner of development of teeth or their inorganic nature, and the histological and molecular structure of the various tissues. The relative permanence of teeth is of great importance to the palaeontologist, and of ever increasing value in pathological and forensic studies (Taylor, 1971b, c; 1972a, b). As organic structures their morphology is of special interest in various fields, but as very small portions of a much larger organism their relationship thereto must be kept in mind. Subjected, no doubt, as parts to many of the influences causing variation in the whole body, they appear to present also many intrinsically dental characters for varying combinations in their morphology. Is it not presumptuous to have assumed that from a few arbitrary measurements, indifferently designed and more or less repeated on various roughly similar fragments of the bodies of a number of individuals, statistical treatment of "data" will significantly contribute to the unravelling of ethnic relationships? Rather these little structures should be examined with an open mind, and while one marvels that the infinite and intricate variety presented does show consistency within specific limits, it should be remembered nevertheless that this same variety renders teeth incomparable by measurement alone.

CONCLUDING COMMENTS

Variation—Application and Implication

Following an air crash and incineration of victims, identification of remains for insurance or other purposes may be extremely difficult. The finding of even an isolated tooth becomes forensically important if it can be shown that the tooth could have, or could not have, formed part of a particular dentition. Hitherto such determination has depended largely on records obtained from the presumed victim's dentist. If these are limited to the usual brief mention of fillings, extractions and radiographs involving fees for services rendered, they may prove useless as aids to identification, but their value may be greatly enhanced by a little more information. This information should relate to the findings described in the present analysis of morphological variation.

Thus, acceptance or rejection of the recovered tooth as part of a known dentition may be greatly assisted by recognition of the personal characters of the tooth, as distinct from acquired characters. The latter may be the result of operative dentistry, but include also evidence of developmental or late pathology or trauma, wear or abrasion associated with function and habits, as well as evidence of age that may be further supported by sectioning, radiography or microscopic examination. Some of these aspects have been dealt with by Miles (1963), Gustafson (1966), Cameron and Sims (1973), Harvey (1976) and Sopher (1976).

Personal characters of roots (whether long or short, slender or robust, straight or curved, fused or divergent), and of crowns (convexity of profiles, length and acumination of cusps, primary and secondary ridges and grooves), relative size of crown and root, and so on, may be very relevant. One of the main purposes of the present report has been to draw attention to the contribution that can be made to forensic data through these hitherto mostly neglected characters. And not only so, but it has also been shown how to recognize and describe these features. In doing this, a wide field has been explored and the nature and extent of variation effectively demonstrated. At the same time certain concepts of the significance of variation have been reviewed and evaluated, and others suggested as being more in accordance with the knowledge gained through the present analysis.

The forensic importance that may devolve upon a single tooth found in particular circumstances has just been mentioned. The tooth would firstly be identified, and a note made of acquired characters. What might be expected in this respect would vary according to culture and environment during life (Taylor, 1971b, c; 1972a, b). Teeth in a contemporary civilized environment seldom present severe occlusal wear; but malocclusion, extractions and conservative or prosthetic dentistry, as well as home prophylaxis, may collectively or separately greatly increase the evidences of wear in various parts of a tooth. It is because some of these effects are not readily recognized or understood that they have received special attention by the author in shorter papers as well as in the present work.

Some of the dental characters considered in this analysis have been designated in kinds or groups that have facilitated recognition of the scope of morphological variation and of their significance therein.

(a) Type

Type or family characters relate to kinds of teeth such as incisors, canines, premolars and molars. They can distinguish upper teeth from lower; incisal edges and occlusal surfaces; convexity and concavity of outlines and profiles; relation of these to basic geometrical forms; relation of axes of crown or root or whole tooth to profiles; cusps, their number and disposition; occlusal ridges and grooves, their style and location; cervical lines, form and height, as on M and D; roots, number and disposition of branches; root ridges and grooves; root form in transverse section, relation to geometrical forms; angularity and flattening, relation of asymmetry to sidedness.

(b) Personal

These characters tend to be found throughout the dentition of one person and probably bear some relation to that person's somatic type and stature (see also ethnic characters).

They are found in crowns, convexity of surfaces, and enamel characters—smoothness, thickness, etc. (Pickerill, 1912).

Occlusal ridges, primary and secondary grooves and fissures (morphological and histological characters may relate to one another).

Cusps, longer or shorter, acuminate or blunt.

Roots, slender or robust, long or short.

Root elements, tendency towards early or late furcation, or fusion.

Root branches, tendency towards divergence or otherwise.

(c) Imposed

These characters arise from anatomical relationships at the time of formation of the crown or root of a tooth. (Some, in roots, might equally be classed as acquired characters consequent on malocclusion.)

In crowns, the compressed type in upper molars.

In roots, curves or "bends" imposed by relationship to adjacent anatomical structures—nasal fossae, maxillary sinus for upper teeth, and inferior dental and mental canals for lower teeth. For both upper and lower teeth the relation of personal characters of tooth root to variations in extent of sinuses and amount of basal bone is a likely additional factor which may impose root conformity.

A tooth which is obstructed so that it must erupt into malocclusion will present various styles of root curvature imposed upon it during emergence.

(d) Complexity

Additional elements in crown or root or both (such as Opc), complicate the "normal" morphology of a tooth. Tubercles, pits, additional ridges, grooves and fissures, which may or may not be associated with a recognizable Opc, increase tooth complexity.

(e) Acquired

These characters may alter normal morphology during tooth formation, or may modify the form or appearance of the completed tooth. They may result from pathology, trauma, function or personal habits, or combinations of these. Hypoplastic enamel may be caused by an exanthematous illness, or by an abscessed deciduous tooth. Caries may be combined with the injury of dilaceration (Fig. 6-38 *d*). The many forms of tissue loss (wear, abrasion, fracture etc.) are acquired characters, as also are the depositions of stain and calculus, and hypercementosis. Among pathological effects are resorption in permanent teeth, and dental caries. Treatment by restorations, by extraction of teeth, with or without prosthetic replacements, all lead to discernible characters in remaining teeth. A mutilated dentition is one where decay or extractions or other conditions are followed by malocclusion through drifting of teeth, and there may be a variety of sequelae. The deflected emerging tooth, erupting to malocclusion with a curved or twisted root (Fig. 6-20 *c,d,f*), has been mentioned under imposed characters, but the result may also be regarded as an acquired character. So also is the effect of orthodontic treatment, as in Figure 6-36 *a,b*.

(f) Ethnic

It does seem that there are ethnic characters in teeth but, as with some bodily physical characters, they are difficult to establish either qualitatively or quantitatively. They may be recognized as a tendency to be present, according to the degree in which they occur, as for example the "shovel" character in incisors. But whether their wide dispersal in an ethnic sense reflects the degree of miscegenation, or the potential for diversification in dental development which has here been recognized as variation, one cannot say. Pickerill (1912, p. 57) showed differences in enamel thickness at the cervices of Maori and European molar teeth, but does not appear to have established that the difference was in fact an ethnic character rather than merely selected examples of variation within the species. Be that as it may, a study of many specimens within an ethnic group can develop in the observer a "feeling" for that material. Whether this comes mainly from familiarity with the morphological and acquired characters of the teeth themselves, or from the dentitions in their relations to the skulls, or from a combination of these, is perhaps questionable. One does however reach the stage when, on being handed a specimen of unknown origin, he can say that it might well belong to a group with which he is familiar, or, alternatively, that he would not expect to find a similar specimen within that group.

Returning to the recording and implications of the data that can be obtained from a tooth, and their application to assist in personal identification or in dental forensics, can it be said that the tooth could, or could not, have formed part of a dentition concerning which certain records are available?

With the tooth identified, notes should be made of its type characters as also its personal and acquired characters as indicated in this study, so that they may be checked against the dentist's records, and the report completed. It goes without saying that examination of the tooth should be thorough, for there are pitfalls for the unwary. Severe wear of a tooth is obvious, but its explanation in unusual positions may require some clinical or ethnological knowledge. Lack of this may also result in overlooking light wear which nevertheless can appreciably alter morphological characters of a tooth. For example, very little wear on the cusp tip of a canine tooth can alter its apparent character from acuminate to rounded. But the reverse can also take place, as was shown in Figure 5-7 *c,d,e*. In the second example the tooth may have erupted with a rounded cusp, but now has two straight shoulders meeting at an obtuse angle. The important point here is that the character of the cusp has been quite changed, although the amount of tooth substance lost was so little that the presence of these facets could easily be overlooked. Harvey (1976) describes a case where very small areas of hypoplasia on the cusp tips of canines were significantly related to bite marks on a murder victim.

It has been reasonable sometimes to generalize, as with references to upper or lower teeth, to incisors or canines, to single-rooted or multi-rooted teeth, to premolars or molars and so on, but most statements must carry some qualification or restriction. Again, since there is so much to consider under a particular heading, the force of a generalization may be lost in subsequent detail. For this reason discussion of variation in each kind of tooth was not necessarily restricted to details applicable only to that tooth. Early in some chapters, later in others, consideration has been given to aspects of variation that had already been mentioned, but which in the later context were again relevant, or served to add emphasis to the earlier discussion.

In some earlier chapters suggestions were given in detail for identification and description of particular teeth and it should not be difficult to adapt the procedure for other teeth. While this report has been concerned primarily with variation, it is also a contribution to forensic odontology. Indeed the descriptive and graphic details presented all have a direct application in that field, and emphasize the potential value of data that could easily be recorded by dentists through their daily work, without sophisticated equipment. To make these better records, although beyond the practitioner's own immediate needs, might well be regarded by that profession as obligatory, since their training and opportunity for such a service is unique.

Variation and Taxonomy

The great amount of work and technical skill represented by the photographs of endocasts presented by Korenhof (1960) has enriched our knowledge of the initial morphology of occlusal features of upper molar teeth. It is likely that some descriptions in the present work would have been modified if similar casts had been available, because the comparison of endocasts and occlusal surfaces shows how the morphology of those features has changed from the beginning of calcification to their completion. The relation of this early morphology to the final form of crown and root of the whole tooth is not known, nor is even the external morphology of the teeth whose endocasts were made. The making of endocasts (or their equivalent by solution of enamel) for mature teeth must destroy the material studied, or greatly reduce the number of teeth that could be studied. Deductions from endocasts of crowns can at best therefore be based on a fraction of essential information. The method of the present study permits much more complete data to be obtained from very many more teeth, and this appears a sound basis for descriptive morphological analysis of variation. The results appear also to be a reasonable basis for doubting the validity of some hypotheses concerning evolutionary significance, when they are based on data from too few teeth about which too little can be ascertained.

Thus one might well review hypotheses based on fossils of the "precursors" of man and his "relations." Where is the evidence that variation as here presented is something new? Indeed there is increasing evidence to support the notion that there has always been variation. Williams (1914) established that the three basic types and their combinations so clearly seen in man are similarly demonstrable in anthropoids. It follows surely that they must be found also in primitive man, if only there were sufficient material with dental morphological details not removed by wear. This is important.

We have shown that normal variation is wide, and no tooth is typical in an ethnic sense. Why then should a dentition or skull, or part of either, be accorded special generic or specific status because it has different details? These differences may well be variations within a normal range, though somctimcs with fcatures suggesting long isolation or special function. Without a broader base taxonomy may tumble.

Anomaly, Atavism or Variation

In the earlier stages of the study it was intended to omit "anomalous" teeth from analysis of variation. When dealing with upper molars, however, it was realized that a high proportion of them could be regarded as containing additional elements. Since there were so many gradations or intermediate examples of some characters, exclusion of these teeth would have led to very inadequate coverage of the material. As the writer had the opportunity to make good some of the deficiencies that were noted concerning published textbooks and atlases of dental anatomy, he undertook the difficult task of analysis of these variations.

Because of the numbers, it was possible to select apparently different varieties and yet find also many cases that appeared related to them. This suggested that classification should not be highly definitive but broadly based. It followed that if there were gradations or links connecting many variations, their occurrence pointed to the operation of a capacity or potential for variation which was still within genetic control as to specific type, basic and personal characters. Alternative hypotheses have explained such variations as atavistic and have been supported by examples presenting a character that was reminiscent of a character found in a fossil specimen.

The data presented may be taken to discredit the atavistic hypotheses on two main counts: Firstly, because an alternative explanation is available; secondly, because it implies a dismal failure of Nature. To elaborate the second, it would be necessary to concede that Nature is earnestly trying to resurrect a few details (which themselves may have been fortuitous occurrences through operation of the same potential for variation), and failing miserably in most cases to come anywhere near the mark. Such failure is incompatible with the otherwise precise genetic control of specific characters.

Scope and Method—Evaluation

Although the range of variation in style and in degree is so great, it is inevitable that among the infinite number of teeth many seem to be similar. Closer examination always reveals differences. As similarities are limited, so also are conclusions that may be drawn from them, and in doing this the differences may not be excluded. Indeed they are in some ways more important, for against them may be tested various hypotheses which have had no better support than a relatively few selected cases.

The wide basis of the present study and the outlines drawn to scale have together produced visible and accurate evidence from more specimens than previously attempted. The method has enabled immediate comprehension of the characters discussed and has established guidelines to enable teeth to be described easily, yet in more effective detail than the inadequate presentation in textbooks of dental anatomy.

It has been shown that teeth can be described without measurement and that variation is comprehensible without complicated formulae in statistical terms, which are incomprehensible to the great majority of people, and of only imaginary significance to others. It has also been demonstrated that individual teeth or groups of teeth *in situ* are unsuitable for measurement, firstly because the morphology of a tooth is lacking in precise anatomical landmarks, and secondly because of the nature of variation. This makes it impossible for any particular tooth, or hypothetical average, to be acceptably representative of its kind or of any ethnic group.

With the number of teeth studied and the methods employed a wide net has been cast, and the big catch of variations has been given detailed analysis. Many cases of dental variation, often by virtue of unusual size or morphology, as in third molars, have hitherto been grouped under a vague classification as anomalies. Illustration of an individual specimen, with the honour of a published account of its surgical removal, or its relegation to a dental museum, seldom extends beyond description. Discussion of the significance of the tooth as part of a human dentition has been difficult because of its apparently unique morphology and of the lack of an available dental atlas or analysis of variation.

It is believed that this lack will be largely overcome through the present work, for many of the formerly neglected or misunderstood forms are shown to have their place within normal variation. One might reasonably concede that some of the more extreme cases could be called "aberrant," for that term at least rescues them from relegation to the realms of anomalies where they would be denied an acceptable place in the Creation. It is certain that many are not products of pathology, although sometimes the line of demarcation is not clear. Moreover it must be conceded that in some cases a pathological condition might have influenced the direction of development of an aberrant specimen.

Reference has just been made to the many similarities as well as differences that contribute to the study of variation. It is not contradictory to say that both are present in a particular case because there are many characters, and there are degrees of development; so that some characters may be prominent and some less so or relatively insignificant. Teeth may be similar in some characters such as number of cusps and root branches, relative or actual size of crown and root, or convexity and curvatures of these; and yet teeth may be quite different as regards primary and secondary occlusal grooves and ridges. Alternatively, crowns may be similar but the roots may present differences in number or divergence of root branches or in position of the furcation, in curvature or sturdiness or style of apex, and so on.

Out of the bewilderment of possibilities, all of which may be expected to "turn up" if the search is sufficiently extensive, an important fact does emerge. We have established that in regard to association of styles or of degrees of variation, whether in crown or root, in the teeth of one dentition, or in corresponding teeth of related persons, there is no pattern of consistency. The nearest that we have found in the way of exception to this rule relates to personal characters, where, for example, the teeth of one dentition may tend to have greater or less convexity of crown surfaces, or slender or sturdy or long roots.

The lack of consistency referred to relates rather to branching or fusion of roots, to position of furcation of roots, presence of additional elements in crown or root, style of such elements, degree of their development, position in the tooth, and so on. There may be a surprise awaiting the dental surgeon who has not made a radiograph before extracting teeth (and even sometimes when he has). Thus an extracted tooth may be found to have a certain character of root, but its companion on the other side may not have such, or *vice versa.* This particular character may well be one that calls for modification in the surgeon's technique if complications are to be avoided, and so he must be constantly alert and prepared.

As for the implications of the finding that there is no pattern of consistency in the association of various aspects of variation, elaboration is necessary in two respects. The first is to justify it. The preceding paragraphs partly summarize the finding, but the whole of this study supports it. The second is to comment on its significance.

The haphazard occurrence and almost infinite range and variety of association of so many characters do not support the contention that some variations are an expression of a kind of genetic memory. On the contrary, the more one becomes aware of what does occur, the stronger is the conviction that collectively these differences testify rather to an inherent potential (within specific and some other limitations) for growing tissues to diversify.

In addition to rejection of the genetic memory as explanation of variation, one may add the equally unacceptable notion that some other particular manifestations of variation have a prophetic significance regarding the direction of human evolution.

The great number of characters possessed by any tooth and subject to variation have been demonstrated; also the lack of consistency in degree of their development and of their association with most other characters has been shown. It follows that within the bounds of species and type of tooth there is a degree of permutation and combination of characters. The results do not lend themselves to precise classification in any way, but how to recognize and describe them has been seen, so that the overall picture is not one of confusion but rather of an orderly diversification.

It is this diversity of dental characters that is part of the normal variation that makes people of particular interest as individuals, while retaining other more or less "exclusive" characters that serve to distinguish them as members of a particular ethnic group.

No dental characters have been found that are exclusive in this way, although there is a tendency for some, such as the so-called "shovel" incisor, to be more easily recognized in some groups (Moorrees, 1957). Certain conclusions have been made in the present report regarding the significance of dental characters because of their range and nature. Their diversity also has been shown to have a very definite and useful application in the forensic field.

Teeth are like fingerprints—everyone is different. As with fingerprints, there are characters and details that do not change through life. Unlike those of fingerprints, some dental characters persist indefinitely after death. There are more teeth than digits and they present many more characters. Some of these are personal characters in that they may be recognized in other teeth of the same dentition, and many dental characters may be recognized by naked-eye examination without any assistance from sophisticated equipment. Much useful data therefore can readily be obtained from teeth. Teeth, like fingerprints, are individual, but teeth are infinitely more eloquent.

Appendix 1

TOOTH DESIGNATIONS: THE FDI SYSTEM

THE GREATER PART of this report, including the figures, was completed before the two-digit system of tooth designation proposed by the special committee on uniform dental recording of the Fédération Dentaire Internationale (Leatherman, 1971) was introduced. It was not practicable to change the system used in the already completed parts of the work, and therefore the long-accepted graphic system of notation has been retained throughout.

The graphic system gives a number to permanent teeth (1 to 8, in each quadrant), and a letter (A to E, or a to e) to deciduous teeth, always starting from the central incisor. The quadrant is indicated graphically by a right angle within which the number of the tooth is placed. The horizontal line distinguishes between an upper or lower tooth, and the vertical part of the right angle indicates left or right. The right angle indicates the quadrant as seen when facing the person. Thus the symbol 2⌉ refers to the lower right second incisor, and 6⌋ is the upper right first permanent molar. For left teeth, ⌈3 is the lower canine and ⌈8 is the lower third molar, and so on.

In the two-digit system, permanent teeth are numbered as before, and deciduous teeth are similarly numbered (1 to 5) in each quadrant. Instead of using the graphic right angle lines to indicate upper or lower, and left or right teeth, a number is allocated to each quadrant. This quadrant number is placed before the tooth number, and it is essential to remember this order to avoid confusion. It is also essential to memorize the order in which the eight quadrants (for permanent and deciduous teeth) are numbered.

The FDI system facilitates clerical counting of operations for institutions or state departments, and no doubt it will be favoured where sophisticated facilities are available to the specialist worker, but its disadvantages should be obvious to the scientist. There are many possibilities for designation of a quite different tooth from the one intended, through accidental reversal of the digits. Such errors would easily be overlooked, for the system bears no visual check. These mistakes could be accepted into a data bank and the resulting error pass undetected.

This two-digit system is further vulnerable to human error through difficulty in learning and reading it, for it lacks consistency in the sequence numbering of quadrants. Thus in the upper jaw, right precedes left, but in the lower jaw left precedes right.

Examples of confusion arise from accidental reversal of digits. For example, the symbols 14 and 41 designate respectively the upper right first premolar and the lower right central permanent incisor. Similarly, 28 and 82 designate the upper left third molar and the lower right second deciduous incisor.

The graphic system has a precise visual impact concerning type and position of the designated tooth, the only likely error being an occasional confusion of left and right. It has the advantages of being both simple and consistent. As a result it is easy to learn and to read, and will convey a clearer message to a wider field of readers.

The following is to assist those who are more familiar with one system than with the other:

R		L
	Upper | Upper	
	Lower | Lower	

becomes

1	2
4	3

for permanent teeth

and

5	6
8	7

for deciduous teeth.

TOOTH DESIGNATION CONVERSION TABLE

Permanent Teeth

	(upper right)								(upper left)							
Graphic	8⌋	7⌋	6⌋	5⌋	4⌋	3⌋	2⌋	1⌋	⌊1	⌊2	⌊3	⌊4	⌊5	⌊6	⌊7	⌊8
F D I	18	17	16	15	14	13	12	11	21	22	23	24	25	26	27	28
F D I	48	47	46	45	44	43	42	41	31	32	33	34	35	36	37	38
Graphic	8⌉	7⌉	6⌉	5⌉	4⌉	3⌉	2⌉	1⌉	⌈1	⌈2	⌈3	⌈4	⌈5	⌈6	⌈7	⌈8
	(lower right)								(lower left)							

Deciduous Teeth

	(upper right)					(upper left)				
Graphic	E⌋	D⌋	C⌋	B⌋	A⌋	⌊A	⌊B	⌊C	⌊D	⌊E
F D I	55	54	53	52	51	61	62	63	64	65
F D I	85	84	83	82	81	71	72	73	74	75
Graphic	E⌉	D⌉	C⌉	B⌉	A⌉	⌈A	⌈B	⌈C	⌈D	⌈E
	(lower right)					(lower left)				

Appendix 2

IDENTIFICATION OF TOOTH SURFACES

In both text and figures, tooth surfaces are referred to by capital letters: M = mesial, O = occlusal, D = distal, B = buccal, L = lingual, P = palatal (= lingual of an upper tooth). These letters, on diagrams and in figures generally, assist in orientation of the tooth and in identification of the surface illustrated. Further identification is provided by the symbols explained in Appendix 1. Mesial and distal surfaces are collectively referred to as approximal or proximal surfaces, but no symbol is used for these terms.

The letters L and R are used for left and right, but no confusion is likely to arise from the use of L also to indicate lingual.

The symbols M-D and B-P are used for "mesial to distal dimension or diameter" and "buccal to palatal dimension or diameter" respectively. When a lower tooth is referred to it is necessary to use B-L instead of B-P.

Appendix 3

SULCUS, GROOVE, FISSURE

Black (1901) complained that "the words sulcus, groove and fissure are often used as if they were synonymous and interchangeable, which has given rise to much confusion." He then describes and defines the terms fossa, sulcus, groove, fault, fissure and developmental and supplemental grooves (Op. cit. pp. 11-13).

In dental anatomy and anthropology, and in dentistry, the terms "groove" and "fissure" are very frequently used, and "fossa" and "sulcus" less often; but seldom are any of them used with the conciseness of meaning desired by Black. Admittedly, some fogginess persists around these terms, probably because the features concerned do not readily fit into precise definitions that may be mutually exclusive. Our familiar occlusal groove or fissure would evidently be "sulcate groove," "sulcate fissure," or "sulcate fault" in Black's terminology. Presumably, then, the corresponding feature of two teeth must bear one of these names but not necessarily the same one in each case. In actual fact, however, it is easy to find a tooth where more than one of these terms could be applied to different parts of the same feature. The difficulty in choosing the correct term thus appears to depend, in part, on ability to recognize histological as well as anatomical characters, an unnecessarily fine distinction in the great majority of instances. The claim that differences can be determined by use of a fine probe or explorer this author rejects emphatically, as there would still be variable factors apart from the impossibility of maintaining an explorer point of standard fineness and taper. It will therefore be accepted that the terms "fissure" and "groove" are reasonably interchangeable and convenient, and that almost all risk of confusion will be avoided if such terms as buccal, occlusal, developmental, etc., are added when it seems advisable.

Appendix 4

THE SUPPORTING COLLECTION

IN ADDITION to a collection of comparative dental anatomy and human skeletal material, the writer has a large collection of extracted teeth, the great majority of which are from European New Zealanders, but a few could be of Maori origin or from a racial mixture. These were obtained, mostly in Wellington but also from Auckland and other parts of New Zealand, between 1927 and 1947, without records of age, sex or race. Subsequently there were additions from the writer's own conservative practice.

Illustrations for the present work are mostly from teeth selected for morphological integrity, mounted on cards in small groups either from one person or to illustrate a particular character. Other major groups comprised deciduous teeth and aspects of pathology.

In the ten chapters there are 267 figures which contain 218 diagrams and also 2,549 outlines drawn to scale. These outlines represent 1,715 teeth, mostly from the mounted portion of the collection. This comprises 773 cards (in 19 series) on which 4,642 teeth have been mounted. A few illustrations are taken from unmounted teeth or from skeletal fragments, or from radiographs of teeth *in situ* in living persons.

The smaller collection of teeth from the writer's own practice is accompanied by relevant data (history or radiograph, sex, and often age, especially where the teeth were premolars removed for orthodontic reasons). Apart from the 4,642 teeth just mentioned which were mounted and allocated to the various series, there are some 2,913 permanent teeth which have been sorted and studied, so there are at least 7,555 in the dental anatomy group.

The collection of deciduous teeth remains largely unexploited. These total approximately 4,314 and would fall into two main groups. Many have perfect or nearly perfect crowns, and they had either been shed naturally, or shedding had been "assisted," to remove obstruction to an erupting tooth or to alleviate irritation. Others constitute a unique group for the study of root form, fusion and divergence of root branches, and of the great variety in style of root resorption.

What might be called applied anatomy in removal of deciduous teeth is a small field, but it can present difficulties. Dealing with these difficulties has been assisted by looking over this material. Invariably these teeth had been extracted because of pulp involvement or alveolar abscess, for in the earlier years of the New Zealand School Dental Service unsaveable deciduous teeth were commonly found at the time of initial treatments in new patients. Before long, a policy of earlier treatment, as well as preventive and conservative measures, gained control of the situation, so that for many years now the children mostly have had functional deciduous, or mixed, dentitions in clean mouths. Thus it would not now be possible in this country to collect so many deciduous teeth with complete, or only partly resorbed, roots.

There is a large number of teeth (few of them deciduous) that have been selected for their evident direct involvement or association with pathological conditions. In many cases there are two or more similarly affected teeth, and often these comprise groups from individuals. There are at least 150 of these groups with 551 teeth. The pathology collection also includes 202 deciduous teeth (of which 42 have been sectioned, and 5,142 loose permanent teeth (of which 236 have been sectioned). The total for the pathology collection therefore is not less than 5,895 teeth. The writer hastens to add that he does not propose to report on these, nor on the deciduous collection, even if he should happen to be reincarnated.

There are mounted teeth on 220 cards which have not been allocated to a series, making a total of 993 cards in the collection. Teeth mounted in series (4,642), plus teeth in the rest of the collection (8,909 permanent and 4,314 deciduous), amount to a grand total of not less than 17,865 teeth. These, however, do not comprise the whole background to the report, nor was the latter limited to academic studies. In addition there has been the vast multitude of human teeth examined in teaching and field work, as well as the rich experience associated with years of clinical practice.

Appendix 5

RELATION OF CUSP TIP AND CERVICAL CREST TO ROOT AXIS IN LOWER CANINES

THIS TABLE refers to outlines of teeth which are examples of the varieties represented by the diagrams of Figure 5-28 and discussed in the text on p. 195. The letters M and D designate whether the tooth is seen from mesial or distal. The "turn-around" contours in broken lines in those outlines are not included here. For example, in Group 1, style *a*, the reference M 5-22 *g* is to the mesial contour given in Figure 5-22 *g*.

Style	Group 1	Group 2	Group 3
a	M 5-22 *g*	M 5-19 *b*	Not
		M 5-25 *a*	applicable
b	M 5-20 *e*	M 5-5 *f*	D 5-5 *c*
	M 5-21 *d*	M 5-9 *c*	D 5-5 *d*
		M D 5-16 *b*	D 5-5 *e*
		M 5-19 *c*	M 5-8 *d*
		M 5-19 *f*	D 5-9 *b*
		M 5-21 *a*	D 5-10 *d*
		M 5-22 *b*	M 5-10 *f*
		M 5-22 *g*	M 5-22 *c*
		D 5-24 *f*	D 5-24 *e*
		D 5-26 *d*	M 5-25 *d*
c	Not	M 5-8 *c*	M 5-1 *b*
	applicable	M 5-21 *c*	M 5-9 *e*
		M 5-25 *c*	M 5-17 *c*
			M 5-20 *c*
			M 5-21 *e*

Appendix 6

THE PILTDOWN PAPER

REFERENCES HAVE BEEN made in this work to the author's "Piltdown" paper which was read at the Meeting of The Australian and New Zealand Association for the Advancement of Science in January 1937 at Auckland. That paper (Taylor, 1937b) was the writer's first report on dental morphology, and the principles established therein were demonstrated from plaster casts of the fragments, and of the generally accepted restoration of the whole skull by Smith Woodward (1918). That those principles were soundly based was confirmed many years later when tests on the actual fragments confirmed their fraudulent association (Weiner et al., 1953; Weiner and Oakley, 1954).

The writer's arguments in the Piltdown paper are the primordial base on which the present report has been developed. The widened application of recognizable morphological asymmetry has shown its importance in determination of sidedness and positive identification of teeth or parts thereof.

The 1937 paper presented proof for the first time that the Piltdown canine tooth was an upper tooth and not a lower, as placed in the restoration. It showed further that the rest of the hypothetical dentition could never have existed.

The story of the finding of the fragments near Piltdown Common in Sussex (Dawson and Woodward, 1918) and of their subsequent incorporation in a restoration as Piltdown Man is well documented, and by 1918 the Piltdown literature had amounted to about 120 papers by fifty authors.

The following extracts are taken verbatim from the 1937 paper, and the accompanying figures are selected from the "lantern slides" shown on that occasion. They comprise portions of the argument that are most relevant to the present report on variation in morphology.

Further, I will demonstrate that the actual tooth which was found subsequently does not confirm the conclusion that the canine teeth should interlock in the true ape-fashion, for such conclusion ignores the alternative possibility that the canine teeth may have overlapped in a true human-fashion often seen in modern man. Again it will be shown that the surface of wear produced on modern teeth may resemble closely that on the Piltdown tooth.

Smith Woodward (1918) gives excellent illustrations of the Piltdown fragments and very interesting comparisons. I must however draw attention to the different directions of the axes of the crowns of the canine teeth in the compared jaws of the ape and of the Piltdown restoration (Fig. 5 of the "Guide" as below). The cusp tips as a result are in quite different positions as in Figure 6. Again, in the comparison of the occluded jaws it is evident that the canines of the Piltdown restoration do not interlock in the manner depicted as "the true ape-fashion" (Figs. 1 and 7). These figure numbers are from the British Museum Guide (Woodward, 1918).

The restored form of the upper canine tooth and its manner of occlusion are hypothetical, and in both respects it is abnormal. I believe these dental abnormalities in the restoration have resulted from an error of judgment whereby the canine tooth fragment was regarded as the lower right tooth instead of the upper left.

I find that others also have expressed the opinion that the canine tooth is an upper left, but that it belonged to a species of chimpanzee instead of to the cranial fragments. Among these are Miller (1915, 1918), Osborn (1915) and Gregory (1914).

In order to establish the claim regarding the identity of the tooth it will be necessary to consider the fundamental difference between upper and lower teeth in general and between upper and lower canines in particular. The Piltdown tooth will then be studied in regard to the characters discussed.

Basic Features of Form in Upper and Lower Teeth

In most mammals there are certain features that distinguish upper teeth from lowers, features that are associated with normal occlusion. In the human series differentiation is made easily when the normal tooth presents more than one cusp or root, but with canine teeth it may be more difficult. After a close study of great numbers of teeth, I find that even though variations in size and form are the rule, upper and lower canine teeth have their own morphological characters. These characters are so constantly present that they may be regarded as basic.

Since function is similar in both the upper and lower canines, these characteristic features are associated primarily with the normal relationship of the teeth during function, and they also bear a relation to the structure and variations of neighbouring anatomical parts. It is well known that in normal occlusion the tips of the upper incisors and canines, and the buccal cusps of the upper premolars and molars, rest outside the corresponding parts of the lower teeth. In connection with this fact it is customary to state that the upper teeth are arranged in a larger curve than are the lower teeth. This is usually considered sufficient explanation of the overlapping, but since it is only partly true it is unsatisfactory from a scientific point of view. The relative size of the arches of the jaw varies according to the part of the tooth considered, and the variations are due partly to the directions of the long axes of the teeth and partly to the relation of the cusps to these axes.

I find that the buccal and lingual cervices of upper and lower teeth normally lie in vertical relationship to each other, and yet it is known that the cusp tips are not so related but interdigitate so that the buccal cusps of the upper teeth occlude outside the buccal cusps of the lower teeth. Similarly, the upper incisors and canines overlap the lowers. It is important to understand how this interdigitation is possible in the presence of a vertical relationship of the cervices. It is then much easier to distinguish between upper and lower teeth.

In the posterior teeth the apparent overlapping of the upper arch beyond the lower follows from the varying position of the cusp tips in regard to the long axes of the teeth (Fig. 7, part 3). The condition may be described by saying that the buccal surface of the lower tooth "slopes in" more from cervix to occlusal than does the lingual, and that in the upper tooth the greater slope is on the lingual surface.

In both the upper and the lower canines

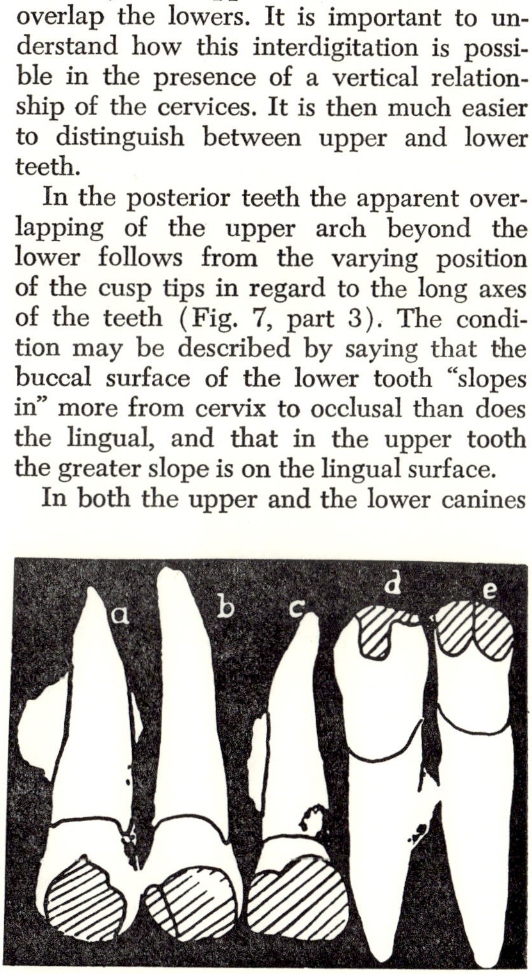

Figure 1. *a,b,c,* lingual view of upper human canines showing the areas of attritional wear, shaded, confined to the lingual surface. *d, e,* labial view of lower canines showing the areas of attritional wear, shaded, confined to the labial surface. The different proportions of the crowns of upper and lower canines are apparent in these teeth, and in Figure 2 *d,e*.

the curvature of the labial and lingual surfaces, and the position of the cusp with regard to the long axis of the tooth, correspond to the condition just described for the molars. This can be seen best by examining the profile of the tooth (Fig. 7, part 2). Again, the broken lines show the vertical relationship of the labial and lingual cervices. In both teeth a line has been drawn from the tip of the cusp to the root apex, and the thick lines show that in the lower tooth this axial line is nearer the lingual, whereas in the upper tooth it is nearer the labial surface.

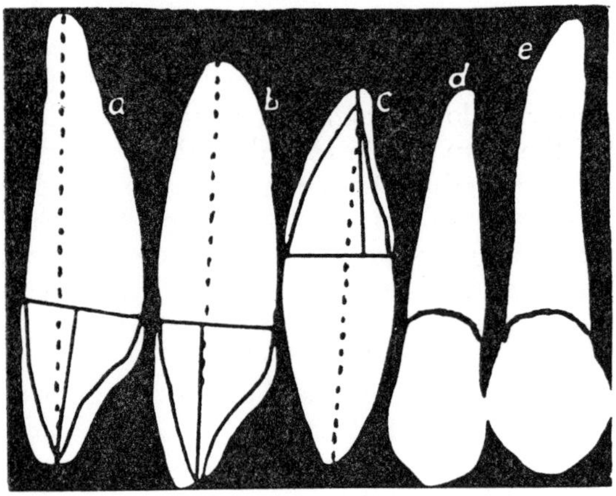

Figure 2. Human canine teeth illustrating characteristic differences between uppers and lowers. *a,b,* upper canines in labio-lingual longitudinal section. The axial line from cusp to apex (broken line) is nearer to the labial surface than to the lingual. A line has been drawn joining labial and lingual cervix, and a perpendicular to this line has been drawn from the cusp tip. The perpendicular cuts the cervical line nearer the labial side. *c,* lower canine similarly sectioned. The arc-like curve from cusp to apex is obvious. The axial line is nearer to the lingual surface. The amelo-dentinal junction has been marked in these three teeth. In *a* and *b* the enamel tip has been worn off. The characteristics just described in these three teeth should be compared with the diagrams of Figure 6 (part 1), 7 (part 2). *d,e,* labial views of lower and upper canines respectively, with the cervix marked. Compare the relatively long slender lower crown with the relatively short broad crown characteristic of the upper, and in *e* note the slight distal curve of the root, so commonly found in these teeth.

Without having drawn or visualized the axial line to the apex, the same fact may be observed by examination of the crown of the tooth alone. From the cusp tip a perpendicular is taken to a line joining the labial and lingual cervices (Fig. 6, part 1). This line is cut by the perpendicular in different proportions in different teeth but almost invariably the shorter portion is toward the labial in the upper tooth and toward the lingual in the lower tooth. The positions of axis and perpendicular in actual teeth may be verified in the photographs (Fig. 2 *a,b,c*). In cases of attrition or wear of the teeth, if the perpendicular is made to pass through the most prominent edge of each tooth, the difference noted between upper and lower teeth is even greater (Fig. 6, part 2).

The crown of a lower canine is relatively long and slender compared with the shorter and more thickset upper crown (Fig. 2 *d,e*). The upper tooth has a more definite lingual cingulum and a labial longitudinal ridge from cusp to cervix. Recognition of all these differences enables one to distinguish between upper and lower canines.

If one looks at an upper canine, end-on, it will be found that the outline is not symmetrical. Outlines for right and left canines (from the same subject) obtained in this way are shown in the photographs (Fig. 3 *f,g*). In this case each cusp has been ground off to facilitate focussing of the camera on the desired region of the teeth. The details of these outlines are shown more clearly in the diagrams (Fig. 5). For the right canine the parts corresponding to the various tooth surfaces have been named. In the lower figures the curves representing these surfaces have been reduced to straight lines for clarity regarding their relative lengths. It will be observed that the labial outline has two components, the angle between them representing the ridge that extends longitudinally from cusp-tip to cervix. In the present instance the important features of the outline are the parts corresponding to the mesial and distal surfaces. It is clear that the mesial surface is wider than the distal. This has been emphasized by marking more thickly along the mesial the equivalent width of the distal side.

The significance of the different widths of these parts is that it enables one positively to identify and distinguish between the mesial and distal surfaces. Thus, even though the root be broken off and the crown modified by attrition, one may determine to which side of the mouth the tooth belonged. At the cervix the outline is similar except that the angle between the labial and distal surfaces is less prominent, and the outline as a whole is more nearly elliptical.

In most lower canines it will be found that the labial outline in profile forms an arc from cusp to apex, exclusive of the small subsidiary labial bend sometimes found at the apex. The axial line forms the chord of the arc, and the lingual outline of the root for the greater part of its length is often parallel to the axial line (Figs. 2 *c*, and 7, part 2). In the upper canine the whole root may show a distal curve (Figs. 2 *e*, and 1 *a,b,c*) and/or some degree of labial curvature. These curves are associated with the proximity of the root to the nasal fossa and orbit and with variations in the form of the maxillary antrum.

The Production of Attritional Wear on Canine Teeth

In order to understand the various forms of attritional faceting or wear that may be produced in these teeth it is necessary to study their interrelationship both in occlusion and also during the movements of incision and mastication. The usual overlap when at rest in occlusion varies from less than one third to about one half of the length of the crown of the tooth, but it may be greater. The movements that initiate attrition are mostly incisive and take place in the direction indicated by the arrow-heads (Fig. 7, part 1).

In the early stages attritional wearing will be limited to this area of occlusal contact. Later, owing to the loss of tooth substance in this region and to obliteration of the cusps in the posterior teeth, the occlusal plane may become so modified that the anterior teeth tend to acquire an edge-to-edge bite. Before this rather advanced stage is reached, particularly where the overbite is deep, attritional faceting on the incisors and canines is at a steep angle. It commences parallel to the occluding surfaces and gradually becomes more

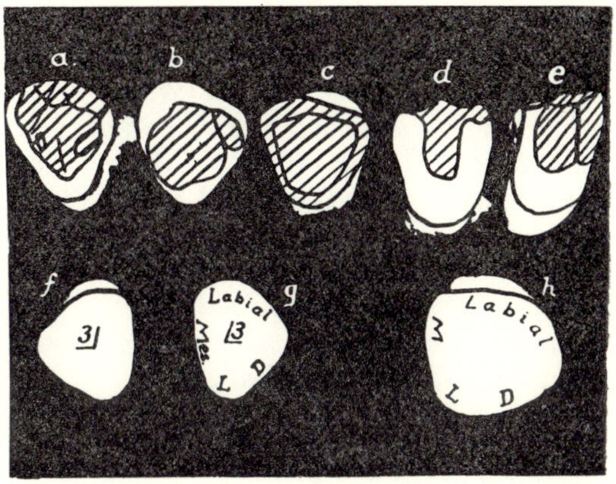

Figure 3. *a,b,c,* occlusal view of upper canine teeth showing the attritional facets, shaded, confined entirely to the lingual surface. (These are the same teeth as in Fig. 1 *a,b,c.*) In tooth *c* the amount of wear and the area involved closely resemble that found in the Piltdown tooth. *d,e,* occlusal view of lower canines showing the attritional facets, shaded, the wear being confined to the labial surface. (These are the same teeth as in Fig. 1 *d,e*). *f,g,* right (3|) and left (|3) upper canines from one person, with the acuminate region of crown removed. These show the "mirror image" symmetry of one to the other, and their individual bilateral asymmetry which enables distinction to be made between left and right teeth. See also Figure 5. *h,* cast of the Piltdown tooth similarly sectioned. The resemblance to the form of |3 is more apparent when the section is made nearer the cervix as in Fig. 4 *e*. M = mesial, D = distal, and L = lingual surface.

nearly horizontal as shown by the dotted lines in the same figure (see also Fig. 6, part 2). There is often a tendency to produce notching of the upper tooth towards the cervical end of the facet. This may be produced by lateral masticatory movements with the mandible in the fully retruded position. The lingual edge of the facet in the lower tooth facilitates the notching of the upper, but when the loss of tooth substance has become excessive, or where the overbite is deep, attritional wear extends to the cingulum of the upper tooth (Fig. 6, part 3).

An important point to note is that at first the wear on the upper tooth with normal overbite is confined to the lingual surface of the crown tip, whereas in the lower tooth it is confined to the labial surface. Also, it will be seen that during most of the stages of attritional wearing, the upper tooth continues to show more wear on the lingual side, while the lower tooth shows it more on the labial side (Fig. 1, and Fig. 3 *a-e*). The attritional plane becomes more nearly horizontal as the edge-to-edge condition is acquired. With a deep overbite this condition may be acquired in a modified form or not at all.

The Relation of Attrition to Occluson in Canine Teeth

In the mammalian dentition it is usual for the lower canine to occlude partly with the upper canine and partly with the upper lateral incisor. This may be associated with an overlap, or there may be a diastema so that the lower canine fits between these teeth. In man the overlapping arrangement is found. In apes, and in other animals with prehensile canines, where the lower canine fits into a space between the upper canine and an incisor, attrition wears away the distal surface of the lower canine and the mesial surface of the upper canine (Fig. 7 of Museum Guide, Woodward, 1918). In man, however, it has been shown that the surfaces affected are the labial of the lower and the lingual of the upper canine. An upper canine worn only on the lingual could not have been associated with a diastema. The Piltdown canine is an upper and is worn in that way; *therefore the diastema given to the restoration cannot be accepted.*

The Occlusion of the Canines in the Piltdown Restoration

In the Piltdown restoration now under discussion considerable attritional wear is found in the tip and on the mesio-labial surface of the hypothetical upper canine, and on the lingual surface of the lower canine. Further, the teeth are set with their crowns so nearly end to end that in the unworn state no other teeth than the canines could have met in occlusion. The restored relationship of these teeth is therefore a malocclusion, and represents a condition that is unlikely to have occurred on account of its instability and the traumatic effects that would inevitably follow. Again, let us suppose that the restored canine occlusion was accepted tentatively; the restorer has postulated the presence of a diastema but presented an arrangement in which there is nothing for a diastema to accommodate. Both features together we could not accept, and I have already shown that it is impossible to accept either of them. The restored occlusion of the canines is quite different from the edge-to-edge bite so often acquired in the later stages of attrition, but the incisors have been given that edge-to-edge occlusion. The presence of both varieties of occlusion in the same mouth appears incompatible.

It seems evident, therefore, that the form or arrangement, or both, of the canines in this restoration is incorrect. But only the lower canine was one of the fragments found, so it follows that the form and position of the upper canine are hypothetical. I have already expressed the opinion that the tooth found is not a lower canine but an upper canine. If this is realized as a fact it will be found that the difficulties regarding attrition and occlusion

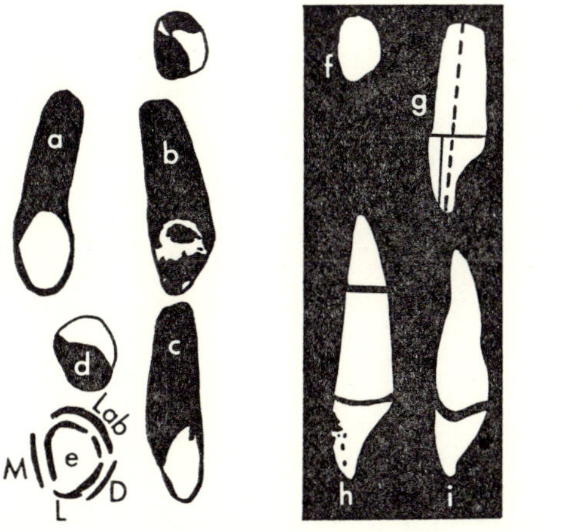

Figure 4. *a-h,* the Piltdown tooth (casts). *i,* natural tooth. *a,* labial view of the tooth showing the root curve to the distal. *b,c,* lingual view *(b)* showing extent of attritional wear, and mesial view *(c)*. *d,* occlusal view of the crown of the tooth, the dark portion being the worn surface. *e,f,* outline of the Piltdown tooth, sectioned approximately at the cervix, to show the bilateral asymmetry which enables the tooth to be identified as belonging to the left side. (See also Fig. 3 *f,g,h* and Fig. 5.) *h,* cast of the Piltdown tooth with the tip restored to the form it could have presented when complete. The line of the truncated root has been marked, also the approximate position of the cervix. *Note.* Owing to loss of enamel from the original tooth, exact determination of the cervix was difficult. The position does not appear to be precisely indicated by the staining differences. *i,* a large modern upper canine human tooth which approaches the Piltdown tooth in size.

disappear. Thus it is desirable that the Piltdown tooth be studied critically for the features already described as basic characters of upper and lower canines.

Description of the Piltdown Tooth

There is no doubt that the Piltdown tooth is a canine rather than an incisor or a premolar. Not only has much of the crown been lost through attritional wear, but also the end of the root is missing (Fig. 4 *a,b,c*) . . .

The amount of attrition indicates that the tooth was in use for a considerable time so that it appears more likely to be a mature and broken tooth than one whose root is incomplete through immaturity. In either case, I feel it is reasonable to suggest that the root, when complete, would have resembled the restoration I have made (Fig. 4 *h*).

From the cast available it could not be determined whether the cusp tip had been broken off or worn off, but since it makes no difference to the argument of this paper, the manner of its loss is not important.

When the position of the axial line is examined it is found to lie definitely nearer to the labial outline, indicating that the tooth is an upper (Fig. 4 *g*). It may be objected that the incomplete root makes this determination impossible, but I claim that the direction of the root gives sufficient guide to the position of the apex in this case. Also, I have shown that the same feature of position of axial line may be determined without the presence of the root, but by examination of the crown only. Again by this test it is found that the tooth resembles an upper canine and not a lower. It may be objected further that, owing to attrition, the apparent position of the cusp tip is not the real position. That may be so, but it has been shown that attrition does not alter the fact that the cusp tip is nearer the labial side; indeed it makes the fact more obvious. A similar argument, *mutatis mutandis,* applies to a lower tooth as regards the effect of attrition on position of the axial line.

In the Piltdown canine the facet is confined almost entirely to the lingual surface and extends from the cusp tip almost to the cervix. The more usual position of the facet has already been illustrated. Thus, the fact that in the Piltdown tooth attrition has reached the lingual cingulum without much loss of substance from the cusp tip, suggests that either the overbite in occlusion was greater than usual or the axes of upper and lower canines were set more obliquely to one another than is usually the case. The probable relationship of the canines to one another has been illus-

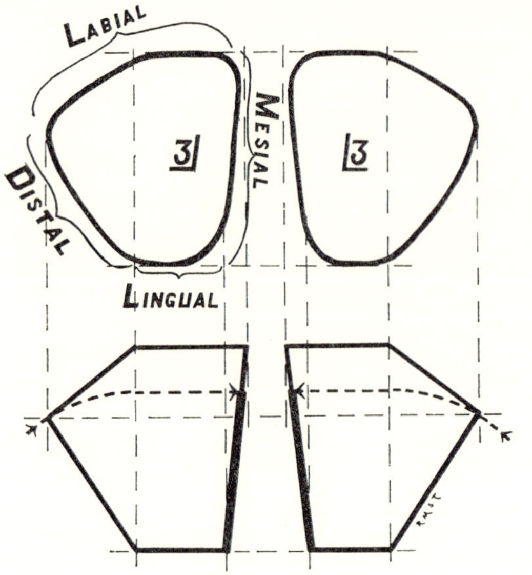

Figure 5. *Upper Figures.* Diagrams representing outlines of sections through the crowns of upper canines near the cervix. The labial and lingual surfaces can be identified, but the diagrams show that mesial and distal surfaces may also be distinguished. The mesial surface is wider than the distal and therefore a tooth may be recognized as left or right. *Lower Figures.* The differences noted above are made more apparent by representing the various surfaces with straight-line outlines. The labial outline has two components meeting to represent the labial ridge. The thickened part of the mesial outline represents the equivalent length of the distal outline. Compare with Figure 3 *f,g*.

trated. In this diagram the form of the lower canine is hypothetical (Fig. 6, part 3).

The position of the facet and the amount of tooth substance lost give an indication of the nature of the masticatory movements that caused attritional wear. Where the overbite is normal, the tips of the incisors and canines may soon be worn off, but it has been shown that one surface of the tooth is affected more than another. This inequality is reduced as wear proceeds, especially where the edge-to-edge bite is acquired. In other words the labial portion of the upper tooth wears more quickly than the lingual portion. The explanation appears to lie in the fact that during the acts of incision and mastication there is more frictional force applied to the incisal portion of the facet and a reduction of force as the jaws reach the position of rest. The incisal portion of the facet, moreover, is more frequently subjected to friction during this act. In the lower tooth the conditions are different because since the lower tooth is the one that moves, the tip is subjected to wear at almost all stages of the movements.

The evidence provided by the canine suggests that the Piltdown individual had not acquired an edge-to-edge bite, but possessed a deep overbite in the anterior teeth, namely the incisors and canines. I believe that the nature of the overbite was modified through its association with some

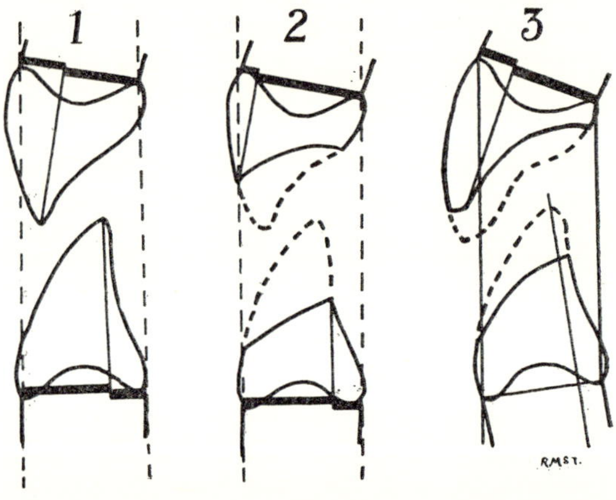

Figure 6. *Part 1.* Normal vertical relationship of crowns of upper and lower canines, and different positions of their cusps associated therewith. Perpendiculars have been drawn from the cusp tips to lines joining labial and lingual cervices in each case. In the upper tooth this line is cut nearer the labial surface, but nearer the lingual surface in the lower. *Part 2.* Where tooth substance has been lost by attrition, the differences just described are accentuated. *Part 3.* The probable relationship of the Piltdown canine teeth. The lower tooth is hypothetical in form, but the upper tooth is drawn from that considered in the present paper. The broken lines show the loss of tooth substance by attrition. Note that while the cervices are in vertical relationship the axes of the tooth are more oblique.

degree of prognathism that must have been present.

Evidence as to the mandibular movements possible is not confined to the canine teeth. Fortunately, two lower molars and one glenoid fossa are intact, and show close resemblance to the corresponding features observed in modern human skulls. That protrusive and lateral movements were possible cannot be doubted. The presence of both would have facilitated obliteration of the cusps and production of the flattened occlusal surface observed in each molar. It may be necessary to explain how protrusive movements could assist in flattening the molars when a deep overbite of the anterior teeth was present. I submit that these conditions would be compatible when the axes of upper and lower anterior teeth are set somewhat obliquely to one another, as shown in Figure 6, part 3. This diagram should be contrasted with Figure 6, part 1, or Figure 7, part 2. If such obliquity of axes existed in the Piltdown individual, it is probable that the front of the arch was not rounded as in the restoration but flattened, the canines forming the angles of the arch. The notion that the canines were so placed is further supported by the position of the attritional facet in regard to the labial surface of the tooth found.

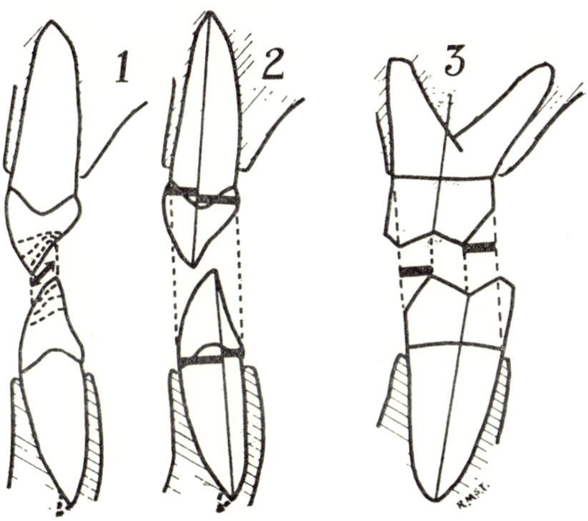

Figure 7. *Part 1.* Distal view of left upper and lower canines to illustrate the initiation and development of attritional faceting in cases of normal slight overbite leading to an edge-to-edge bite. *Part 2.* The relation of upper and lower canines to one another (apart from mesio-distal interdigitation) and the relation of the axial lines to the labial and lingual outlines of these teeth. *Part 3.* The vertical relationship of right upper and lower first molars (apart from mesio-distal interdigitation). This diagram shows how, in the presence of vertical relationship of the cervices, there is bucco-lingual interdigitation of the cusps. This relationship is made possible by the fact that the lower buccal cusps and the upper lingual cusps are "set in" as shown by the short thick lines. The curved outlines of the crowns have been represented by straight lines.

In the restoration the amount of protrusive and of lateral movement is very limited unless the teeth are separated. Therefore, such an occlusion could not have produced flattening of the molars. Similarly, neither the lingual attrition attributed to the lower canine nor the form of attrition given to the hypothetically restored incisors could have been produced by this occlusion.

The evidence so far considered shows that the hypothetically restored occlusion is incompatible with certain features of the known parts of the dentition, particularly as regards the canine teeth. It has been found that the attritional facet is by form and position similar to that normally found in upper canines but not in lowers. As regards the morphological characters of the whole tooth, it is found that the crown is thickset and shows a prominent labial longitudinal ridge. When observed in profile the axial line and the cusp tip are nearer to the labial than to the lingual surface. A transverse section at the cervix shows a broad oval which is characteristic in its form and asymmetry (Fig. 4 *e*). In these features the tooth is again found to resemble an upper canine and not a lower. The asymmetry of the transverse section both at the cervix and in the crown resembles closely the corresponding sections of modern upper left canines. The root curves to the distal, and here again the tooth resembles a left upper canine (Fig. 4 *a,b*). Attempts to place it as a lower right canine by the curve of the root fail, on account of the resulting position of the crown. Similarly, the tooth cannot be placed as a lower right, using the crown as a guide, on account of the resulting position of the root.

By every test, therefore, the tooth contrasts with a lower right canine but corresponds with a normal upper left canine, and there is no alternative but to regard it as such. The tooth is larger than those seen in modern Europeans, but so also are the molars, and its proportionate size is to be expected (Fig. 4 *h,i*) . . .

References

Alexandersen, V. (1963). Double-rooted human lower canine teeth, *in* Brothwell, D. R. (ed.) *Dental anthropology*. Oxford, Pergamon, p.235.

Armitage, B. (1971). Three-rooted first premolars and their genetic and anthropological significance. *Br. Dent. J. 130,* 245-246.

Barnicoat, C. R. (1957). Wear in sheep's teeth. *N.Z. Jl Sci. Technol. 38A,* 583.

Barnicoat, C. R. (1959). Wear in sheep's teeth. VI. Chemical composition of teeth of grazing sheep. *N.Z. Jl Agri. Res. 2,* 1025-1040.

Barnicoat, C. R., and Hall, D. M. (1960). Attrition of incisors of grazing sheep. *Nature, Lond. 185,* 179.

Black, G. V. (1901). *Descriptive anatomy of the human teeth.* 4th ed., Philadelphia, S. S. White Dental Manufacturing Co.

Brash, J. C. (1924). The growth of the jaws and palate, in *The growth of the jaws, normal and abnormal, in health and disease.* London, Dental Board of the United Kingdom, p.37.

Broca, P. (1879). Instructions relatives à l'étude anthropologique du système dentaire. *Bull. Soc. Anthrop. Paris* (3) *2,* 128-163.

Brodie, A. G. (1934). Present status of knowledge concerning movement of the tooth germ through the jaw. *J. Am. Dent. Ass. 21,* 1830-1838.

Cameron, J. M., and Sims, B. G. (1973). *Forensic dentistry.* Edinburgh, Churchill-Livingstone.

Carter, A. M. (1914). The problem of root variation and curvature. *Aust. J. Dent. 18,* 15-24, 55-62, 96-104, 128.

Christiansson, H., Hedegard, B., Lewin, T., Anders, N., and Sarnäs, K. V. (1967). Skeletal remains at the Russian settlement at Russekeila in West Spitzbergen. *Acta Odont. Scand., Suppl.* 43.

Cryer, M. H. (1901). *Studies of the internal anatomy of the face.* Philadelphia, S. S. White Dental Manufacturing Co.

Dahlberg, A. A. (1963). Analysis of the American Indian dentition, *in* Brothwell, D. R. (ed.) *Dental anthropology.* Oxford, Pergamon, p.156.

Dawson, C., and Woodward, A. S. (1914). Supplementary note on the discovery of a palaeolithic human skull and mandible at Piltdown (Sussex). *Q. Jl Geol. Soc. Lond. 70,* 82-93.

Dempster, W. T., Adams, W. J., and Duddles, R. A. (1963). Arrangement in the jaws of the roots of the teeth. *J. Am. Dent. Ass. 67,* 779-797.

Dietz, V. H. (1944). A common dental morphotropic factor: the Carabelli cusp. *J. Am. Dent. Ass. 31,* 784-789.

Every, R. G. (1960). The significance of extreme mandibular movements. *Lancet, ii,* 37-39.

Fanning, E. A. (1961). A longitudinal study of tooth formation and root resorption. *N.Z. Dent. J. 57,* 202-217.

Goh, S. W. (1957). Variations in the morphology of mandibular premolar roots. *Br. Dent. J. 102,* 311-314.

Goose, D. H. (1963). Dental measurements in anthropological studies, *in* Brothwell, D. R. (ed.) *Dental anthropology.* Oxford, Pergamon, p.130.

Gregory, W. K. (1914). The dawn man of Piltdown, England. *Am. Mus. J. 14,* 189-200.

Gustafson, G. (1966). *Forensic odontology.* London, Staples Press.

Harvey, W. (1976). *Dental identification and forensic odontology.* London, Kimpton.

Herbst, E., and Apffelstaedt, M. (1930). *Malformations of the jaws and teeth.* London, Oxford Univ. Press.

Korenhof, C. A. W. (1960). *Morphogenetical aspects of the human upper molar.* Utrecht, Uitgeversmaatschappij Neerlandia.

Laws, A. J. (1971). Prevalence of canal irregularities in mandibular incisors: a radiographic study. *N.Z. Dent. J. 67,* 181-186.

Leatherman, G. (1971). Two-digit system of designating teeth—FDI submission. *Aust. Dent. J. 16,* 394.

Lee, K. W., Lee, E. C., and Poon, K. Y. (1968). Palato-gingival grooves in maxillary incisors. A possible predisposing factor to localised periodontal disease. *Br. Dent. J. 124,* 14-18.

Lunt, D. A. (1954). A case of taurodontism in a modern European molar. *Dent. Rec. 74,* 307-312.

McNulty, E. C., Lear, C. S. C., and Moorrees, C. F. A. (1968). Variability in lip adaptation to changes in incisor position. *J. Dent. Res. 47,* 537-547.

Manson, J. D. (1968). *A comparative study of the post-natal growth of the mandible.* London, Kimpton, p.120.

Massler, M., and Schour, I. (1958). *Atlas of the mouth in health and disease.* 2nd ed. Chicago, Amer. Dent. Assoc.

Massler, M., Schour, I., and Poncher, H. G. (1941). Developmental pattern of the child as reflected in the calcification pattern of the teeth. *Am. J. Dis. Child. 62,* 33-67.

Mead, A. D. (1966). *Richard Taylor, missionary tramper.* Wellington, Reed.

Miles, A. E. W. (1954). Malformations of the teeth. *Proc. R. Soc. Med. 47,* 817-826.

Miles, A. E. W. (1963). The dentition in the assessment of individual age in skeletal material, *in* Brothwell, D. R. (ed.) *Dental anthropology.* Oxford, Pergamon, p.191.

Miles, A. E. W., and West, W. H. (1954). The relationship of the mandibular third molar to the mandibular canal. *Dent. Practnr, 4,* 370-375.

Miller, G. S. (1915). The jaw of Piltdown man. *Smithson. Misc. Collns, 65,* 1-31.

Miller, G. S. (1918). The Piltdown jaw. *Am. J. Phys. Anthrop. 1,* 25-52.

Moorrees, C. F. A. (1957). *The Aleut dentition.* Cambridge, Harvard Univ. Press.

Muhlreiter, E., and De Jonge Cohen, Th.E. (1928). *Anatomie des menschlichen Gebisses.* 5 Aufl. Leipzig, Felix.

Mummery, J. H. (1924). *The microscopic and general anatomy of the teeth, human and comparative.* 2nd ed. London, Humphrey Milford, p.371.

Osborn, H. F. (1915). Review of the Pleistocene of Europe, Asia and Northern Africa. *Ann. N.Y. Acad. Sci. 26,* 215-315 (pp. 286-287 on Piltdown man, *Eoanthropus dawsoni*).

Pickerill, H. P. (1912). *The prevention of dental caries and oral sepsis.* London, Bailliere, Tindall and Cox.

Rosenberg, M. N. (1972). An evaluation of the incidence and amount of apical resorption and dilaceration occurring in orthodontically treated teeth having incompletely formed roots at the beginning of Begg Treatment. (Thesis abstract in *Am. J. Orthod. 61,* 524.)

Rouiller, C. H., Huber, L., and Rutishauser, E. (1952). La structure de la dentine: étude comparée de l'os et de l' ivoire au microscope électronique. *Acta Anat. 16,* 16-28.

Schour, I., and Massler, M. (1940). Studies in tooth development: the growth pattern of the human teeth. *J. Am. Dent. Ass. 27,* 1778-1793; 1918-1931.

Schour, I., and Massler, M. (1944). Chronology of the development of the dentition, *in* Brauer, J. C., Higley, L. B., Massler, M., and Schour, I. *Dentistry for children.* 2nd ed. Philadelphia, Blakiston (1950), pp.50-51.

Schroeter, C. (1966). *The dentition of man; an atlas of tooth morphology.* Seattle, Univ. Washington Press.

Sicher, H. (1960). *Oral anatomy.* 3rd ed. St. Louis, Mosby.

Sissons, H. A. (1956). The growth of bone, *in,* Bourne, G. H. (ed.) *The biochemistry and physiology of bone.* New York, Academic Press, pp.443-474.

Sopher, I. M. (1976). *Forensic dentistry.* Springfield, Thomas.

Suzuki, M., and Sakai, T. (1960). A case of buccolingually compressed mandibular second premolar in the Japanese. *J. Anthrop. Soc. Japan, 68,* 119-123.

Taylor, R. M. S. See the schedule of publications at the end of this list.

Tomes, Sir J. (1887). *A system of dental surgery.* 3rd ed. London, Churchill.

van Reenen, J. F. (1967). *Evolutionary trends in the human dentition.* Johannesburg, Witwatersrand Univ. Press.

Wallace, J. A. (1975). Did La Ferrassie I use his teeth as a tool? *Curr. Anthrop. 16,* 393-401.

Warwick, R. (1950). The relation of the direction of the mental foramen to the growth of the human mandible. *J. Anat. 84,* 116-120.

Weiner, J. S., Oakley, K. P., and Le Gros Clark, W. E. (1953). The solution of the Piltdown problem. *Bull. Br. Mus. Nat. Hist. A. Geol. 2,* 139-146.

Weiner, J. S., and Oakley, K. P. (1954). The Piltdown fraud: available evidence reviewed. *Am. J. Phys. Anthrop. 12,* 1-7.

Wickham, N. E. (1968). Teeth apart: Bruxism. *Bull. N.Z. Soc. Periodont. 25,* 10-21.

Williams, J. L. (1914). A new classification of human tooth forms; with special reference to a new system of artificial teeth. *J. All. Dent. Socs. 9,* 1-52.

Williams, R. (1967). *You are extraordinary.* New York, Random House.

Woodward, A. S. (1918). *A guide to the fossil remains of man in the Department of Geology and Palaeontology in the British Museum (Natural History).* 2nd ed. London, British Museum.

LIST OF PUBLICATIONS BY THE AUTHOR

1927

Case of fracture of both jaws. *N.Z. Dent. J. 24,* 3-5.

1934

Maori foods and methods of preparation. *N.Z. Dent. J. 30,* 88-96.

1937

(a) Dental disease in relation to public health. *N.Z. Dent. J. 33,* 72-82.

(b) (By title only) The dentition of the Piltdown fossil man (Eoanthropus dawsoni) from a new aspect. *Rep. Aust. N.Z. Ass. Advmt. Sci. 23,* 201, 245. Here reprinted as Appendix 6.

(c) The dental condition and diet of the Maoris of Maungapohatu Village, Urewera. (With J. L. Saunders.) Report of the Director-General of Health. Appendix C, 7-9. N.Z. Govt. Printer. (Reprinted as 1938a, q.v.)

1938

(a) The dental condition and diet of the Maoris of Maungapohatu Village, Urewera. (With J. L. Saunders) *N.Z. Dent. J. 34,* 92-96.

(b) Health we have not. Why not? *N.Z. Dent. J. 34,* 281-287.

1941

2nd ed. Contributor to: Dental Caries—findings and conclusions on cause and control. Research Commission of American Dental Association, New York, 1941, p.217.

1947

(a) Health service (oral) for children. *Dent. J. Aust. 19,* 161-168.

(b) The N.Z. school dental service. *Aust. J. Dent. 51,* 20-25.

(c) Gum conditions in a Maori area. *N.Z. Sch. Dent. Serv. Gaz. 7,* 11, 15.

(d) Aborigine and Maori. *J. Polynes. Soc. 56,* 163-172.

1948

(a) Aborigine and Maori. *Dent. Mag. Oral Top. 65,* 169-177 (Ref. 1947d reprinted, with illustrations added).

(b) Report on a survey of Australian school children and young Aborigines. *Aust. Dent. Congr. Proc. 11,* 537-544. (On p.539, between 5th and 4th lines from the bottom of page, the typesetter has missed two lines of text.)

1949

(a) Dental caries in children of Northern Territory, Australia. *Dent. J. Aust. 21,* 123-137.

(b) Anthropology and modern life. *N.Z. Sci. Rev. 7,* 63-64.

1955

Maori midden and skeleton at Waimamaku. *J. Polynes. Soc. 64,* 165-167.

1962

(a) The human palate. *Acta Anat. Suppl.* 43.

(b) Non-metrical studies in the human pal-

ate and dentition in Moriori and Maori skulls. Part I. *J. Polynes. Soc. 71,* 83-100.
(c) Non-metrical studies in the human palate and dentition in Moriori and Maori skulls. Part II. *J. Polynes. Soc. 71,* 167-187.

1963
(a) Cause and effect of wear in teeth. *Acta Anat.* 53, 97-157.
(b) Review of *Introduction to physical anthropology,* laboratory manual by Kelso and Ewing. *J. Polynes. Soc. 72,* 301.

1966
Review of *Bones, bodies and disease,* by Calvin Wells. *Newsl. N.Z. Archaeol. Ass. 9,* 39.

1968
(a) Gemination in a lower molar. *N.Z. Dent. J. 64,* 113-115.
(b) North Cape Notes. *Newsl. N.Z. Archaeol. Ass. 11,* 39-49.
(c) Review of *A comparative study of the post-natal growth of the mandible,* by J. D. Manson. *N.Z. Dent. J. 64,* 279-281.

1969
(a) Variation in form of human teeth: I. An anthropologic and forensic study of maxillary incisors. *J. Dent. Res. 48,* 5-16.
(b) Variation in form of human teeth: II. An anthropologic and forensic study of maxillary canines. *J. Dent. Res. 48,* 173-182.
(c) Review of *Cranial and post-cranial skeletal remains from Easter Island,* by R. I. Murrill. *J. Polynes. Soc. 78,* 144-145.

1970
(a) Dilaceration of incisor tooth crowns—report of two cases. *N.Z. Dent. J. 66,* 71-79.
(b) On adding life to years. *Bull. N.Z. Soc. Periodont.* 29, 1-5.
(c) Fern root planes. *N.Z. Dent. J. 66,* 248-251.
(d) Fellowship "Down Under." *Rotarian, 117,* 28-30.

1971
(a) Applied anatomy in tooth brushing. *Acta Anat. 79,* 300-304.
(b) Dental report on archaeological material from Tonga. *Aust. Dent. J. 16,* 175-181.
(c) Assault or accident. *Br. Dent. J. 131,* 419-420.
(d) Dilaceration of incisor tooth crowns—report of two cases. *Yb. Dent.* 75-77 (Ref. 1970a reprinted.)

1972
(a) Terminal hypoplasia in tooth roots. *Bull. Grpmt. Int. Rech. Scient. Stomat. 15,* 97-106.
(b) A Maori mortal combat weapon. *Man, 7,* 141-145.

1973
(a) Notes on the *mere pounamu. Newsl. N.Z. Archaeol. Ass. 16,* 133-134.
(b) Applied anatomy in tooth brushing. *Yb. Dent.* 454-455 (Ref. 1971a reprinted).

1975
The significance of tooth wear in Polynesians—a review. *J. Dent. Ass. S. Afr. 30,* 241-244.

1976
The significance of tooth wear in Polynesians—a review. *Ann. Dent. 35,* 5-11 (Ref. 1975 reprinted).

Author Index

Subject Index

Note: Page numbers will generally identify the major discussion of a tooth type, such as canine, molar, etc., e.g.: maxillary premolars, pp. 47-88. The reader is referred to the list of contents on pp. xix-xxiii for this advantage, although it should be noted that there will be other references to the various tooth types throughout the book.